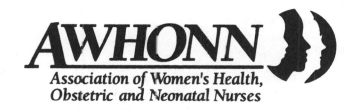

AWHONN
*Association of Women's Health,
Obstetric and Neonatal Nurses*

High-Risk and Critical Care Intrapartum Nursing

SECOND EDITION

Lisa K. Mandeville, RN, MSN
Administrative Director
Women's Patient Care Center
Associate in Obstetrics
Vanderbilt University
Nashville, Tennessee

Nan H. Troiano, RN, MSN
Co-Director, Critical Care Obstetrics
Department of Obstetrics and Gynecology
Division of Maternal–Fetal Medicine
Jefferson Medical College
Thomas Jefferson University
Philadelphia, Pennsylvania

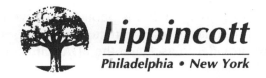

Lippincott
Philadelphia • New York

Acquisitions Editor: Jennifer Brogan
Coordinating Editorial Assistant: Susan V. Barta
Production Manager: Helen Ewan
Production Service: Michael Bass & Associates
Compositor: Andrea Reider
Printer/Binder: Victor Graphics, Inc.
Second edition

9 8 7 6 5 4 3 2 1

Library of Congress Cataloging-in-Publication Data

AWHONN's high-risk and critical care intrapartum nursing / edited by Lisa K. Mandeville, Nan H. Troiano.
— 2nd ed.
    P. cm.
    Rev ed. of: High-risk intrapartum nursing. c1992.
    Includes bibliographical references and index.
    ISBN 0-397-55467-2
    1. Maternity nursing. 2. Pregnancy—Complications—Nursing. 3. Labor (Obstetrics)—Complications—Nursing. I. Mandeville, Lisa K. II. Troiano, Nan H. III. Association of Women's Health, Obstetric, and Neonatal Nurses. IV. High-risk intrapartum nursing. V. Title: High risk and critical care intrapartum nursing.
    [DCLM: 1. Pregnancy Complications—nursing. 2. Maternal–Child Nursing—methods. 3. Critical Care—in pregnancy. 4. Pregnancy, High-Risk. 5. Labor Complications—nursing. 6. Delivery—nursing.
WY 157.3 A963 1999]
RG951.H537 1999
610.73'—DC21
DNLM/DLC
for Library of Congress   98-21938
                                                                                                             CIP

Care has been taken to confirm the accuracy of the information presented and to describe generally accepted practices. However, the authors, editors, and publisher are not responsible for errors or omissions or for any consequences from application of the information in this book and make no warranty, express or implied, with respect to the contents of the publication.

The authors, editors, and publisher have exerted every effort to ensure that drug selection and dosage set forth in this text are in accordance with current recommendations and practice at the time of publication. However, in view of ongoing research, changes in government regulations, and the constant flow of information relating to drug therapy and drug reactions, the reader is urged to check the package insert for each drug for any change in indications and dosage and for added warnings and precautions. This is particularly important when the recommended agent is a new or infrequently employed drug.

Some drugs and medical devices presented in this publication have Food and Drug Administration (FDA) clearance for limited use in restricted research settings. It is the responsibility of the health care provider to ascertain the FDA status of each drug or device planned for use in their clinical practice.

CONTRIBUTORS

Julie M. R. Arafeh, RN, MSN
Advanced Practice Nurse
Harvey, Troiano, and Associates, Inc.
Houston, Texas

Suzanne McMurtry Baird, RN, MSN
Instructor in the Practice of Nursing
Clinical Placement Coordinator
Vanderbilt University School of Nursing
Nashville, Tennessee
Senior Consultant, Critical Care Obstetrics
Harvey, Troiano, and Associates, Inc.
Houston, Texas

Jamie Caldwell, RNC, MSN
Perinatal Clinical Nurse Specialist,
Mercy Health Care
Sacramento, California

Jane B. Daddario, RNC, MSN
Assistant Professor of the Practice of Nursing
Specialty Director, Women's Health Nurse
    Practitioner Program
Vanderbilt University
School of Nursing
Nashville, Tennessee

Karen Dorman, RN, MS
Research Coordinator
Division of Maternal-Fetal Medicine
Baylor College of Medicine
Houston, Texas

Susan B. Drummond, RN, MSN
Clinical Nurse Specialist
Department of Obstetrics and Gynecology
Division of Maternal Fetal Medicine
Vanderbilt University Medical Center
Nashville, Tennessee

Kathryn B. Flynn
Women's Health Nurse Practitioner
Division of Ob/Gyn Nursing and Maternal
    Fetal Medicine
University of Rochester
Strong Memorial Hospital
Rochester, New York

Shirley M. Griffith, RNC, MSN
Perinatal CNS and Women's Health Nurse
    Practitioner
Maternal Fetal Care P.C.
Stamford, Connecticut

Carol J. Harvey, RNC, MS
Chief Executive Officer
Harvey, Troiano, and Associates, Inc.
Houston, Texas

Mildred G. Harvey, RNC, MSN
Obstetrical Clinical Nurse Specialist
Perinatal Nursing Consultant
Senior Consultant, Harvey, Troiano, and
    Associates, Inc.
Houston, Texas

Marykay Hill, RN, BSN
Perinatal Nurse Coordinator
Family Center Program
Methadone Maintenance and Drug
    Rehabilitation
Thomas Jefferson University Hospital
Philadelphia, Pennsylvania

Marion Jones, RN, MSN
Manager of Clinical Operations
New Hanover Regional Medical Center
Wilmington, North Carolina

Jo M. Kendrick, RNC, MSN, CDE
Manager, Nurse Practitioner Services
Department of Obstetrics and Gynecology
University of Tennessee Medical Center
Knoxville, Tennessee

Theresa Leicht, RNC, MSN
Clinical Nurse Specialist
Labor and Delivery
The University of Texas Medical Branch at
    Galveston
Galveston, Texas

Carol Jean Luppi, RNC, BSN
Co-Chair, Critical Care Obstetric Nursing Team
Harvard University/Brigham and Women's
    Hospital
Boston, Massachusetts

Lisa K. Mandeville, RN, MSN
Administrative Director
Women's Patient Care Center
Associate in Obstetrics
Vanderbilt University
Nashville, Tennessee

Kathryn A. May, DNSc, RN, FAAN
Professor and Director, School of Nursing
University of British Columbia
Vancouver, British Columbia, Canada

Susan Pozaic, RNC, MS, CRNP
Women's Health Nurse Practitioner
Student Health
University of Pennsylvania
Philadelphia, Pennsylvania
Consultant
Harvey, Troiano, and Associates, Inc.
Houston, Texas

Donna Jean Ruth, RNC, MSN
Instructor, Maternal-Child Nursing
Aquinas College
Nashville, Tennessee
Staff Nurse
Labor and Delivery and Critical Care Obstetrics
Vanderbilt University Medical Center
Nashville, Tennessee

Sheron J. Salyer, MSN, RNC
Doctoral Student
Vanderbilt University School of Nursing
Nashville, Tennessee

Patricia M. Sauer, RNC, MSN
Clinical Nurse Specialist, Labor and Delivery,
    High Risk Obstetrics
Northside Hospital
Atlanta, Georgia

Judy V. Schmidt, EdD, RNC
Assistant Professor
Perinatal Nurse Practitioner Program
    Coordinator
Nell Hodgson Woodruff School of Nursing
Emory University
Atlanta, Georgia

Diane M. Shannon, RN, MSN
Perinatal Clinical Nurse Specialist
Thomas Jefferson University Hospital
Philadelphia, Pennsylvania

Melissa C. Sisson, RN, MN
Director of Women's Services
Northside Hospital
Atlanta, Georgia

Nancy Surratt Townsend, RN, MSN
Clinical Nurse Specialist/Research Nurse
Department of Obstetrics and Gynecology
Division of Maternal-Fetal Medicine
Vanderbilt University Medical Center
Nashville, Tennessee

Nan H. Troiano, RN, MSN
Co-Director, Critical Care Obstetrics
Department of Obstetrics and Gynecology
Division of Maternal-Fetal Medicine
Jefferson Medical College
Thomas Jefferson University
Philadelphia, Pennsylvania

Eda M. Uckan, RNC, MSN
Director of Clinical Research
Chairman's Research Division
Department of Obstetrics and Gynecology
University of Texas Medical Branch
Galveston, Texas

FOREWORD

As perinatal nurses, we are fortunate to work in a speciality area where the majority of patients are healthy, experience uncomplicated pregnancies and births, and welcome to their family a healthy newborn. Nonetheless, we must always be prepared for the mother who is experiencing a high-risk pregnancy with a potential for a less than optimum perinatal outcome. This book is for nurses practicing in all intrapartum settings. While it may be a common perception that high-risk patients are cared for only at large specialty care facilities, the fact is that every nurse working in an intrapartum setting encounters women with high-risk pregnancies.

There is a possibility that women with high-risk pregnancies may increase in number. As our society changes, many women postpone childbearing. Because chronic diseases increase as women age, there is a potential that these women's risk factors for pregnancy will increase as well. Advances in health care have provided some women with chronic diseases the opportunity to bear a child who previously would not have considered or survived a pregnancy. And the lifestyle of women who are chemically dependent also increases the number of high-risk pregnancies. Perinatal nurses must be prepared to address the challenges of these high-risk pregnancies in the intrapartum setting.

It is with deep appreciation that we thank the editors, Lisa Mandeville and Nan Troiano, and each of the contributors to this second edition for providing perinatal nurses this valuable resource. Each member of the team has up-to-date knowledge and expertise in specific areas of high-risk and critical care intrapartum nursing.

Patsy Kennedy, RNC, WHNP
1998 AWHONN President

DISPLAY

The Association of Women's Health, Obstetric and Neonatal Nurses

The Association of Women's Health, Obstetric and Neonatal Nurses (AWHONN), an organization comprised of 22,000 healthcare professionals, promotes excellence in nursing practice to improve the health of women and newborns. Through dynamic programs, services and community outreach, AWHONN strives to enrich not only the health and well-being but the lives of women and newborns.

Significant challenges continue to face nurses who provide care for pregnant women during the intrapartum period. It is a dynamic profession in a dynamic period of time.

Arguably the most apparent challenge is meeting the healthcare needs of an increasingly diverse patient population. It is still true that most pregnant women are without identified risk factors and proceed through pregnancy, labor, delivery, and the postpartum period without problems. Thus, obstetric nursing care remains focused on a wellness-oriented framework. However, as anyone who has ever practiced within the specialty can attest, acute complications may develop at any time without regard for a woman's "identified" risk status. At the other extreme is a growing number of pregnant women identified as high-risk for development of serious sequelae during pregnancy. Because of the complex nature of certain conditions and the concomitant risk of perinatal morbidity or mortality, some women within this group require obstetric critical care. In addition to the unique physiologic needs of high-risk and critically ill pregnant women, psychosocial and cultural needs must also be identified and integrated into an individualized plan of care for these patients and their families.

Providing care to high-risk and critically ill pregnant women and their families within the current healthcare delivery system poses additional challenges. Efforts to reform health care have attempted to address the concepts of quality patient care and cost containment. Debate will no doubt continue regarding both the effectiveness and wisdom of some reform measures. However, many experienced nurses who provide care "at the bedside" find it difficult to herald the gains without also acknowledging changes that impact their ability to give the type of care their patients need. Short staffing is a recurrent theme in many units. Decreased institutional support for continuing professional education is common as is the elimination of nursing positions traditionally focused on staff orientation and education. Seemingly just at the point we were ready to accept that it was impossible for every obstetric nurse to have the knowledge and skills commensurate with every patient situation, we found ourselves faced with fewer nurses to care for a more diverse patient population. Even use of terms such as "intrapartum," "high-risk," and "critical care," each of which implies a categorical boundary for either the patient or the nurse, may be questionable.

This edition of *High-Risk and Critical Care Intrapartum Nursing* is reflective of these and other challenges. Not only have chapters from the previous edition been updated but additional subjects have been included that address the need for an expanded knowledge base in the obstetric healthcare setting. The first section is devoted to discussion of foundations for practice. Maternal and fetal physiologic principles are included as well as a description of unique psychosocial issues related to high-risk obstetric care. The second section presents information on the use of critical care technology during pregnancy. We hope this information proves useful for nurses caring for critically ill obstetric patients in a labor and delivery setting as well as for those providing consultation for such patients on other services. The third section has been expanded significantly to address the issue of application of concepts to clinical practice. The fourth section includes resources in the form of sample procedures, protocols, collaborative paths, and documentation tools.

We are grateful for the overwhelmingly positive feedback from the first edition. Such response confirmed our belief in the need for such a resource and helped direct us along the path to the second edition. We are in debt again to a wonderful group of contributing authors for sharing their expertise and time. It has been a pleasure to work with these colleagues, AWHONN, and Lippincott on this project.

Lisa K. Mandeville
Nan H. Troiano

CONTENTS

PART

I

Foundations for Practice

CHAPTER 1

Physiologic Changes During Pregnancy

Mildred G. Harvey

Appreciation of the normal adaptations to pregnancy and recognition of abnormal findings on assessment are fundamental in the management of normal as well as high-risk and complicated pregnancy. Numerous maternal alterations to the pregnancy state have an impact on parameters of health status, and many values that are normal during pregnancy differ from those in the nonpregnant state. As the maternal body makes necessary adjustments for the developing uteroplacental–fetal unit, the functioning of almost every organ system is affected.

The myriad of physiologic adaptations begin soon after conception, then continue to expand and evolve throughout the remaining weeks of pregnancy, labor, delivery, and puerperium. Control of the majority of alterations is hormonal, either directly or through secondary effects. However, a few adaptations result from the presence and mechanical effects of the enlarging uterus and growing fetus.

Information in this chapter will focus on normal anatomic and physiologic changes that impact major organ systems. Normal adaptations are interrelated and complex among systems. These changes may exacerbate preexisting medical conditions or even contribute to the development of high-risk status during pregnancy in some women. The quick and accurate interpretation of findings of a physical assessment is basic to nursing expertise; therefore, information provided in this chapter should be helpful to the clinician.

CARDIOVASCULAR SYSTEM

The most profound and dramatic changes during pregnancy involve the cardiovascular system. Complex adaptations are necessary to meet the challenge of evolving maternal changes in physiologic functioning, to promote the growth and development of the uteroplacental–fetal unit and to allow for blood loss at time of delivery. Adaptations include both hemodynamic and anatomic alterations. Hemodynamic alterations produce a "high-flow, low-resistance hemodynamic state," with changes in blood volume, heart rate, stroke volume, cardiac output, systemic vascular resistance (SVR), and arterial blood pressure. These alterations can be further affected by gestational age, maternal position, pain, labor, and peripartum blood loss. See Table 1-1 for a synopsis of changes in the cardiovascular system.

Anatomic

The progressively enlarging uterus elevates the diaphragm and displaces the heart upward and to the left to produce a slight anterior rotation of the heart on its long axis. A slight, lateral move of the apex of the heart is produced and the apex beat or apical impulse, termed the point of maximum intensity (PMI), becomes

TABLE 1-1. Cardiovascular Changes in Pregnancy

Parameter	Pregnancy	Nonpregnancy	Change (Percent)
Cardiac Output (liters/minute)	6.2 ± 1.0	4.3 ± 0.9	+ 43% by 36–38 wks
			+ 22% by 8 wks
Stroke Volume			+ 32% by 20–24 wks
Blood Volume			+ 48% (1570 ml)
Plasma Volume			+ 45–50% (1200–1300 ml)
RBC Mass			+ 20–30% (250–450 ml)
Mean Arterial BP (mm Hg)	86 ± 8	90 ± 6	–10%
Systolic BP			Decreases 5–10 mm Hg
Diastolic BP			Decreases 10–15 mm Hg
Systemic Vascular Resistance (SVR) (dyne/s/cm$_{-5}$)	1210 ± 266	1530 ± 520	–21%
Pulmonary Vascular Resistance (PVR) (dyne/s/cm$_{-5}$)	78 ± 22	119 ± 47	–34%
Heart			Displaced to left & upward
PMI			Located 4th ICS & lateral
Heart Rate	83 ± 10	71 ± 10	+ 17%

audible in the fourth intercostal space rather than the fifth space, lateral rather than medial to the mid-clavicle line (Walters & Lim, 1975). Increased blood volume during gestation produces a slight left ventricular hypertrophy that does not alter left ventricular function in normal pregnancy (Clark et al., 1989; Katz et al., 1978). Enein and colleagues (1987) reported that a slight degree of benign pericardial effusion accompanies normal pregnancy, may increase the cardiac silhouette on x-ray, and increases the difficulty in diagnosing moderate cardiomegaly during pregnancy. Pregnancy can produce changes in the electrocardiogram, including a left axis deviation of the QRS complex due to displacement of the heart (Walters & Lim, 1975), nonspecific S-T segment, and T-wave abnormalities (Shabetai, 1994).

Auscultatory changes produced by the increase in circulating blood volume are so extensive they would be considered abnormal in the nonpregnant state. Cutforth and MacDonald (1966) utilized serial phonocardiograms on 50 normal pregnant women at various stages of gestation to identify normal auscultatory changes. Normal changes in heart sounds during pregnancy are listed in Display 1-1.

Two types of functional murmurs are produced by the hyperdynamic state of pregnancy. The first is a pulmonary systolic murmur that is heard loudest at the right intercostal space. The second is a supraclavicular systolic murmur produced by increased blood flow in the brachiocephalic trunks.

Heart Rate

A progressive increase in maternal heart rate, apparent by the seventh week, produces a 20% increase by the third trimester, so that the mean heart rate increases 15 to 20 bpm. Table 1-1 shows increase of 12 bpm (Lee & Cotton, 1991). Wilson and associates' (1980) sequential study of heart rate changes related to maternal position found a similar progressive rise in rate in

DISPLAY 1-1

Normal Changes in Heart Sounds During Pregnancy

1. Exaggerated splitting of S_1 with increased loudness in both S_1 and S_2.
2. Longer intervals between mitral and tricuspid components of S_1.
3. No changes in S_2 until 30 weeks gestation.
4. No definite changes in the aortic and pulmonary elements of S_2, and a loud, easily heard S_3 by 20 weeks.
5. Less than 5% have a fourth heart sound.
6. 95% develop a systolic murmur at 22 weeks. This intensifies during inspiration in some or with expiration in others, and disappears after delivery.
7. 20% have a soft diastolic murmur heard transiently.
8. 10% have continuous murmurs from increased breast vasculature.

S_1 = First heart sound
S_2 = Second heart sound
S_3 = Third heart sound

three positions studied. Higher rates occurred when standing, median rates when sitting, and lower rates in the supine position. Heart rate in the supine position had increased 22.7 bpm by 36 weeks. Rises in heart rate in all positions reached a plateau at 32 weeks.

Katz and colleagues (1978) proposed that maternal tachycardia is due to hypervolemia and blood volume overload present during gestation, in conjunction with hormonal influences. Heart rate may vary during labor in response to anxiety, uterine contractions, pain, position changes, analgesics, type of delivery, and anesthetics. Heart rate decreases dramatically following delivery, with a reported 15% decrease in heart rate at one hour postpartum (Ueland &

Hansen, 1969b). Heart rate decreases 20% by 2 weeks postpartum (Robson et al., 1987b) and returns to the prepregnant levels by 6 weeks postpartum (Walters & Lim, 1975).

Blood Volume

Maternal blood volume increases markedly. In Pritchard's classic study (1965) of 50 normal women with a singleton pregnancy, the degree of hypervolemia showed a wide variation among subjects and ranged from an increase as small as 20% to an increase as high as 100%. An important finding in this investigation was that absolute increase in blood volume was directly correlated to the number of fetuses. Pritchard further found that women showed a tendency for the same plasma volume pattern to be repeated in successive pregnancies. This study reported the average increase in total blood volume for a singleton pregnancy is 1570 ml, a 48% increase over prepregnancy values (Pritchard, 1965). Maternal hypervolemia for twin gestations is greater than for the singleton pregnancy and the same study noted that twin pregnancies resulted in an average increase in blood volume of 1960 ml, an increase of 51%. Rovinsky and Jaffin's (1965) study also noted a progressive rise in blood volume for twin gestations that reaches a level of 28% above prepregnancy values at 21 to 24 weeks gestation to a peak increase of 59% at 37 to 40 weeks gestation. Triplet pregnancies show an even greater increase. A recent study confirms the early findings. Capeless and Clapp (1989) reported a rapid increase in blood volume during pregnancy, with a 22% increase by 8 weeks gestation that continued to increase progressively to a maximum 45% increase by 32 to 34 weeks gestation that was maintained until after delivery.

The expansion in total blood volume results from an increase in both plasma volume and red blood cell mass. Onset of increase in plasma volume occurs early, at 6 to 8 weeks gestation. Clapp and associates (1988) reported an 11% increase in maternal plasma by 7 weeks gestation. The increase reaches a plateau by approximately the thirty-second week of gestation and is maintained until delivery (Lund & Donovan, 1967; Metcalfe et al., 1981). Plasma volume measures 1200 to 1300 ml greater than nonpregnant plasma volume (Hytten & Leitch, 1971), a 45 to 50% increase.

Red cell volume increases 250 to 450 ml over prepregnant red cell volume, a 20 to 32% increase. Increase in red cell mass begins later in pregnancy and continues longer than does the increase in plasma volume. In addition, the progressive increase in red cell mass occurs at a slower rate than the plasma volume increase. Expansion in red cell volume is related to an increase in red cell production and not to prolongation of red cell life (Pritchard 1965).

Hemodilution results from the disproportionate increases in plasma and red cell volumes, as plasma volume increases 45 to 50%, and red cell volume increases only 20 to 30%. Hemodilution produces a decrease in hemoglobin and hematocrit concentrations; thus, physiologic anemia of pregnancy occurs, even in women with normal iron and folate stores (Hytten & Leitch, 1971). Plasma volume reaches its plateau around 30 to 32 weeks with maximal hemodilution, which is the time anemia is most pronounced. An increase in erythropoiesis without further expansion of plasma volume occurs at the same time, and the anemia improves in the last weeks of pregnancy. The stimulus for increased maternal erythropoiesis is placental production of chorionic somatomammotropin, progesterone, and possibly prolactin (Jepson, 1968).

The hypervolemia produced during normal pregnancy is beneficial for optimum pregnancy outcome. This importance is emphasized by reports of poor outcomes in pregnancies with decreased blood volume, such as pregnancies complicated by preeclampsia or IUGR (Clark et al., 1994). Hypervolemia serves to meet metabolic demands of the uteroplacental–fetal unit, to protect the mother and, therefore, the fetus. Hypervolemia compensates for impaired venous return and decreased cardiac output during the mother's daily activities, involving numerous position changes. It also prepares the mother for the normal blood loss that accompanies delivery and the early puerperium.

Although the exact physiology that produces blood volume expansion is unknown, and several theories have attempted to explain the process, two long-standing theories remain today. Burwell's studies in 1936 and 1938 proposed that the low-resistance uteroplacental circulation acts as a functional arteriovenous shunt and causes vascular volume expansion. The second theory proposes that the physiologic mechanism responsible for pregnancy hypervolemia is related to hormonal changes (Biglier & Forsham, 1961; Tapia et al., 1973). Which precedes the other, volume expansion or hormonal changes? This is a question for debate today, as Metcalfe and colleagues (1981) questioned whether venous relaxation due to the action of progesterone on the smooth muscle in the wall of the vessels accommodates the increased volume of blood and/or blood volume expansion occurs to compensate for this increase in vascular capacity.

Cardiac Output

Cardiac output (CO) reflects the functional capacity of the heart to maintain a satisfactory blood pressure and to adequately perfuse organ systems and is the most important assessment of the cardiovascular system. CO is defined as the volume of blood ejected by the left ventricle in one minute. It is reported in liters per minute and is determined by four factors: preload, afterload, contractility, and heart rate. All four components coordinate efforts to maintain adequate cardiac output. See Chapter 4 for a detailed discussion of cardiac output and related hemodynamic assessments.

There are now data to support that cardiac output increases as early as 10 weeks gestation and peaks at 30 to 50% over prepregnancy values by the latter part of the second trimester (Clark et al., 1994). Capeless and Clapp (1989) reported that increase in cardiac output begins very early in pregnancy with a 22% increase by 8 weeks gestation.

Optimizing maternal cardiac output is important when caring for a pregnant woman, but is especially so when making assessments. Right lateral or left lateral positions promote optimum cardiac output. Positioning the mother in a way that decreases cardiac output can initiate a compensatory mechanism that vasoconstricts the peripheral circulation to shunt peripheral blood to the central circulation. Peripheral circulation includes the skin, renal system, gastrointestinal (G-I) tract, pulmonary vasculature, and reproductive system. Decreasing maternal cardiac output can therefore decrease perfusion to multiple organ systems, including the reproductive system. If supine positioning is necessary during the last trimester, a wedge placed under a hip or manual displacement of the uterus to one side should be performed to prevent a reduction in maternal cardiac output with a resultant potential decrease in fetal perfusion.

Cardiac output increases 40 to 50% at rest during pregnancy, so the normal value for cardiac output at term is 6 to 7 liters per minute rather than the 4 to 5 liters per minute that is normal for the nonpregnant state (Clark et al., 1989). Clark and associates (1989) used pulmonary artery catheterization to assess cardiac output in the left lateral recumbent position. Using the thermodilution technique, 10 healthy primiparas were studied between 36 and 38 weeks gestation to determine normal values for pregnancy. This study reported a 43% increase in cardiac output during pregnancy in the left lateral recumbenty position.

Cardiac Output Changes During Labor

Labor produces significant cardiovascular changes. Ueland and Hansen (1969a, 1969b) found that cardiac output increased 15.3% in the first stage and 49% in the second stage, primarily because of an increase in stroke volume in their study of 23 laboring women. However, women in the study were in the supine position and received no sedation or regional anesthesia. Lee and associates (1989), correcting for the variables of maternal position and influence of pain, used M-mode and pulsed-Doppler echocardiography to noninvasively evaluate the effects of uterine contractions on cardiac output during labor. Women in the study were in the left decubitus position and received epidural anesthesia. They reported an 11% increase in cardiac output during uterine contractions related to an increase in left ventricular stroke volume. The increase in cardiac output with contractions could not be completely

abolished by relief of pain, as there is a 300 to 500 ml autotransfusion from the uterus to the maternal circulation with each contraction (Monga & Creasy, 1994). This increases the risk for women with borderline cardiac reserve or cardiac disease to develop congestive heart failure at this time. The pain stimulus from uterine contractions during labor can trigger the release of catecholamines that increase heart rate and further increase cardiac output. Robson and associates (1987a) utilized Doppler ultrasound and cross-sectional echocardiography for serial maternal cardiac output measurements during labor. The magnitude of contraction-induced cardiac output changes increased with the progression of labor presumably due to the augmentation in preload from repetitive uterine contraction. Robson and colleagues found the following:

Labor Status	Cardiac Output Increase
≤ 3 cm dilated	17%
4–7 cm dilated	23%
≥ 8 cm dilated	34%

Lower cardiac output in women receiving epidural anesthesia is attributed to the decrease in pain perception, in combination with the sympathetic effect of peripheral vasodilation that reduces preload and thereby reduces cardiac output.

Systemic and Pulmonary Vascular Resistance

Clark and associates (1989) found that systemic vascular resistance (SVR) decreases 21%, accompanied by a more dramatic decrease in pulmonary vascular resistance (PVR) of 34%. SVR is a measure of the tension (pressure) required for the ejection of blood into the systemic circulation (left afterload). PVR is a measure of the tension (pressure) required for the ejection of blood into the pulmonary circulation (right afterload).

The decrease in SVR seems to be related to both hormonal and mechanical factors. Peripheral vasodilation, produced by the hormonal effects of estrogen, progesterone, and local prostaglandins

(Greiss & Anderson, 1970; Symonds, 1983) in conjunction with the major low vascular resistance circulation developed by the uteroplacental circulation, are factors that reduce cardiac output (Lee & Cotton, 1991). Uterine veins undergo a great increase both in size and number during gestation, with a resultant decrease in uterine vascular resistance. The resultant low pressure network utilizes a large portion of the maternal circulation (Hytten & Leitch, 1971).

As vascular tone in peripheral vessels decreases, peripheral vasodilation is produced to accommodate increased blood flow to the skin and the kidneys. The decreased SVR reflects a decreased mean arterial pressure (MAP). The previously mentioned study by Clark and associates (1989) found the mean SVR in late pregnancy to be 1210 ± 266 dyne/ sec./cm^{-5}, in comparison to the nonpregnant mean of 1530 ± 520 dyne/sec/cm^{-5}.

The decrease in PVR reflects the increased vascular reactivity in the pulmonary circulation. The vascular tone of vessel walls in the pulmonary vasculature decreases and a low resistant pulmonary circulation results. The same study reported that mean PVR in late pregnancy is 78 ± 22 dyne/sec/cm,$^{-5}$ in comparison to the nonpregnant mean of 119 ± 47.0 dyne/sec/cm^{-5}.

Clark and colleagues (1989) found no increase in pulmonary capillary wedge pressure or central venous pressure in late pregnancy as compared with the nonpregnant state, although marked increases in intravascular volumes were present. This finding reflects that the decreased SVR and PVR allow both systemic and pulmonary circulations to accommodate higher volumes at normal vascular pressures.

Blood Pressure

Systolic and diastolic blood pressures decrease in the first trimester of pregnancy, reach their lowest levels during the second trimester, and then gradually rise toward the prepregnancy level by term (Clark et al., 1994). Systolic pressure decreases 5 to 10 mm Hg from the nonpregnant value, and the diastolic pressure decreases progressively to nearly a 10 to 15 mm Hg decrease by 28 to 32 weeks gestation. This results in an

increase in pulse pressure (Wilson et al., 1980). Mean arterial blood pressure decreases by approximately 10% as early as the seventh week of pregnancy (Clapp et al., 1988).

Etiology of blood pressure (BP) changes during gestation is related to hormonal and cardiovascular adaptations. Peripheral vasodilation and increased cardiac output are found earlier in pregnancy than gestational hypervolemia (Lee & Cotton, 1991). The increase in cardiac output does not completely compensate for the decreased SVR, which may explain the decrease in BP apparent as early as the first trimester.

BP measurements are very sensitive to maternal position. Wilson and colleagues (1980) observed that lowest BP readings were obtained with the gravida in the left lateral decubitus position. They reported an increase of approximately 14 mmHg when subjects were turned to the supine position. However, supine hypotension syndrome is possible if the woman remains supine; therefore, this position was used only briefly for study purposes. There is a difference of 10 to 12 mm Hg in BP readings between the superior and inferior arms in the lateral recumbent position. The superior arm will have the lower reading and the dependent arm will have the higher reading because of hydrostatic principles. Consistency in BP measurements is necessary to determine actual changes. When documenting BP assessments it is important to note maternal position with the reading.

It is especially important to establish a baseline BP value during the first weeks of gestation to facilitate early recognition of developing complications (Villar et al., 1989). BP values can be affected by activity and anxiety, and are likely to increase with uterine contractions. Increased blood volume of pregnancy increases the difficulty in determining Korotkoff's phase 5 (the point the sound disappears) of the diastolic pressure. The sound may be heard all the way to zero. If this occurs, Korotkoff's phase 4 (the point of muffling) may be included in the documentation of the BP reading: for example, 120/60/12 (Villar et al., 1989).

Hypertension during pregnancy is a serious complication, and the clinician is alert for early signs of this problem. A sustained rise of 30 mm Hg systolic and 15 mm Hg diastolic in BP assessments over baseline value may be indicative of pregnancy-induced hypertension, as well as other findings. An in-depth discussion of this complication and correlated nursing assessments is included in the chapter on hypertension and pregnancy.

Colloid Osmotic Pressure

Hemodynamic adaptations during pregnancy include a decrease in the plasma colloid osmotic pressure (COP). The osmotic pressure of a fluid is a relative property and can be demonstrated when two solutions of differing colloid concentrations are separated by a semipermeable membrane (Moise & Cotton, 1991). Molecules unable to pass through a semipermeable membrane are termed colloids, and those that pass are crystalloids. In hemodynamics, the semipermeable membrane is the capillary membrane and the colloid molecules are the plasma proteins: albumin, globulin, and fibrinogen.

Fluid transport between the plasma and interstitial compartment takes place at the capillary level across the semipermeable capillary membrane. The COP is the gradient controlling whether fluid remains inside the capillary or passes through the membrane into the interstitial space. Colloids in the plasma exert the force to keep fluid inside the capillary, which is measured as the colloid osmotic pressure (COP); the force that moves fluid across the membrane is the capillary hydrostatic pressure, and is measured as the pulmonary capillary wedge pressure (PCWP). The lower the COP and the higher the PCWP, the more likely that pulmonary edema will develop due to a lower COP-to-PCWP gradient.

Plasma concentration of albumin is the largest and most significant colloid. Albumin is twice the plasma concentration of globulin and 15 times that of fibrinogen; thus, changes in the concentration of albumin are most significant. The hemodilution state of normal pregnancy progressively reduces the plasma albumin concentration about 10 grams/liter below the prepregnancy level by term (Fadnes & Øian,

1989). This produces a steady decrease in COP values during pregnancy, with a nadir at approximately 34 to 36 weeks gestation. Such a reduction in the COP should lead to a movement of fluid from the intravascular compartment to the interstitial compartment; however, a steady state is maintained by the balance of the reduced peripheral resistance versus the increase in capillary pressure (Valenzuela, 1989). See Table 1-2 for COP values, including those at prepregnancy, pregnancy, and postpartum stages.

The complication of pregnancy-induced hypertension (PIH) produces lower COP values than values for the normotensive pregnancy. Etiology for a lower COP was previously thought due to proteinuria that accompanies PIH (Chesley, 1978). More recent studies (Bhatia et al., 1987; Øian et al., 1986) propose that capillary damage produced by PIH alters capillary permeability to plasma proteins and thus reduces the COP. Therefore, PIH produces decreased COP values as a result of loss of serum proteins across capillary membranes, in combination with proteinuria (Clark et al., 1994).

Venous Pressure

Although venous pressure remains unchanged in the upper extremities during pregnancy, there is a progressive increase in venous pressure in the lower extremities as pregnancy advances. The increase in lower extremity venous pressure is mainly due to hydrostatic forces of vasodilation, enhanced blood volume,

TABLE 1-2. Colloid Osmotic Pressure Values	
Stage	Value
Prepregnancy	25.4 ± 2.3 mm Hg
Pregnancy	22.4 ± 0.5 mm Hg
Postpartum	15.4 ± 2.1 mm Hg
PIH delivery	17.9 ± 0.7 mm Hg
PIH postpartum	13.7 ± 0.5 mm Hg

and compression of pelvic veins and inferior vena cava by the enlarging uterus (Monga & Creasy, 1994).

A more prominent venous bed is present during pregnancy, as a result of peripheral vasodilation. Enlarged, superficial veins are readily seen over the entire body. Vasodilation increases venous compliance that peaks in the last trimester, so that hemodynamic adaptations can be accommodated. The increased compliance contributes to such a decrease in the velocity of venous blood flow that venous stasis may result (Monga & Creasy, 1994).

Dependent edema is common during the last half of pregnancy as a result of two physiologic actions. First, an increase in venous pressure occurs in the lower extremities when the pregnant woman stands or sits upright. This positioning increases the capillary pressure in the lower legs as the gravid uterus exerts pressure on major veins in the abdomen and pelvis. Second, there is a decrease in colloid oncotic pressure during normal pregnancy. These two actions facilitate fluid shift from the capillaries to the extravascular space with a resultant dependent edema (Pritchard & MacDonald, 1980). Pedal edema worsens when the gravid woman is erect and busy with daily activities, but is greatly alleviated after rest in the lateral position, as this position eliminates uterine compression on abdominal and pelvic veins so that extravascular fluid is mobilized into the systemic circulation.

Plasma volume regulation and transcapillary fluid balance are the result of many complex mechanisms. Plasma renin activity and aldosterone levels increase during gestation to promote sodium retention and an increase in total body water. Tubular sodium reabsorption rises with gestation, and approximately 900 mEq of sodium are retained along with an increase of 6 to 8 liters of total body water, two thirds of which is extracellular (Lindheimer & Katz, 1975).

Cardiac Symptoms in Pregnancy

The profound and complex hemodynamic changes of normal pregnancy can mimic cardiac disease and increase the difficulty in diagnosing cardiovascular disease. As pregnancy progresses, many women report dyspnea, dizzy spells, easy fatigue, the need for additional pillows for sleep, and feeling lightheaded. Normal physical findings include dependent edema that worsens as pregnancy advances, distended neck veins, transient crackles in the lower lung fields, hyperventilation, palpitations, and even slight cardiomegaly. Systolic murmurs, mammary flow murmurs, and venous hums are common.

However, the clinician should be alert for complaints of severe dyspnea, syncope with exertion, hemoptysis, paroxysmal nocturnal dyspnea, or chest pain on exertion. These are NOT normal for pregnancy, and suggest a cardiac problem. These symptoms necessitate immediate further evaluation (Shabetai, 1994).

Postpartum Hemodynamics

Hemodynamic changes that occur in the postpartum period may fluctuate significantly as they reflect results of blood loss sustained at delivery and the body's compensation to peripartum hemorrhage. Pritchard and colleagues (1962) reported their measurement of blood loss to be 505 ml with vaginal delivery and 1028 ml with cesarean delivery. They also found that normal pregnant women could lose up to 30% of antepartum blood volume with little change in postpartum hematocrit or blood pressure.

Ueland (1976) studied the differences in blood volume and hematocrit changes between vaginal delivery and selective cesarean delivery with serial measurements of venous hematocrit and blood volume. He reported the average blood loss with vaginal delivery to be 610 ml, and 1030 ml with cesarean delivery. After vaginal delivery blood volume steadily decreased from the first hour postpartum until the third postpartum day, whereas blood volume remained fairly stable following cesarean delivery. In both groups, blood loss measured 1000 ml by the third postpartum day, regardless of mode of delivery.

However, differences in hematocrit changes were noted in this same study. With a vaginal delivery one half of the blood volume loss occurs during delivery, while the remaining loss is caused by diuresis, as evidenced by a rise in hematocrit of 5.2%. In contrast, with a cesarean delivery the entire blood loss occurs during surgery as evidenced by a drop in the hematocrit of 5.8%.

Postpartum diuresis normally occurs between the second and fifth postpartum days, and is the physiologic mechanism to excrete the increase in extracellular fluid that is accumulated during pregnancy (Cunningham et al., 1989). Chesley and associates (1959) were the first to observe that during the first postpartum week there is a decrease of 2 liters in the extracellular fluid compartment that accounted for 3 kilograms of weight loss. Hankins and colleagues (1984) noted in a group of 8 eclamptic women with invasive hemodynamic monitoring that if women did not have significant diuresis by 48 to 72 hours, they produced elevated wedge pressures comparable to pulmonary edema and that the wedge pressures normalized following diuresis. Therefore, mobilization of the extracellular fluid is normal following delivery and if diuresis does not occur, the woman is at increased risk for developing pulmonary edema.

The postpartum period is a high cardiac output state. A large increase in venous blood return to the heart occurs as a result of (1) shunting of blood from the uteroplacental unit to the intravascular space, (2) loss of the heavy, gravid uterus and associated pressure on the vena cava, and (3) the mobilization of extravascular fluid into the intravascular space (Clark et al., 1994). Ueland and Hansen (1969b) reported that by one hour postpartum, cardiac output had increased 49% above intrapartum values, with a stroke volume increase of 67% above baseline values; while heart rate had decreased 15%. During this same period no significant changes in blood pressure were noted.

Studies of the return of cardiac output values to the prepregnancy state show a wide variation in time, with most reports showing the time required for this to be from 2 to 4 weeks postpartum. Ueland (1976) reported blood volume returns to nonpregnant values by 6 weeks postpartum. Metcalfe (1985) found cardiac output still elevated approximately 18 to 29% over prelabor values at 4 to 5 days postpartum. Robson and

associates (1987b) reported a 33% decrease in cardiac output at 2 weeks postpartum from prelabor values, attributed to a 20% decrease in heart rate and an 18% decrease in stroke volume. This same study reported that cardiac output, stroke volume and left ventricular mass continued to decline for 24 weeks after delivery, but that most of the decrease had occurred by 12 weeks. A study by Capeless and Clapp (1991) also showed that end-diastolic volume, cardiac output, and stroke volume had not returned to prepregnancy values by 12 weeks postpartum.

Colloid osmotic pressure (COP) decreases significantly in the first 24 hours postpartum. Cotton and associates (1984) showed a COP value of 15.4 ± 2.1 mm Hg postpartum as compared to a COP value of 21.0 mm Hg ± 2.1 during labor. See Table 1-2 for normal COP values. Etiology for the large decrease in COP in the immediate postpartum period includes several propositions: (1) supine positioning during labor and delivery, (2) blood loss at time of delivery, (3) administration of large amounts of crystalloid intravenous fluids during labor and delivery, and (4) mobilization of extravascular fluid to the intravascular space.

RESPIRATORY SYSTEM

Pregnancy necessitates numerous adaptations in the respiratory system so that a functional system is established for adequate oxygen delivery to mother and fetus, along with the elimination of carbon dioxide. Oxygen consumption increases progressively during gestation to meet the surge in oxygen requirements as fetal needs multiply with growth and development, along with an increase in maternal metabolism and growth. Significant changes occur in lung volume, capacities, ventilation and acid-base balance as a result of mechanical and biochemical factors.

Interpretation of data obtained with assessment of respiratory status is an important step in the nursing process. A review of the definitions of lung volumes and lung capacities that are commonly used in assessment of respiratory physiology may be helpful. See Display 1-2 for definitions of lung volumes and capacities.

Anatomic

The increase in blood supply to peripheral tissues during gestation results in hyperemia of capillaries in the nose, nasopharynx, larynx, and tracheobronchial tree. Nasal congestion is common, nosebleed occurs easily, and edema of the larynx can produce voice changes (Bonica, 1967). The hyperemia narrows passages, necessitating care if manipulation of the upper airway is indicated. Too forceful suctioning, forceful placement of airway adjuncts, or careless laryngoscopy may result in bleeding and trauma (Gutsche, 1979). A smaller 6.5 to 7.0 mm cuffed endotracheal tube is often recommended, rather than the usual 8 mm size, whenever endotracheal intubation is necessary as edema is usually present in the area of the false cords.

Increased intra-abdominal pressure from the enlarging uterus elevates the diaphragm approximately 4 cm above the nonpregnant level. This decreases lung length and increases intrathoracic pressure (Pritchard & MacDonald, 1980). In compensation, the transverse and anteroposterior diameters of the chest increase by 2 cm as the lower rib cage flares out. The substernal angle widens 50%, from 70 degrees in the first trimester to 105 degrees at term (Bonica, 1967), and the thoracic cage circumference increases 5 to 7 cm. These anatomic alterations facilitate maintenance of overall volume in the lungs and seem to be a result of hormonal, as well as mechanical influences, as alterations in chest configuration begin early in gestation before upward pressure from the uterus is possible. However, uterine enlargement becomes the main factor in late pregnancy (Pritchard & MacDonald, 1980).

Respiratory compensations necessary to counteract effects of elevation of the diaphragm on the lungs include:

1. Compensatory increase in chest circumference
2. Change from abdominal to thoracic breathing
3. Relaxation of smooth muscle in the tracheobronchial tree
4. Increase in minute ventilation

DISPLAY 1-2

Definitions of Lung Volumes and Capacities

1. **Vital Capacity**—the maximum volume of gas that can be expired after a maximum inspiration. Does not include the residual volume.

2. **Tidal Volume**—the volume of gas that is exchanged with each breath.

3. **Minute Ventilation**—the volume of gas expired per minute.

4. **Functional Residual Capacity**—the volume of gas that remains in the lungs at the end of a normal expiration. (Expiratory reserve volume plus residual volume).

5. **Inspiratory Capacity**—the maximum volume of air that can be inspired from the resting expiratory level.

6. **Residual Volume**—the volume of gas remaining in the lungs at the end of maximal expiration. Does not include the anatomical dead space of the trachea and bronchial tree.

7. **Inspiratory Reserve Volume**—maximum amount of air that can be inspired, beyond the normal tidal inspiration.

8. **Expiratory Reserve Volume**—maximum amount of air that can be expired from the resting end-expiratory position.

9. **Resting End-Expiratory Position**—the position of the chest at the end of quiet expiration.

Breathing becomes diaphragmatic. However, the enlarging uterus does not impede diaphragmatic excursion, as it actually increases 1 cm to 2 cm (Gabbe et al., 1986). The rapid, deep breathing that is normal for pregnancy enhances gas anesthesia, as it facilitates a more rapid induction and recovery from inhalation anesthesia (Bonica, 1967).

Physiologic

See Figure 1-1 for an illustration of respiratory changes during pregnancy, labor, and the postpartum period.

Tidal volume and minute ventilation increase during gestation, while residual volume, expiratory reserve volume, and functional residual capacity decrease. Dead space, closing capacity, and closing volume do not change.

A relative hyperventilation of pregnancy begins in the first trimester and increases 42% by term (Cugell et al., 1953). The hyperventilation appears to result from increased progesterone levels that accompany gestation (Clark et al., 1994). A progressive increase in minute ventilation begins in the first trimester and at term is 48% above prepregnancy levels (Prowse & Gaensler, 1965). This increase is accomplished mainly by an increase in tidal volume. Oxygen consumption increases 21% and the Basal Metabolic Rate (BMR) increases 14%. Respiratory rate is essentially unchanged, as it only increases from 14 to 15 breaths per minutes (Bonica, 1967). The relatively greater increase in minute volume over oxygen consumption or BMR is attributed to an increase in tidal volume (Prowse & Gaensler, 1965), which increases from 450 ml/min before pregnancy to 600 ml/min at term (Bonica, 1967).

As oxygen consumption increases in conjunction with the increase in elimination of carbon dioxide, ventilation must increase to meet the demands for pregnancy; thus, hyperventilation results. The ventilation in liters for each 100 ml of oxygen consumption is persistently raised to produce a reduction in alveolar and arterial carbon

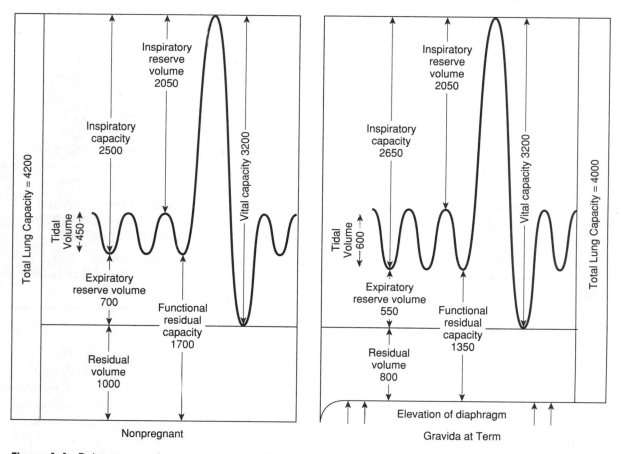

Figure 1-1. Pulmonary volumes and capacities during pregnancy, labor, and postpartum period. From *Principles and Practice of Obstetric Analgesia and Anesthesia* (p. 24), by J. J. Bonica, 1967, Philadelphia: F. A. Davis. Copyright by Lea & Febiger. Reproduced with permission from J. J. Bonica.

dioxide tension (Bonica, 1967). See Table 1-3 for arterial blood gas values during pregnancy.

During active labor, especially the transition phase and pushing efforts during second stage, ventilation may increase as much as 300% compared to the nonpregnant state because of hyperventilation in response to pain (Gutsche, 1979). Pain relief such as epidural anesthesia or breathing techniques taught in prepared childbirth class can help prevent maternal alkalemia during this part of labor.

Arterial Blood Gases

Arterial oxygen tension in pregnant women increases to mean values ranging from 106 to 108 mm Hg in the first trimester to 101 to 104 mm Hg by the third trimester (Templeton & Kelman, 1976; Anderson et al., 1969). A postural effect on arterial oxygen tension at term has also been reported, with higher values in the sitting position and a moderate hypoxemia in the supine position (Awe et al., 1979). The resting maternal arterial carbon dioxide tension (PaCO2) is below 30 mm Hg (Clark et al., 1994). Maternal acid-base balance is maintained by the compensatory decrease in serum bicarbonate of about 4 mEq/liter (from 26 to 22 mEq/l).

The lowered maternal PaCO2 produces a concentration gradient across the placenta to facilitate elimination of fetal carbon dioxide (Pritchard & MacDonald, 1980). High pregnancy levels of progesterone and estrogen produce an increase in the values of maternal 2,3 diphosphoglycerate. This results in a right shift in the maternal oxyhemoglobin dissociation curve with a decrease in the affinity of maternal hemoglobin to oxygen. Fetal hemoglobin has an increased affinity for oxygen. Gas exchange of oxygen and carbon dioxide across the placenta is regulated by a change in the oxygen affinity of the maternal and fetal hemoglobin (double Bohr effect). The lower maternal PaCO2 maximizes oxygen exchange from the maternal and fetal circulation as it increases the amount of oxygen released to the fetal tissue at any given time (Bauer et al., 1969). A thorough discussion of concepts related to fetal oxygenation is presented in Chapter 2.

Normal arterial blood gas values for pregnancy in comparison with nonpregnancy values are

TABLE 1-3. Arterial Blood Gas Values (ABG'S)

Parameter	Pregnancy	Prepregnancy
pH	7.40–7.45	7.35–7.45
pO_2 (mm Hg)	104–108	80–100
pCO_2 (mm Hg)	27–32	35–42
Bicarbonate HCO_3 (mEq/L)	22	26

listed in Table 1-3. Note that normal arterial blood gas values for pregnancy reflect the state of chronic compensated respiratory alkalosis. Thus, the pregnant woman will develop respiratory acidosis and metabolic acidosis more rapidly than a woman in the nonpregnant state.

Lung Volumes

Tidal volume increases from 450 ml/min before pregnancy to 600 ml/min at term, a 40% increase (Bonica, 1967). As the enlarging uterus elevates the diaphragm, functional residual capacity (FRC) progressively decreases to 18% below prepregnancy values (Cugell et al., 1953). FRC is the volume of gas that mixes with the inhaled air of each breath. Because tidal volume increases 40% and FRC decreases 18%, an increased volume of inhaled air is mixed with a smaller volume of residual air in the lungs. Thus, there is a more efficient mixing and exchange of the gases during the pregnant state (Gutsche, 1979).

However, the decreased FRC lowers oxygen reserve and hypoxia can occur rapidly during gestation, even with only a short period of apnea. The increased oxygen consumption that accompanies pregnancy further enhances the rapid development of hypoxia with a short period of apnea (Bonica, 1967). Increased airway resistance does not accompany the reduction in FRC during pregnancy. A reduction in FRC results in less distended lungs. Less distended lungs usually produce smaller airways with smaller lumen. However, increased progesterone levels during gestation relax the bronchial smooth muscle, so that decreased airway resistance is present during gestation (Bonica, 1967).

Oxygen Consumption

A progressive increase in oxygen consumption occurs as pregnancy advances. Studies have reported that oxygen consumption increases 20% during the last weeks of pregnancy when the gravid woman is at rest (Baldwin et al., 1977; Hytten & Leitch, 1971; Pernoll et al., 1975). One half of this increase is used by the fetus and placenta, and one half by the maternal body. Oxygen consumption is proportionally increased in multiple gestation (Hytten & Leitch, 1971). Oxygen consumption further increases during labor. There is a 300% increase with each uterine contraction during the transition phase of labor, and pushing efforts require an additional 200% increase in oxygen consumption (Gutsche, 1979).

HEMATOLOGIC SYSTEM

Increased blood volume during gestation is a result of an increase in volume of both plasma and erythrocytes. The usual pattern is an initial rise in plasma volume, followed by an increase in the volume of erythrocytes. Pregnancy is also a state of hypercoagulation, with an increase in fibrinogen and clotting factors and suppressed fibrinolysis, in preparation for normal blood loss at delivery.

Plasma Volume and Red Blood Cell Mass

The progressive increase in maternal plasma volume is detectable as early as 6 weeks gestation, with levels rising rapidly to reach a peak around 32 to 34 weeks gestation that plateaus until delivery (Lund & Donovan, 1967). The increase in erythrocyte volume begins around 10 weeks gestation and increases steadily until term. However, these increases are disproportionate, as the rise in plasma volume is greater than the rise in erythrocyte volume. Although the plasma volume increase is larger, there is a considerable rise in the volume of circulating erythrocytes (red blood cell mass) that averages

450 ml, an increase of 45% (Cunningham et al., 1993). The expansion in erythrocyte volume is related to an increase in red blood cell production rather than to prolongation of red blood cell life (Pritchard, 1965).

The increase in red blood cell mass begins later and continues longer than the increase in plasma volume, with a progressive increase at a slower rate than the rate of plasma volume increase. During the last half of pregnancy, the mean life of maternal erythrocytes is shorter because the rate of red cell production exceeds that of destruction, resulting in a larger percentage of young, immature red blood cells in the plasma. As the mean cell volume increases, red blood cells become more spherical with a decreased diameter and increased thickness (Cunningham et al., 1993). After 20 weeks gestation, moderate erythroid hyperplasia is present in the bone marrow and the reticulate count is slightly elevated because of increased maternal plasma erythropoietin levels, which increase two- to threefold. Red cell counts decrease from nonpregnant values of $4.6 \times 10^6/mm^3$ to $3.88 \times 10^6/mm^3$ at 36 weeks gestation (Meyer, 1983).

When first released from the bone marrow, red cells are their largest; therefore, an increased number of immature red cells requires more space and thus the volume increases. This type of erythrocyte has an increased concentration of 2,3-diphosphoglycerate that decreases the oxygen affinity and facilitates the dissociation of oxygen from hemoglobin for placental transfer to fetal hemoglobin (Bauer et al., 1969).

Despite the augmented erythropoiesis, concentrations of hemoglobin and red blood cells decrease slightly. Whole blood viscosity decreases. The plasma volume increase of 50% and red cell volume increase of only 20% is disproportional and produces a decreased packed cell volume (PCV), or hematocrit during pregnancy. A relative anemia of pregnancy occurs even in women with normal iron and folate stores (Hytten & Leitch, 1971). As plasma volume reaches its plateau around 30 to 32 weeks with maximal hemodilution, the anemia is most pronounced, and then improves as red cell production increases and plasma volume plateaus. Hemoglobin and hematocrit decrease 15%, with an overall hematocrit in the second trimester of 33.4% (range 31.9 to 36.5%), and 33.8% in the third trimester (range 31.9 to 36.5%) (Anderson, 1989).

Iron supplementation during pregnancy makes a significant difference in red cell volume. Hytten and Leitch (1971), reported an increase in red cell volume of only 250 ml without iron supplementation, whereas the increase in red cell volume was 400 to 500 ml with iron supplementation. A landmark study in which iron was readily available for maternal erythropoiesis (Pritchard & Hunt, 1958) found the average hemoglobin concentration at term to be 12.5 g/dl. Only 6% of participants had a hemoglobin concentration below 11.0 g/dl.

Thus, a hemoglobin concentration below 11.0 g/dl in late pregnancy is abnormal and is usually caused by iron deficiency anemia and should not be attributed immediately to hypervolemia of pregnancy (Cunningham et al., 1993).

White Blood Cells

Pregnancy is associated with an increase in the neutrophil count that begins during the second month (Laros, 1994). The total white blood cell (WBC) count increases because of the increase in neutrophil polymorphonuclear leucocytes (Fleming, 1975). The blood leukocyte count varies during gestation, with a mean WBC count in the first trimester of 9500/mm³, whereas the normal range is 3000 to 15,000/mm³. The mean increases further to 10,500/mm³, with a range of 6000 to 16,000/mm³ during the second and third trimesters. During labor the count may rise to 20,000 to 30,000/mm³ in the noninfected patient (Pitkin & Witte, 1979). The count returns to nonpregnant levels by the end of the first week postpartum.

Platelets

As pregnancy progresses there is a moderate decrease in the number of platelets per unit volume (Pitkin & White, 1979) that is thought to be a result of increased platelet consumption throughout normal pregnancy (Fay et al., 1983). The platelet count remains within the normal range for the nonpregnant state of 150,000 to 400,000/mm³ even with the progressive decline in the platelet count throughout pregnancy, and the rise of the platelet count in the early puerperium (Pitkin & White, 1979). The mean platelet count in early pregnancy (less than 20 weeks) is 275,000/mm³, and in late pregnancy (greater than 35 weeks) the mean count is 260,000/mm³ (Gerbasi et al., 1990).

Blood Coagulation

Pregnancy has been called a "hypercoagulative state" because of the increase in several blood coagulation factors that enhance coagulation and thrombosis. Levels of factors XII, IX, VII, X, VIII, V, and fibrinogen increase during gestation. Plasma fibrinolytic activity is depressed as a result of placental inhibitors, but returns to normal following delivery (Bonnar et al., 1969). Placental separation releases tissue thromboplastin into the circulation, increasing the risk of thrombosis (Bonnar, 1981). See Chapter 13 for a detailed description of this topic.

Fibrinogen levels begin a profound increase by the twelfth week of gestation and reach a concentration about 50% above prepregnancy values, with an average of about 450 mg/dl in late pregnancy. The range is 300 to 600 mg/dl. Levels of 600 mg/dl have been observed related to the increased synthesis that occurs during pregnancy (Meyer, 1983).

Significant increases occur in concentrations of factor VII (proconvertin), factor VIII (antihemophilic globulin), factor IX (plasma thromboplastin component or Christmas factor), and factor X (Stuart–Prower factor). Usually the levels of factor II (prothrombin) only increase slightly. In contrast, a decrease in factors XI (plasma thromboplastin antecedent) and XIII (fibrin-stabilizing factors) occur, probably because of consumption at the placental site.

Bleeding time, prothrombin time, and partial thromboplastin time are essentially unchanged and remain within normal limits, mainly a result of the increased blood volume and hemodilution that accompanies normal pregnancy. Postpartum diuresis causes concentration of clotting factors as extra plasma volume is excreted. This increases the risk for development of deep vein thrombosis or thromboembolism during the puerperium period (Gerbasi et al., 1990)

Renal System

Striking hemodynamic and hormonal changes during normal pregnancy alter renal physiology immensely. Thus, significant changes are seen in laboratory and diagnostic test results and increase the risk of erroneous interpretation of said test results. In addition, the normal changes in the renal system during pregnancy actually increase the risk for development of urinary tract infections.

Anatomic

There is a slight increase in renal size and weight, a result of increased renal blood flow, vascular volume, and interstitial volume (Beydoun, 1985). Kidney length increases approximately 1 cm (Bailey & Rolleston, 1971), and renal volume increases approximately 30% (Christensen et al., 1989).

More significant is the dilation of the urinary collecting system that occurs in 80% of pregnancies (Monga & Creasy, 1994). Beginning in the first trimester, the renal calyces, pelves, and ureters dilate to produce a physiologic hydroureter of pregnancy. Schulman and Herlinger (1975) reported that calyceal and ureteral dilation occur more frequently on the right side (three fourths of cases) than on the left side (one third of cases), with the degree of calyceal dilation greater on the right, at 15 mm, than on the left, at 5 mm.

The primary etiology for the physiologic hydronephrosis and hydroureter of pregnancy seems to be obstruction or compression of the ureters by the enlarging uterus and ovarian vein plexus. This theory is supported as ureteral dilation is rarely present beyond the pelvic brim, and tapering of the ureters as they cross the common iliac artery can be seen with ultrasound (MacNeily et al., 1991). This mechanical theory is further supported by the fact that the dominance of changes occur on the right side. An earlier theory suggested that a hormonal influence was also a factor because dilation begins by the tenth week of gestation, as well as the mechanical compression that occurs later, and the dilation continues throughout pregnancy and into the puerperium (Hytten & Leitch, 1971).

Right-sided preponderance occurs as the right ureter is more dilated than the left ureter, thought to be a result of the following: (1) dextrorotation of the gravid uterus; (2) the right ovarian vein with its multiple branches crosses the right ureter, whereas the left ovarian vein parallels the left ureter; (3) the sigmoid colon, located on the left side contributes to the dextrorotation of the uterus to further compress the ureter on the right side; or (4) the protective, cushioning effect exerted by the sigmoid colon. An additional suggestion has been the greater kinking of the right ureter as it crosses the iliac vessels at the pelvic brim (Beydoun, 1985).

Dilation of the urinary collecting system produces significant consequences, including an increase in ascending urinary tract infections, difficulty in interpreting radiologic tests of the urinary tract, and renal function tests. The dead space, or capacity of the ureters to increase related to dilation, and the entire collecting system may have a volume of 200 ml in late pregnancy. This potential dead space can significantly affect evaluation of changes in renal function during pregnancy. In addition, the increased volume of urine in the dilated ureters and renal pelvis slows urine flow, increasing the risk of urinary tract infections (Hytten & Leitch, 1971). Within the first week of delivery, renal volume returns to normal (Christensen et al., 1989), but hydronephrosis and hydroureter may last for as long as 3 to 4 months following delivery (Fried et al., 1983).

Lindheimer and Katz (1975), reported that physiologic hydroureter of pregnancy is characterized by a marked increase in the diameter of the ureteral lumen, accompanied by hypotonicity and hypomotility of its musculature. Microscopic changes in the ureters include hyperplasia of the longitudinal smooth muscle and inflammatory edema. Sala and Rubi (1967) studied ureteral contractility during gestation and found that normal rhythmic contractions and extended periods of relaxation in the ureters are not diminished during pregnancy. However, a decrease in the mean contractile pressure in the lower part of the ureter occurs during pregnancy.

This decrease in pressure results in a larger volume of urine contained in the collecting system, with a slower flow of urine. Stasis, or urinary stagnation, ensues. Because of the stasis, additional time is required for urine to reach the bladder after being formed. Urine clearance test results are not as accurate as in the nonpregnant state. Test results may reflect the prolonged time necessary for substances in the glomerular filtrate to reach the bladder. The increased risk for urinary tract infections is another result of the stagnation of urine, as the urine is rich in nutrients during pregnancy and is an excellent medium for bacterial growth.

After the fourth month of pregnancy, the enlarging uterus, in conjunction with the hyperemia of pelvic organs and the hyperplasia of the muscle and connective tissue, elevates the bladder trigone and causes thickening of the posterior margin. This process continues until the end of pregnancy and produces marked deepening and widening of the trigone.

Controversies exist with reports of studies in regard to changes in urinary bladder pressures and capacities during gestation. Whereas one study reported a hypotonic, flaccid bladder during pregnancy with decreased pressures and increased capacity near term (Beydoun, 1985), another study found that urinary bladder pressure doubled between the first and third trimesters of pregnancy, indicating a decrease in bladder capacity (Iosif et al., 1980). Iosif and colleagues found that to compensate for reduced bladder capacity, uretheral length and intrauretheral closure pressure increased 20% to preserve urinary continence, but stress incontinence increases during pregnancy.

Toward the end of pregnancy, especially with the multipara when the presenting part engages prior to the onset of labor, the entire base of the bladder is displaced anteriorly and superiorly. This changes the normal bladder surface from a normal convex shape into a concave one, greatly increasing the difficulties in diagnostic or therapeutic procedures. Pressure from the term uterus on the bladder can interfere with drainage of blood and lymph from the bladder base, making the bladder base edematous, easily traumatized, and susceptible to infection (Davidson, 1985).

Renal Function

Effective renal plasma flow, used as an index of renal blood flow, increases markedly by 60 to 80% over prepregnancy values by the middle of the second trimester, then falls to 50% above prepregnancy values in the third trimester (Dunlop, 1981; Hytten & Leitch, 1971). Renal plasma flow (RPF), like cardiac output, was significantly higher when the gravida was in the left lateral recumbent position than in the sitting, standing, or supine position. This reflected maximal venous return to the heart in the left lateral position (Davidson & Dunlop, 1984; Ezimokhai et al., 1981). *Note:* These studies did not include measurements in the right lateral position. Clark and associates (1991) were first to report results with right lateral positioning. Today, "lateral" positioning is used by the clinician to promote optimum renal plasma flow, as well as optimum cardiac output.

The glomerular filtration rate (GFR) is estimated by the evaluation of either inulin or creatinine clearance. Inulin determination is more accurate, as inulin is cleared only by the glomerulus, whereas creatinine is excreted by the tubules as well as the glomerulus. Although creatinine clearance measurements are usually higher than the actual GFR, creatinine clearance is an easier test to perform and is usually used clinically to determine the approximate GFR, as the test has a good clinical correlation in the normal range. However, if a disease condition is present that will give grossly false results for the creatinine clearance test, inulin clearance measurements are often used to determine the actual GFR (Brinkman, 1989).

The GFR increases progressively in normal pregnancy to parallel the progressive increase in systemic blood volume. The increase begins as early as 6 weeks gestation, with a peak of 50% over prepregnancy values by the end of the first trimester (Davidson & Dunlop, 1984). There are little data on the evaluation of GFR after 36 weeks gestation, however GFR does not seem to decrease at term (Monga & Creasy, 1994). Creatinine clearance is therefore increased during pregnancy with rates of 110 to 150 ml/min. Kalousek and associates (1969) found this rate to have a circadian variation, with maximal excretion between 1400 and 2200 hours and lowest excretion between 0200 and 1000 hours. The increment in RPF is initially greater than the rise in the GFR; therefore, the filtration fraction (GFR/RPF) decreases until the third trimester or pregnancy. At this time a decrease in RPF results in the return of the filtration fraction to prepregnancy values of 1/5 (Davidson & Dunlop, 1984).

As a result of the increased GFR during pregnancy, which occurs without any concomitant increase in production of urea or creatinine, there are decreased serum creatinine and urea concentrations during gestation (Davidson et al., 1981). Serum creatinine levels decrease from the nonpregnant level of 0.83 mg/dl to 0.73 mg/dl by the end of the first trimester, with levels of 0.58 in the mid second trimester, and to 0.50 mg/dl in the latter weeks of pregnancy (Monga & Creasy, 1994). Immediately after delivery, 24-hour creatinine clearance increases profoundly to parallel the increased blood volume associated with the autotransfusion that occurs in the fourth stage of labor. The marked diuresis that accompanies the early puerperium eliminates the extra fluid and creatinine clearance values return to nonpregnant levels by the sixth day postpartum (Davidson, 1985).

The blood urea nitrogen level decreases from the prepregnancy value of 12.0 mg/dl to values of 11 mg/dl in the first trimester, 9 mg/dl in the second trimester, and 10 mg/dl in the third trimester as a result of the increased GFR (Monga & Creasy, 1994).

Serum uric acid levels decrease in early pregnancy, reaching the lowest levels of 2.0 to 3.0 mg/dl by 24 weeks gestation. Uric acid levels then begin to rise and reach the nonpregnant levels by the end of gestation (Lind et al., 1984).

Renal Tubular Function

The increase in maternal plasma volume and interstitial fluid space results in a hypervolemia that challenges the renal system. Renal excretory responses must be modified for the kidney to retain adequate water and electrolytes.

Renal Sodium

Renal sodium is the prime determinant of volume homeostasis, and the net reabsorption of sodium during pregnancy is a dynamic process. The increase in the glomerular filtration rate and increase in renal plasma flow are the primary factors in the increased natriuresis that is normal for pregnancy. Each day approximately 20,000 mEq to 30,000 mEq of sodium are filtered through the kidneys. Other factors promoting sodium excretion include hormones and posture. Despite these forces, there is a gradual accumulation of approximately 950 mEq of sodium in the fetus, placenta, and maternal intravascular and interstitial compartments during the pregnancy (Lindheimer, 1980). Two to six mEq of sodium are reabsorbed each day to meet fetal and maternal needs (Davidson, 1985).

The change in tubular reabsorption represents the largest renal adjustment that occurs during gestation (Davidson, 1985). Plasma sodium decreases slightly during gestation as a result of water retention in excess of solute (Davidson et al., 1981). Balance is made difficult by opposing factors.

Factors that promote sodium excretion during pregnancy are

1. Increased GFR and RPF
2. Elevated progesterone levels
3. Atrial natriuretic factor
4. Increased antidiuretic hormone (ADH)
5. Decreased plasma albumin
6. Vasodilatory prostaglandins
7. Decreased vascular resistance

Increased secretion during pregnancy of factors that promote sodium reabsorption are

1. Aldosterone
2. Estrogens
3. Deoxycorticosterone

Volume Homeostasis

The normal increase in body weight during pregnancy can be as much as 30 to 35 pounds, with an increase in body water accounting for two thirds of this increased weight. The extracellular space gains 6 to 7 liters and the intracellular space gains approximately 2 liters. Plasma volume expansion accounts for 25% of the increase in extracellular water; the rest is attributed to interstitial fluid (Hytten, 1981b).

As water content is retained, plasma osmolarity decreases 10 mOsm/kg from the prepregnancy value of 289 ± 2.1 mOsm/kg to the normal pregnancy value of 280.9 ± 2.1 mOsm/kg. Plasma sodium levels decrease slightly, from the prepregnancy value of 140.3 ± 1.7 mM/liter to the pregnancy value of 136.6 ± 1.5 mM/liter. Plasma urea levels also decrease from the prepregnancy value of 4.9 ± 0.9 mM/liter to the pregnancy value of 2.9 ± 0.5 mM/liter (Davidson et al., 1981).

All components of the renin-angiotensin-aldosterone system are elevated during gestation. The increase in aldosterone concentrations begins in the first trimester and increases progressively until term, with a similar pattern in the increase in renin-substrate. Estrogens stimulate the liver production of renin-substrate. This results in increased renal production of renin, which peaks at 32 weeks gestation. A rise in renin causes increased conversion of angiotensinogen to angiotensins I and II (Wilson et al., 1980). The normal pregnant woman has a markedly reduced sensitivity to the hypertensive effects of angiotensin. The main response during pregnancy to the elevated levels of angiotensin is to stimulate increased aldosterone production and thereby promote sodium reabsorption.

Posture affects sodium excretion. A reduction in renal blood flow and GFR occurs in both supine and upright positions, reducing the excretion of water and sodium. The upright position triggers an extracellular shift of fluid to the legs to cause a relative decrease in central blood volume. Renin is then released to stimulate angiotensin to stimulate aldosterone secretion. Aldosterone enhances renal tubular reabsorption of sodium to reduce urinary excretion of sodium and water, and thereby the kidney is able to maintain volume homeostasis. This response is more exaggerated in the supine position (Pritchard & MacDonald, 1980).

Venous return from the legs is reduced in both the supine and upright positions. The inferior vena cava and descending aorta can be compressed by the gravid uterus in the supine position; the common iliac veins can be compressed by the uterus in the upright position. Compression of these vessels can decrease cardiac output and drop the arterial blood pressure. The result is compensatory renal vasoconstriction with decreased renal blood flow, which reduces glomerular filtration. Thus, the excretion of water and electrolytes is reduced (Pritchard & MacDonald, 1980).

Diurnal Pattern

Large amounts of fluid are retained during waking hours, when the pregnant woman is upright and engaged in usual daily activities. For this reason, dependent edema commonly develops. Fluid retention increases urine concentration as the day progresses. During sleep, especially in the lateral recumbent position, the retained fluid is mobilized into the systemic circulation and excreted. As nocturia develops, urine concentration decreases. Therefore, evening urine specimens during pregnancy are more accurate for urine concentration tests to determine tubular function than are early morning specimens (Kalousek et al., 1969).

Glucose

Glucose excretion increases during pregnancy by 10 to 100 times prepregnancy values so that glycosuria is frequently present even with normal blood glucose levels. Glycosuria is related to impaired reabsorption by the collecting tubule and Henle's loop of increased filtered glucose that misses proximal convoluted tubular reabsorption (Bishop & Green, 1981). Because the tubular maximum for glucose reabsorption does not change during pregnancy, glucose that exceeds the reabsorption capacity is excreted in the urine (Davidson, 1985).

There are three clinically important aspects for the clinician as follows:

1. Glycosuria does not necessarily denote diabetes mellitus during pregnancy.
2. Urine glucose testing cannot accurately monitor the pregnant woman with diabetes mellitus.
3. Glycosuria predisposes the pregnant woman for urinary tract infections.

Amino Acids

The increased GFR, in combination with the inability of the tubules to increase reabsorption, result in a selective amino aciduria, where three distinct patterns of amino acid excretion are present during pregnancy. Excretion patterns are as follows (Brinkman, 1989):

1. Glycine, histidine, threoine, serine, and alanine: Begin to increase in early pregnancy, double by 16 weeks gestation, then continue a progressive increase until delivery.
2. Lysine, crystine, taurine, phenylalanine, leucine, and tyrosine: Double by 16 weeks, then plateaus or decrease in the last one half of pregnancy.
3. Asparagine, glutamic acid, methionine, isoleucine, ornithine, and arginine: Unchanged with pregnancy.

The mechanism for this selective amino aciduria is not known. There is a controversy as to whether renal excretion of albumin decreases (Misiani et al., 1991), or remains stable (Wright et al., 1987) during normal pregnancy, as studies report different findings.

Urinary protein excretion increases in normal pregnancy. Normal protein excretion in the urine is less than 300 mg; therefore, proteinuria in pregnancy is not considered significant until protein excretion exceeds 300 mg in 24 hours (Davidson, 1985).

Bicarbonate

The hyperventilation and hypocarbia that accompany pulmonary adaptations during pregnancy cause an increase in the urinary excretion of bicarbonate. This produces a slight increase in the urine pH.

GASTROINTESTINAL SYSTEM

A variety of problems and complaints can develop from normal alterations in gastrointestinal function during pregnancy. In addition, pregnancy-induced hormonal and metabolic alterations may affect preexisting gastrointestinal disease. See Display 1-3 for a partial listing of women at increased risk for nutritional problems during pregnancy.

Anatomic

As pregnancy advances, positioning of the stomach and intestines is altered by the enlarging uterus, changing the angle of the gastroesophageal junction. This may displace the lower esophageal sphincter into the thorax and cause incompetence of the gastroesophageal pinchcock mechanism so that stomach contents enter the esophagus passively. Therefore, the pregnant woman is prone to passive regurgitation and aspiration during general anesthesia or periods of unconsciousness from any cause (Gutsche, 1979). Delayed gastric emptying and intestinal transit times during pregnancy are a result of hormonal and/or mechanical factors. A longer time is necessary for emptying the stomach, gastric acid secretion increases in the third trimester, and the risk for pulmonary aspiration further increases.

Clinical reports that peptic ulcer disease improves during pregnancy are common (Scott, 1994). In 1971, Hytten and Leitch proposed that the reduced symptoms were due to a reduction in acid secretion during pregnancy. When studied over the course of gestation, research has found that gastric acid secretion is reduced in the first and second trimesters, but increases significantly in the third trimester over nonpregnant values (Murray et al., 1957) and significantly increases during lactation (Hunt & Murray, 1958).

Gutsche's study (1979) found that women in labor have greater than 25 ml of gastric fluids, with a pH less than 2.5, even after an overnight fast. This puts laboring women at high risk for regurgitation and aspiration of highly acidic gastric contents. Antacids may be prescribed during labor, or prior to delivery to decrease the risk for acid aspiration syndrome if aspiration of gastric contents occurs.

Metabolism

Remarkable changes in metabolic homeostasis occur during normal pregnancy to promote fetal growth, maturation, and survival. Pregnancy has

DISPLAY 1-3

Risk Factors that May Lead to Nutritional Problems

- Significant deviation of prepregnancy weight from ideal
- Inadequate or excessive weight gain during pregnancy
- Age: Under 15, or over 35 years
- Multiple gestation
- Obstetrical history of problems, especially prior low-birth-weight infant
- Medical history of chronic illness
- Obstetrical problems with current pregnancy
- Substance abuse/Chemical dependency
- Eating disorders, including allergies, intolerances, and pica
- Psycho-social factors that limit or affect nutrition adequacy
- Abnormal laboratory findings: low hemoglobin value, abnormal blood glucose value, proteinuria, ketonuria

Normal pregnancy is also characterized by hyperinsulinemia and progressive insulin resistance. As pregnancy advances and maternal levels of glucose decrease, increased mobilization of free fatty acids and ketones occur. In the presence of hyperinsulinemia, peripheral tissues are able to utilize free fatty acids and ketones for energy; thus, more glucose is available for fetal needs. Normal pregnant women maintain a very narrow euglycemic range with a mean 24-hour plasma glucose level of 84 ± 10 mg/dl, with marked hyperinsulinemia (Felig, 1977). During sleep, the nonfeeding nighttime hours, the plasma glucose level falls progressively as the fetus continues to feed. Mean values for fasting blood glucose values decrease by 11 mg/dl as pregnancy enters the third trimester.

During the latter half of pregnancy, pancreatic reserve is stressed by the insulin-antagonist effects of rising levels of placental human chorionic somatomammotropin (HCS), prolactin, and maternal cortisol and glucagon. These effects have been described as "accelerated starvation" during the fasting state and "facilitated anabolism" after feeding (Freinkel et al., 1985). Whenever fasting is prolonged during pregnancy, ketonemia rapidly appears (Bender & Chickering, 1985). Ketones readily cross the placenta into the fetal circulation; therefore, the fetus is at risk for ketonemia when the pregnant woman fasts longer than 10 to 12 hours (Freinkel et al., 1985).

Common Problems

Nausea and Vomiting

Nausea and vomiting often occur in the first half of pregnancy. The onset typically is between the first and second missed menstrual periods and continues to about 14 to 16 weeks. Symptoms vary from a slight nausea on awakening in some women to persistent and frequent vomiting throughout the day in other women. Nausea and vomiting are usually worse in the morning, but may continue throughout the day.

The etiology of pregnancy-induced nausea and vomiting is not fully understood. Human

been termed a diabetogenic state because insulin resistance increases during gestation. In the early weeks of gestation, maternal carbohydrate metabolism is affected when elevated estrogen and progesterone levels stimulate pancreatic B-cell hyperplasia, which stimulates insulin secretion. Increased glycogen storage and increased utilization of peripheral glucose also occurs. Hepatic glucose production and maternal fasting blood glucose levels decrease. Glucose and amino acids are continuously transferred from the maternal circulation to the fetus for growth and development. These combined effects create a relative hypoglycemia in normal pregnancy (Felig, 1977).

chorionic gonadotropin (HCG) has been suggested as the cause because levels are increased at the same time that nausea and vomiting are most common. Also, levels of HCG are much higher in cases of hydatidiform mole than in normal pregnancy, and nausea and vomiting are more severe in molar pregnancies. However, Soules and associates (1980), and Depue and colleagues (1987) found no relationship between maternal serum HCG levels and the degree of nausea and vomiting, either in the normal or molar pregnancy.

The pregnant woman has a more acute sense of taste and smell because of hyperemia of the mucous membranes in the nasopharynx. Odors of fried foods, coffee, and perfumes may become offensive, and may precipitate nausea and vomiting in the early weeks of pregnancy. During the first trimester, the acute sense of taste that develops during pregnancy can contribute to the nausea. After the nausea is alleviated, the enhanced palate may add to the enjoyment of food and facilitate adequate weight gain.

Emotional factors probably contribute to the severity of nausea and vomiting. The goal of the clinician is to minimize the discomfort until the symptoms are relieved after the first trimester. Relief measures include frequent small feedings, stopping short of satiation, and avoiding as much as possible those foods that seem to precipitate nausea and vomiting. Other suggestions include consumption of a dry, carbohydrate food such as crackers upon awakening and before sitting up in the morning, or consumption of something sweet such as fruit or fruit juice, and the avoidance of spicy foods with strong odors (Harvey & Moretti, 1993).

Severe nausea and vomiting with the inability to retain any food and clinical findings of dehydration are cause for concern. The fetus is at risk for ketonemia when the pregnant woman fasts longer than 10 to 12 hours (Freinkel et al., 1985). Glucose administration may be indicated until oral feedings are retained.

Most women respond to support and counseling, and it is rare for vomiting to become so severe that dehydration, electrolyte and acid-base disturbances, and starvation become serious problems.

Heartburn

Heartburn (pyrosis) is common during pregnancy and is probably caused by reflux of acidic gastric contents into the lower esophagus. The altered position of the stomach, in combination with relaxation of the lower esophageal sphincter and delayed gastric-emptying time, are factors in the occurrence of heartburn. The increased intragastric pressure, with decreased intraesophageal pressure compounds the problem (Hytten, 1981a). Heartburn is described as a painful, retrosternal burning sensation. Relief measures include frequent, smaller meals of bland foods, and waiting at least 2 hours after eating before lying down. Antacid preparations may be prescribed (Harvey & Moretti, 1993).

Constipation

Constipation is a common problem during pregnancy because of decreased motility of the colon, increased water absorption from the colon, and mechanical pressure from the enlarging uterus. Relief measures include a high fiber diet, adequate fluid intake, exercise, and the establishment of regular bowel habits (Harvey & Moretti, 1993). Flatulence is also a common problem in pregnancy related to decreased motility in the intestinal tract along with the mechanical pressure of the enlarging uterus. Relief measures include the avoidance of gas-forming foods, increased physical activity, and development of regular bowel habits (Harvey & Moretti, 1993).

Hemorrhoids

Many factors contribute to the development of hemorrhoids in late pregnancy and the early puerperium. These include hyperemia of all organs in the pelvis, accompanied by mechanical obstruction by the enlarged uterus. This produces venous engorgement and increased pressure on the hemorrhoidal vein, which may be aggravated by constipation. Hemorrhoids can be especially severe after a prolonged second stage of labor when extended pushing efforts are necessary. Prevention of constipation does much to prevent hemorrhoids. Other relief measures include hot sitz baths, application of a local anesthetic ointment, and avoidance of standing or sitting in one position for long periods of time. The condition usually improves rapidly following delivery (Harvey & Moretti, (1993).

Weight Gain

The evaluation of weight gain and the pattern of weight gain are important in determining fetal as well as maternal status. Increased maternal metabolism and the added nutritional needs for fetal growth and development necessitate increased energy intake during pregnancy. Both prepregnancy body mass index and incremental weight gain during pregnancy are determinates of the adequacy of fetal growth (IOM, 1990). Women who are underweight prior to pregnancy or women with an inadequate weight gain during gestation are at increased risk of delivering an infant weighing less than 2500 grams. Women who are overweight prior to pregnancy or women who gain an excessive amount of weight during pregnancy are at increased risk of delivering a macrosomic infant (Abrams, 1994). Some studies suggest an association between weight gain, prepregnancy body mass index and preterm delivery (IOM, 1990; Abrams et al., 1989).

Abrams and Laros (1986) found the impact of maternal weight gain on birth weight decreases as prepregnancy weight for height increases. Therefore, different amounts of weight gain are recommended by the Institute of Medicine according to prepregnancy weight for height values, or body mass index (BMI) (IOM, 1990).

See Table 1-4 for these weight gain recommendations during pregnancy.

Although the recommended weight gain for the woman with a normal BMI is 25 to 35 pounds, additional factors influence recommendations for weight gain during pregnancy. Young adolescents and African-American women are advised to have weight gain goals at the upper ends of their recommended ranges. Women less than 62 inches tall are recommended to have weight gain goals at the lower ends of their target ranges. The recommended weight gain is greater for multiple gestation, ranging 35 to 40 pounds.

Obese women are at increased risk for both maternal complications and fetal mortality (Abrams, 1994). There are insufficient data for exact weight gain recommendations for this group of patients. The weight gain goal of 15 pounds conservatively compensates for the estimated weight of the products of conception. Due to the risks and uncertainties, individual dietary assessment and nutritional counseling should be offered to all obese pregnant women. Because total weight gain cannot be ascertained until delivery, clinicians must depend upon the rate and pattern of weight gain to manage a pregnancy. The cumulative energy cost of pregnancy has been calculated as 80,000 additional calories over prepregnancy requirements, or 300 extra calories per day (NAS, 1989). The usual weight gain pattern for the gravida with an average BMI shows a gain of 2 to 4 pounds for the first trimester, followed by a steady gain of

TABLE 1–4. Recommendations for Weight Gain During Pregnancy

Body Mass Index (BMI)	Recommended Weight Gain
Low BMI	28 to 40 pounds
Normal BMI	25 to 35 pounds
High BMI	15 to 25 pounds
Obese Women	15+ pounds
Multiple Gestation	35 to 45 pounds

From "Maternal Nutrition," by B. Abrams, 1994, in R. K. Creasy and R. Resnick, *Maternal–Fetal Medicine: Principles and Practice,* 3rd ed. Philadelphia: W. B. Saunders.

approximately 1.0 pound per week during the second and third trimesters.

Pica

Occasionally the craving to eat nonnutritive or inedible materials, including laundry starch, clay, or even dirt, may develop during pregnancy. Poor weight gain or refractory anemia may indicate pica is being practiced. Although the craving for nonnutritive foods seems to be the result of cultural influences rather than hunger, ingestion of starch (ammylophagia) or clay (geophagia) is most common in lower socioeconomic groups (Cunningham et al., 1993), especially in the southern states. In the United Kingdom, the most common form of pica is coal. Soap, toothpaste and ice pica have also been reported in numerous areas of the world (Cruikshank & Hays, 1986).

It is questionable whether or not the iron deficiency anemia in pregnant women is the cause or effect of pica. Some studies suggest that pica is triggered by iron-deficiency anemia, including the report by Pritchard and MacDonald (1980), which concluded that women with severe iron-deficiency anemia seemed to crave nonfood substances. In addition, Minnich and associates (1968) found that clays from Turkey, the state of Mississippi, and the state of Georgia impaired iron absorption. Other studies do not support this premise, as Talkington and associates (1970) reported that clays from the state of Texas and "Argo Gloss Starch"® did not significantly reduce iron absorption.

HEPATIC SYSTEM

The position of the gravid uterus in the third trimester causes the liver to rotate to a more superior and posterior position during pregnancy. Marked displacement of the liver to the right reduces the usual dullness to percussion. The size of the liver does not change significantly during pregnancy; thus, a palpable liver usually indicates disease. Hepatic blood flow increases because of increased circulating blood volume, but remains at 24 to 35% of cardiac output. Excess circulating volume is redistributed through the portal veins and vena cava, and in more than one half of normal pregnant women is seen with endoscopy as engorgement of the esophageal veins (Fagan, 1994). Normal pregnant women frequently develop spider angiomata and palmer erythema, seen in the nonpregnant individual with acute liver failure. These skin changes disappear after delivery.

Alterations in liver function during pregnancy are so significant that normal serum values for liver function tests would be suggestive of liver disease in the nonpregnant patient state (Bynum, 1977; Combes & Adams, 1972). See Table 1-5 for normal trends in liver function tests during pregnancy.

Heat-stable alkaline phosphatase isozymes are produced by the placenta, beginning in the first trimester and increasing progressively until term. They combine with hepatic stores to cause a progressive rise in serum alkaline phosphatase activity that reaches values 2 to 4 times greater than nonpregnant values (Sadovsky & Zuckerman, 1965). Levels are higher with multiple gestation and preeclampsia (Tindall, 1975). Following delivery, levels decrease gradually and reach prepregnancy values about 3 weeks postpartum (Sandusky & Zuckerman, 1965).

Serum cholesterol levels double by the end of pregnancy, along with the values of most other lipids (Tindall, 1975). Serum concentration of many proteins produced by the liver rise due to elevated estrogen levels. Ceruloplasmin concentrations also increase in response to estrogen, as do the binding proteins for corticosteroids, sex steroids, thyroid hormone, and vitamin D (Cruikshank & Hays, 1986). Fibrinogen levels increase 50% by the end of the second trimester.

The hemodilution, associated with normal pregnancy, produces a progressive decrease in serum albumin and total protein levels. Albumin values decrease to levels of 3 gm/dl during gestation from the prepregnancy level of 4.3 gm/dl. The decrease in albumin causes a fall in total serum protein concentration, but values remain above 6 gm/100 ml (Combes & Adams, 1972). Most globulins increase progressively throughout gestation. The fall in serum albumin and rise

Test	Values in Pregnancy
TABLE 1–5. Normal Values for Liver Function Tests in Pregnancy	
INCREASE	
Total alkaline phosphatase	Progressive to 2–4 x greater by term
Globulins, alpha and beta	Progressive to term
Lipids	Progressive to term
Fibrinogen	50% by second trimester
Ceruloplasmin	
Transferrin	
DECREASE	
Serum albumin	Progressive to term
Total protein	Progressive to term
Globulins, gamma	Minor decrease, or unchanged
Albumin to globulin ratio	Progressive to term
UNCHANGED	
Serum bilirubin	
Serum transaminase	
Aspartate aminotransferase (AST/SGOT)	
Alanine aminotransferase (ALT/SGPT)	
Prothrombin time	
5-Nucleotidase	
Gamma glutamyl transpeptidase (GGT, or Gamma-GT)	

in serum globulins cause a decrease in the albumin to globulin ratio (Combes & Adams, 1972).

The use of the dye bromsulphthalein (BSP) to study liver function is impaired during pregnancy as the liver decreases its ability to excrete this dye by 27% in the last one half of pregnancy. The liver also increases its capacity to store the dye by 122%. Values for excretion and storage return to normal soon after delivery.

Intrahepatic Cholestasis of Pregnancy (IHCP)

Intrahepatic cholestasis of pregnancy (IHCP), a result of liver retention and accumulation of bile related to increased levels of estrogens and progesterones, is the most common liver disorder unique to pregnancy. IHCP is characterized by generalized pruritis that usually develops after 30 weeks gestation, becomes progressively severe to term, and disappears within days following delivery (Fagan, 1994). This pruritis has been termed "pruritis gravidarum" and is caused by a deposition of bile salts in the skin (Lunzer et al., 1986). Bynum (1977) reported the severity of itching correlated with the levels of bile salts in the serum. Itching of trunk, palms, and soles of feet can be severe, especially at night, and produce insomnia and fatigue. Anorexia, malaise, epigastric discomfort, and dark urine are common. Jaundice may develop 2 to 4 weeks after the onset and resolves rapidly after delivery.

Management includes reassurance that the disorder will resolve itself after delivery as well as paliative measures. Frequent cornstarch baths, soothing ointments, and avoidance of perfumed soaps and toiletries are recommended. Oral cholestyramine use is somewhat controversial. Shaw and associates (1982) reported disappointing results, whereas Lunzer and colleagues (1986) found the drug helpful to reduce the discomfort of itching. Administration of vitamin K throughout the time the drug is used, and especially at the time of delivery, is recommended to prevent hemorrhage.

Gallbladder

A progressive increase in gallbladder size occurs during pregnancy. The gallbladder is compressed and brought into a horizontal position by the enlarging uterus (Bartoli et al., 1984). It becomes hypotonic and distended, with increases in residual and fasting volumes in late pregnancy. Mean diameter of the common bile duct is greater in pregnant women than in nonpregnant women (Radberg et al., 1989). Emptying is slowed and incomplete, as the residual volume left in the gallbladder after a meal is larger during pregnancy than in the nonpregnant state. Radberg and associates (1989) reported that causation was the relaxation effect on smooth muscle of progesterones and that the progesterones and trophic factors induce gallbladder hypertrophy.

Cholesterol gallstone formation is more common in women than in men in all populations. The incidence is further increased for pregnant women and women taking steroid contraceptives (Braverman, 1980). Abnormal gallbladder function during pregnancy, including incomplete emptying and larger residual volume of cholesterol crystals (Braverman, 1980), in conjunction with increased levels of ovarian hormone (Bartoli et al., 1984), contribute to the formation of cholesterol gallstones during pregnancy.

Acute cholecystitis is the second most common nonobstetrical surgical condition in pregnancy, after appendicitis. Diagnosis and management of acute cholecystitis and biliary obstruction during pregnancy are the same as in the nonpregnant state. Classic complaints are pain in the right upper quadrant, perhaps radiating to the back, and nausea and vomiting. Weight loss, intolerance to fatty foods, and fever are common (Fagan, 1994). General medical management includes bed rest, no oral feeding (NPO), intravenous fluids, and antibiotics. After ruling out other problems, surgical intervention is usually indicated.

REFERENCES

Abrams, B. (1994). Maternal nutrition. Chapter 11. In R. K. Creasy & R. Resnik (Eds.), Maternal–fetal medicine: Principles and practices (3rd ed.). Philadelphia: W. B. Saunders.

Abrams, B. F., & Laros, R. K. (1986). Prepregnancy weight, weight gain, and birth weight. American Journal of Obstetrics and Gynecology, 154, 503.

Abrams, B., Newman, V., Kay, T., & Parker, J. (1989). Maternal weight gain and preterm delivery. Obstetrics and Gynecology, 74, 577.

Anderson, G. J., James, G. B., Mathers, N. P., et al. (1969). The maternal oxygen tension and acid-base status during pregnancy. Journal of Obstetrics and Gynaecology British Commonwealth, 76, 16.

Anderson, H. M. (1989). Maternal hematologic disorders. Chapter 45. In R. K. Creasy & R. Resnik (Eds.), Maternal–fetal medicine: Principles and practice (2nd ed.). Philadelphia: W. B. Saunders.

Awe, R. J., Nocotra, M. B., Newsom, T. D., et al. (1979). Arterial oxygenation and alveolar-arterial gradients in term pregnancy. Obstetrics and Gynecology, 53, 182.

Bailey, R. R., & Rolleston, G. L. I. (1971). Kidney length and ureteric dilation in the puerperium. Journal of Obstetrics and Gynaecology British Commonwealth, 78, 55.

Baldwin, G. R., Moorthi, D. S., Whelton, J. A., & MacDonnell, K. F. (1977). New lung functions and pregnancy. American Journal of Obstetrics and Gynecology, 127(3), 235.

Bartoli, E., Calonaci, N., & Nenci, R. (1984). Ultrasonography of the gallbladder in pregnancy. Gastrointestinal Radiology, 9, 35.

Bauer, C., Ludwig, M., Ludwig, I., & Bartels, H. (1969). Factors governing the oxygen affinity of human adult and foetal blood. Respiratory Physiology, 7, 271.

Bender, H. S., & Chickering, W. R. (1985). Minireview: Pregnancy and diabetes: The maternal response. Life Science, 37, 1.

Beydoun, S. N. (1985). Morphologic changes in the renal tract in pregnancy. Clinical Obstetrics and Gynecology, 28(2), 245.

Bhatia, R. K., Bottoms, S. F., Saleh, A. A., et al. (1987). Mechanisms for reduced colloid osmotic pressure in preeclampsia. American Journal of Obstetrics and Gynecology, 157, 106.

Biglier, E. G., & Forsham, P. H. (1961). Studies on the expanded extracellular fluid and the responses to various stimuli in primary aldosteronism. American Journal of Medicine, 30, 564.

Bishop, J. H. V., & Green, R. (1981). Effects of pregnancy on glucose reabsorption by the proximal convoluted tubule in the rat. Journal of Physiology, 319, 271.

Bonica, J. J. (1967). Principles and practice of obstetric analgesia and anesthesia: Vol. 1: Fundamental considerations. Philadelphia: F. A. Davis.

Bonnar, J. (1981). Venous thromboembolism and pregnancy. Clinical Obstetrics and Gynecology, 8, 455–473.

Bonnar, J., McNichol, G. P., & Douglas, A. S. (1969). Fibrinolytic enzyme system and pregnancy. British Medical Journal, 3, 387–389.

Braverman, D. Z., Johnson, M. L., & Kern, F., Jr. (1980). Effects of pregnancy and contraceptive steroids on gallbladder function. New England Journal of Medicine, 302(7), 362.

Brinkman, C. R., III (1989). Biologic adaptations to pregnancy. Chapter 38. In R. K. Creasy & R. Resnik (Eds.), Maternal-fetal medicine: Principles and practice (2nd ed.) Philadelphia: W. B. Saunders.

Burwell, C. S. (1936). The influence of pregnancy on the course of heart disease. Southern Medical Journal, 29, 1194.

Burwell, C. S., Strayhorn, W. D., Flickinger, D., et al. (1938). Circulation during pregnancy. Arch Internal Medicine, 62, 979.

Bynum, T. E. (1977). Hepatic and gastrointestinal disorders in pregnancy. Medical Clinic of North America, 61(1), 129.

Capeless, E. L., & Clapp, J. F. (1989). Cardiovascular changes in early phase of pregnancy. American Journal of Obstetrics and Gynecology, 165, 883.

Chesley, L. (1978). Hypertensive disorders of pregnancy (p. 115). New York: Appleton-Century-Crofts.

Capeless, E. L., & Clapp, J. F. (1991). When do cardiovascular parameters return to their preconception values? American Journal of Obstetrics and Gynecology, 165, 883.

Chesley, L. C., Valenti, C., & Uichano, L. (1959). Alterations in body fluid compartments and exchangeable sodium in early puerperium. American Journal of Obstetrics and Gynecology, 77, 1054.

Christensen, T., Klebe, J. G., Bertelsen, V., et al. (1989). Changes in renal volume during normal pregnancy. Acta Obstetrica Gynaecoligica Scandinavica, 68, 541.

Clapp, J. F., Seaward, B. L., Sleamaker, R. H., et al. (1988). Maternal physiologic adaptations to early human pregnancy. American Journal of Obstetrics and Gynecology, 156, 1456.

Clark, S. L., Cotton, D. B., Hankins, G. D. V., & Phelan, J. P. (1994). Handbook of critical care obstetrics. Oxford: Blackwell Scientific.

Clark, S. L., Cotton, D. B., Lee, W., et al. (1989). Central hemodynamic assessment of normal term pregnancy. American Journal of Obstetrics and Gynecology, 161(6), 1439.

Clark, S. L., Cotton, D. B., Pivarnik, J. M., et al. (1991). Position change and central hemodynamic profile during normal third trimester pregnancy and postpartum. American Journal of Obstetrics and Gynecology, 164, 883–887.

Combes, B., & Adams, R. H. (1972). Disorders of the liver in pregnancy. Chapter 6. In N. S. Assali & C. R. Brinkman III, Pathophysiology of gestation: Vol. I. Maternal disorders. New York: Academic.

Cotton, D. B., Gonik, B., Spillman, T., & Dorman, K. F. (1984). Intrapartum to postpartum changes in colloid osmotic pressure. American Journal of Obstetrics and Gynecology, 149, 174.

Cruikshank, D. P., & Hays, P. M. (1986). Maternal physiology in pregnancy. Chapter 5. In S. G. Gabbe, J. R. Niebyl, & J. L. Simpson (Eds.), Obstetrics: Normal and problem pregnancies. New York: Churchill Livingstone.

Cugell, D. W., Frank, N. R., Gaensler, E. A., et al. (1953). Pulmonary function in pregnancy. I.

Serial observations in normal women. American Rev Tuberc, 67, 568.

Cunningham, F. G., MacDonald, P. C., & Gant, N. F. (1989). The puerperium. In Williams obstetrics (18th ed., p. 251). New York: Appleton-Century-Crofts.

Cunningham, F. G., MacDonald, P. C., Gant, N. F., et al. (1993). Maternal adaptations in pregnancy. Chapter 8. In Williams obstetrics (19th ed.). New York: Appleton-Century-Crofts.

Cutforth, R., & MacDonald, C. G. (1966). Heart sounds and murmurs in pregnancy. American Heart Journal, 71(6), 741.

Davidson, J. M. (1985). The physiology of the renal tract in pregnancy. Clinical Obstetrics & Gynecology, 28(2), 257.

Davidson, J. M., & Dunlop, W. (1984). Changes in renal hemodynamics and tubular function induced by normal human pregnancy. Seminars in Nephrology, 4, 198.

Davidson, J. M., Vallotton, M. B., & Lindheimer, M. D. (1981). Plasma osmolarity and urinary concentration and dilution during and after pregnancy. British Journal of Obstetrics and Gynaecology, 88, 472.

Depue, R. H., Bernstein, L., Ross, R. K., Judd, H. I., & Henderson, B. E. (1987). Hyperemesis gravidarium in relation to estradiol levels, pregnancy outcome, and other maternal factors: A seroepidemiologic study. American Journal of Obstetrics and Gynecology, 156, 1137.

Dunlop, W. (1981). Serial changes in renal haemodynamics during normal human pregnancy. British Journal of Obstetrics and Gynaecology, 88, 1.

Enein, M., Zina, A. A. A., Kassem, M., & El-Tabbakh, G. (1987). Echocardiography of the pericardium in pregnancy. Obstetrics and Gynecology, 69, 851.

Ezimokhai, M., Davidson, J. M., Phillips, P. R., et al. (1981). Non-postural serial changes in renal function during the third trimester. British Journal of Obstetrics and Gynaecology, 88, 465.

Fadnes, H. O., & Øian, P. (1989). Transcapillary fluid balance and plasma volume regulation: A review. Obstetrics & Gynecologic Survey, 44(11), 769.

Fagan, E. A. (1994). Diseases of liver, biliary system, and pancreas. Chapter 58. In R. K. Creasy & R. Resnik (Eds.), Maternal–fetal medicine: Principles and Practices (3rd ed.). Philadelphia: W. B. Saunders.

Fay, R. A., Hughes, A. O., & Farron, N. T. (1983). Platelets in pregnancy: Hyperdestruction in pregnancy. Obstetrics and Gynecology, 61(2), 238.

Felig, P. (1977). Body fuel metabolism and diabetes in pregnancy. Medical Clinic of North America, 61(1), 43.

Fleming, A. F. (1975). Haematological changes in pregnancy. Clinical Obstetrics and Gynecology, 2(2), 269.

Fried, A. Woodring, J. H., & Thompson, T. J. (1983). Hydronephrosis of pregnancy. Journal of Ultrasound Medicine, 2, 255.

Freinkel, N., Dooley, S. L., & Metzger, B. E. (1985). Care of the pregnant woman with insulin-dependent diabetes mellitus. New England Journal of Medicine, 313, 96.

Gabbe, S. G., Niebyl, J. R., & Simpson, J. L. (Eds.). (1986). Obstetrics: Normal and problem pregnancies. New York: Churchill Livingstone.

Gerbasi, F. R., Bottoms, S., Farag, A., & Mammen, E. F. (1990). Changes in hemastasis activity during delivery and the immediate postpartum period. American Journal of Obstetrics and Gynecology, 162(5), 1158.

Greiss, F., C., & Anderson, S. G. (1970). Effect of ovarian hormones on the uterine vascular bed. American Journal of Obstetrics and Gynecology, 107, 829.

Gutsche, B. B. (1979). Maternal physiologic adaptations during pregnancy. In S. M. Schnider & G. Levinson, Anesthesia for obstetrics. Baltimore: Williams and Wilkins.

Hankins, G. D. V., Wendel, G. D., Cunningham, F. G., et al. (1984). Longitudinal evaluation of hemodynamic changes in eclampsia. American Journal of Obstetrics and Gynecology, 150, 506.

Harvey, M. G., & Moretti, M. L. (1993). Maternal adaptations to pregnancy. Chapter 13. In R. A. Knuppel & J. E. Drukker (Eds.), High-risk pregnancy: A team approach (2nd ed.). Philadelphia: W. B. Saunders.

Hunt, J. N., & Murray, F. A. (1958). Gastric function in pregnancy. Journal of Obstetrics and Gynaecology British Commeonwealth, 65, 78.

Hytten, F. E. (1981a). The alimentary system. In F. Hytten & G. Chamberlain (Eds.), Clinical physiology in obstetrics. Oxford: Blackwell Scientific.

Hytten, F. E. (1981b). Weight gain in pregnancy. In F. Hytten & G. Chamberlain (Eds.), Clinical physiology in obstetrics. Oxford: Blackwell Scientific.

Hytten, F. E., & Leitch, I. (1971). The physiology of human pregnancy (2nd ed.). Oxford: Blackwell Scientific.

IOM (Institute of Medicine), Committee on Nutritional Status During Pregnancy and Lactation. (1990). National academy of sciences, nutrition during pregnancy. Washington, DC: National Academy Press.

Iosif, S., Ingermarsson, I., & Ulmsten, U. (1980). Urodynamics studies in normal pregnancy and in puerperium. American Journal of Obstetrics and Gynecology, 137, 696.

Jepson, J. H. (1968). Endocrine control of maternal and fetal erythropoiesis. Canadian Medical Association Journal, 98, 844.

Kalousek, G., Hlavecek, C., Nedoss, B., et al. (1969). Circadian rhythms of creatinine and electrolyte excretion in healthy pregnant women. American Journal of Obstetrics and Gynecology, 103, 856.

Katz, R., Karliner, J. S., & Resnik, R. (1978). Effects of a natural volume overload state (pregnancy) on left ventricular performance in normal human subjects. Circulation, 58, 434.

Kerr, M. G. (1965). The mechanical effects of the gravid uterus in late pregnancy. Journal of Obstetrics and Gynaecology British Commonwealth, 72, 513.

Laros, R. K. (1994). Maternal hematologic disorders. Chapter 53. In R. K. Creasy & R. Resnik. Maternal–fetal medicine: Principles and practice (3rd ed.). Philadelphia: W. B. Saunders.

Lee, W., & Cotton, D. B. (1991). Cardiorespiratory changes during pregnancy. Chapter 1. In S. L. Clark, D. B. Cotton, G. D. V. Hankins, & J. P. Phelan, Critical care obstetrics (2nd ed.). Oxford: Blackwell Scientific.

Lee, W., Rokey, R., Miller, J., & Cotton, D. (1989). Maternal hemodynamic effects of uterine contractions by M-mode and pulsed-Doppler echocardiography. American Journal of Obstetrics and Gynecology, 161(4), 974.

Lees, M. M., Taylor, S. H., Scott D. B., et al. (1967). A study of cardiac output at rest throughout pregnancy. Journal of Obstetrics and Gynaecology British Commonwealth, 74, 319.

Lind, T., Godfrey, K. A., & Otum, H. (1984). Changes in serum uric acid concentrations during normal pregnancy. British Journal of Obstetrics Commonwealth, 91, 128.

Lindheimer, M. D., (1980). Current concepts of sodium metabolism and use of diuretics in pregnancy. Contemporary OB/GYN, 15, 207.

Lindheimer, M. D., & Katz, A. I. (1975). Renal changes during pregnancy: Their relevance to volume homeostasis. Clinical Obstetrics and Gynecology, 2(2), 345.

Linhard, J. (1915). Uber das minutevolumens des herzens bei ruhe und bei muskelarbeit. Plugers Arch, 161, 233. Quoted in S. L. Clark, D. B. Cotton, G. D. V. Hankins, & J. P. Phelan. (1991). Critical care obstetrics (2nd ed., p. 9). Oxford: Blackwell Scientific.

Lund, C. J., & Donovan, J. C. (1967). Blood volume during pregnancy. American Journal of Obstetrics and Gynecology, 98(3), 393.

Lunzer, M., Barnes, P., Byth, K., & O'Halloran, M. (1986). Serum bile acid concentrations during pregnancy and their relationship to obstetric cholestasis. Gastroenterology, 91, 825.

Mabie, W. C., DiSessa, T. G., Crocker, L. G., et al. (1994). A longitudinal study of cardiac output in normal human pregnancy. American Journal of Obstetrics and Gynecology, 170, 849–856.

MacNeily, A. E., Goldenberg, S. L., Allen, G. J. J., et al. (1991). Sonographic visualization of the ureter in pregnancy. Journal of Urology, 146, 298.

Metcalfe, J. (1985). Oxygen supply and fetal growth. Journal of Reproductive Medicine, 30, 301.

Metcalfe, J., McAnulty, J. H., & Ueland, K. (1981). Cardiovascular physiology. Clinical Obstetrics and Gynecology, 24(3), 693.

Meyer, J. E. (1983). Clinical chemistry. Chapter 9. In R. S. Abrams & P. Wexler (Eds.), Medical care of the pregnant patient. Boston: Little, Brown.

Minnich, V., Okcuoghi, A., Tarcon, V., et al. (1968). Pica in Turkey, II. Effect of clay upon iron absorption. American Journal of Clinical Nutrition, 21, 78.

Misiani, R., Marchesi, D., Tiraboschi, G., et al. (1991). Urinary albumin excretion in normal pregnancy and pregnancy-induced hypertension. Nephron, 59, 416.

Moise, K. J. Jr, & Cotton, D. B. (1991). Colloid osmotic pressure and pregnancy. Chapter 2. In S. L. Clark, D. B. Cotton, G. D. V. Hankins, & J. P. Phelan (Eds.), Critical care obstetrics (2nd ed.). Oxford: Blackwell Scientific.

Monga, M., & Creasy, R. K. (1994). Cardiovascular and renal adaptation to pregnancy. Chapter 46. In R. K. Creasy & R. Resnik (Eds.), Maternal-fetal medicine: Principles and Practices (3rd ed.). Philadelphia: W. B. Saunders.

Murray, F. A., Eishine, J. P., & Fielding, J. (1957). Gastric secretion in pregnancy. Journal of Obstetrics and Gynaecology British Empire, 64, 373.

NAS (National Academy of Sciences). (1989). National research council, food and nutrition board: Recommended dietary allowances (10th ed.). Washington, DC.

Øian, P., Maltau, J. M., Noddeland, H., & Fadnes, H. O. (1986). Transcapillary fluid balance in preeclampsia. British Journal of Obstetrics and Gynaecology, 93, 235.

Pernoll, M. L., Metcalfe, J., Schlenker, T. L., et al. (1975). Oxygen consumption at rest and during exercise in pregnancy. Respiratory Physiology, 25, 285.

Pitkin, R. M., & Witte, D. L. (1979). Platelet and leukocyte count in pregnancy. Journal American Medical Association, 242(24), 2696.

Pritchard, J. A. (1965). Changes in blood volume during pregnancy and delivery. Anesthesiology, 26(4), 393.

Pritchard, J. A., Baldwin, R. M., Dickey, J. C., & Wiggins, K. M. (1962). Blood volume changes in pregnancy and the puerperium. II. Red blood cell loss and changes in apparent blood volume following vaginal delivery, cesarean section, and cesarean section plus total hysterectomy. American Journal of Obstetrics and Gynecology, 84, 1271.

Pritchard, J. A., & Hunt, C. F. (1958). A comparison of the hematologic responses following the routine prenatal administration of intramuscular, and oral iron. Surgical Gynecology and Obstetrics, 106, 516.

Pritchard, J. A., & MacDonald, P. C. (1980). Williams obstetrics (16th ed.). New York: Appleton-Century-Crofts.

Prowse, C. M., & Gaensler, E. A. (1965). Respiratory and acid-base changes during pregnancy. Anesthesiology, 26, 381.

Radberg, G., Asztely, M., Cantor, P., et al. (1989). Gastric and gallbladder emptying in relation to the secretion of cholecystokinin after a meal in late pregnancy. Digestion, 42, 174.

Robson, S. C., Dunlop, W., Boys, R. J., & Hunter, S. (1987a). Cardiac output during labor. British Medical Journal, 295, 1169.

Robson, S. C., Hunter, S., Moore, M., & Dunlop, W. (1987b). Haemodynamic changes during the puerperium: A Doppler and M-Mode echocardiographic study. British Journal of Obstetrics and Gynaecology, 94, 1028.

Robson, S. C., Hunter, S., Boys, R. J., & Dunlop, W. (1989). Serial study of factors influencing changes in cardiac output during human pregnancy. American Journal of Physiology, 256, H1060.

Rovinsky, J. R., & Jaffin, H. (1965). Cardiovascular hemodynamics in pregnancy: Blood and plasma values in multiple pregnancy. American Journal of Obstetrics and Gynecology, 93(1), 1.

Rubler, S., Damani, P. M., & Pinto, E. R. (1977). Cardiac size and performance during pregnancy estimated with echocardiography. American Journal of Cardiology, 40, 534.

Sadovsky, E., & Zuckerman, H. (1965). An alkaline phosphatase specific to normal pregnancy. Obstetrics and Gynecology, 26(2), 211.

Sala, N. L., & Rubi, R. A. (1967). Ureteral function in pregnant women: II. Ureteral contractility during normal pregnancy. American Journal of Obstetrics and Gynecology, 99(2), 228.

Schulman, A., & Herlinger, H. (1975). Urinary tract dilation in pregnancy. British Journal of Radiology, 48, 638.

Scott, L. D. (1994). Gastrointestinal disease in pregnancy. Chapter 57. In R. K. Creasy & R. Resnik (Eds.), Maternal–fetal medicine: Principles and practice (3rd ed.). Philadelphia: W. B. Saunders.

Shabetai, R. (1994). Cardiac diseases. Chapter 47. In R. K. Creasy & R. Resnik (Eds.), Maternal–fetal medicine: Principles and practice (3rd ed.). Philadelphia: W. B. Saunders.

Shaw, D., Frohlich, J. Wittmann, B. A., et al. (1982). A prospective study of 18 patients with cholestasis of pregnancy. Ameriçan Journal of Obstetrics and Gynecology, 142, 621.

Soules, M. R., Hughes, C. L., Garcia, J. A., et al., (1980). Nausea and vomiting of pregnancy: Role of human chorionic gonadotropin and 17-hydroxyprogesterone. Obstetrics and Gynecology, 55, 696.

Symonds, F. M. (1983). Renin-angiotensin system in normal and hypertensive pregnancy. In P. J. Lewis, S. Moncada, & J. O'Grady (Eds.), Prostacyclin in pregnancy (p. 91). New York: Raven Press.

Talkington, K. M., Gant, N. F., Scott, D. E., & Pritchard, J. A. (1970). Effect of ingestion of starch and some clays on iron absorption. American Journal of Obstetrics and Gynecology, 108, 262.

Tapia, H. R., Johnson, C. E., & Strong, C. G. (1973). Effect of oral contraceptive therapy on the reninangiotensin system in normotensive and hypertensive women. Obstetrics and Gynecology, 41, 643.

Templeton, A., & Kelman, G. R. (1976). Maternal blood-gases, (PAO_2-PaO_2), physiologic shunt, and VD/VT in normal pregnancy. British Journal of Anaesthesiology, 48, 1001.

Tindall, V. R. (1975). The liver in pregnancy. Clinical Obstetrics and Gynecology, 2(2), 441.

Ueland, K., & Hansen, J. M. (1969a). Maternal cardiovascular dynamics II: Posture and uterine contractions. American Journal of Obstetrics and Gynecology, 103(1), 1.

Ueland, K., & Hansen, J. M. (1969b). Maternal cardiovascular dynamics III: Labor and delivery under local and caudal analgesia. American Journal of Obstetrics and Gynecology, 103(1), 8.

Ueland, K., Novy, M. J., Peterson, E. N., & Metcalfe, J. (1969). Maternal cardiovascular dynamics IV: The influence of gestational age on the maternal cardiovascular response to posture and exercise. American Journal of Obstetrics and Gynecology, 104(6), 856.

Ueland, K. (1976). Maternal cardiovascular dynamics VII: Intrapartum blood volume changes. American Journal of Obstetrics and Gynecology, 126(6), 671.

Valenzuela, G. J. (1989). Is a decrease in plasma oncotic pressure enough to explain the edema of pregnancy? American Journal of Obstetrics and Gynecology, 161(6), 1624.

Villar, J., Pepke, J., Markush, L., et al. (1989). The measuring of blood pressure during pregnancy. American Journal of Obstetrics and Gynecology, 161(4), 1019.

Walters, W. A. W., & Lim, Y. L. (1975). Blood volume and haemodynamics in pregnancy. Clinical Obstetrics and Gynecology, 2(2), 301–320.

Wilson, M., Morganti, A. A., Zervoudakis, J., et al. (1980). Blood pressure, the renin-aldosterone system and sex steroids throughout normal pregnancy. American Journal of Medicine, 68, 97.

Wright, A., Steeke, P., Bennet, J. R., et al. (1987). The urinary excretion of albumin in normal pregnancy. British Journal of Obstetrics and Gynaecology, 94, 408.

CHAPTER 2

Fetal Adaptation

Eda M. Uçkan and Nancy Surratt Townsend

The complex and unique physiology of the fetal cardiovascular system allows for the necessary growth and development of the fetus. An intimate understanding of these processes in conjunction with maternal physiologic adaptations during pregnancy provide the clinician with the necessary foundation for optimal care of the mother and fetus.

FETAL CARDIOVASCULAR PHYSIOLOGY

Fetal blood flow patterns and oxygen delivery differ fundamentally from those of the adult. Conceptualization of fetal circulation has evolved from mammalian animal models, particularly those of fetal sheep. Such investigation has shown this unique system's ability to promote fetal growth and development via high flow rates in attempt to counteract overall decreased levels of circulating partial pressure of oxygen (PO_2).

A brief comparison between fetal and adult circulation reveals that adult blood is oxygenated by the lungs and ejected from the left ventricle, perfusing all major organs with complete separation of oxygenated and deoxygenated blood. Cardiac output is the singular result of outflow from the left ventricle. Fetal blood, by contrast, is oxygenated by the placenta and ejected from both left and right ventricles with each supplying mainly the upper and lower body, respectively, with multiple mixing points of oxygenated and deoxygenated blood (Bristow, Rudolph, & Itskovitz, 1981; Edelstone & Rudolph, 1979; Peeters et al., 1979). Cardiac output is a result of combined right and left ventricular outflow. The interdependence of these dissimilar circulations further contributes to the complexities of parturition and care of the high-risk mother and fetus. Figure 2-1 outlines significant maternal and fetal cardiovascular differences.

Circulation

Fetal circulation has unique anatomic and physiologic properties. Edelstone and Rudolph (1979) describe fetal circulation as an altered blood flow with intercommunicating pathways and preferential streaming patterns to provide optimal delivery of oxygenated umbilical venous blood to the fetus.

Oxygenated blood returns to the fetus through the umbilical vein of the placenta. It branches to the left lobe of the liver and empties in the inferior vena cava, where it combines with less oxygenated blood in the heart. Studies outline streaming tracts that diminish the mixture of oxygenated and deoxygenated blood in the fetal circulation (Bristow et al., 1983; Peeters et al., 1979). This preferential streaming also promotes more oxygenated blood to be direct-

32

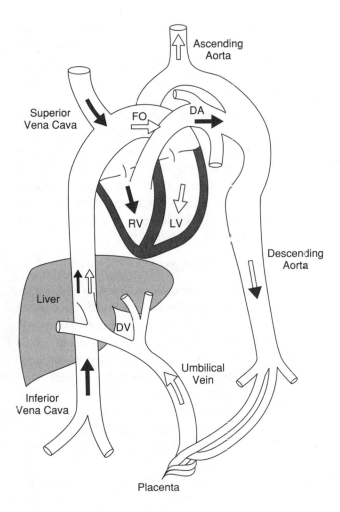

Figure 2-1. Fetal circulation.

The right and left fetal ventricles function in parallel rather than in series as a result of shunting within the fetal heart. Right ventricular outflow, approximately 65% of total cardiac output, primarily supplies the peripheral circulation and is recirculated back to the placenta for gas exchange. Left ventricular outflow perfuses the brain and myocardium representing approximately 35% of total cardiac output. Blood ejected from the left heart is well oxygenated (approximately 60%) as opposed to the relatively desaturated output of the right heart. Such preferences in perfusion allow the more highly saturated left ventricular output to increase in times of stress, thereby selectively directing blood flow to the heart and brain while redirecting flow from nonvital end organs.

An overwhelming 40% of total fetal cardiac output is directed to the placental circulation for gas exchange and returned to the heart for organ perfusion. The fetus utilizes a distinct mechanism of blood flow distribution and redistribution to end organs based on arterial oxygen content (Peeters et al., 1979). Blood is systematically shunted to the central nervous system and heart during periods of decreased arterial oxygen content. Umbilical venous blood flow is increased and thus matched to the oxygen requirements of the fetus without any changes in maternal delivery of blood to the placenta. This is accomplished by the ability of the fetus to maintain a high degree of mean systemic blood pressure to increase blood flow from the umbilical vein. Fetal heart rate, not an increase in stroke volume, is the main fetal compensatory mechanism under these circumstances. Data suggest that fetal heart function is at or near capacity and exhibits a limited ability to alter cardiac output in response to stress (Gilbert, 1980). Although fetal circulation is able to compensate for hypoxia, this window of balance is quite limited. Therefore, optimizing maternal blood and oxygen delivery to the placenta is crucial to overall fetal well-being.

ed across the foramen ovale to the left atrium and ultimately to myocardial and cerebral tissue. Blood with less oxygen saturation is preferentially directed to the lower body and back to the placenta for reoxygenation.

Cardiac Output

Once it becomes functional, the fetal heart is a remarkably effective pump and the combined ventricular cardiac output has been reported at approximately 450 ml/kg/min (Friedman, 1972). In comparison to adult cardiac output, the fetus delivers significantly more blood and oxygen per unit of body weight (Jones et al., 1977). A constant return of umbilical venous blood to the heart ultimately allows for this elevated cardiac output.

Regulation

The fetus meets its oxygen demands via complex neural and hormonal responses that allow for maintenance of blood pressure, heart rate, and distribution of blood flow. Interactions between these responses favor a redistribution of cardiac output in the face of fetal stress. Regulation is accomplished through baroreceptors, chemoreceptors, and neural and hormonal mediators.

Baroreceptors located in the aortic arch and in the carotid sinus are sensitive stretch receptors that detect changes in arterial pressure and play a role in the overall stabilization of the fetal circulation (Itskovitz, 1983; Hanson, 1988). These receptors cause changes in fetal heart rate in response to increases and decreases in fetal blood pressure. Tachycardia is induced to compensate for decreased blood pressure that may be precipitated by hemorrhage or venous occlusion. With large blood pressure drops, however, bradycardia ensues.

Chemoreceptors, present in the medulla oblongata, carotid bodies, and aortic bodies respond to conditions of asphyxia with changes in oxygen and carbon dioxide tension. Although their exact role in the fetus is unclear, the net result of hypoxia or hypercapnia is bradycardia and hypertension (Parer, Kreuger, & Harris, 1980). Chemoreceptor stimulation rather than baroreceptor stimulation might be the primary cause of the increased vagal activity and bradycardia, which accompanies fetal hypoxemia (Lewis et al., 1980).

Autonomic nervous system control of the heart begins very early in fetal development. Sympathetic stimulation of alpha-adrenergic and beta adrenergic innervation results in tachycardia, augmented myocardial contractility, and increased arterial blood pressure. Innervation is in the sinoatrial node, atrioventricular node, and within the arterioles of the fetal circulation. Cardiac beta-adrenergic stimulation is responsible for increased heart rate and contractility in addition to increased pulmonary and myocardial flow. Peripheral alpha-adrenergic stimulation mediates vasoconstriction of the renal and mesenteric circulations with a resulting increase in blood pressure.

Parasympathetic innervation is via the vagus nerve and elicits an inhibitory effect of the fetal heart rate. The interplay between decreased fetal heart rate caused by parasympathetic innervation and increased heart rate resulting from sympathetic innervation is responsible for the beat-to-beat variability demonstrated via electronic fetal monitoring.

Many factors contribute to the regulation of fetal circulation. Circulating catecholamines play a role in the fetal stress response later in gestation. Prostaglandins contribute to cerebral blood flow in the presence of hypoxemia and arginine vasopressin produces vasoconstriction to peripheral organs while redistributing blood flow in the face of hypoxia.

Fetal Oxygen Transport

The transport of oxygen from the atmosphere to fetal tissues is accomplished through a series of progressively decreasing partial pressures of oxygen (PO_2) from mother to fetus (Rankin et al., 1971). Overall transport is driven by a gradient of oxygen pressure that favors fetal oxygen consumption. Despite an end result of decreased PO_2, the fetus thrives in an environment of aerobic metabolism. Figure 2-2 details this process.

Exchange of maternal oxygen to umbilical circulation occurs across the semipermeable membrane of the placenta. There is no continuous direct communication between maternal and fetal blood, however, the placenta acts as a venous equilibrator to enhance optimal fetal gas exchange. Equilibration occurs across unidirectional channels between maternal and intervillous blood and fetal capillary blood. As illustrated in Figure 2-3, maternal blood has a higher PO_2 than that of fetal blood. While approaching the venous end of these channels, maternal PO_2 decreases and fetal PO_2 increases so that both are equal. Fetal PO_2 does not exceed that of maternal PO_2, and the total transfer of oxygen is a relatively inefficient process (Rankin et al., 1971). As noted, average umbilical venous PO_2 levels are significantly lower than maternal arterial PO_2. This accounts for fetal PO_2 values of approximately 25 to 30 torr. Therefore, optimal maternal oxygenation and blood flow to the uterus and placenta are crucial to fetal tissue perfusion. Oxygen uptake and consumption by fetal tissue are reported to be considerably higher per

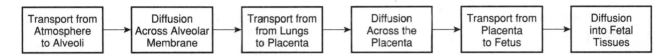

Figure 2-2. Transport of oxygen to fetus.

unit of body weight than in the adult model (Battaglia & Meschia, 1986). The following fetal adaptations enable transport of large amounts of oxygen for tissue consumption in the fetus.

Oxygen delivery is a function of oxygen content and cardiac output. Oxygen content is based upon the ability of the blood to hold and release oxygen. It is a function of the quantity of hemoglobin available for oxygen binding, the affinity for binding of oxygen, overall saturation of hemoglobin with oxygen, and oxygen dissolved within the circulating plasma. Although all are important, quantity of hemoglobin can have a significant impact on oxygen content and intrauterine fetal transfusion has been utilized to maintain adequate levels of hemoglobin in pathologic fetal conditions.

Hemoglobin within fetal red blood cells has a higher affinity for oxygen than adult hemoglobin. There is a leftward shift in the fetal oxyhemoglobin dissociation curve (Figure 2-4) relative to the adult, thus increasing oxygenation at any given oxygen tension. This high affinity allows for binding of oxygen to hemoglobin molecules at very low concentrations of PO_2, such as

those represented in the umbilical venous flow. This further enables the red blood cells to circulate through the placenta and become highly saturated with oxygen.

Crucial to the delivery of oxygen to fetal end organs is an effective method of transportation. This is accomplished by the cardiac output and as previously mentioned is significantly elevated in the fetus. Comparatively, oxygen delivery may reach 2 to 3 times that of the adult per unit of body weight and compensates for low circulating PO_2 values. The aforementioned regulatory mechanisms of fetal circulation contribute to this elevated baseline.

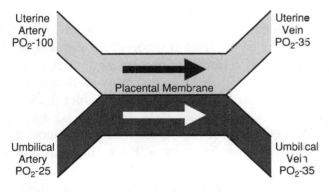

Figure 2-3. Model of venous equilibration.

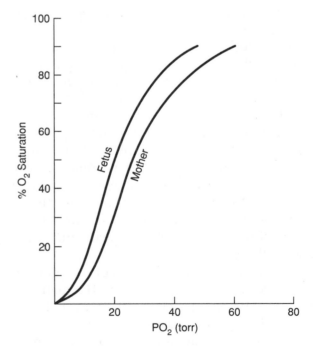

Figure 2-4. Maternal and fetal oxyhemoglobin dissociation curves.

FETAL RESPONSES TO ACUTE HYPOXEMIA

Circulatory and Metabolic Responses

Much has been learned about fetal responses to acute hypoxemia through chronically catheterized fetal lamb models. With decreasing amounts of umbilical venous oxygen, the fetus enters three stages of acute hypoxemia (Peeters et al., 1979). The first stage is characterized by the fetal ability to compensate for up to a 50% reduction in oxygen content. Fetal cardiac output is redistributed to the heart, brain, and adrenal glands. This is accomplished by vasoconstriction of the peripheral organs and decreased vascular resistance of the fetal brain, heart and adrenal glands. This flow redistribution results in decreased oxygen delivery to the periphery (Cohn, Sacks, Heyman, & Rudolph, 1974; Peeters et al., 1979; Reid et al., 1991). In this first stage, the fetus is not in a life-threatening state. However, further decreases of oxygen content may not be tolerated.

If hypoxemia progresses, the fetus enters a second stage, the chief component of which is anaerobic metabolism. If the oxygen supply is not restored in a timely manner, lactic acid will accumulate, eventually resulting in a base deficit and metabolic acidemia. There is some evidence suggesting that the cardiovascular response to hypoxia is influenced by blood pH. In one study on newborn lambs, cardiac output reportedly fell to approximately 60% of control following a drop in pH to 7.11 (Fisher, 1986). In any event, further compensatory decreases in blood flow to nonvital organs and tissues will occur, in an attempt to maximize blood flow to the heart and brain. This shift of blood flow in favor of the heart and brain allows these organs to receive available oxygen and to maintain oxygen consumption in the face of hypoxia (Fisher, Heymann & Rudolph, 1982; Jones et al., 1977). Even if oxygen delivery is decreased, the fetal tissues in this second stage are still able to extract more oxygen from hemoglobin in order to meet the high and fixed oxygen demands of the brain

and heart (Gu, Jones, & Parer, 1985; Wilkening & Meschia, 1983; Rurak et al., 1990).

If hypoxia is severe or prolonged, the fetus will enter what is known as a delivery-dependent state. At this point, the fetus is no longer able to increase oxygen extraction from available sources in order to meet tissue demands. Thus, tissue oxygenation becomes dependent on oxygen delivery. The cerebral vascular resistance cannot decrease further in response to the increasing hypoxemia, and thus cerebral blood flow can no longer be augmented. With the progressive reduction in oxygen delivery, the uptake of oxygen falls (Field et al., 1990). Perfusion of the priority organs can no longer be maintained, and, because lactate efflux from the brain is relatively slow, central nervous system damage may occur (Parer, 1994). Fetal death is the endpoint of this degree of hypoxia.

Neurohormonal Responses

These compensatory mechanisms to hypoxia are mediated by several neurohormonal factors. As the partial pressure of oxygen decreases, both the chemoreceptors and baroreceptors are stimulated. This stimulation causes sympathetic and parasympathetic responses. The fetal heart rate decreases prior to any change in fetal blood pressure, suggesting that chemoreceptor activation occurs before baroreceptor activation (Parer, Krueger, & Harris, 1980). Parasympathetic discharge mainly results in decreased fetal heart rate due to a vagal effet on the sinoatrial (SA) node. The sympathetic response is manifested by a cardiac beta-adrenergic response (increased heart rate/contractility) and a peripheral alpha-adrenergic response (vasoconstriction).

Arginine vasopressin (AVP) plays an important role in the fetal compensatory cycle. This hormone is released in response to changes in either maternal or fetal osmolality or decreases in fetal intravascular volume or fetal blood pressure (Weitzman et al., 1978; Leake et al., 1978; Ervin et al., 1986; Rurak, 1979). The changes in blood flow mediated by AVP are similar to the hemodynamic changes noted in an acute hypoxemic fetus (Ervin, Ross, Leake, & Fisher, 1992; Irion, Mack, & Clark, 1990).

Hypoxia may cause an increase in fetal renin activity (Nakamura, Ayres, Gomez, & Robillard, 1985). However, unlike in the adult model, fetal angiotensin II and aldosterone do not increase in relation to changes in renin activity (Robillard & Nakamura, 1988).

Other factors in the fetal compensatory response to hypoxia include secretion of adreno-corticotropic hormone (ACTH) and cortisol (Brooks & Challis, 1992; Ozollins, Young, & McMillin, 1992). Fetal plasma catecholamine levels are also known to increase in response to hypoxia. The initial fetal blood pressure elevation during a hypoxemic episode corresponds to an increase in norepinephrine secretion. However, plasma norepinephrine levels decline after about 5 minutes of hypoxemia. Conversely, adrenal epinephrine secretion starts gradually, but levels persist during longer periods of hypoxia (Cohn, Piasecki, & Jackson, 1982).

Fetal Heart Rate Responses

One of the most commonly used methods of intrapartum evaluation of fetal well-being is electronic fetal heart rate (FHR) monitoring (Freeman, Garite, & Nageotte, 1991). This method may be used to indirectly detect developing fetal hypoxia, thus allowing prompt intervention to avoid acidosis and neurologic injury. Specific FHR patterns may be identified as a result of hypoxia (Parer & Livingston, 1990). A brief overview of FHR patterns follows.

Late decelerations of the FHR are attributed to a decrease in fetal oxygenation caused by a decrease in uterine blood flow (Damron, Chaffin, & Anderson et al., 1994). Hon (1959) was one of the first to describe the pathophysiology of late decelerations. This late deceleration pattern is thought to have both reflex and hypoxic components. Work by Martin and colleagues (1979) helped clarify the physiologic mechanisms involved in FHR responses to hypoxemia. In their sheep model, they proposed that late decelerations are primarily reflex changes with nonacidemic hypoxia. They demonstrated that, when fetal oxygenation decreased, chemoreceptor-mediated fetal hypertension occurred. Furthermore, they suggested

that in the presence of hypoxia severe enough to cause acidemia, late decelerations are reflective of myocardial depression. Harris and colleagues (1982) also demonstrated that late decelerations can result from vagal reflex mechanisms or hypoxia-induced myocardial depression.

The loss of fetal heart rate variability may often suggest fetal hypoxia, though other factors, such as maternal drug administration or congenital anomalies, may be responsible. Even if periodic patterns of the FHR tracing are nonreassuring, the presence of good beat-to-beat variability is usually reassuring (Paul et al., 1979; Boehm, 1977; Hammacher, Huter, Bokelmann, & Werners, 1968). During early fetal hypoxia, the general increase in autonomic tone causes an increase in both short- and long-term variability. Mild hypoxia causes adrenergic stimulation and fetal hypertension. This fetal hypertension then causes fetal baroreceptor stimulation and a reflex vagal discharge (Druzen, Ikenoue, Murata et al., 1979). However, prolonged and severe fetal hypoxia with acidemia results in decreased FHR variability, presumably related to ther central nervous system effects of hypoxia and acidosis (Freeman, Garite, & Nageotte, 1991). Parer (1983) suggested that FHR decelerations indicate intermittent asphyxial "stresses," whereas the collective influence of these stresses on the fetal physiologic compensatory mechanisms is determined by the decrease or loss of FHR variability, signifying a cumulative oxygen debt and decompensation. Therefore, the presence of FHR variability is indicative of CNS or myocardial (or both) normoxia, whereas its decrease, in the presence of nonreassuring patterns, suggest hypoxia (Parer & Livingston, 1990).

Marked variability (more than 25 bpm) may be representative of a shifting PO_2 and PCO_2 relationship mediated by the baro- and chemoreceptors. Unless repetitive decelerations accompany this exaggerated variability, there is generally no significant change in fetal oxygenation (Reiss, Gabbe, & Petrie, 1996).

Fetal tachycardia, though often caused by factors such as maternal fever, drug administration, or fetal cardiac anomalies, may be caused by hypoxia. A prolonged fetal tachycardia that could be abolished with beta-adrenergic blockade has been described by Jones & Ritchie (1983). This indicates that the increase in the baseline FHR was the result of a prolonged increase in sympathetic activity (Nijland et al., 1995). Because tachycardia represents increased sympathetic and/or decreased parasympathetic tone, it may be associated with diminshed FHR variability. Most cases of fetal tachycardia, especially in the term fetus, are not reflective of compromise (Freeman, Garite, & Nageotte, 1991). The likely mechanism is chemoreceptor-stimulated beta-adrenergic activity. Therefore, if there is no obvious explanation for fetal tachycardia, hypoxia must be the suspected cause of the changes in autonomic tone.

When the FHR baseline is less than 110 bpm, fetal bradycardia is present. When uteroplacental flow is reduced, both oxygen transport to the fetus and carbon dioxide transport from the fetus are restricted. Both hypoxemia and hypercapnia may cause fetal bradycardia (Hanson, 1988; Boekkooi, Baan, Teitel, & Rudolph, 1992). The usual effect of acute hypoxemia on the FHR is transient bradycardia followed by a delayed return to baseline (Cohn, Sachs, Heymann, & Rudolph, 1974; Giussani et al., 1993). This is caused by a rapid decrease in fetal oxygen delivery, which activates the fetal chemoreceptors. Then a reflex slowing of the FHR occurs. However, in a study on fetal lambs, when maternal FIO_2 was lowered in a stepwise manner bradycardia was noticed in only one of nine subjects. This may have been related to failure of the gradual reduction of PO_2 to evoke a chemoreceptor response (Nijland et al., 1995). Fetal bradycardia can be seen in patients treated with beta-blockers, prolonged maternal hypoglycemia, maternal hypothermia, congenital fetal heart block (i.e., in cases of maternal autoimmune disease), or fetal panhypopituitarism with brain stem injury (Reis & Dodson, 1996; Freeman, Garite, & Nageotte, 1991; Marsh, Lagrew, Cook, & Lavery, 1987). If the bradycardia is associated with good variability, the practitioner may be reassured.

A sinusoidal FHR pattern, though rare, may be of clinical significance. The baseline FHR is usually in the normal range, but demonstrates a smooth pattern of uniform long-term variability with an amplitude of 5 to 20 bpm that resembles a sine wave. Short-term variability is absent. This type of pattern is often associated with fetal anemia. The physiologic basis for the sinusoidal pattern is not clear, but some investigators feel that it represents abnormal neurologic control of the FHR that may result from anemia or hypoxia (Reiss, Gabbe, & Petrie, 1996). A report by Elliott and colleagues (1980) suggested that tissue hypoxia may be relieved by raising the hemoglobin concentration. They showed that the sinusoidal pattern observed in an anemic fetus was also noted in the neonate. This heart rate pattern, which did not respond to adequate neonatal oxygenation, disappeared following neonatal blood transfusion.

When evaluating fetal cardiac arrhythmias, the practitioner should first be certain that there is no electrical or mechanical interference. Such interference is frequently referred to as "artifact." Therefore, confirmation of secure electrical connections is warranted. In addition, if a direct fetal ECG electrode (FSE) is utilized, one must be certain that the connecting wires are firmly applied to the fetus, and that the wires to the maternal leg plate are secure. Fetal cardiac arrhythmias may be of clinical significance; in fact, some have even been associated with fetal compromise. Sustained fetal tachycardia at a rate above 200 bpm may lead to heart failure and hydrops and thus warrants investigation (Reiss, Gabbe, & Petrie, 1996). If complete fetal heart block is present, the baseline FHR is usually in the range of 50 to 70 bpm.

INTRAUTERINE RESUSCITATION

Fetal Oxygen Delivery

When there is evidence or suspicion of diminished oxygen delivery to the fetus, the clinician must first conduct a careful assessment of maternal oxygenation status. In some situations of nonreassuring fetal status, delivery may be the chosen treatment option. In other scenarios, the maternal condition may not tol-

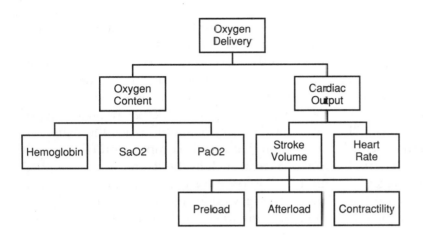

Figure 2-5. Components of the oxygen delivery process.

erate the hemodynamic stresses of active labor or operative intervention. In situations of extreme prematurity, extrauterine life may pose a greater risk to the fetus than would continued intrauterine life. In these situations, the clinician must attempt to optimize maternal and fetal oxygen delivery. Oxygen delivery involves both oxygen content and cardiac output. In order to accurately assess and intervene where necessary, attention must be paid to all components of the oxygen delivery process. (For a graphic representation of these components, see Figure 2-5).

Maternal/fetal oxygenation depends on blood flow, as pregnancy is normally a state of high flow with low resistance. Maternal cardiac output and uterine blood flow must be optimized. If maternal cardiac output is impaired, uterine blood flow will likewise be impaired, thus leading to a reduction in fetal cardiac output and oxygen delivery. Oxygen delivery is directly proportional to cardiac output; if cardiac output falls by 50%, so does oxygen delivery. Conversely, doubling cardiac output doubles oxygen delivery (Hankins, 1991). Therefore, attention must be given to the components of cardiac output: volume status, vascular resistance, and ventricular performance. In some instances, this will require pulmonary artery catheterization to assess and optimize cardiac function (Thorp & Cefalo, 1991). Avoidance of the supine position and the potential for subsequent vena caval compression is another essential measure in maintaining oxygen delivery.

Oxygen content is the other critical element of oxygen delivery. The clinician must assess maternal hemoglobin levels, as the majority of oxygen transported in blood is bound to hemoglobin. Because anemia dramatically diminishes the oxygen-carrying capacity of blood, replacement with packed red blood cells may be a necessary element of intrauterine resuscitation. Damaged red blood cells, such as those that have undergone hemolysis in the disease process of hemolysis, elevated liver enzymes, and low platelets (HELLP syndrome), may be less able to bind oxygen molecules and carry them to the tissues. Therefore, one must assess both the quantity and quality of hemoglobin. In addition, maternal acidosis or fever may shift the oxyhemoglobin dissociation curve to the right, thus decreasing the affinity of hemoglobin for oxygen. Such cases of decreased affinity lower the oxygen-carrying capacity of hemoglobin molecules, as they do not attract oxygen to the binding sites when affinity is low. Thus, when the hemoglobin molecules reach the tissue level, oxygen availability is decreased.

Nursing Interventions

The observant nurse who detects subtle signs of impaired oxygen delivery may avert catastrophe. In other scenarios, prompt aggressive intervention will minimize morbidity. The first, and most simple, is to wedge the patient onto her left or right side, thus shifting the gravid uterus off of the inferior vena cava and aorta. Compression of the inferior vena cava and aorta may decrease cardiac output and/or uteroplacental perfusion. Lateral positioning will enhance blood return to the maternal heart, augment maternal preload, increase maternal cardiac output, and improve uteroplacental perfusion. Thus, when maternal cardiac output is optimized, improved oxygen delivery to both mother and fetus will result.

Volume resuscitation may be another nursing intervention if volume status is impaired. This intervention is aimed at enhancing maternal preload and cardiac output. Fluid volume deficit and the need for replacement may be assessed noninvasively by measurement of intake and output, skin turgor/temperature, heart sounds, heart rate, blood pressure, and urine specific gravity. More precise quantification of volume status may be made through invasive hemodynamic monitoring. The pulmonary capillary wedge pressure provides information about the volume of blood in the left side of the heart. A less specific mode of central volume assessment is the central venous pressure.

Hypotension threatens both mother and fetus by decreasing oxygen availability to both. Uterine blood vessel tone is decreased, and maternal cardiac output is also reduced related to hypotension, thus leading to decreased uterine blood flow. Hypotension reduces maternal oxygen delivery by decreasing venous blood return to the heart, and thus decreasing cardiac output. The resultant reduction in maternal cerebral blood flow is of particular concern. When hypotension is recognized promptly and treated effectively, very little, if any, untoward effects accrue to either mother or fetus (Hawkins, Chestnut, & Gibbs, 1996, p. 436). If the fetus is chronically compromised, however, hypotension can result in further compromise. Treatment of hypotension starts with prophylaxis, especially when the patient is undergoing regional anesthesia such as an epidural block. An intravenous infusion of crystalloid solution is usually administered prior to regional anesthesia to prevent hypotension associated with decreased systemic vascular resistance. Glucose-containing solutions, which easily cross the placenta, should be avoided because of the potential side effect of neonatal hypoglycemia. The nurse should place the patient in a position that avoids compression of the aorta or vena cava, such as the lateral side-lying position. If this position is not practical, the nurse may place a wedge under the patient's left or right hip in order to displace the uterus and avoid lower central vessel compression. If these simple measures are not sufficient, vasopressor agents may be ordered and administered. Ephedrine, the drug of choice in obstetric anesthesia, produces peripheral vasoconstriction without reducing uterine blood flow (Briggs & Garite, 1991; Patterson, 1984). Other vasopressor agents should be used with caution because of the potential vasoconstrictive effect on uterine blood flow. Alpha-adrenergic agents such as phenylephrine are generally avoided, although the potential risks must be weighed against expected therapeutic benefits. In the presence of cardiopulmonary arrest, the full range of cardiotonic and vasopressor agents may be utilized in an effort to resuscitate the mother (Daddario & Johnson, 1992).

If fetal oxygen delivery is impaired by uterine hyperstimulation, astute nursing surveillance and intervention are critical. If an oxytocic agent is infusing, the infusion rate should be decreased or discontinued. This intervention is aided by the short half-life of oxytocin. In addition, the nurse may administer a tocolytic medication, such as brethine, in order to correct uterine tetany. Brethine is a betamimetic agent, which works by stimulating both the beta1 and beta2 adrenergic receptors. The desired effect relates to beta2 properties, specifically smooth muscle relaxation in the uterus. This is accomplished by decreasing the availability of calcium in the smooth muscle contraction process. Ongoing assessment should include uterine activity, fetal responses, and maternal hemodynamic status.

Supplemental oxygen, when administered to the mother, may be of benefit in the intrauterine resuscitation process. If the mother's PO_2 is decreased, the fetus is at risk for decreased oxygenation. Large increases in the PO_2 of maternal-inspired air ultimately results in increased oxygen content in the fetus (Thorp & Cefalo, 1991, p. 110). Once the uterine venous oxygen content is increased (as a result of the increase in maternal PO_2 and thus uterine venous oxygen content), the uterine arterial PO_2 rises. It is important to note that the uterine arterial PO_2 will not increase as much as the uterine venous PO_2. This is because these changes take place at different points on the oxyhemoglobin dissociation curve. Because the fetus is operating on the steep portion of the oxyhemoglobin dissociation curve, small changes in fetal PO_2 result in proportionately larger changes in oxygen content. In like manner, decreasing the maternal arterial PO_2 below 60 mm Hg results in a dramatic reduction in fetal oxygen content. Therefore, it is imperative that the mother's PO_2 be maintained above 60 mm Hg. Optimal maternal PO_2 would be in the range of 104–108 mm Hg in order to maintain the normal diffusion gradient. Many high-risk and critically ill pregnant women require supplemental oxygen in order to maintain adequate maternal/fetal oxygenation.

Amnioinfusion is a method of intrauterine resuscitation that may be considered for patients with variable decelerations, oligohydramnios, or meconium-stained amniotic fluid (Ouzounian & Paul, 1996). There is considerable evidence to support the use of this simple technique for improving pregnancy outcome and for reducing the incidence of cesarean delivery for nonreassuring fetal status in such patients (Strong, Hetzler, & Paul, 1990; Strong, Hetzler, Sarno & Paul, 1990; Nageotte et al., 1991; Schrimmer, Macri, & Paul, 1991; Wenstrom & Parsons, 1989; Macri et al., 1992). Umbilical cord compression secondary to oligohydramnios may impede blood flow, increase vessel resistance, and possibly lead to fetal hypercarbia and and hypoxemia. In addition, amnioinfusion may have a beneficial impact through a dilutional or irrigational effect inpatients with thick meconium-stained amniotic fluid, or in cases where microorganisms

have invaded the amniotic cavity (Dye, Aubry, Gross, & Artal, 1994; Ouzounian & Paul, 1996). Although most investigators have used normal saline as the infusate, Puder and colleagues (1994) documented no difference between normal saline and Ringer's lactate with respect to neonatal outcome. Furthermore, warmed and room-temperature saline have been compared, as have infusion pumps. Both have been shown to make no difference in terms of neonatal outcome (Nageotte et al., 1991; Glantz & Letteney, 1996). In the face of ominously nonreassuring fetal heart rate patterns, delaying delivery to perform amnioinfusion is not recommended (Ouzounian & Paul, 1996). The nurse should carefully assess the infusate volume and intrauterine pressure in order to avoid uterine overdistension and tetany.

Prior to initiating intrauterine resuscitation, the nurse should prepare the patient and others in her support system emotionally, especially as the family may lack sufficient knowledge to interpret the situation accurately. Parents sometimes become fearful about potential loss, which, in fact, may be unlikely. Therefore, an assessment of the family's knowledge of the procedure, the rationale for its use, how the procedure is performed, and the anxiety level related to the procedure should be conducted. Then the nurse may proceed with appropriate teaching and environmental control.

FETAL SURVEILLANCE

Uteroplacental function and the intrauterine environment is evaluated in order to assess the risk of fetal death and investigate the potential for fetal acid-base imbalance during the high-risk pregnancy. The most common tests are maternal assessment of fetal activity, the nonstress test (NST), the biophysical profile, the contraction stress test, Doppler flow studies, and fetal scalp blood sampling. Fetal pulse oximetry, a relatively new assessment modality, will also be discussed.

Maternal assessment of fetal activity is the most simple method for antepartum testing. In general, the presence of fetal movement is a reassuring sign of fetal health (Druzin & Gabbe, 1996). Many studies have been conducted in the area of third trimester fetal body movements. Patrick and colleagues (1982) showed that the fetus spends 10% of its time generating gross body movements, and that thirty of these movements occur each hour. In that same study, the researchers noted the longest period without fetal movements in a normal fetus was approximately 75 minutes. The fetus makes fine body movements as well as gross gestures, i.e., limb extension, hand grasping, and sucking. However, the mother is usually unable to perceive such movements. In fact, the mother is able to perceive only about 70 to 80% of gross fetal movements (Druzin & Gabbe, 1996). Although absence of fetal activity is not directly indicative of fetal compromise, it is known that fetal activity is sensitive to a decrease in oxygenation. In a sheep model, Natale and colleagues (1981) demonstrated that a small fall in fetal PO_2 was associated with a cessation of limb movements. Therefore, absence or decrease in fetal activity requires further assessment.

Several methods have been used to monitor fetal activity. One popular technique, described by the work of Pearson and Weaver (1976), is the Cardiff Count-to-Ten chart. This method involves teaching the patient to start counting fetal movement in the morning and to record the time of day when the tenth movement has been observed. She is instructed to notify her obstetric care provider if she does not perceive 10 movements in 12 hours, or if it takes longer each day to reach 10 movements. Depending on assessment of the patient's educational or motivational level, the care provider may elect to modify this test. Regardless of the technique chosen, the nurse must carefully explain the procedure, the rationale for fetal activity assessment, and parameters for notifying the obstetric care provider.

The nonstress test (NST) is the most widely applied technique for antepartum evaluation (Druzin & Gabbe, 1996). This method is "based on the assumption that a fetus with an intact central nervous system and in whom there is adequate oxygenation will exhibit transient fetal heart rate (FHR) accelerations in response to fetal movement" (Lake, 1992). A reactive test is one in which there are two accelerations of 15 beats-per-minute amplitude that last at least 15 seconds within a 10- to 20- minute period. If the fetus is suspected to be in a sleep state, a vibroacoustic stimulation device may be applied to the maternal abdomen in an attempt to awaken the fetus. If the NST is nonreactive, further evaluation is indicated. Clark and colleagues (1989) modified the NST by adding a single one- to two-second sound stimulation applied to the maternal abdomen, if no spontaneous acceleration was noted within 5 minutes of beginning the NST. In addition, all patients received assessment of amniotic fluid volume. In this series, there were no unexpected antepartum fetal deaths in 5973 tests. Clark and colleagues also noted that the use of sound stimulation resulted in a significant shortening of testing time.

The biophysical profile (BPP) is an assessment method that incorporates the NST, fetal movement, fetal breathing movements, fetal tone, and amniotic fluid volume. Each parameter is assessed by signifying a score of zero to 2, with 2 being the normal evaluation. The BPP correlates well with fetal acid-base status, as documented by Vintzileos and colleagues (1987). In a study of 124 patients, they documented that fetuses with BPP scores of 8 or above had mean arterial pH's of 7.28. In this series, only two of the fetuses were acidotic, while the fetuses with scores of 4 or less had a mean pH of 6.99. All fetuses in the group with low BPP scores were acidotic. Furthermore, it has been suggested that a nonreactive NST and absent fetal breathing are the first signs of fetal compromise, whereas absent body movement and tone are associated with more advanced degrees of fetal compromise (Vintzileos & Knuppel, 1994).

The contraction stress test (CST), also known as the oxytocin challenge test (OCT), examines the fetal response to uterine contractions. This test is based on the intrapartum fetal monitoring principle that a fetus with uteroplacental insufficiency will demonstrate late decelerations in response to hypoxia. The test should begin with initial assessment of the fetal heart rate baseline and uterine activity/resting tone. This initial assessment period should last approximately 10 to 20 minutes. In some cases, spontaneous uterine activity will be adequate, whereas others will require additional uterine stimulation. An adequate CST requires moderate-intensity uterine contractions, each lasting 40 to 60 seconds, with three contractions in a 10-minute period. If necessary, additional uterine stimulation may be achieved via breast stimulation or intravenous oxytocin infusion (Druzin & Gabbe, 1996). Most clinicians agree on the negative and positive OCT criteria first outlined by Freeman in 1975. He described a negative OCT as one in which there are no late decelerations appearing on the FHR tracing with adequate uterine contractions present. A positive OCT is one in which persistent late decelerations occur with the majority (greater than 50%) of contractions in the absence of uterine hyperstimulation. Other terms have more recently been used in clinical practice such as "equivocal" or "suspicious" to describe a test where an occasional late deceleration is present. Because negative CSTs have been consistently reported with good fetal outcomes, negative results may permit caregivers to safely prolong high-risk pregnancies.

Doppler velocimetry is a noninvasive method of quantifying placental resistance to blood flow (Bruner, Gabbe, Levy, & Arger, 1993). The premise of this method is that the frequency of reflected sound is proportional to the speed of red blood cells as they move through a vessel. Thus, Doppler velocimetry analyzes arterial waveforms in an attempt to evaluate fetuses at risk for increased peripheral resistance and subsequent hypoxia. It is through this mode of fetal surveillance that qualitative assessment of umbilical arterial waveforms can be made. With proper performance technique, one can assess flow velocity within a vessel. Forward flow of blood occurs during normal systolic and diastolic phases, the latter indicating resistance in

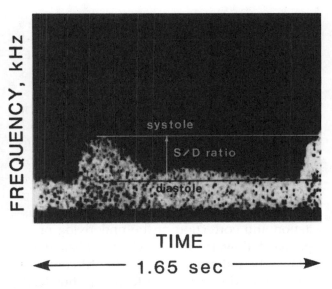

Figure 2-6. Doppler ultrasound flow velocity waveform.
(Courtesy of Joseph P. Bruner, MD)

the placental bed. Increased peripheral resistance is indicated by decreased, absent, or, in severe cases, reverse end-diastolic flow. One index of flow assessment is the peak systolic/diastolic (S/D) ratio (see Figure 2-6). As the diastolic flow increases the S/D ratio decreases. Conversely, as peripheral resistance increases, diastolic flow decreases, resulting in an increased S/D ratio. Marked increases in the S/D ratio, when compared with previous S/D ratios in the same patient, may indicate a fetus at increased risk of compromise (Devoe, Gardner, Dear, & Faircloth, 1992). When intrauterine growth retardation has been diagnosed, an abnormal S/D ratio may be more predictive of neonatal morbidity than the NST (Trudinger, Cooke, Jones, & Giles, 1986). On the other hand, in a study comparing three surveillance modes in a general high-risk population, Devoe and colleagues (1990) found that the nonstress test was more powerful than amniotic fluid measurements or Doppler velocimetry when used as "stand-alone" screening tests. Doppler velocimetry seems to be most reliable in conditions predisposing to IUGR, such as hypertensive disorders, collagen vascular diseases, or other diseases in which vasospasm plays a major role. It is also a valuable technique for follow-up of pregnancies with a diagnosis of IUGR or in multiple gestation pregnancies where growth discordancy is present (Druzin & Gabbe, 1996).

Fetal acid-base balance may be assessed via scalp sampling in the intrapartum period. Because nonreassuring fetal heart rate tracings may be indicative of fetal acidosis, the collection of fetal capillary blood for pH and gas/buffer evaluation may alert caregiveres to fetal compromise. In some instances, intrauterine resuscitation and correction of the underlying problem may follow. In other cases, immediate delivery may be indicated. Umbilical cord compression may lead to a drop in fetal pH, thus leading to accumulation of carbon dioxide and respiratory acidemia. In the face of uteroplacental insufficiency, fetal oxygenation may be impaired, thus leading to anaerobic energy production, lactic acidosis, and a drop in pH. The nurse may assist in obtaining a scalp pH sample by first providing anticipatory guidance, and then by placing the patient in the dorsal lithotomy or lateral Sims position. A cone-shaped speculum is placed in the vagina so that the fetal presenting part is visualized. Following identification of a puncture site, avoiding the suturelines or fontanelles, the caregiver will clean the site with a sponge. In some cases a layer of silicone will be spread over the site in order to smooth the fetal hair and to provide a smooth surface on which a globule of fetal capillary blood may form. The scalp is then punctured by a small scalpel. A heparinized capillary tube will be used to collect the fetal blood for analysis. Following scalp sampling, pressure should be applied to the site until there is no bleeding. Many institutions have the capability to analyze the sample in the Labor & Delivery suite. However, if immediate processing is not possible, the blood sample should be protected from coagulation by placing a "flea" (a small piece of metal) in the capillary tube. A magnet ring is then placed around the capillary tube and slowly moved from one end of the sample to the other in order to move the "flea" and thus prevent clot formation. In addition, sealing clay should be placed on each end of the tube.

A trend of serial pH determinations correlates with the clinical scenario and is more important than a value of a single value of pH and gas parameters (Druzin & Gabbe, 1996). Various studies have established normal ranges for umbilical artery pH and blood gas values (Thorp, Sampson, Parisi, & Creasy, 1989; Zalar & Quilligan, 1975; Yeomans et al., 1985). Traditionally, a low umbilical arterial pH has been defined as less than 7.20 (Wible, Petrie, Koons, & Perez, 1982; ACOG, 1995). However, as suggested by Thorp and colleagues (1989), this level may be arbitrarily high, and may range as low as 7.10. Furthermore, the incidence of asphyxia-related newborn complications are observed below a certain pH with a metabolic component to the acidemia and with a low 5-minute Apgar score. Thus, it is uncommon to document significant neonatal adverse sequelae until the pH drops below 7.10. That value may be as low as 7.00 (Goldaber et al., 1991; Winkler et al., 1991).

Intrapartum fetal oxygen saturation monitoring is an emerging tool that has potential for clinical use. Pulse oximetry, a standard of care in many adult and neonatal critical care settings, as well as during administration of anesthesia, measures the fraction of light transmitted through tissues using two different light wavelengths. Through spectrophotometry, the photodetector in the pulse oximeter measures light as it passes through tissue. Then, the measured ratios of red to infrared light are converted to a value of percent saturation (SpO_2) (Dildy, Clark, & Loucks, 1996). Animal studies have suggested that the critical value, that is the percent SpO_2 below which pathologic fetal acid base changes occur, is approximately 30%. In these studies, the risk of hypoxia increased if the SpO_2 dropped below 30% or stayed significantly below 30% for long periods of time (Oeseburg et al., 1992; Nijland et al., 1995; Richardson, Carmichael, Homan, & Patrick, 1992). Human data have shown that, in a group of women undergoing vaginal delivery with normal neonatal outcomes, the fetal SpO_2 values were generally greater than 30% (Dildy et al., 1994). This new technology may potentially aid caregivers in managing difficult cases, such as fetal arrhythmias, in which the FHR tracing is nonreassuring or uninterpretable (van den Berg, Nijhuis, & Jongsma, 1993; Dildy, Loucks, & Clark, 1993). If safety, efficacy, and cost issues are resolved through randomized controlled clinical trials, intrapartum fetal oxygen saturation monitoring could be a major advance in obstetrics (Dildy, Clark, & Loucks, 1996).

Other adjunctive technologies are being tested, including fetal ECG interpretation. For several years, researchers have analyzed the fetal ECG signal to determine whether changes in morphology would correlate to fetal and/or neonatal outcome (Harvey, 1997). Analysis of the PR interval as an adjunct to EFM has been compared to EFM alone. The researchers reported a decreased need for follow-up fetal scalp sampling to identify the hypoxemic fetus (Van Wijngaarden et al., 1996).

The intrapartum nurse must be skilled in fetal assessment. Knowledge of maternal–fetal physiology, pathophysiology, and assessment techniques will help the nurse to accurately assess clinical scenarios, develop a plan of care, and guide interventions in order to promote optimal outcomes.

REFERENCES

Acheson, G. H., Dawes, G. S., & Mott, J. C. (1957). Oxygen consumption and the arterial oxygen saturation in fetal and newborn lambs. Journal of Physiology, 135, 623–642.

ACOG, American College of Obstetricians & Gynecologists. (1995). Umbilical artery blood acid-base analysis, Technical Bulletin #216 (November). Washington, DC: ACOG.

Ball, R. H., Espinosa, M. I., Parer, J. T., Alon, E., Vertomman, J., & Johnson, J. (1994). Regional blood flow in asphyxiated fetuses with seizures. American Journal of Obstetrics and Gynecology, 170(Pt. 1), 156–161.

Ball, R. H., & Parer, J. T. (1992). The physiologic mechanisms of variable decelerations. American Journal of Obstetrics and Gynecology, 166(6, Pt. 1), 1693–1689.

Ball, R. H., Parer, J. T., Caldwell, L. E. & Johnson, J. (1994). Regional blood flow and metabolism in ovine fetuses during severe cord occlusion. American Journal of Obstetrics and Gynecology, 171(6), 1549–1555.

Battaglia, F. C., & Meschia, G. (1986). An Introduction to Fetal Physiology. New York: Academic Press.

Bocking, A. D., White, S. E., Homan, J., & Richardson, B. S. (1992). Oxygen consumption is maintained in fetal sheep during prolonged hypoxaemia. Journal of Developmental Physiology, 17(4), 169–174.

Boehm, F. H. (1997). FHR variability: Key to fetal well-being. Contemporary OB/GYN, 9, 57–68.

Boekkooi, P. F., Baan, J., Jr., Teitel, D., & Rudolph, A. M. (1992). Chemoreceptor responsiveness in fetal sheep. American Journal of Physiology, 263(1, Pt. 2), H162–167.

Briggs, G. G., & Garite, T. J. (1991). Effects on the fetus on drugs used in critical care. In S. L. Clark, D. B. Cotton, G. D. V. Hankins, & J. P. Phelan (Eds.), Critical care obstetrics (2nd ed., pp. 704–718). Cambridge, MA: Blackwell Scientific.

Bristow, J., Rudolph, A. M., Itskovitz, J., & Barnes, R. (1983). Hepatic oxygen and glucose metabolism in the fetal lamb. Journal of Clinical Investigation, 71(1), 96–102.

Brooks, A. N., & Challis, J. R. (1992). Adrenocorticotrophin responses to hypoxaemia in fetal sheep are sustained in the presence of naloxone. Journal of Developmental Physiology, 17(5), 221–225.

Bruner, J. P., Gabbe, S. G., Levy, D. W., & Arger, P. H. (1993). Doppler ultrasonography of the umbilical cord in normal pregnancy. Southern Medical Journal, Journal of the Southern Medical Association, 86(1), 52–55.

Clark, S. L., Sabey, P., & Jolley, K. (1989). Nonstress testing with acoustic stimulation and amniotic fluid volume assessment: 5973 tests without unexpected fetal death. American Journal of Obstetrics and Gynecology, 160(3), 694–697.

Cohn, H. E., Piasecki, G. J., & Jackson, B. T. (1982). The effect of beta-adrenergic stimulation on fetal cardiovascular function during hypoxemia. American Journal of Obstetrics and Gynecology, 144(7), 810–816.

Cohn, H. E., Sacks, E. J., Heymann, M. A., & Rudolph, A. M. (1974). Cardiovascular responses to hypoxemia and acidemia in fetal lambs. American Journal of Obstetrics and Gynecology, 120(6), 817–824.

Daddario, J. B., & Johnson, G. (1992). Trauma in pregnancy. In N. H. Troiano & L. K. Mandeville (Eds.), High risk intrapartum nursing. Philadelphia: J. B. Lippincott.

Damron, D. P., Chaffin, D. G., Anderson, C. F., & Reed, K. L. (1994). Changes in umbilical arterial and venous blood flow velocity waveforms during late decelerations of the fetal heart rate. Obstetrics and Gynecology, 84, 1038–1040.

Devoe, L. D., Carlton, E., & Prescott, P. (1995). Neural network prediction of nonstress test results: How often should we perform nonstress tests? American Journal of Obstetrics and Gynecology, 173(4), 1128–1131.

Devoe, L. D., Gardner, P., Dear, C., & Castillo, R. A. (1996). The diagnostic values of concurrent nonstress testing, amniotic fluid measurement, and Doppler velocimetry in screening a general high-risk population. American Journal of Obstetrics and Gynecology, 163(3), 1040–1048.

Devoe, L. D., Gardner, P., Dear, C., & Faircloth, D. (1992). The significance of increasing umbilical artery systolic-diastolic ratios in third-trimester pregnancy. Obstetrics and Gynecology, 80(4), 684–687.

Dildy, G. A., Clark, S. L., & Loucks, C.A. (1996). Intrapartum fetal pulse oximetry: Past, present, and future. American Journal of Obstetrics and Gynecology, 175(1), 1–9.

Dildy, G. A., Loucks, C. A., & Clark, S. L. (1993). Intrapartum fetal pulse oximetry in the presence of fetal cardiac arrhythmia. American Journal of Obstetrics and Gynecology, 169(6), 1609–1611.

Dildy, G. A., van den Berg, P. P., Katz, M., Clark, S. L., et al. (1994). Intrapartum fetal pulse oximetry: Fetal oxygen saturation trends during labor and relation to delivery outcome. American Journal of Obstetrics and Gynecology, 171(3), 679–684.

Druzen, M., Ikenoue, T., Mutata, Y., et al. (1979). A possible mechanism for the increase in FHR variability following hypoxemia. Presented at the 26th Annual Meeting of the Society for Gynecological Investigation, San Diego, CA, March 23.

Druzin, M. L., & Gabbe, S. G. (1996). Antepartum fetal evaluation. In S. G. Gabbe, J. R. Niebyl, & J. L. Simpson (Eds.), Obstetrics: Normal & problem pregnancies (3rd ed. pp. 327–367). New York: Churchill-Livingstone.

Dye, T., Aubry R., Gross, S. & Artal, R. (1994). Amnioinfusion and the intrauterine prevention of meconium aspiration. American Journal of Obstetrics and Gynecology, 171(6), 1601–1605.

Elliott, J. P., Modanlou, H. D., O'Keeffe, D. F., & Freeman, R. K. (1980). The significance of fetal and neonatal sinusoidal heart rate pattern: Further clinical observations in Rh incompatibility. American Journal of Obstetrics and Gynecology, 138(2), 227–230.

Ervin, M. G., Ross, M. G., Leake, R. D., & Fisher, D. A. (1992). V1- and V2-receptor contributions to ovine fetal renal and cardiovascular responses to vasopressin. American Journal of Physiology, 262(4, pt. 2), R636–643.

Ervin, M. G., Ross, M. G., Youseff, A., Leake, R. D., & Fisher, D.A. (1986). Renal effects of ovine fetal arginine vasopressin secretion in respone to maternal hyperosmolality. American Journal of Obstetrics and Gynecology, 155(6), 1341–1347.

Fisher, D. J. (1986). Acidemia reduces cardiac output and left ventricular contractility in conscious lambs. Journal of Developmental Physiology, 8(1), 23–31.

Fisher, D. J., Heymann, M. A., & Rudolph, M.A. (1982). Fetal myocardial oxygen and carbohydrate consumption during acutely induced hypoxemia. American Journal of Obstetrics and Gynecology, 242, H 657.

Field, D. R., Parer, J. T., Auslender, R. A., Cheek, D. B., et al. (1990). Cerebral oxygen consumption during asphyxia in fetal sheep. Journal of Developmental Physiology, 14(3), 131–137.

Freeman, F. C., & Meschia, G. (1986). An Introduction to Fetal Physiology. New York: Academic Press.

Freeman, K. S., Carite, T., & Nagoette, K. (1991). Fetal heart rate monitoring (2nd ed.) Baltimore: Williams & Wilkins.

Freeman, R. K. (1975). The use of the oxytocin challenge test for antepartum clinical evaluation of uteroplacental respiratory function. American Journal of Obstetrics and Gynecology, 121(4), 481–489.

Friedman, W. F. (1972). The intrinsic physiologic properties of the developing heart. Progress in Cardiovascular Diseases, 15(1), 87–111.

Gilbert, R. D. (1980). Control of fetal cardiac output during changes in blood volume. American Journal of Physiology, 238(1), H80–86.

Giussani, D. A., Spencer, J. A. D., Moore, P. J., Bennet, L., & Hanson, M. A. (1993). Afferent and efferent components of the cardiovascular reflex responses to acute hypoxia in term fetal sheep. Journal of Physiology, 461, 531–449.

Glantz, J. C., & Letteney, D. L. (1996). Pumps and warmers during amnioinfusion: Is either necessary? Obstetrics and Gynecology, 87(1), 150–155.

Goldaber, K. G., Gilstrap, L. C., III, Leveno, K. J., Dax, J. S., & McIntire, D. D. (1991). Pathologic fetal acidemia. Obstetrics and Gynecology, 78, 1103–1107.

Gu, W., Jones, C. T., & Parer, J. T. (1985). Metabolic and cardiovascular effects on fetal sheep of sustained reduction of uterine blood flow. Journal of Physiology, 368, 109–129.

Hammacher, K., Huter, K. A., Bokelmann, J., & Werners, P. H. (1968). Foetal heart frequency and perinatal condition of foetus and newborn. Gynaecologia, 166, 348–360.

Hankins, G. D. V. (1991). Acute pulmonary injury and respiratory failure during pregnancy. In S. L. Clark, D. B. Cotton, G. D. V. Hankins, & J. P. Phelan (Eds.), Critical care obstetrics (2nd ed., pp. 340–370). Cambridge, MA: Blackwell Scientific.

Hanson, M. A. (1988). The importance of baro- and chemoreflexes in the control of the fetal cardiovascular system. Journal of Physiology, 10(6) 491–511.

Harris, J. L., Krueger, T. R., & Parer, J. T. (1982). Mechanisms of late decelerations of the fetal heart rate during hypoxia. American Journal of Obstetrics and Gynecology, 144(5), 491–496.

Harvey, C. J. (1997). Coming to terms: Electronic fetal monitoring update. Lifelines, 1(3), 42–44.

Hawkins, J. L., Chestnut, D. H., & Gibbs, C. P. (1996). Obstetric anesthesia. In S. G. Gabbe, J. R. Niebyl, & J. L. Simpson (Eds.), Obstetrics: Normal and problem pregnancies (3rd ed., pp. 425–468). New York: Churchill-Livingstone.

Hon, E. H., (1959). Observations of pathologic fetal bradycardia. American Journal of Obstetrics and Gynecology, 77, 1084–1099.

Hooper, S. B., (1995). Fetal metabolic responses to hypoxia. Reproduction, fertility & development, 7(3), 527–538.

Irion, G. L., Mack, C. E., & Clark, K. E. (1990). Fetal hemodynamic and fetoplacental vascular response to exogenous arginine vasopressin. American Journal of Obstetrics and Gynecology, 162(4), 1115–1120.

Itskovitz, J., LaGamma, E. F., & Rudolph, A. M. (1983). The effect of reducing umbilical blood flow on fetal oxygenation. American Journal of Obstetrics and Gynecology, 145(7), 813–818.

Jensen, A., & Berger, R. (1991). Fetal circulatory responses to oxygen lack. Journal of Developmental Physiology, 16(4), 181–207.

Jensen, A., Hohman, M., & Kunzel, W. (1987). Dynamic changes in organ blood flow and oxygen consumption during acute asphyxia in fetal sheep. Journal of Developmental Physiology, 9(6), 543–559.

Jones, C. T., & Ritchie, J. W. K. (1983). The effects of adrenergic blockage on fetal response to hypoxia. Journal of Developmental Physiology, 5, 211–222.

Jones, M. D., Sheldon, R. E., Peeters, L. L., Meschia, G., Battaglia, F. C., & Makowski, E. L. (1977). Fetal cerebral oxygen consumption at different levels of oxygenation. Journal of Applied Physiology, 43(6), 1080–1084.

Krebs, H. B., Petres, R. E., Dunn, L. J., Jordaan, H. V., & Segreti, A. (1979). Intrapartum fetal heart monitoring: I. Classification and prognosis of fetal heart rate patterns. American Journal of Obstetrics and Gynecology, 133(7), 762–772.

Lake, M. L. (1992). Prolonged pregnancy. In L. K. Mandeville & N. H. Troiano (Eds.), High risk intrapartum nursing (pp. 83–89). Philadelphia: J. B. Lippincott.

Leake, R. D., Weitzman, R. E., Effros, R. M., Siegel, S. R., & Fisher, D. A. (1979). Maternal fetal osmolar homeostasis: Fetal posterior pituitary autonomy. Pediatric Research, 13(7), 841–844.

Lewis, A. B., Donovan, M., & Platzker, A. C. (1980). Cardiovascular responses to autonomic blockade in hypoxemic fetal lambs. Biology of the Neonate, 37(5–6), 233–242.

Macri, C. J., Schrimmer, D. B., Leung, A., Paul, R. H., et al. (1992). Prophylactic amnioinfusion improves outcome of pregnancy complicated by thick meconium and oligohydramnios. American Journal of Obstetrics and Gynecology, 167(1), 117–121.

Manning, F. A., Morrison, I., Lange, I. R., Harman, C. R., & Chamberlain, P. F. (1985). Fetal assessment based on fetal biophysical profile scoring: Experience in 12,620 referred high-risk pregnancies. American Journal of Obstetrics and Gynecology, 151(3), 343–350.

Marsh, T. D., Lagrew, D. C., Cook, L. N., & Lavery, J. P. (1987). Unexplained fetal baseline bradycardia in congential panhypopituitarism. American Journal of Obstetrics and Gynecology, 156(4), 977–979.

Martin, C. B. Jr., de Haan, J., van der Wildt, B., Jongsma, H. W., Dieleman, A., & Arts, T. H. (1979). Mechanisms of late decelerations in the fetal heart rate. A study with autonomic blocking agents in fetal lambs. European Journal of Obstetrics, Gynecology, & Reproductive Biology, 9(6), 361–373.

May, K. (1992). Psychosocial implications of high risk intrapartum care. In L. K. Mandeville & N. H. Troiano (Eds.), High risk intrapartum nursing (pp. 41–51). Philadelphia: J. B. Lippincott.

Nageotte, M. P., Bertucci, L., Towers, C. V., Lagrew, D. L., & Modanlou, H. (1991). Prophylactic amnioinfusion in pregnancies complicated by oligohydramnios: A prospective study. Obstetrics and Gynecology, 77(5), 677–680.

Nakamura, K. T., Ayres, N. A., Gomez, R. A., & Robillard, J. E. (1985). Renal responses to hypoxemia during renin-angiotensin system inhibition in fetal lambs. American Journal of Physiology, 294(1, Pt. 2), R116–124.

Natale, R., Clewlow, F., & Dawes, G. (1981). Measurement of fetal forelimb movements in the lamb in utero. American Journal of Obstetrics and Gynecology, 140(5), 545–551.

Nelson, K. B., Dambrosia, J. M., Ting, T. Y., & Grether, J. K. (1996). Uncertain value of electronic fetal monitoring in predicting cerebral palsy. New England Journal of Medicine, 334(10), 613–618.

Nijland, R., Jongsma, H. W., Nijhuis, J. G., van den Berg, P. P., & Oeseburg, B. (1995). Arterial oxygen saturation in relation to metabolic acidosis in fetal lambs. American Journal of Obstetrics and Gynecology, 172(3), 810–819.

Oeseburg, B., Ringnalda, B. E. M., Crevels, J., & Jongsma, H. W. (1992). Fetal oxygenation in chronic maternal hypoxia; what's critical. In W. Erdmann & D. F. Bruley (Eds.), Oxygen transport to tissue: Vol. 14 (pp. 499–502). New York: Plenum Press.

Ouzounian, J. G., & Paul, R. H. (1996). Role of amnioinfusion in contemporary obstetric practice. Contemporary OB/GYN (August issue, pp. 36–57).

Ozolins, I. Z., Young, I. R., & McMillen, I. C. (1992). Surgical disconnection of the hypothalamus from the fetal pituitary abolishes the corticotrophic response to intrauterine hypoglycemia or hypoxemia in the sheep during late gestation. Endocrinology, 130(5), 2438–2445.

Parer, J. T. (1994). Fetal cerebral metabolism: The influence of asphyxia and other factors. Journal of Perinatology, 14(5), 376–385.

Parer, J. T. (1983). Handbook of fetal heart rate monitoring. Philadelphia: W. B. Saunders.

Parer, J. T., Kruger, T. R., & Harris, J. L. (1980). Fetal oxygen consumption and mechanisms of heart rate response during artificially produced late decelerations of fetal heart rate in sheep. American Journal of Obstetrics and Gynecology, 136(4), 478–482.

Parer, J. T., & Livington, E. G. (1990). What is fetal distress? American Journal of Obstetrics and Gynecology, 162(6), 1421–1427.

Patrick, J., Campbell, K. Carmichael, L. Natale, R., & Richardson, B. (1982). Patterns of gross fetal body movements over 24-hour observation intervals during the last 10 weeks of pregnancy. American Journal of Obstetrics and Gynecology, 142(4), 363–371.

Patterson, R. M. (1984). Trauma in pregnancy. Clinical Obstetrics & Gynecology, 27(1), 32–37.

Paul, R. H., Suidan, A. K., Yeh, S. Y., Schifrin, B. S., & Hon, E. H. (1975). Clinical fetal monitoring. VII: The evaluation and significance of intrapartum baseline fetal heart rate variability. American Journal of Obstetrics and Gynecology, 123(2), 206–210.

Pearson, J., & Weaver, J. (1976). Fetal activity and fetal well being: An evaluation. British Medical Journal, 1, 1305.

Peeters, L. L., Sheldon, R. E., Jones, M. D., Jr., Makowski, E. L., & Meschia, G. (1979). Blood flow to fetal organs as a function of arterial oxygen content. American Journal of Obstetrics and Gynecology, 135(5), 637–646.

Puder, K. S., Sorokin, Y., Bottoms, S. G., et al. (1994). Amnioinfusion: Does the choice of solution adversely affect neonatal eletrolyte balance? Obstetrics and Gynecology, 84(6), 956–959.

Rankin, J. H., Meschia, G., Makowski, E. L., & Battaglia, F. C. (1971). Relationship between uterine and umbilical venous PO2 in sheep. American Journal of Physiology, 220(6), 1688–1692.

Reid, D. L., Parer, J. T., Williams, K., Darr, D., Phernetton, T. M., & Rankin, J. H. G. (1991). Effects of severe reduction in maternal placental blood flow on blood flow distribution in the sheep fetus. Journal of Developmental Physiology, 15, 183–188.

Reis, M. J., & Dodgson, H. W. (1996). Maternal hypothermia and persistent fetal bradycardia during the intrapartum process. JOGNN, 25(8), 674–680.

Reiss, R. E., Gabbe, S. G., & Petrie, R. H. (1996). Intrapartum fetal evaluation. In S. G. Gabbbe, J. R. Niebyl, & J. L. Simpson (Eds.), Obstetrics: Normal and problem pregnancies (pp. 397–424). New York: Churchill-Livingstone.

Richardson, B. S., Carmichael, L., Homan, J., & Patrick, J. E. (1992). Electrocortical activity, electroocular activity, and breathing movements in fetal sheep with prolonged and graded hypoxemia. American Journal of Obstetrics and Gynecology, 167(2), 553–558.

Robillard, J. E., & Nakamura, K. T. (1988). Neurohormonal regulation of renal function during development. American Journal of Physiology, 254(6, Pt. 2), F771–779.

Rurak, D. W. (1979). Plasma vasopressin levels during haemorrhage in mature and immature fetal sheep. Journal of Developmental Physiology, 1(1), 91–101.

Rurak, D. W., Richardson, B. S., Patrick, J. R., Carmichael, L. & Homan, J. (1990). Oxygen consumption in the fetal lamb during sustained hypoxaemia with progressive acidemia. American Journal of Physiology, 258(5, Pt. 2), R1108–1115.

Schrimmer, D. B., Macri, C. J., & Paul, R. H. (1991). Prophylactic amnioinfusion as a treatment for oligohydramnios in laboring patients: A prospective, randomized trial. American Journal of Obstetrics and Gynecology, 165(4, Pt. 1), 972–975.

Strong, T. H., Jr., Hetzler, G., & Paul, R. H. (1990). Amniotic fluid increase after amnioinfusion of a fixed volume. American Journal of Obstetrics and Gynecology, 162(3), 746–748.

Strong, T. H., Jr., Hetzler, G., Sarno, A. P., & Paul, R. H. (1990). Prophylactic intrapartum amnioinfusion: A randomized clinical trial. American Journal of Obstetrics and Gynecology, 162(6), 1370–1375.

Thorp, J. M., & Cefalo, R. C. (1991). Maternal-fetal physiological interactions in the critically ill pregnant patient. In S. L. Clark, D. B. Cotton, G. D. V. Hankins, & J. P. Phelan (Eds.), Critical care obstetrics (2nd ed., pp. 102–111). Cambridge, MA: Blackwell Scientific.

Thorp, J. A., Sampson, J. E., Parisi, V. M., & Creasy, R. K. (1989). Routine umbilical cord gas determinations. American Journal of Obstetrics and Gynecology, 161(3), 600–605.

Trudinger, B. J., Cook, C. M., Jones, L., & Giles, W. B. (1986). A comparison of fetal heart rate monitoring and umbilical artery waveforms in the recognition of fetal comporomise. British Journal of Obstetrics & Gynecology, 93(2), 171–175.

van den Berg, P. P., Nijhuis, J. G., & Jongsma, H. W. (1993). Intrapartum fetal surveillance with pulse oximetry in complete fetal heart block (CHB)—A case report. American Journal of Obstetrics and Gynecology, 1(1), 341 (abstract).

Van Wijngaarden, W. J., Sahota, D. S., James, D. K., Farrell, T., Mires, G. J., Wilcox, M., & Chany, A. (1996). Improved intrapartum fetal survillance with PR interval analysis of the fetal electrocardiogram: A randomized trial showing a reduction in fetal blood sampling. American Journal of Obstetrics and Gynecology, 174(4), 1295–1299.

Vintzileos, A. M., Gaffnew, S. E., Salinger, L. M., et al. (1987). The relationship between fetal biophysical profile and cord pH in patients undergoing cesarean section before the onset of labor. Obstetrics and Gynecology, 70(2), 196–201.

Vintzileos, A. M., & Knuppel, R. A. (1994). Multiple parameter biophysical testing in the prediction of fetal acid-base status. Clinics in Perinatology, 21(4), 823–848.

Weitzman, R. E., Fisher, D. A., Robillard, J. E., Erenberg, A., Kennedy, R., & Smith, F. (1978). Arginine vasopressin response to an osmotic stimulus in the fetal sheep. Pediatric Research, 12(1), 35–38.

Wenstrom, K. D., Andrews, W. A., & Maher, J. E. (1995). Amnioinfusion survey: Prevalence, protocols, and complications. Obstetrics and Gynecology, 86(4, pt. 1), 572–576.

Wenstrom, K. D., & Parsons, M. T. (1989). The prevention of meconium aspiration in labor using amnioinfusion. Obstetrics and Gynecology, 73(4), 647–651.

Wible, J. L., Petrie, R. H., Koons, A., & Perez, A. (1982). The clinical use of umbilical cord acid-base determinations in perinatal surveillance and management. Clinics in Perinatology, 9, 387–397.

Wilkening, R. B., & Meschia, G. (1983). Fetal oxygen uptake, oxygenation, and acid-base balance as a function of uterine blood flow. American Journal of Physiology, 244(6), H749–755.

Winkler, C. L., Hauth, J. C., Tucker, J. M., Owen, J., & Brumfield, C. G. (1991). Neonatal complications at term as related to the degree of umbilical artery acidemia. American Journal of Obstetrics and Gynecology, 164(2), 637–641.

Yeomans, E. R., Hauth, J. C., Gilstrap, L. C., III, et al. (1985). Umbilical cord pH, PCO_2, and bicarbonate following uncomplicated term vaginal deliveries. American Journal of Obstetrics and Gynecology, 151(6), 798–800.

Zalar, R. W., Jr., & Quilligan, E. J. (1975). The influence of scalp sampling on the cesarean section rate for fetal distress. American Journal of Obstetrics and Gynecology, 135(2), 239–246.

CHAPTER 3

Psychosocial Implications of High-Risk Intrapartum Care

Katharyn A. May and Sheron J. Salyer

A significant minority of childbearing women and their families experience complications that require high-risk perinatal management. Conditions once regarded as beyond effective perinatal management are now more or less routinely managed in hospitals across the country. Recent advances in perinatal care have changed the appearance and function of conventional labor and delivery units, such that they now are specialized intensive care units with all of the attendant technological supports.

As a result, nursing responsibilities in the care of the high-risk patient and her family during the intrapartum period have expanded dramatically. As is often the case, this rapid change in practice is reflected in an emphasis on technological aspects of care, both in the nursing literature and in continuing education efforts. Although this focus is essential, it is insufficient alone. The psychosocial needs of the family experiencing a high-risk labor and birth are urgent and complex, and fall almost exclusively within the nurse's realm of responsibility.

The unique psychosocial needs of the high-risk intrapartum patient are universally acknowledged in the nursing literature. Truly expert clinicians are recognized as those who address these needs as an intrinsic part of their care. Clinicians use a kind of shorthand when describing care for such patients: "We know good support when we

see it, and we know when it's needed." However, it is unclear how we come to know these things. Effective psychosocial support of the high-risk intrapartum patient is still largely a product of the individual nurse's personal style and clinical trial-and-error.

Effective psychosocial care is difficult to teach and even more difficult to measure or document, because it has been inadequately described and studied. Clinical and research literature in perinatal nursing remains relatively silent on the *specifics* of providing specialized psychosocial care to high-risk patients and their families during the critical intrapartum period. Statements like "the nurse should provide sensitive and caring support" are far too general to provide clear direction. Many questions remain unanswered: What is effective support? What does it look like? When is such support needed? Under what conditions? How do we know it makes a difference?

Without more specificity, documentation of patient needs and necessary nursing resources, instruction on how to provide psychosocial care, and validation of the effectiveness of psychosocial care in the intrapartum period is hampered. Although psychosocial nursing care is not well described and is even less understood from a research perspective, research indicates that psychological distress in the perinatal period can have lingering effects on individual and

51

family well-being (Mercer, Ferketich, May, & DeJoseph, 1987; Mercer, 1990). Further, it is clear that the dramatic and sometimes frightening intrapartum period can leave lasting impressions. It can enhance or inhibit the family's ability to integrate the birth experience into their lives, and made it difficult then to move on to productive parenthood or to resolution of their perinatal loss, if that is the end result (Grossman, 1988; May & Sollid, 1984; Parke & Beitel, 1988).

This chapter will first review the growing research literature on psychosocial implications of at-risk childbearing, with a focus on causes and effects of distress in the perinatal period. Nursing responsibilities for psychosocial assessment and support during the intrapartum period will be then be outlined, and expected outcomes for psychosocial nursing care will be proposed.

Given the lack of a well-developed body of research on the psychosocial aspects of high-risk labor and birth, these recommendations for specific assessment and intervention strategies should be seen only as guidelines against which to evaluate current practice. Much more focused attention by clinicians and researchers is needed before specific recommendations for psychosocial care of the high-risk intrapartum patient and family can be proposed with confidence.

CAUSES AND EFFECTS OF PSYCHOLOGICAL DISTRESS IN THE PERINATAL PERIOD

The transition to parenthood is a stress-producing process involving adaptation by both partners, even under the most favorable of circumstances (Belsky & Pensky, 1988). Several studies have reported that families who have higher levels of potentially disruptive stress during pregnancy are also more likely to go on to develop perinatal complications (Lederman, 1986; Norbeck & Tilden, 1983; O'Hara, Rehm, & Campbell, 1983). The evidence is not sufficiently strong to suggest that high levels of preexisting psychosocial stress *cause* perinatal complications. However, nurses must be alert to the possibility that the high-risk intrapartum patient and her family are not only dealing with the situational stressor of a high-risk condition, but also may be carrying a stress burden from preexisting stressors.

Preexisting Sources of Perinatal Stress

Information about the family's level of psychosocial adaptation during pregnancy may be available to the labor and delivery nurse only at the most general level, in anecdotal information on the prenatal record, for example, "pregnancy unplanned," "spousal conflict during pregnancy," "questionable social support available to mother," or "maternal ambivalence about pregnancy." Admittedly, such factors are not within the scope of nursing management in the intrapartum period, even if there was sufficient documentation about the patient's psychosocial status. However, there is growing research evidence that preexisting distress and the effects of cumulative life stress can also directly affect individual and family well-being in the perinatal period.

Anxiety, Depression, and High Perinatal Risk

Anxiety and depression are emotional states that can be thought of as distress responses to stress. Some anxiety and depression are normal in both partners during the childbearing year, because such a major life event demands changes in relationships and lifestyle. However, several studies link higher levels of emotional distress during pregnancy with poorer perinatal outcomes as well as poorer family functioning in the childbearing years (Barnett & Parker, 1986; Lederman, 1986; Norbeck & Tilden, 1983; O'Hara et al., 1983; Paarlberg, Vingerhoets, Passchier, Dekker, & Van Geijn, 1995). Mercer and others found anxiety and depression were higher among parents experiencing a high-risk pregnancy than they were among those with a normal pregnancy, as would be expected; however, half of high-risk women and almost one third of their mates demonstrated mood disturbance at levels suggestive of clinical depression (Mercer et al., 1987; Mercer, 1990). Clearly, many families can be expected to enter the high-risk intrapartum experience with depleted emotional resources, especially if they have been coping with a high-risk pregnancy.

Self-Esteem and Adaptation to At-Risk Childbearing

Several studies have focused on maternal self-esteem as a factor that may predict how a woman adapts to the reality of at-risk childbearing. In a study of women hospitalized for a high-risk pregnancy, low maternal self-esteem, high negative life stress, low social support, and an inadequate or absent mate relationship were predictive of high obstetric risk (Curry & Snell, 1985).

Self-esteem may not necessarily be of great importance in isolation, but it may have more significance when taken into account with other aspects of the family's situation. For example, the results of a longitudinal study of women experiencing a high-risk pregnancy and birth showed that women with high self-esteem who experienced intimacy with spouse and friends were more likely to feel well supported as though they coped well with this stress (Hobfoll, Nadler, & Leiberman, 1986) . Women with low self-esteem but adequate spousal support fared almost as well as women with high self-esteem. However, women with low self-esteem who had high intimacy with their own family of origin but not with spouse or friends reported they felt less well-supported, experienced more significant levels of depression, and coped less well with an at-risk birth. Perhaps low self-esteem in a childbearing woman contributes to a certain isolation and a reluctance to distance self from the family of origin. When an at-risk pregnancy results, the woman in this situation may perceive that she is getting insufficient support from those around her. This situation may characterize many young mothers who require high-risk perinatal care today.

High-Risk Pregnancy as a Prelude to High-Risk Labor and Delivery

In a now classic paper, Cohen (1979) identified four factors that contributed to maladaptation in

pregnancy and the neonatal period: previous adverse experience in childbearing, conflicts or problems in support systems, inadequate preparation for childbearing or childrearing and maternal health concerns. Most, if not all, of these factors may have been present during pregnancy in a woman who now presents requiring high-risk intrapartum care.

Further, if prescribed antepartal care has required the family to make major adjustments, such as loss of maternal employment, activity restriction, or multiple hospitalizations, the nurse can assume that the family enters the intrapartum experience with a high level of preexisting stress. Support systems may be strained or depleted due to demands during pregnancy (May, 1993). Assets the family usually relies upon to cope with stress, such as a satisfactory marital relationship, may not be optimal because of the challenge of coping with the high-risk pregnancy. Financial worries may be overwhelming if there has been a loss of maternal employment during pregnancy and the family now faces the prospect of a high-risk delivery and neonatal course (May, 1994). These factors may be pushed into the background as the family copes with immediate events; however, the sum total of these stressors may result in a family system with barely adequate coping resources with which to deal with labor and birth.

Effect of High Perinatal Risk on Parent–Fetal/Infant Attachment

An issue frequently raised about the impact of high-risk childbearing is the possible effect on the process of parent–fetal/newborn attachment. The construct of maternal–fetal attachment, addressed in the research literature first by Cranley (1983), suggests that feelings of connection to and protectiveness of the unborn arise for both parents prior to delivery, and factors such as self-esteem, emotional balance, and satisfaction in primary relationships (most often the mate relationship) are thought to enhance this emotional bond.

Kemp and Page (1987) examined the relationship between at-risk pregnancy and maternal–fetal attachment in a population of 54 low-risk and 32 high-risk pregnant women. Women who experienced a high-risk pregnancy demonstrated lower self-esteem than their low-risk counterparts, but no differences were found in maternal–fetal attachment. A subsequent study of over 500 high- and low-risk pregnant women and their partners found, as expected, that levels of prenatal attachment are consistently higher in women than in their partners (Mercer et al., 1988). However, similar to Kemp and Page, these investigators found that a high-risk pregnancy requiring hospitalization had no effect on prenatal attachment. Further, this study also showed that factors such as self-esteem, anxiety, depression, or marital satisfaction did not contribute substantially to prenatal attachment in low-risk women and their partners, or in high-risk women.

In addition, the relationship between prenatal and postbirth attachment is still not clear. Mercer and associate found that levels of prenatal attachment were not predictive of postbirth attachment in high-risk women or their partners (Mercer, Ferketich, May, De Joseph, & Sollid, 1988). Factors that appear to contribute to postbirth attachment in parents with a high-risk pregnancy include negative life events, stress during pregnancy, self-esteem and sense of parental competence, low levels of depression, and higher perceived social support.

Thus, the consequences of a high-risk pregnancy and birth on the process of prenatal and postbirth attachment are as yet poorly understood, and clearly more research is needed before specific interventions can be recommended. At this point in the development of perinatal nursing practice and research, it may be productive to direct nursing time and energy toward control of environmental stressors, to assist parents to reframe expectations, and to support positive family coping, as these factors may contribute to greater emotional balance and positive adaptation in the postbirth period.

In addition, although preexisting psychological stress may be associated with the development of perinatal complications, the more important issue for nursing is the recognition that high-risk intrapartum patients may already have depleted their coping resources during pregnancy and face the probability of an at-risk birth with this deficit. Even when the pregnancy has been relatively stress-free, the diagnosis of "at-risk" in the intrapartum period creates a storm of frightening possibilities with which families must grapple. When complications arise, all members of the family should be considered to be "at risk" for psychological distress. One source of immediate distress for high-risk childbearing families is the loss of emotional security when their own expectations for a normal birth are not met. This is worsened when the professionals caring for them respond rapidly to an at-risk condition that is difficult for parents to see and comprehend.

Shifting Expectations in the Intrapartum Period

One of the first consequences of an at-risk intrapartum situation is the loss of the expected and hoped-for normal birth. When long-held expectations for birth are not met, and when families find themselves in situations unlike any they have experienced before, a period of adaptation is required during which the family reorients to their changed circumstances. Clearly, the most appropriate psychosocial care can be rendered only if the nurse recognizes what the parents' expectations were, and how rapidly they may be able to adapt to the new situation.

For the well prepared, highly educated couple experiencing a "premium pregnancy," expectations for birth may be quite specific and may have focused on "options" such as use of a birthing room, avoidance of analgesia, and the presence of family and other support people. For them, control of the experience—more particularly, the avoidance of medical intervention—may have been an important expectation, because the health of mother and baby was largely assumed (Perez, 1995).

The reality of an at-risk birth introduces a sense of being helpless and out-of-control, and reduces the usefulness of their coping strategies, which had been focused on achieving a "normal" (i.e., low-intervention) birth. Such parents may very quickly recognize when things are "not normal," but they may not be able to "shift gears" to concentrate on new priorities as rapidly as their level of mastery and preparation might suggest (May & Sollid, 1984).

Other families who are not as well educated or as well prepared for childbirth will still respond to unmet expectations in the face of an at-risk birth, although perhaps in different ways. Interventions, such as a cesarean delivery, may be viewed positively in and of themselves (Cummins, Scrimshaw, & Engle, 1988; Sandelowski & Bustamante, 1986). However, an at-risk situation introduces new and complicated explanations from professionals, sudden separation from family, and frightening new experiences. In both cases, parents may resist the efforts of professionals to deal with the at-risk condition or may deny an at-risk condition exists. This behavior may be interpreted as overly controlling, obstructionist, or uninformed. However, what is more likely to be occurring in both of these cases is that parents have not yet shifted to a new set of expectations, already held by professionals, which focuses on doing what is necessary to achieve a positive outcome in the face of increased risk.

Adjusting to Crisis Management: A Major Stressor for Families

In the high-risk intrapartum situation, professionals and parents often adapt at different speeds and respond to different crises. Under the best of circumstances, parents have a limited repertoire of knowledge and experiences with which to cope with childbirth. They adapt to the current situation with difficulty and are unable to anticipate *what may happen* because adapting to *what is* requires all of their available energy. Professionals, on the other hand, adapt more quickly to changed circumstances because of their broader knowledge and experience, and move quickly to anticipate what may happen.

Unfortunately, the professional's ability to anticipate sometimes creates rather than diminishes the family's distress, because it widens the gap between what the professional is responding to and what the family is experiencing. As professionals project forward to prevent problems, even as they are dealing with existing ones, they sometimes forget that parents are adapting at a slower pace.

In addition, it is sometimes difficult to determine whether professionals are responding to an actual emergency in which seconds count, or the potential emergency that the professional knows may arise and that can be prevented. In an actual emergency, quick and efficient action is needed, and some aspects of sensitive care must be sacrificed for the sake of effective crisis management. However, when the situation has worsened but no crisis yet exists, professionals nevertheless may still shift into crisis management. This shift occurs rapidly and far outpaces the family's ability to take in and process what is happening to them. An overly brisk transition to crisis management on the part of professionals has been aptly called "treating provider anxiety" or more graphically, "the stormtrooper approach to obstetrics."

The "stormtrooper approach" is characterized by a number of occurrences: rushed or absent explanation of the situation to the woman and her family; no allowance for private discussion before a family decision is required or for privacy of any sort; a pressured quality in interactions, arbitrary and often unnecessary separation of the father or support person from the mother without appropriate follow-up; and (perhaps more common in teaching hospitals) twice as many bodies in the patient's room than are required to manage the situation.

This brisk shift to crisis management may occur without conscious thought and is based on the best of intentions. However, it is not without significant negative consequences. Some of the more disturbing memories and sense impressions parents carry away from the experience of an at-risk birth are those created by unthinking application of "stormtrooper" obstetrics (May & Sollid, 1984) . Women experiencing unexpected cesarean births report that things "suddenly started moving very fast," with "lots of people in the room, telling (me) what to do"; that moment was intensely frightening and long remembered. Could necessary tasks have been completed with fewer people in the room, with a few moments of quiet while one person gave instructions? How much of the "hurry" was necessary, and how much was a consequence of caregiver anxiety? Fathers routinely spent periods waiting alone during high-risk intra-partum care. Was separation really necessary? In all but the most acute emergencies (which in reality are relatively rare), a more deliberate approach to care and provision of sensitive support is possible, and may save patient and family considerable emotional distress.

Saving the family unnecessary distress in the face of an at-risk birth is an important nursing concern. Thus, reducing the environmental stress on families by actively managing the pace at which families are forced to adapt to the professional's mode of crisis management is an appropriate nursing intervention. This is not merely a nicety; with the emergence of an at-risk condition, the patient and family should be supported in redirecting their energy to coping with the potential for serious loss.

Fear of Intrapartum Loss

During a complicated pregnancy, fear of potential loss is clearly a stressor affecting women and their families (Cohen, 1979; Curry & Snell, 1985; Mercer, 1990). It is reasonable to assume that this fear also operates in the context of high-risk intrapartum care. Perinatal complications create the potential for varying degrees of loss: loss of the normal desired labor and birth, loss through maternal or fetal/neonatal injury, loss of life.

Whereas professionals understand the gradations of risk and the margins of safety associated with complications, parents and family usually do not have sufficient knowledge to make those distinctions. Because they lack sufficient knowledge to interpret the situation accurately, sometimes parents become fearful about potential loss that, in fact, is unlikely. For example, parents may interpret signs of increasing concern about fetal well-being as indications of a life-threatening complication, even when the objective risk is low and the problem can be managed with relative safety.

The nurse should remember that each parent brings a different set of concerns and expectations to the high-risk labor and delivery experience. If her physiological condition is unimpaired, the laboring woman is usually primarily concerned about the unborn. The mother is often acutely aware of subtle changes in professional behavior, and will sometimes conclude that her unborn is in significant jeopardy, when professionals are only mildly concerned. However, medications, labor sensations, or physiological changes may limit the mother's perceptual field and dampen the intensity of her response. The father's anxiety level is likely to be high enough to make him exquisitely sensitive to environmental cues. However, his primary concern is usually his partner's well-being. Thus, based on what he sees unfolding before him, a father may conclude that his partner's life is in serious danger even though it is the unborn who is primarily at risk. In a large study of families in which the woman was hospitalized for complications of late pregnancy, fathers expressed fear of "leaving the hospital alone" in situations where, objectively speaking, only the fetus was at significant risk (Mercer et al., 1987). The urgency of actions surrounding an at-risk birth communicated a diffuse sense of danger to these fathers, leading them to fear greatly for their partners' lives, even when the condition being treated was fetal distress or preterm labor, in which maternal risk is relatively low.

Unfortunately, limited research attention has been paid to families' experiences of high-risk labor and birth irrespective of actual loss, and to levels of emotional distress families experience during the process of high-risk intrapartum care. This is probably the result of the pressures of high-intensity care, the necessary concentration of maternal/fetal-neonatal survival, and the tendency to focus on situations such as poor neonatal outcome or perinatal demise as the only situational model for high emotional distress.

However, there is evidence to suggest that the long-term consequences of situational distress, even when maternal/neonatal outcomes are "good," may be detrimental to individual and family well-being. Pioneering studies, such as those by Tilden and Lipson (1982), and Cranley, Hedahl, and Pegg (1983) have already documented that women may require months for the process of resolving grief and loss from a cesarean delivery. Even though outcomes may be excellent, for many women the emotional impact of an at-risk delivery is not reduced. The same may be true for an increasing number of men, as more men become actively involved in the process of labor and birth. May and Sollid (1984) found that fathers were sometimes plagued with lingering guilt about "failing their partners" when an unexpected cesarean delivery was required. They worried that their relationships with their infants were damaged because they "didn't bond" with their newborns immediately after delivery.

Helping the family to focus their concerns about the at-risk situation without allowing them to become overwhelming is a nursing responsibility in the intrapartum period. The nurse usually has enough information about preexisting family stressors, objective maternal/fetal risk, and the immediate situational factors affecting the family to provide reassurance, modify environmental stressors, and help the family focus its energy on achieving the best possible outcome. The following section addresses strategies for assessment and intervention in regard to psychosocial needs of the high-risk intrapartum patient and her family.

PSYCHOSOCIAL ASSESSMENT AND INTERVENTION WITH THE HIGH-RISK PATIENT

Ideally, a plan of care for a family facing an at-risk labor and delivery should be developed as a collaborative effort between the woman and her partner, their physician, and the nursing personnel who will have intrapartum responsibilities for care, and should be prepared well in advance of the anticipated delivery date. This plan should address the physical and psychological needs of the pregnant woman and her family, and the needs of the healthcare professionals responsible for intrapartum management Comport & Seng, 1997; Jordon & Pugh, 1996; Roth, Riley, & Cohen, 1992). Such an approach gives the pregnant woman and her family an opportunity to develop realistic expectations for their intrapartum experience (Gilbert & Harmon, 1993).

When optimal prenatal care has been provided, the woman and her partner facing an at-risk birth will have an accurate understanding of the anticipated sequence of events. General information on how intrapartum care will likely unfold in the context of an at-risk delivery (i.e., continuous fetal monitoring, need for close monitoring of maternal vital signs) will have been given well in advance of delivery and supplemented with information on what will be required to manage the woman's specific risk condition (i.e., intrapartum insulin management of diabetes, cardiac monitoring for heart disease).

The woman and her family will also have been taught some problem-solving skills to help them appraise and respond to a range of experiences associated with high-risk labor and birth. For instance, teaching the couple how to ask specific questions of their care providers during rapidly changing events will increase their ability to clarify their understanding and to reframe their birth experience as it unfolds. This kind of preparation helps the woman and her partner maintain emotional equilibrium in the midst of the rapid changes typical of a high-risk birth and often enables them to feel a sense of participation in the process, even when events seem increasingly out of their control. (Gilbert & Harmon, 1993; Roth et al., 1992).

Assessing Psychosocial Status

A growing body of research suggests that psychosocial information collected systematically during prenatal care and made available to the intrapartum nurse can be used to benefit the woman with high-risk pregnancy during labor and birth. When intrapartum nurses have access to information about the family's adaptation to a high-risk pregnancy, they can individualize plans of care to build on family strengths and provide support in key areas (May & Mahlmeister, 1994). For instance, Radin and associates (1993) found that nursing care incorporating specific attention to emotional aspects of prenatal care can influence birth outcomes; when psychological data collected prenatally was used in intrapartum nursing care, patients experienced shorter labors, reduced incidence of forceps or vacuum extraction, and significantly fewer cesarean deliveries.

It is likely that these outcomes occur because an awareness of psychological strengths in the family, such as coping and stress management skills, communication skills, important social relationships and religious and cultural needs, allows the nurse to intervene in ways that enhance the family's ability to manage stress and uncertainty in the intrapartum period (Haggerty, 1996; Stainton, 1992; Stainton, 1994). Further, the provision of individualized and continuous emotional support during labor has been associated with a decrease in cesarean births (Kennell, Klaus, McGrath, & Hinckley, 1991; Radin, Harmon, & Hanson, 1993), shorter labors (Hetherington, 1990; Kennell et al., 1991), increased maternal sense of control and decreased use of analgesia during labor (Hodnett & Osborn, 1989; McNiven, Hodnett, & O'Brien-Pallas, 1992).

Unfortunately, prenatal care and intrapartum care of at-risk women is not always well integrated, and the provision of supportive nursing care in the intrapartum period is not always guaranteed. In many cases, although there is usually systematic collection and documentation of physiological data throughout pregnancy, assessment and documentation of the woman's psychological adaptation are not always recorded in a systematic fashion. Often, the only documentation on psychological adaptation appears in cases where patients exhibit extreme attitudes or behaviors (i.e., the patient is "non-compliant," or expresses expectations and goals for childbirth that are dramatically different from those of care providers).

Even when information on psychosocial adaptation during pregnancy is recorded, intrapartum nurses are usually forced to rely on information gathered and interpreted by others regarding levels of family stress and adaptation during pregnancy to formulate an initial plan of intrapartum care. A more thorough assessment of psychosocial needs of high-risk intrapartum patients and their families becomes a significant nursing challenge, as the nurse must simultaneously assess physiologic status and establish a working relationship with the family and with the rest of the professional team caring for them.

Although the intrapartum nurse's attention is largely focused on assessing the physiological and psychological condition of the laboring woman and her partner, the nurse should also be alert to cues that parents are emotionally tied to the fetus and should acknowledge expressions of that attachment, when present. Positive responses to fetal movement, or physical evidence of the fetus (ultrasound images, fetal heart rate tracings), reference to the fetus by name, or positive verbalizations are evidence of an established bond.

Although the presence of such cues is reassuring, it is important to remember that their absence is *not* compelling evidence of a poor bond, and intervention to "enhance bonding" during this period may be ill-advised. Parental behavior in regard to the unborn will be profoundly influenced by previous obstetric events (especially a previous loss), personality traits, cultural factors, and the intense nature of the intrapartum experience.

Unfortunately, for some couples, the intrapartum period will be the only opportunity they will have to parent a living child. Thus, when there is a fetal/neonatal loss or one is clearly imminent, the nurse's assessment regarding the couple's responses to the stress of labor and birth and strength of the bond between parents and newborn will be valuable in shaping a new plan of care for the grieving family.

Other families find the adjustment from a strong attachment to the fantasized newborn to acceptance of the actual newborn difficult after the stresses of a high-risk labor and birth. The intrapartum nurse's impressions of the nature of the parental bond can provide information useful to care providers working with families during the neonatal period, especially if the newborn's status is unstable.

Intervening with Psychosocial Stress and Distress

If information is unavailable about the woman and her family's skills at managing stress and uncertainty and the woman is in stable condition, the nurse must gather information about individual and family responses to the stresses of labor quickly and under rapidly changing conditions. The nurse can begin by discussing ways in which the family has responded to similar situations in the past, and can encourage them to use strategies that were successful then and that may be of assistance in this situation.

Supporting the Mate Relationship

Patterns of association between the quality of the mate relationship, self-esteem, and anxiety and depression in high-risk pregnancies may substantially contribute to the eventual adaptation of the woman and her family after an at-risk birth (Ferketich & Mercer, 1990; Ferketich & Mercer, 1994; Mercer, 1990; Mercer & Ferketich, 1994). These indicators may also be useful in the intrapartum setting to identify families with the greatest need for psychosocial support during an at-risk birth. The nurse should note whether the mate relationship seems well established and secure. If there is expression of mutual concern, a desire to remain together, and some ability on the part of each partner to meet the other's emotional needs in this stressful situation, it is likely that the relationship is providing an important level of support for the laboring woman. In this case, nursing interventions may focus on supporting that closeness, monitoring fatigue and worry in the partner, and substituting for that support when separation of the partners is necessary.

If the nurse senses the partners are not able to support each other emotionally during this crisis, it may be useful to consider whether the situation can be improved through specific nursing interventions. For instance, if it appears that the woman and her partner lack information about strategies for coping with labor, the nurse can offer basic information on techniques that may be useful, and can evaluate whether the partner can assist the woman in using these techniques. Breathing techniques, visual imagery, massage techniques, effleurage, and counterpressure can all be adapted and taught successfully to women and their partners during a high-risk labor experience (Hetherington, 1990).

If long-standing disagreements or ongoing tension appear to be present, the nurse can anticipate that the partner relationship may not be an optimal source of support for the woman.

In this situation, the nurse may need to assess whose presence is most supportive and reassuring to the laboring woman in this situation, while also supporting the needs of the partner. It must be remembered that research shows women usually identify a sense of comfort from their mate's presence that is separate from the types of physical care or comforting he may be able to provide (Kennell et al., 1991). Thus, the nurse may need to consider how to optimize the mate's positive contribution while controlling or minimizing any negative effects.

The intrapartum nurse should observe how the woman and her mate respond to changes in the labor situation and to interactions with care providers. For instance, couples who have prepared carefully for an at-risk birth often have a clear understanding of goals to be achieved and may be at risk for judging themselves too harshly against performance expectations. In this situation, it may be useful to provide praise for appropriate coping, but also to help the couple identify the need to "stay flexible" and to reframe expectations within what is possible. The nurse may notice that some couples respond favorably to reassurance about their ability to cope with labor, that is, such comments appear to calm them. Others respond more favorably to specific instructions and praise for their efforts, requiring the nurse to remain in a teaching or coaching relationship with the woman and her partner, while others choose to rely more heavily on direct support from the nurse with the mate in a less active role.

Helping the Family Reframe the Intrapartum Experience

In order to cope with and adjust to the stress of a high-risk labor and birth and the crisis situations that can result, the nurse can help the couple focus on reframing the experience, a process in which one first states their understanding of the current situation, and then seeks to understand what is changing or has changed and what those changes mean. The couple can be encouraged to restate what they understood to be the situation and then what they heard about changes ("I heard you say..."), to clarify what was said ("I'm not sure I understood...") and then to explore the meaning of the situation. If necessary, the nurse can guide the woman and her partner through this process, allowing the couple a clearer understanding of the physician's perceptions of the situation and the implications of new information to the woman and the fetus. Once the couple understands this new assessment of the situation, they can then move to exploring the risks and benefits of any proposed changes in the plan of care. The couple should be encouraged to ask, or guided through, such questions as: "What are the benefits of this plan for me and for my baby? What are the risks? Are there alternatives? How quickly must a decision be made?" (Thorne, 1993a).

Learning how to reframe a situation in this way enables families to remain part of the decision-making process, even in the rapidly changing context of a high-risk birth (Robinson, 1996; Thorne, 1993b). Some families will choose to exercise this level of participation, while others will delegate decisions to their healthcare providers (Angst & Deatrick, 1996). By using this technique to assist families to understand their situation as it changes, the nurse can ensure they have as much or as little information as they choose, and can remain as actively involved in decision making as they want to be.

Managing Anxiety and Fear

Intervening with anxiety and fear during high-risk labor involves essentially the same processes as those employed in a low-risk birth. However, the nurse should also recognize that the latent fears of loss and injury experienced by any laboring couple become real and ominous under circumstances of at-risk childbearing (DeVore, 1990). The nurse should carefully explain and reinforce information about the nature of emerging threats and how professionals plan to deal with them. It is unwise to assume that parents understand information previously explained. Instead, the nurse should look for ways to assess understanding, reinforce positive points, and correct misconceptions (i.e., "You remember that your wife's condition is stable—what we are concerned about right

now is that the baby's heart rate appears to be slowing" [Driscoll, 1996]).

High levels of anxiety or depression may be hinted at in the prenatal record, in notes regarding lack of partner support or involvement, missed prenatal visits or unexplained delays in seeking care, difficulty in meeting typical demands of pregnancy, or extremes in vigilance (very high or very low) about physical signs or symptoms or about fetal well-being. Worrisome signs in the intrapartum period may include extreme distancing or withdrawal of the mate from the situation, expressions of helplessness or emotional outbursts from the woman or mate unrelated to the course of labor, or blaming the baby for the at-risk situation or for disruption in the relationship. The nurse should consider these signs that the woman and her partner may require intensive and continuous emotional support to cope with the labor and birth experience; in this situation, continuity of nursing care and careful attention to supportive and clear communication with both partners is of considerable importance.

Managing Environmental and Emergent Stressors

Perhaps the most important area for nursing action in the psychosocial care of the high-risk intrapartum patient is in the control of the environment and the stressors therein. The nurse must be assertive in exerting control over the patient's environment. The number of personnel and the number of entrances and exits from the patient's room can be kept to a safe minimum. Care and procedures can be clustered to avoid constant interruptions. The nurse should be especially vigilant to help patient and family cope with the rapidity of change and the behavioral changes demonstrated in providers as they adapt to clinical needs.

When conditions are changing rapidly, the nurse should periodically step back and see how the patient and family are responding, and then step back in to ask "what can I do to help you right now?" Using the same reframing technique, the nurse can state her appraisal of the family's situation, ask for clarification, point out changes in the situation, and explore possibilities for effective response. When they are over-whelmed in a crisis situation, couples will frequently need assistance in identifying what is happening, what can be ignored or merely watched, and what must be responded to and in what ways.

In particular, the nurse should avoid "flying into action" with equipment and procedures without preparing the patient with a brief explanation of what has changed and the interventions that will be used to manage the situation. Other care providers should be reminded to do likewise. Giving patient and family a few moments in which to adjust before the action resumes may be a valuable key in helping them maintain their equilibrium. Also, "nursing the equipment" rather than the patient and family is a constant threat in rapidly changing situations and must be guarded against.

The physical environment should be viewed from the family's eyes as much as possible. Even in an intensive care environment, there is usually room for the patient to make choices about sounds, lighting, and arrangement of bedside space. However, patient choice is only possible if someone asks about preferences and then intervenes to honor them. Within safe practice limits, allowing the woman on continuous monitoring to sit in a bedside chair or offering self-regulated epidural anesthesia can increase a woman's sense of control over her environment.

Finally, the nurse must remember that, even within the context of high-risk intrapartum care, the focus of care is the family, not the obstetrical or medical complication. When intrapartum care is offered to a high-risk family, there are in reality three patients requiring nursing care: the woman, the unborn, and the woman's significant other. Family-centered care is even more important for high-risk patients than for their low-risk counterparts (Stainton, 1994). At every opportunity, the nurse should ask: "What can I do to support this family's well-being right now?" Appropriate interventions may include ensuring flexibility with visitors within safe limits, assigning some temporary and intensive support for a father who is at his own emotional limits, avoiding unnecessary and arbitrary separation of mates (even if it means challeng-

ing hospital policy), and teaching family members how to help each other focus their energy effectively.

Such work is difficult. The nurse should also be sensitive to the fact that others must assist at times and that others may have insights into what may help a particular patient at a particular time. Consultation on psychosocial care is as important as consultation on physical or technical aspects of care, yet nurses sometimes hesitate to ask for help in this arena.

Nurses also may be hesitant to communicate their observations and their plans of psychosocial care to other healthcare providers, because it seems "not as important" as information about a patient's obstetric and medical status. Although it may be understandable, such hesitation suggests a worrisome lack of regard for the documented importance of psychological factors in human health and well-being. There is clear and compelling evidence that optimal maternal and neonatal outcomes require careful attention to psychosocial aspects of labor and birth; therefore, it is a nursing responsibility to ensure that emotional comfort and security of the family are addressed in the context of high-risk intrapartum care.

Expected Outcomes of Psychosocial Care

Evaluating outcomes of intrapartum care in the psychosocial arena is notoriously difficult because of the absence of reliable ways to measure comfort and distress, the constant and sometimes rapid changes in patient condition, and the absence of well-defined protocols for nursing care for emotional distress. The challenge is made even more difficult by the overlay of an at-risk birth with the attendant threats to life and well-being. Although focused research on the process and outcomes of intrapartum nursing care is still rather limited, there is growing evidence that the quality of nursing care in regard to psychosocial needs contributes directly to maternal and neonatal outcomes.

Appropriate attention to the emotional needs of the woman and her family has been shown not only to improve birth outcomes, but also to influence patient satisfaction with the childbirth experience. It is clear that, regardless of how birth experiences unfolded, women who reported that they had caring intrapartum nurses who responded to them as individuals had more positive impressions of their birth experiences than those who reported otherwise (Brown & Lumley, 1994). A systematic review of randomized controlled trials of labor and birth care completed in the Cochrane Collaborative Data Base shows compelling evidence that emotional and psychological support during labor contributes to optimal perinatal outcomes (Enkin, Keirse, Renfrew, & Neilson, 1995).

Despite this evidence, analysis of current patterns of intrapartum nursing practice suggests that a very small percentage of nursing work focuses on this aspect of practice. In a study of intrapartum nursing activities by Gagnon and Waghorn (1996), 47.6% of activities were indirect (i.e., nurses were not in the patient's room) and only 6.1% of activities were in supportive care. Again, of the activities included in supportive care, half of the time was spent in instructional or educational activities and less than 20% was spent in providing emotional support. In a similar study by McNiven and associates (1992), only 9.9% of intrapartum nursing activities were spent in providing supportive care to laboring patients. Of the supportive care that was offered, most fell into categories of "gathering and providing information" (6.65%). Emotional support accounted for 2.6% of the nursing activities, while physical comfort measures and advocacy were nearly absent at 0.3% of activities respectively.

Nurses caring for high-risk women and their families in the intrapartum period should carefully evaluate their clinical practice in terms of the type, amount, and effectiveness of the emotional support they offer. The following nursing actions in the context of high-risk intrapartum care suggest outcomes against which care can be judged and toward which progress can be made:

- Verify that the patient and family understand the at-risk condition and the significance of changes in that condition for the woman and fetus.
- Ensure that patient and family are informed of changes in condition and encourage them to ask questions of staff.

- Seek information from prenatal care providers on which to base psychosocial support interventions.
- Assess for evidence of preexisting cumulative stress and provide supportive care as indicated.
- Encourage the patient to express emotional distress and provide supportive care as needed.
- Assess patient–family responses to psychosocial interventions and evaluate and modify plans of care to optimize family coping and minimize distress.
- Limit environmental stressors in keeping with patient-family wishes and safe standards of care.

The challenge of providing sensitive and effective psychosocial care in the context of high-risk labor and birth is great, but the benefits of such nursing care are so clear for women and their families. As Tomlinson and associates (1996, p. 335) wrote: "The need for help during the stress of labor and delivery can contribute to openness to intervention and acceptance of support beyond the hospital stay. In this way, supportive interventions that may seem trivial may have far-reaching effects." Meeting the needs of women and their families through the blending "high tech/high touch" is the essence of intrapartum nursing care, and it is with high-risk patients and their families that nursing can demonstrate the best it has to offer.

References

Angst, D., & Deatrick, J. (1996). Involvement in health care decisions: Parents and children with chronic illness. Journal of Family Nursing, 2(2), 174–194.

Barnett, B., & Parker, G. (1986). Possible determinants, correlates and consequences of high levels of anxiety in primiparous mothers. Psychological Medicine, 16, 177–185.

Belsky J., & Pensky, E. (1988). Marital change across the transition to parenthood. In R. Palkowitz & M. Sussman (Eds.), Transitions to parenthood. New York: Haworth Press.

Brown, S., & Lumley, J. (1994). Satisfaction with care in labor and birth: A survey of 790 Australian women. Birth, 21(1), 4–13.

Cohen, R. (1979). Maladaptation to pregnancy. Seminars in Perinatology, 3, 15–24.

Comport, K., & Seng, J. (1997). Aortic stenosis in pregnancy: A case report. JOGNN, 26(1), 67–77.

Cranley, M. (1983). Development of a tool for the measurement of maternal attachment during pregnancy. Nursing Research, 30(6), 281–284.

Cranley, M., Hedahl, K., & Pegg, S. (1983). Women's perceptions of vaginal cesarean deliveries. Nursing Research, 32(1), 10–16.

Cummins, L., Scrimshaw, S., & Engle, P. (1988). Views of cesarean birth among primiparous women of Mexican origin in Los Angeles. Birth, 15(3), 164–168.

Curry, M., & Snell, B. (1985). Antenatal hospitalization: Maternal behavior and the family. (Final report, DHHS, HRSA, Division of Nursing, Nursing Research Support Section, Grant #1, RO1 NU 00939).

DeVore, N. (1990). Maternal psychosocial adaptations to high risk pregnancy. In B. Buckley (Ed.), High risk maternity nursing manual. Baltimore: Williams & Wilkins.

Driscoll, J. (1996). Psychosocial adaptation to pregnancy and postpartum. In K. R. Simpson & P. A. Creehan (Eds.), AWHONN's perinatal nursing. Philadelphia: Lippincott.

Enkin, M., Keirse, M., Renfrew, M., & Neilson, J. (1995). Effective care in pregnancy and childbirth: A synopsis. Birth, 22(2), 101–110.

Ferketich, S., & Mercer, R. (1990). Effects of antepartal stress on health status during early motherhood. Scholarly Inquiry for Nursing Practice, 4(2), 127–149.

Ferketich, S., & Mercer, R. (1994). Predictors of paternal role competence by risk status. Nursing Research, 43(2), 80–85.

Gagnon, A., & Waghorn, K. (1996). Supportive care by maternity nurses: A work sampling study in an intrapartum unit. Birth, 23, 1–6.

Gilbert, E., & Harmon, J. (1993). Psychologic adaptations. In E. Epstein & B. Copland (Eds.), Manual of high risk pregnancy and delivery (pp. 100–112). St. Louis, MO: Mosby-Year Book.

Grossman, R. (1988). Strain in the transition to parenthood. In R. Palkowitz & M. Sussman (Eds.), Transitions to parenthood. New York: Haworth Press.

Haggerty, L. (1996). Assessment parameters and indicators in expert intrapartal nursing decisions. JOGNN, 25(6), 491–499.

Hetherington, S. (1990). A controlled study of the effect of prepared childbirth classes on obstetric outcomes. Birth, 17, 86–91.

Hobfoll, S., Nadler, A., & Leiberman, J. (1986). Satisfaction with social support during crisis: Intimacy and self-esteem as critical determinants. Journal of Personality and Social Psychology, 51(2), 296–304.

Hodnett, E., & Osborn, R. (1989). Effects of continuous intrapartum professional support on childbirth outcomes. Research in Nursing and Health, 12, 289–297.

Jordon, E., & Pugh, L. (1996). Pregnancy after cardiac transplantation: Principles of nursing care. JOGNN, 25(2), 131–143.

Kemp, V., & Page, C. (1987). Maternal prenatal attachment in normal and high-risk pregnancies. JOGNN, 16(3), 179–184.

Kennell, J., Klaus, M., McGrath, S., & Hinckley, C. (1991). Continuous emotional support during labor in a U.S. hospital. Journal of the American Medical Association, 256, 2197–2201.

Lederman, R. (1986). Maternal anxiety in pregnancy: Relationship to fetal and newborn health status. Annual Review of Nursing Research: For Nursing Practice, Management, and Education, 4, 3–19.

May, K. (1993). Impact of preterm labor on families. (Final report, National Institutes of Health, National Institute of Nursing Research, Grant # RO1-NR 02377).

May, K. (1994). Impact of preterm labor and maternal activity restriction on the expectant father. JOGNN, 23(3), 246–253.

May, K., & Mahlmeister, J. (1994). Maternal and neonatal nursing: Family-centered care. Philadelphia: J. B. Lippincott.

May, K., & Sollid, D. (1984). Fathers' responses to unanticipated cesarean delivery. Birth, 11, 87–95.

McNiven, P., Hodnett, E., & O'Brien-Pallas, L. (1992). Supporting women in labor: A work sampling study of the activities of labor and delivery nurses. Birth, 19, 1, 3–9.

Mercer, R. (1990). Parents at risk. New York: Springer.

Mercer, R., & Ferketich, S. (1994). Predictors of maternal role competence by risk status. Nursing Research, 43(1), 38–43.

Mercer, R., Ferketich, S., May, K. & DeJoseph, J. (1987). Antepartal stress: Effect on family health and functioning. (Final report, National Cancer for Nursing Research, Grant #5 RO1 NR01064-03).

Mercer, R., Ferketich, S., May, K. DeJoseph, J., & Sollid, D. (1988). Further exploration of maternal and fetal attachment. Research in Nursing and Health, 11, 83–95.

Norbeck, J., & Tilden, V. (1983). Life stress, social support, and emotional disequilibrium in complications of pregnancy: A prospective multivariate study. Journal of Health and Social Behavior, 24, 30–46.

O'Hara, M., Rehm, L., & Campbell, S. (1983). Postpartum depression: A role for social network and life stress variables. Journal of Nervous Mental Disease, 171, 336–341.

Paarlberg, K., Vingerhoets, A., Passchier, J., Dekker, G., & Van Geijn, H. (1995). Psychosocial factors and pregnancy outcome: A review with emphasis on methodological issues. Journal of Psychosomatic Research, 39(5), 563–595.

Parke, R., & Beitel, A. (1988). Disappointment: When things go wrong in the transition to parenthood. In R. Palkowitz & M. Sussman (Eds.), Transitions to parenthood. New York: Haworth Press.

Perez, P. (1995). When the birth plan changes. [Special Issue]. Childbirth Instructor, 22–24.

Radin, T., Harmon, J., & Hanson, D. (1993). Nurses' care during labor: Its effect on the cesarean birth rate of healthy, nulliparous women. Birth, 20(1), 14–21.

Robinson, C. (1996). Health care relationships revisited. Journal of Family Nursing, 2(2), 152–173.

Roth, C., Riley, B., & Cohen, S. (1992). Intrapartum care of a woman with aortic aneurysms. JOGNN, 21(4), 310–317.

Sandelowski, M., & Bustamante, R. (1986). Cesarean birth outside of the natural childbirth culture. Research in Nursing and Health, 9, 81–88.

Stainton, M. (1992). Mismatched caring in high-risk perinatal situations. Clinical Nursing Research, 1, 34–49.

Stainton, M. (1994). Supporting family functioning during a high-risk pregnancy. Maternal Child Nursing, 19, 24–28.

Thorne, S. (1993a). Trust and confidence. In S. Thorne (Ed.), Negotiating health care: The social context of chronic illness. Newbury Park, CA: Sage.

Thorne, S. (1993b). Relationships with health care providers. In S. Thorne (Ed.), Negotiating health care: The social context of chronic illness. Newbury Park, CA: Sage.

Tilden, V., & Lipson, J. (1982). Cesarean childbirth: Variables affecting psychological impact. Western Journal of Nursing Research: An International Forum for Communication, 3, 127–132.

Tomlinson, P., Bryan, A., & Esau, A. (1996). Family-centered intrapartum care: Revisiting an old concept. JOGNN, 25(4), 331–337.

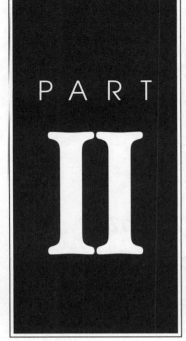

PART

II

Critical Care Adjuncts

CHAPTER
4

Invasive Hemodynamic Monitoring in Obstetrics

Nan H. Troiano

Invasive hemodynamic monitoring is a significant adjunct often used in the care of critically ill patients. Data obtained from such devices enhance the ability of the critical care nurse to assess the patient's hemodynamic and oxygen transport status, formulate nursing diagnoses, develop and implement an appropriate plan of care, and evaluate patient responses over time.

Irrespective of the location at which care is provided, the obstetric nurse caring for the critically ill pregnant woman should understand principles associated with invasive hemodynamic monitoring and interpretation of data. This chapter reviews fundamental principles related to invasive central hemodynamic monitoring during pregnancy. More thorough discussion of clinical application to specific patient problems is presented elsewhere in this book.

CARDIAC ANATOMY AND PHYSIOLOGY

Delivery of adequate oxygen, nutrients, and other vital substances in the blood to tissues is necessary for cellular function that sustains life. The cardiovascular system is responsible for pumping these substances through the vascular bed by contraction of the heart. Normal cardiac anatomy is depicted in Figure 4-1.

Atria are low-pressure chambers that serve as reservoirs of blood for the ventricles. The right

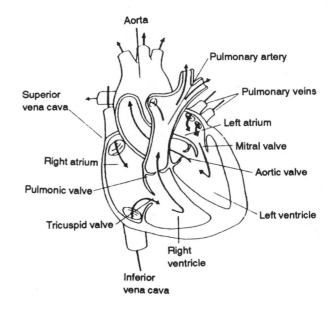

Figure 4-1. Normal cardiac anatomy (arrows indicate normal path of circulation).

atrium receives venous blood via the superior and inferior vena cavae and coronary sinus from the systemic bed. The left atrium receives oxygenated blood returning to the heart from the pulmonary bed via the four pulmonary veins. Approximately 70–80% of blood flows passively from the atria to the ventricles during early ventricular diastole, known as protodiastole. During the later phase, the atria contract and pump an additional 20–30% of blood into the ventricles. Loss of atrial systole, also referred to as "atrial kick," in an otherwise normal heart usually has only minimal effect. However, in patients with impaired left ventricular filling, left atrial systole is very important and may account for more than 50% of left ventricular filling.

The ventricles provide the force necessary to circulate blood through the lungs and the rest of the body. The right ventricle pumps deoxygenated blood into the pulmonary circulation via the pulmonary artery. The left ventricle much thicker than the right, pumps oxygenated blood into the systemic circulation via the aorta. The left side of the heart functions as a higher pressure system than does the right side. Under normal circumstances, the right ventricle ejects approximately 50–60% of its end-diastolic volume with each cardiac contraction, whereas the left ventricle ejects 60–70%.

Atrioventricular valves consist of the tricuspid valve on the right and mitral valve on the left. During diastole, valve leaflets open, which allows unidirectional blood flow into the respective ventricle. As ventricular pressure increases during systole, valve leaflets close, which prevents retrograde flow. Semilunar valves consist of the pulmonic valve on the right and aortic on the left. Open during ventricular systole, each of these valves allows unidirectional blood flow to the respective arterial outflow tract. Following systole as arterial pressures increase, each valve closes to prevent retrograde flow during diastole.

DETERMINANTS OF CARDIAC OUTPUT

Cardiac output is the amount of blood ejected from the heart per unit of time. It is determined by four variables: preload, afterload, contractility, and heart rate.

Preload

Preload refers to the tension or load on a muscle as it begins to contract. In the context of the cardiovascular system, preload is the length of the ventricular muscle fiber at end-diastole. The principal factor that determines muscle fiber length is the amount of blood in the ventricles at the point of maximal filling. The intrinsic ability of the heart to adapt to increased loads of incoming blood is called Starling's law of the heart. Within certain physiologic limits, the more the heart is filled with blood during diastole, the greater the quantity of blood that will be ejected during systole. Conversely, when the amount of blood returning to the ventricles is diminished, cardiac output may be impaired. For example, this may be evident in the patient with significant blood loss or hypotension who has decreased circulating blood volume or venous return to the heart.

Afterload

Afterload is the resistance or load that opposes ventricular ejection of blood during systole. The right ventricle pumps against pressure or resistance in the pulmonary vasculature, whereas the left ventricle pumps against the higher pressure or resistance in the systemic circulation. In contrast to preload, afterload and cardiac output have an inverse relationship. Within certain physiologic limits, the lower the afterload or resistance applied against the ventricles during systole, the greater the cardiac output. Conversely, patients with clinical conditions such as pulmonary or systemic hypertension, in which pressure in the pulmonary or systemic vessels respectively is increased, are at risk for decreased cardiac output.

Contractility

Contractility, also known as the inotropic state of the heart, is the intrinsic ability of the heart muscle to shorten or develop tension, or both, independent of variations in preload and afterload. Not easily measured in clinical situations, contractility can nonetheless be inferred by a change in cardiac output when afterload and preload remain constant. Under conditions of altered catecholamine production or following administration of medications that alter inotropic response, the Starling curve shifts upward with a higher cardiac output for a given filling pressure. Conversely, with decreased contractility, the heart pumps less well at a given filling pressure. Thus, patients with a compromised heart function at higher pressures under normal conditions have less reserve and are more prone to heart failure when stressed.

Heart Rate

Heart rate affects the strength of myocardial contraction and thus cardiac output. For example, at faster rates the force of contraction is strong, and at slower rates the force is weaker. This intrinsic property of the heart muscle may be attributable to rate-driven variations in sarcoplasmic calcium concentration. It should be noted, however, that increased heart rate also results in decreased diastolic filling time and may thereby decrease preload, and over a period of time, cardiac output. In addition, a pause between heart contractions results in increased force of the next contraction, also known as rest potentiation, which may increase cardiac output. For these reasons, rate-related changes in the force of contraction, preload, and cardiac output interact in a complex manner.

OXYGEN TRANSPORT PHYSIOLOGY

The ability of cells to function normally is dependent on a continuous supply of adequate oxygen. When oxygen transport is impaired, the patient is at increased risk for end-organ dysfunction or failure. Thus, evaluation of oxygen transport is essential in the care of the critically ill patient. Key concepts related to oxygen transport include oxygen content, affinity, delivery, and consumption.

Oxygen Content

Oxygen is transported to the tissues in two ways: dissolved under pressure in plasma and bound to hemoglobin within the red blood cells. The oxygen dissolved in plasma makes up approximately 1–2% of the total oxygen content, whereas oxygen bound to hemoglobin makes up the remaining 98–99%.

The role of hemoglobin in the transport of oxygen is significant. Hemoglobin is composed of four subunits, each consisting of a protein

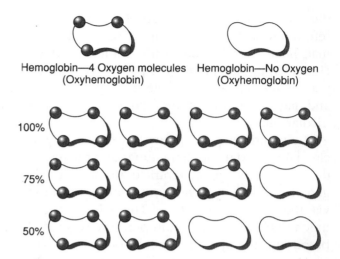

Figure 4-2. Percent saturation of hemoglobin.

chain with a heme group attached to a histidine residue. One molecule of oxygen is loosely bound with one of the six coordinate valencies of each of the heme iron atoms. Thus, each molecule of hemoglobin is associated with four molecules of oxygen. The kinetics of the association are such that all the molecules of oxygen bind at the same rate. When a hemoglobin molecule is combined with oxygen it is called oxyhemoglobin. The saturation of hemoglobin with oxygen is the ratio of oxyhemoglobin to the total amount of hemoglobin that is capable of transporting oxygen. This concept is illustrated in Figure 4-2.

Although it represents only a small fraction of total oxygen content, oxygen dissolved in plasma plays a crucial role. The ability of oxygen to combine with hemoglobin in the lungs, later to be released at the tissue level, is affected by oxygen in the plasma. This reversible binding of hemoglobin to oxygen is an important concept in oxygen transport and allows for the loading of oxygen in the lungs and unloading at the tissue level.

Oxygen Affinity

Affinity refers to the ability of oxygen to combine with hemoglobin. Both the uptake and the release of oxygen by the hemoglobin molecules

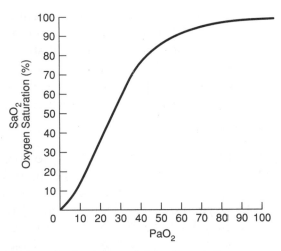

Figure 4-3. Oxyhemoglobin dissociation curve.

are represented visually by the oxyhemoglobin dissociation curve (Figure 4-3).

The curve depicts the relationship between the partial pressure of oxygen (PaO_2) in arterial blood and the saturation of hemoglobin (SaO_2). The sigmoid shape of the normal curve is the result of the increased affinity of hemoglobin for oxygen as more oxygen molecules combine with it, despite large alveolar PO_2 changes (the flat upper portion of the curve) and the rapid unloading of oxygen from hemoglobin, with small changes in PaO_2 (the steep, lower portion of the curve). The position of the curve is defined more precisely by a reference point known as the P_{50}. The P_{50} represents the PaO_2 at which hemoglobin is 50% saturated. Under normal conditions in nonpregnant individuals, the P_{50} is 26.3 mm Hg.

The P_{50} is not fixed in critically ill individuals. If the affinity and P_{50} change, the oxyhemoglobin dissociation curve shifts to the right or left to represent the change. Conditions known to change oxygen affinity are described in Table 4-1. Decreased oxygen affinity, resulting in a right shift in the oxyhemoglobin dissociation curve, means that at any given PaO_2 there is decreased saturation. Thus, oxygen is released more readily to tissues. Conversely, increased oxygen affinity, resulting in a left shift in the curve, means that at any given PaO_2 there is increased saturation. This results in oxygen binding more tightly to hemoglobin.

It should be noted that pregnancy also affects the position of the oxyhemoglobin curve. The maternal curve normally shifts to the right, whereby oxygen is released more quickly from hemoglobin. The fetal curve normally shifts to

TABLE 4-1. Conditions Known to Change Oxygen Affinity to Hemoglobin

Conditions That Alter Affinity	
Increase Affinity (Left Shift)	Decrease Affinity (Right Shift)
High pH	Low pH
Hypothermia	Fever
Decreased $PaCO_2$	Increased $PaCO_2$
Decreased 2,3 DPG	Increased 2,3 DPG
Stored bank blood	Anemia
Hypothyroidism	Chronic hypoxemia
Hypophosphatemia	Hyperthyroidism
Chronic acidemia	Chronic alkalemia
	Some hormones

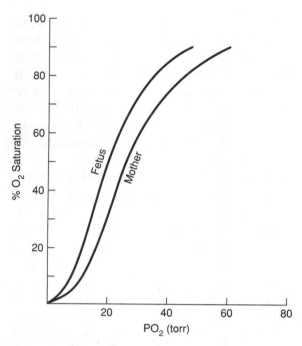

Figure 4-4. Normal maternal and fetal shifts in the oxyhemoglobin dissociation curve.
From <u>Critical Care Obstetrics</u>. (p. 106), by S. L. Clark, D. B. Cotton, G. D. V. Hankins, and J. P. Phelan (Eds.), 1991, New York: Blackwell Scientific Publications. Reproduced with permission

the left resulting in increased affinity of oxygen for hemoglobin. (See Figure 4-4.)

Oxygen Delivery

Oxygen delivery (DO_2) is the amount of oxygen delivered to the tissues per unit of time. The delivery of oxygen from the lungs to the tissues depends on the cardiac output as well as on the content of oxygen in the blood. It should be recalled that cardiac output is dependent on preload, afterload, contractility, and heart rate. The oxygen content is determined by the hemoglobin concentration and the oxygen saturation of the hemoglobin.

Factors that increase cardiac output, such as uterine contractions, increased metabolism, and certain drugs, will also increase DO_2. In addition, factors that increase total oxygen content, such as transfusion of packed red blood cells, increase DO_2. Conversely, factors that decrease cardiac output or total oxygen content decrease DO_2. Such conditions may include hypovolemia, hypoxemia, anemia, and certain drugs. When

oxygen supply is threatened, the body attempts to compensate and maintain delivery to the tissues by first increasing cardiac output. It should be noted that healthy individuals may increase cardiac output severalfold above normal levels in the presence of stressful circumstances.

Oxygen Consumption

Oxygen consumption (VO_2) refers to the amount of oxygen consumed by the tissues each minute. At rest, VO_2 is approximately 25% of the total oxygen delivery. During periods of stress, VO_2 may increase approximately threefold to about 75% of the total oxygen available. Oxygen consumption is increased by numerous conditions, as well as by interventions, therapeutic procedures, and various other stresses. It should be noted that VO_2 also increases significantly during normal pregnancy.

The normal relationship between DO_2 and VO_2 is such that sufficient reserve exists to maintain VO_2 *independent* of DO_2 over a wide range of delivery values. However, situations may develop whereby prolonged decreased DO_2, below some critical threshold, eventually results in a linear fall in VO_2. This is known as *delivery dependent* VO_2 because the amount of oxygen consumed is limited by the amount of oxygen delivered. In such circumstances, VO_2 does not become independent of DO_2 except at very high levels of oxygen delivery, if at all. This pathologic response is related to the fixed oxygen-extraction ratio present in some critically ill patients.

CENTRAL HEMODYNAMIC ASSESSMENT

Invasive hemodynamic monitoring may be accomplished via use of a central venous pressure or pulmonary artery catheter. The description, assessment capabilities, indications, and associated complications for each follows.

Central Venous Pressure Catheter

The central venous pressure (CVP) catheter is a single or multiple lumen catheter advanced through a peripheral or central vein until the tip is in the proximal superior vena cava (Figure 4-5). Central venous access is most commonly obtained during pregnancy via the internal jugular or subclavian vein. The internal jugular vein is preferred by many physicians because of the increased risk of pneumothorax with subclavian attempts during pregnancy.

Use of this catheter permits evaluation of right preload, expressed in mm Hg as central venous pressure, as well as access for administration of fluid or medications. The primary limitation is that right ventricular function may not accurately reflect left ventricular function. Thus, clinical use of the CVP may be misleading and possibly deleterious, in certain clinical situations, to the patient's health. In addition, a CVP catheter does not permit evaluation of data regarding other determinants of cardiac output or oxygen transport parameters. For these reasons, use of a CVP catheter for assessment of hemodynamic function in a critically ill obstetric patient is seldom, if ever, indicated (Clark, Cotton, Hankins, & Phelan, 1994).

Complications related to obtaining central venous access include inadvertent arterial puncture, pneumothorax, and cellulitis at the site of insertion. Although pneumothorax has been reported to occur in 1–5% of a general patient population undergoing central venous catheterization, in a compilation of obstetric and gynecologic patients, Clark and associates observed no pneumothorax when the internal jugular approach was used (Clark, Horenstein, Phelan et al., 1985).

Pulmonary Artery Catheter

The pulmonary artery (PA), or Swan-Ganz, catheter is a balloon-tipped, flow-directed, multiple lumen catheter (Figure 4-6).

The basic, standard PA catheter is a flexible, flow-directed, 7 French polyvinylchloride catheter that contains three lumens and a thermistor bead. Additional catheters are available that provide extra central venous infusion ports, capability for ventricular pacing, evaluation of right ventricular function, continuous mixed venous oxygen saturation assessment, and continuous measurement of cardiac output. The size of these catheters varies depending on the number and type of additional options.

The PA catheter is inserted into the pulmonary artery through a percutaneous intro-

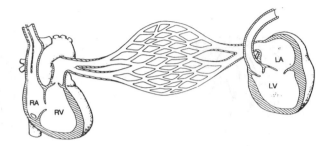

Figure 4-5. Central venous pressure catheter location.
From <u>Hemodynamic Monitoring: Invasive and Noninvasive Clinical Application</u>, by G. O. Darovic, 1987, Philadelphia: W. B. Saunders. Reproduced with permission.

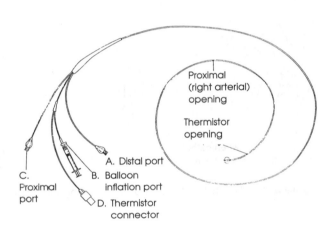

Figure 4-6. Pulmonary artery catheter.

ducer placed in a central vein. Characteristic pressure waveforms may be visualized as the catheter tip passes through various cardiac structures (Figure 4-7). Following insertion, the catheter rests in the pulmonary artery with the balloon tip deflated.

Use of this catheter permits continuous evaluation of pressures of the central vein and pulmonary artery. Intermittent inflation of the balloon permits evaluation of pulmonary capillary wedge pressure. This provides information regarding left preload by simulating closure of the pulmonic valve (Figure 4-8). Intermittent evaluation of cardiac output may also be conducted

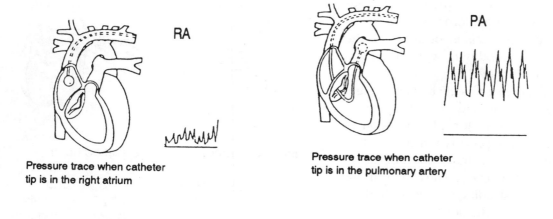

Figure 4-7. Characteristic waveforms during pulmonary artery catheter insertion.

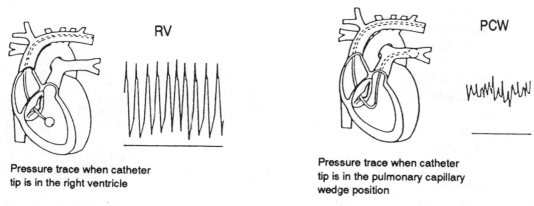

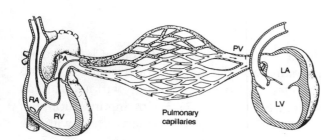

Figure 4-8. Pulmonary artery catheter location during assessment of pulmonary capillary wedge pressure.
From <u>Hemodynamic Monitoring: Invasive and Noninvasive Clinical Application</u>, by G. O. Darovic, 1987, Philadelphia: W. B. Saunders. Reproduced with permission.

utilizing thermodilution technology. Other hemodynamic data may be derived through calculations based on the preceding basic parameters. Normal hemodynamic values during pregnancy, are presented in Table 4-2 (Clark, Cotton, Lee et al., 1989).

Pulmonary artery catheterization is not without risks, but few are life-threatening. Most of these complications are nonspecific and seen with all types of intravascular catheters. However, some are specific to PA catheters. Onset of ventricular dysrhythmias is the most common complication specific to PA catheters. It has been reported to occur, in a nonobstetric patient population, in approximately 50% of insertions when the catheters are passed through the right side of the heart (Marino, 1991). These dys-

TABLE 4-2. Normal Hemodynamic Values in Pregnancy

Parameter	Value and Standard Deviation
Cardiac output (liters/minute)	6.2 ± 1.0
Systemic vascular resistance (dyne/sec/cm^{-3})	1210 ± 266
Pulmonary vascular resistance (dyne/sec/cm^{-5})	78 ± 22
Mean pulmonary artery pressure (mm Hg)	13 ± 2
Pulmonary capillary wedge pressure (mm Hg)	7.5 ± 1.8
Central venous pressure (mm Hg)	3.6 ± 2.5
Left ventricular stroke work index (g/m/m^{-2})	48 ± 6

rhythmias are almost always benign and disappear when the catheter is either advanced into the pulmonary artery or is withdrawn. Rignt bundle branch block may also occur but usually disappears within 24 hours of insertion. Pulmonary artery rupture is a rare complication, with 10 cases reported in the first 10 years of catheter use (Paulson, Scott, & Sethl, 1988).

The American College of Obstetricians and Gynecologists describes indications for use of a pulmonary artery catheter in obstetric patients. These are listed in Table 4-3.

A majority of clinicians who practice in critical care environments believe information provided by the PA catheter is helpful in guiding therapy and improving outcome in selected critically ill patients (Chernow, 1997). However, the impact of PA catheter use on reduction of morbidity and mortality remains controversial. Numerous stud-

ies fail to demonstrate the benefit of PA catheterization (Dolen, 1990; Gore, Goldberg, Spodick et al., 1987; Sibbald & Sprung, 1988). Criticisms of these studies relate to small sample sizes, lack of control groups, discrepancies in severity of illness, and lack of information regarding oxygen transport status. Connors and associates (1996) reported no benefit to right-heart catheterization in the initial care of critically ill patients and, in a summation commentary, questioned whether the Food and Drug Administration (FDA) should impose a moratorium on the use of the PA catheter (Connors, Speroff, Dawson et al., 1996).

A consensus development conference was subsequently sponsored by the Society of Critical Care Medicine and a consensus statement was issued regarding use of the PA catheter in critical care settings (Society of Critical Care Medicine: Consensus Development Conference,

TABLE 4-3. Indications for Invasive Hemodynamic Monitoring in Obstetrics

Severe preeclampsia with refractory oligcria or pulmonary edema

Massive hemorrhage or volume replacement needs

Shock of unknown etiology

Sepsis with oliguria or refractory hypotension

Cardiovascular decompensation during intrapartum or intraoperative periods

Chronic disease during labor or intraoperatively

Pulmonary edema, oliguria, or heart failure refractory to treatment or of unknown etiology

1997). The statement reiterated that, as with other diagnostic modalities, the clinical utility of the PA catheter depends on proper interpretation of the data. The need for additional prospective, randomized studies regarding use of the PA catheter in various disease processes was also noted. With respect to pregnancy, the ACOG guidelines for invasive hemodynamic monitoring were referenced along with a recommendation for further research in the field.

OXYGEN TRANSPORT ASSESSMENT

Technical adjuncts that enhance the ability to assess the oxygen transport status of critically ill patients include the pulse oximeter and continuous mixed venous oxygen saturation (SvO_2) PA catheter.

Pulse Oximetry

Oximetry is an optical method for measuring oxygenated hemoglobin in blood. It is based on the ability of different forms of hemoglobin to absorb light of different wavelengths. Oxygenated hemoglobin (HbO_2) absorbs light in the red spectrum and deoxygenated or reduced hemoglobin (RHb) absorbs light in the near-infrared spectrum. If a light beam composed of red and infrared wavelengths is passed through a blood vessel, the transmission of each wavelength will be inversely proportional to the concentration of HbO_2 and RHb in the blood (see Figure 4-9). The oxygen saturation is then calculated as the ratio of HbO_2 to total hemoglobin in the sample.

This calculation of oxygen saturation uses only two forms of hemoglobin and therefore neglects methemoglobin and carboxyhemoglobin. The cooximeters for in vitro use have multiple wavelengths of light and can detect all forms of hemoglobin. Thus, use of the cooximeter permits evaluation of *fractional* saturation, whereas the type of pulse oximeter used clinically in most patients measures *functional* saturation.

Original oximeters suffered from two limitations. The first related to interference from light absorption by pigments and other tissue elements. The second was the inability to differentiate hemoglobin in the arteries from that in the veins. These limitations were reduced by oximeters that measure light transmission through pulsatile vessels only. These "pulse" oximeters are the type widely utilized in clinical practice today. In addition, the photodetectors in pulse oximeters can sense an alternating light input from arterial pulsations and a steady light input from veins and other nonpulsatile elements. Only the alternating light input is selected for analysis, thus eliminating contribution from other sources. This explains why pulse oximeters are not influenced by tissue thickness or pigments. General indications for use of pulse oximetry in obstetrics are presented in Table 4-4 (Shailer, Harvey, & Guyer, 1992).

Principles of Reflection Spectrophotometry
Fiberoptic catheter oximetry (in vivo)

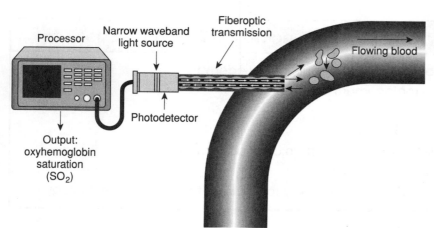

Figure 4-9. Reflective spectrophotometry. From "Continuous Measurement of Blood Oxygen Saturation in the High Risk Patient. Introduction and Historical Perspective," by J. F. Schweiss, 1986, Mountain View, CA: Abbott Critical Care. Reproduced with permission.

Mixed Venous Oxygen Saturation PA Catheter

The venous oxygen saturation (SvO_2), or the percentage of saturation of venous hemoglobin, reflects the overall balance between oxygen delivery and oxygen consumption of perfused tissues. This variable is dependent on the interactions of oxygen transport and consumption. Measurement of SvO_2 is determined by the saturation of hemoglobin in the pulmonary artery, the least oxygenated point in the cardiovascular system. This blood originates from the superior vena cava, the inferior vena cava, and the coronary sinus and reflects a mixture of venous saturation from various organ systems. It is thus called "mixed" venous blood because it represents oxygen saturation of the body, rather than one organ or area.

SvO_2 values may be obtained intermittently or continuously. Intermittent analysis of SvO_2 is made from blood samples obtained from the distal lumen of a standard pulmonary artery catheter. The sample is drawn slowly to prevent blood that has been reoxygenated from being aspirated into the sample.

Continuous measurement of SvO_2 is obtained with a special pulmonary artery catheter, first introduced in 1981 by Abbott Critical Care Systems, Mountain View, California. The catheter is equipped with a fiberoptic light source and receiver to measure pulmonary artery hemoglobin saturation (Figure 4-10). There are now several systems available for the continuous measurement of SvO_2 (Figures 4-11a, and 4-11b). Each system consists of a microprocessor capable of in vitro calibration and memory storage for retroactive correction vis-à-vis a reference calibration. Analysis of the reflected light intensity and calculation of oxyhemoglobin saturation is achieved by the microprocessor. The ratio of saturated and

---

TABLE 4-4. Candidates for Pulse Oximetry in Obstetrics

Patients experiencing or at risk for pulmonary compromise
    Pulmonary edema
    Pulmonary embolus
    Amniotic fluid embolus (anaphylactoid
        syndrome of pregnancy)
    Aspiration
    Acute respiratory distress syndrome
    Dependent on oxygen or ventilator
    After general anesthesia
Patients experiencing or at risk for cardiovascular compromise
    Cyanotic heart disease
    Congestive heart failure
    Cardiomyopathy
    Myocardial infarction
Patients experiencing hypertensive crisis
Patients experiencing or at risk for neurologic emergencies
Patients experiencing drug overdose
Patients experiencing hemorrhage
Patients experiencing disseminated intravascular coagulation (DIC)

Source:

FIBEROPTIC CATHETER

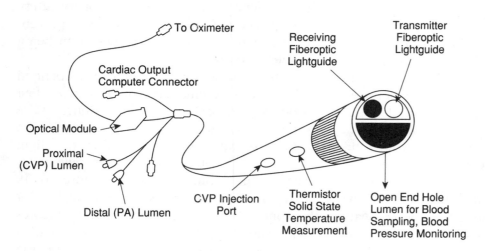

Figure 4-10. Fiberoptic catheter.
Reproduced with permission from Abbott Critical Care. Mountain View, CA.

desaturated hemoglobin is measured and a numeric value is displayed by the monitor. In addition, a continuous recording of SvO_2 may be visualized on the digital display of the monitor (Figure 4-12). The normal value for SvO_2 is between 60% and 80%, though higher values are common during pregnancy secondary to the higher cardiac output state.

SvO_2 monitoring permits more thorough assessment of oxygen transport status in critically ill patients. Specific data that may be obtained with this technology and the formula for calculation of each parameter are presented in Table 4-5.

SvO_2 provides invaluable information to the critical care nurse regarding a patient's oxygen supply at rest and ability to meet oxygen demands during periods of stress. If the patient has physiologic conditions that increase oxygen demand and the oxygen delivery system is marginal in meeting those needs, increasing the oxygen demand with nursing care activities may push the patient beyond physiologic limits. When SvO_2 is decreased, the nurse should consider the increase in oxygen demand that usually accompanies routine care or other clinical conditions (Table 4-6).

Technical Issues During Pregnancy

As the Thunder Project, sponsored by the American Association of Critical Care Nurses, concluded, risk of nonpatency of pressure monitoring lines is greatest in women with short, nonfemoral lines who do not receive other anticoagulants or thrombolytics and have nonheparinized flush solutions (American Association of Critical Care Nurses, 1993). It is important to also note that pregnancy is a hypercoagulable state. Most procoagulant factors including factors V, VII, VIII IX, X, XII, and prothrombin are increased during pregnancy. Fibrinogen also is significantly increased to levels between 400 and 600 mg/dL. Fibrinolysis is prolonged during pregnancy because of a reduction in the levels of antithrombin III and plasminogen activator. For these reasons, it is recommended that all pressure monitoring lines be heparinized when caring for the critically ill pregnant woman. Flush solutions for this patient population usually contain a concentration of between 3 and 5 units of heparin per milliliter of normal saline.

As previously described, cardiac output is most often assessed at the bedside in critical

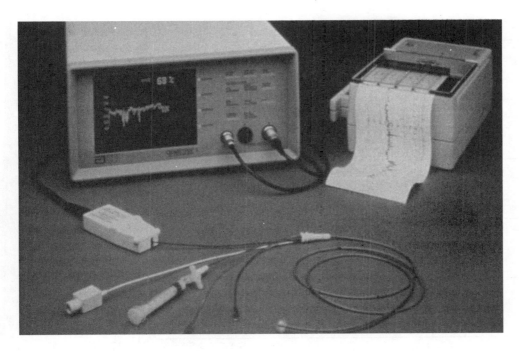

Figure 4-11a. The Oximetrix continuous mixed venous oximetry system showing the fiberoptic catheter, optical module and cable, the processor display unit, and a recorder.
From Abbott Critical Care, Mountain View, CA. Reproduced with permission from Baxter Healthcare Corporation, Edwards Critical-Care Division.

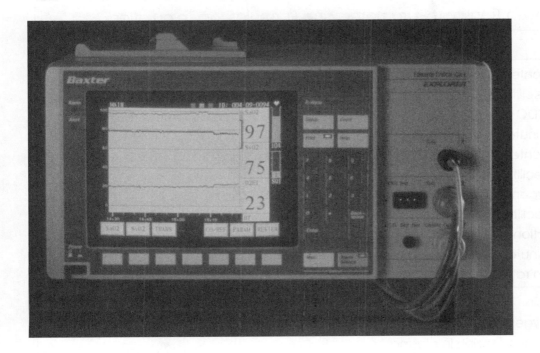

Figure 4-11b. The "Explorer" continuous venous oximeter SvO$_2$ system.
Reproduced by permission from Baxter Healthcare Corporation, Edwards Critical-Care Division.

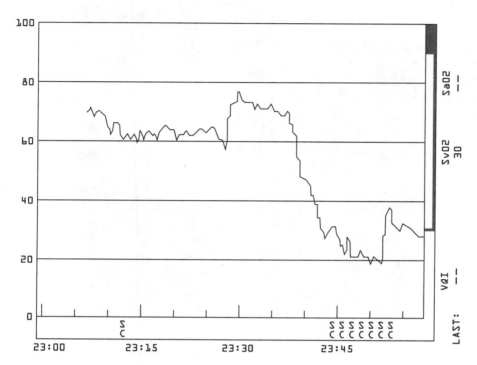

Figure 4-12. Hard copy printout of continuous SvO_2 values. Large drop in SvO_2 values corresponded to suctioning of the patient's endotracheal tube.

TABLE 4-5.	Oxygen Transport Parameters and Formulas for Calculation
Parameter	Formula
Arterial oxygen content (CaO_2) (milliliters per deciliter: ml/dl)	$(1.34 \times Hgb \times SaO_2) + (PaO_2 \times 0.0031)$
Oxygen delivery (DO_2) (milliliters per minute: ml/min)	$CaO_2 \times$ Cardiac Output $\times 10$
Venous oxygen content (CvO_2) (milliliters per deciliter: ml/dl)	$(1.34 \times Hgb \times SvO_2) + (PvO_2 \times 0.0031)$
Arteriovenous oxygen difference ($avDO_2$) (milliliters per deciliter: ml/dl)	$CaO_2 - CvO_2$
Oxygen consumption (VO_2) (milliliters per minute: ml/min)	$avDO_2 \times$ Cardiac Output $\times 10$
Oxygen extraction ratio (O_2ER) (per cent: %)	$VO_2 \div DO_2$

Hgb = hemoglobin
SaO_2 = arterial oxygen saturation
PaO_2 = arterial oxygen tension in plasma
SvO_2 = venous oxygen saturation
PvO_2 = venous oxygen tension in plasma

care settings by use of the thermodilution method. Temperature of the injectate solution is an issue when caring for the critically ill pregnant woman. Favorable correlation exists between room temperature and iced injectate solutions for thermodilution cardiac output assessment in the absence of either low or high cardiac output states. This has been most often defined as an expected cardiac output greater than 4.0 liters per minute but less than 8.0 liters per minute. However, as Wallace describes, correlation is poor in patients with low or high cardiac output states (Wallace & Winslow, 1993). For these reasons, it is recommended that iced injectate be utilized when assessing cardiac output by thermodilution in pregnant women. A schematic representation of an iced injectate, thermodilution cardiac output system is depicted in Figure 4-13. Studies are currently under way to determine the reliability during pregnancy of measurements obtained from pulmonary artery catheters with continuous cardiac output capabilities. No published data are currently available.

INTERPRETATION OF DATA

Interpretation of hemodynamic and oxygen transport data requires knowledge of the normal values and trends during pregnancy and is facilitated by the use of a systematic approach to synthesize complex information. Information obtained by invasive monitoring modalities should always be integrated with information obtained from review of the patient's history, underlying disease processes, clinical physical assessment findings, and laboratory data. It should be noted that abnormalities in centrally obtained hemodynamic and oxygen transport data may precede clinical manifestations. Thus, data may be used in such circumstances to prevent complications.

Hemodynamic Profile

Interpretation of a patient's hemodynamic profile begins with assessment of the cardiac output. This is done to ascertain whether or not the overall amount of blood ejected from the heart per minute is sufficient to meet the patient's current demands. It should be recalled that cardiac out-

TABLE 4-6. Percentage Increase in Resting Oxygen Consumption (VO_2) Associated with Conditions and Activities

Conditions	(%)	Activities	(%)
Fever (each 1° C)	10	Dressing change	10
Fractures (each)	10	Electrocardiogram	16
Agitation	18	Physical exam	20
Chest trauma	25	Visitors	22
Work of breathing	40	Bath	23
Critically ill in emergency room	60	Chest x-ray	25
Severe infection	60	Endotracheal suctioning	27
Shivering	50–100	Nasal intubation	25–40
Sepsis	50–100	Turn to side	31
Head injury, sedated	89	Chest physiotherapy	35
Head injury, not sedated	138	Weight on sling scale	36
Burns	100		

From "Using Continous SvO2 to Assess Oxygen Supply/Demand Balance In the Critically Ill Patient," by K. M. White, 1993, Clinical Issues in Clinical Care Nursing, (4)1, pp. 134–147.

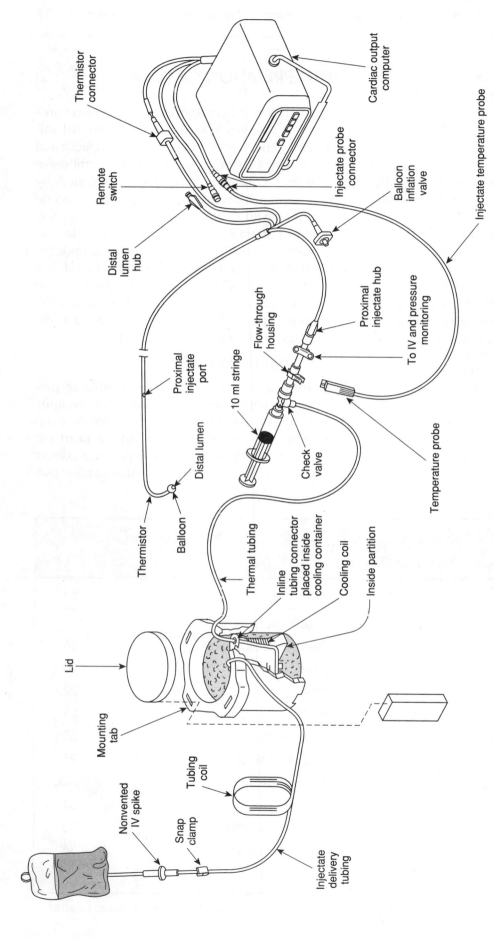

Figure 4-13. Schematic illustration of a closed injectate delivery system (CO-set) for use with cold injectate. Courtesy American Edwards Laboratories, Santa Ana, CA.

put is a significant component to the formula for determining oxygen delivery. If the cardiac output is not sufficient, the patient may exhibit clinical evidence of end-organ dysfunction or failure.

Following assessment of cardiac output, each of the four determinants of cardiac output should be evaluated. Preload, or central volume status, is the first determinant that should be assessed. If discrepancy exists between the right and left preload values, CVP and PCWP respectively, it should be recalled that the left ventricle should be the focus of any evaluation of hemodynamic function in the critically ill pregnant woman. Thus, the PCWP is more helpful in providing information in an acute setting regarding central volume status. At this point, the nurse should be able to determine if the patient is centrally "wet," "dry," or normovolemic. When integrated with knowledge of the patient's underlying disease process, this information is often valuable.

The next determinant that should be assessed is afterload. It should be recalled that afterload is resistance that the ventricles must overcome to eject blood during systole. Alterations in right or left afterload values, PVR and SVR respectively, may represent the cause of a hemodynamic problem or may be indicative of a compensatory response to another problem. For example, a hypertensive patient may have elevated left afterload (SVR) that is causing increased left preload (PCWP) and is thus placing the patient at risk for pulmonary edema. The cornerstone for therapy would be administration of an agent to decrease left afterload. In contrast, a patient who is centrally "dry," as may be present with severe preeclampsia, may be vasoconstricting to compensate for the hypovolemia and decreased cardiac output. The cornerstone for therapy of this patient would be administration of intravascular fluid to expand vascular volume. Administration of an agent in this patient to decrease afterload would be deleterious to her overall condition.

Contractility and heart rate are evaluated next. Left ventricular function, indicated by the LVSWI, is often elevated in critically ill patients. This represents a valuable compensatory response in the healthy heart to alterations in preload and afterload. Contractility is increased in order to main-

tain adequate cardiac output and oxygen delivery. The same is true for elevations in the heart rate. When contractility is decreased, the patient is said to be in left ventricular failure. Most often this indicates loss of a valuable compensatory function and the patient is at significant risk of hemodynamic failure and cardiopulmonary arrest. Interventions are targeted toward inotropic support. This may be accomplished by administration of medications such as dobutamine hydrochloride or by administration of intravascular fluids to optimize preload and thus, ventricular stretch and cardiac output.

Oxygen Transport Data

Following assessment of the hemodynamic profile, the patient's oxygen delivery (DO_2) is evaluated. A determination should be made whether the overall DO_2 is sufficient to meet the demands of the patient. It should be recalled that oxygen demand increases during pregnancy, labor and other stressful circumstances. With certain disease processes, correction of oxygen deficit to specific end organs may require supranormal levels of DO_2. It is important to remember that in calculation of arterial oxygen content (CaO_2), a current hemoglobin is required. Because the amount of oxygen dissolved under pressure in plasma accounts for such a small percentage of the total, in the absence of a current arterial blood gas value, the PaO_2 is often deleted from the calculation formula. If the DO_2 is low, the cause should be ascertained and intervention directed toward correction of the underlying problem. For example, if the cardiac output is normal but the hemoglobin is low, the CaO_2 will also be low, thus producing a low DO_2. Intervention would include transfusion of packed red blood cells to correct anemia.

Next oxygen consumption (VO_2) is assessed in the critically ill patient. It should be recalled that VO_2 is increased in normal pregnancy. Labor and other stressful conditions increase VO_2 further. When VO_2 is increased, it is important to identify possible reasons. (Refer to Table 4-6.) Interventions may include administration of medication to relieve pain or reduce fever. When VO_2 is decreased, it is important to assess the patient for evidence of end organ dysfunction or failure. In the presence of organ failure, oxygen extraction by tissues in that organ is severely impaired or eliminated.

In addition to assessment of oxygen delivery and consumption, it is important to note the amount of oxygen reserve in a patient on an ongoing basis. Routine interventions as well as special procedures should be planned according to the ability of the patient to meet the concomitant increase in oxygen demand.

SUMMARY

Invasive hemodynamic and oxygen transport monitoring devices enhance the ability of the nurse to assess the critically ill pregnant woman (Figure 4-14). Data may be used to plan and implement care as well as to evaluate patient responses to various interventions. However, monitoring equipment alone is not sufficient to improve patient outcome. It is imperative that nurses caring for critically ill pregnant women have a thorough understanding of how to correctly interpret data within the context of pregnancy and to integrate information with the complete clinical picture.

REFERENCES

American Association of Critical Care Nurses. (1993). Evaluation of the effects of heparinized and nonheparinized flush solutions on the patency of arterial pressure monitoring lines: The AACN Thunder Project. <u>American Journal of Critical Care</u>, <u>2</u>, 3–15.

Chernow, B. (1997). A statement by the American College of Chest Physicians and the American Thoracic Society. <u>Chest</u>, <u>111</u>, 261.

Clark, S. L., Cotton, D. B., Hankins, G. D. V., & Phelan, J. P. (Eds.). (1994). The pulmonary artery catheter: Insertion technique and complications. In <u>Handbook of critical care obstetrics</u>. (pp 33–38) Cambridge, MA: Blackwell Scientific Publications.

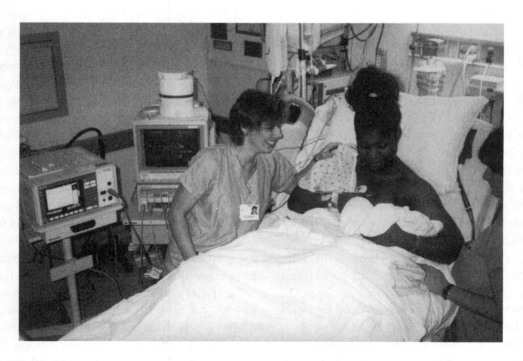

Figure 4-14. Photograph of intrapartum patient with cardiac disease with invasive hemodynamic monitoring.
Photographed at Thomas Jefferson University Hospital; Delivery Room/Critical Care Obstetrics.
Used with patient permission.

Clark, S. L., Cotton, D. B., Lee W. et al. (1989). Central hemodynamic assessment of normal term pregnancy. American Journal of Obstetrics and Gynecology, 161, 1439–1442.

Clark, S. L., Horenstein, J. M., Phelan, J. P. et al. (1985). Experience with the pulmonary artery catheter in obstetrics and gynecology. American Journal of Obstetrics and Gynecology, 152, 374.

Connors, A. F., Jr., Speroff, T., Dawson, N. V. et al. (1996). The effectiveness of right heart catheterization in the initial care of critically ill patients. Journal of the American Medical Association. 18, 889–897.

Dalen, J. E. (1990). Does pulmonary artery catheterization benefit patients with acute myocardial infarction? Chest, 98, 1313–1314.

Gore, J. M., Goldberg, R. J., Spodick, D. H. et al. (1987). A community wide assessment of the use of pulmonary artery catheters in patients with acute myocardial infarction. Chest, 92, 721–727.

Marino, P. L. (Ed.). (1991). The world of the pulmonary artery pressure catheter. In The ICU book (pp. 101–110) Malveryn, PA: Lea and Febiger.

Paulson, D. M., Scott, S. M., & Sethi, G. K. (1988). Pulmonary hemorrhage associated with balloon flotation catheter. Journal of Thoracic and Cardiovascular Surgery, 80, 453–458.

Shailer, T. L., Harvey, C. J., & Guyer, F. (1992). Principles of oxygen transport in the critically ill obstetric patient. Clinical Issues in Perinatal and Women's Health Nursing, 3(3), 392–398.

Sibbald, W. J., & Sprung, C. J. (1988). The pulmonary artery catheter: The debate continues. Chest, 94, 899–901.

Society of Critical Care Medicine: Consensus Development Conference. (1997). Pulmonary artery catheter concensus conference: Consensus statement. New Horizons, 5(3), 175–193.

Wallace, D. C., & Winslow, E. H. (1993, January/February). Effects of iced injectate on cardiac output measurements in critically ill patients with low and high cardiac output. Heart and Lung, 22(1), 55–63.

White, K. M. (1993). Using continuous SvO_2 to assess oxygen supply/demand balance in the critically ill patient. Clinical Issues in Critical Care Nursing, 4(1), 134–147.

CHAPTER 5

Mechanical Ventilation During Pregnancy

Nan H. Troiano and Karen Dorman

Mechanical ventilatory support is an integral component in the delivery of critical care. Increasingly, obstetric critical care nurses face the challenge of caring for women who require mechanical ventilation during pregnancy. Irrespective of the location at which care is to be provided, it is important that nurses caring for such patients understand fundamental principles related to mechanical ventilation, implications of pregnancy, associated complications, and specific nursing care measures.

This chapter reviews indications for intubation and mechanical ventilatory support. Types and modes of both conventional and newer ventilatory adjuncts are presented. Issues related to use during pregnancy as well as specific nursing care measures are also described. Detailed discussion of disease processes during pregnancy that may lead to respiratory failure are presented elsewhere in this book.

INDICATIONS

Patients with refractory hypoxemia or tissue hypoxia who, despite supplemental therapy are unable to ventilate sufficiently, require intubation and mechanical ventilation. Mechanical assistance may be necessary because ventilation is inadequate to control pH, because adequate oxygenation cannot be achieved at a fraction of inspired oxygen (FiO_2) without manipulating the pattern of ventilation, or because activity of the ventilatory muscles places excessive demands for blood flow on an already compromised cardiovascular system. General guidelines for the diagnosis of respiratory failure are presented in Table 5-1. (Clark, Cotton, Hankins, & Phelan, 1994). It should be noted that determination of some of these criteria are based on results of pulmonary function tests, which quantify respiratory function by measuring lung volume during normal and maximal ventilation.

CONVENTIONAL TYPES OF MECHANICAL VENTILATORS

Generally, conventional ventilators used today can be divided into two types, volume-cycled and pressure-cycled, classified according to the mechanism that terminates the inspiratory phase. Both types are positive pressure systems. The specific ventilator selected for use in a given clinical situation may depend on a number of variables including the models available within the hospital and the familiarity or experience level of the patient's physician with one type over another. Irrespective of which type or model is used, a mechanical device used to sustain life is only as good as its design and the health care team using it.

Negative Pressure

Early ventilators were negative pressure systems known as *iron lungs*. The patient's body was encased in an iron cylinder and negative pressure was generated, which enlarged the thoracic cavity. A modification of this system involves a suit or shell that is fitted over the patient's chest with a hose connecting the device to a negative pressure generator. In either model, lung inflation is accomplished by reducing the pressure within the container to below atmospheric pressure. This causes the pressure surrounding the chest to drop below the pressure within the lungs, and the chest rises. The lungs then expand and the pressure within them becomes less than atmospheric. Atmospheric gases are drawn into the lungs until equilibrium between lung pressure and atmospheric pressure is reached. Inspiration then ends. Once subatmospheric pressure surrounding the chest is released, the natural elastic recoil of the thoracic cage and lungs causes lung pressure to exceed atmospheric pressure. Thus, gas leaves the lungs until pressures are again equal.

Negative pressure ventilator systems are advantageous in that they mimic normal respiration. However, such systems are rarely used except in selected out-of-hospital settings.

Positive Pressure
Volume-Cycled

The volume-cycled ventilators are the most frequently used type in adult critical care settings. The basic principle behind this type of ventilator is that once a designated volume of air is delivered to the patient, inspiration is terminated.

At the moment of cycling, the time taken to deliver the volume, the pressure developed in the patient circuit, and the flow rate may all vary from one respiratory cycle to the next. The only parameter that remains constant is the volume.

Traditionally, volume-cycling is accomplished with the use of a double-circuit ventilator (Dupuis, 1986). In these systems, the primary circuit is usually a blower and the secondary circuit comprises a bellows assembly. The volume-cycling mechanism itself can be either pneumatically or electronically operated. Because of rapid advancement in the field of electronics, reliable timing and flow-sensing devices integrated electronically to measure volume are now found in single-circuit, volume-cycled systems.

TABLE 5-1.   Guidelines for the Diagnosis of Respiratory Failure

Parameter	Normal	Intubate
Respiratory rate	12–20	> 35
Vital capacity (ml/kg)	65–75	< 15
FEV_1 (ml/kg)	50–60	< 10
Inspiratory force (cm H_2O)	75–100	< 25
PaO_2 (mm Hg)	104–108	< 70
		mask 0.40
$PaCO_2$ (mm Hg)	27–32	> 55
VD/VT	0.25–0.40	> 0.60

FEV_1 = forced expiratory volume, 1 second
VD/VT = ratio of dead space volume to tidal volume

Use of a volume-cycled ventilator requires the clinician to set the volume, flow, and frequency of air delivered. The primary advantage to this type of system is that despite changes in patient lung compliance, a consistent tidal volume (Vt) will be delivered.

Pressure-Cycled

The pressure-cycled ventilator works on the basic principle that once a preset pressure is reached, inspiration is terminated. At this pressure point, the inspiratory valve closes and exhalation occurs passively. At the moment of cycling, the volume delivered, the time taken to deliver the volume, and the flow rate may all vary from one respiratory cycle to the next. The only nonvariable is the preset cycling pressure. Pressure-cycling mechanisms within the ventilator may be pneumatic, electronic, or a combination of both.

Clinical judgment dictates the cycling pressure selected. Because the patient's lung condition at the time of initiation of ventilatory assistance is not known, there is no simple way of predicting the initial pressure requirements. Once the preliminary settings are made, the patient is connected to the ventilator. The volume delivered at that pressure and flow rate is determined with a volume measuring device. Final adjustments to the cycling pressure and flow rate are then performed based on patient assessment data. If the tidal volume is too low, the cycling pressure is increased. If the tidal volume is too high, the cycling pressure is reduced. Clinically, as a patient's lungs become less compliant, the volume of air delivered to the patient may decrease. Thus, to ensure adequate minute ventilation and to detect changes in lung compliance and resistance, inspiratory pressure, rate, and exhaled tidal volume must be monitored frequently.

Although volume-cycled ventilators remain the most frequently used type in most adult situations, pressure-controlled and time-cycled systems are increasingly chosen in selected cases. Because high volumes and pressures can lead to lung damage, pressure-controlled ventilation allows the clinican to select and control mean airway pressure as well as peak airway pressure. This may be especially beneficial in patients refractory to conventional ventilation or those with acute respiratory distress syndrome.

Time-Cycled

The time-cycled ventilator works under the basic principle that once a preset time is completed, inspiration is terminated. Expiratory time is determined by inspiratory time and rate of breaths per minute. This is expressed as inspiratory to expiratory ratio (I:E ratio). The typical I:E ratio is 1:2.

Time-cycled machines limit the pressure achieved within the system and cause the ventilator to cycle at a preset interval, thereby setting frequency. Tidal volume (Vt) is varied by adjusting the flow rate and inspiratory time, or by setting minute ventilation and frequency. Many ventilators, especially those used in neonatology, are pressure-limited but time-cycled, allowing the delivered Vt to be highly variable.

MODES OF MECHANICAL VENTILATION

The mode of ventilation generally refers to the interaction between the patient's ventilatory effort and mechanical assistance. There are a variety of modes from which to choose once the type of ventilator has been selected. Conventional modes include control, assist control, intermittent mandatory ventilation, synchronized intermittent mandatory ventilation, and continuous positive airway pressure. A schematic representing the ventilatory pattern for each is presented in Figure 5-1 (Troiano & Dorman, 1992).

Control

With controlled mandatory ventilation (CMV), the ventilator delivers a preset Vt a preset number of times per minute. The patient cannot spontaneously ventilate or trigger breaths, thus the machine controls ventilation. Because the patient must have a drive to breathe, this mode is restricted to patients who are apneic as a result of brain damage, sedation, or muscle paralysis. If the patient is conscious or is not paralyzed, this mode can provoke high anxiety and

Mode	Schematic

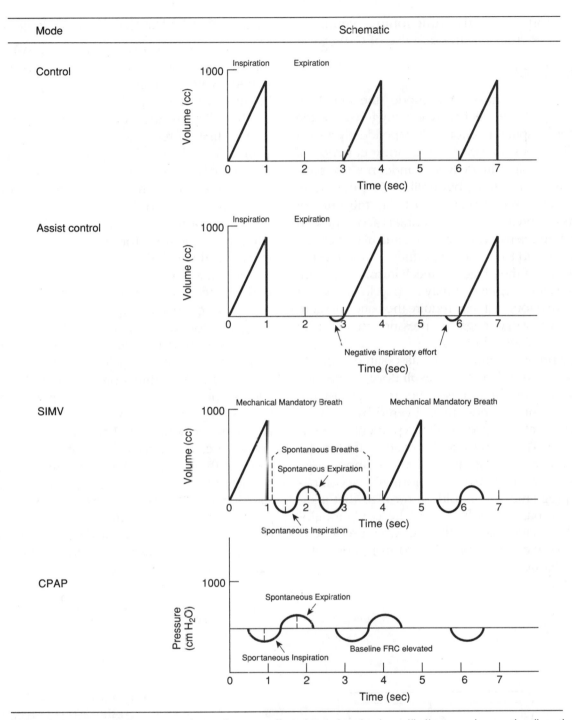

Figure 5-1. Schematic comparison of conventional mechanical ventilation modes and adjuncts.

discomfort. Properly functioning ventilator alarms are crucial to the safe use of CMV.

Assist-Control

In the assist-control (AC) mode, the ventilator delivers a breath either when triggered by the patient's inspiratory effort or independently if such an effort does not occur within a preset period of time. All breaths are delivered under positive pressure by the machine, but unlike CMV, the preset rate can be exceeded by the patient's triggering of additional breaths. This triggering is accomplished by setting a sensitivity detector. Particular attention must be paid to proper adjustment of the level of sensitivity of the triggering mechanism. If the ventilator is too sensitive, it may autocycle. If it is not sensitive enough, it may require the patient to generate very large negative pressure in order to receive additional breaths.

The primary complication associated with this mode of ventilation is respiratory alkalemia. Because every breath, whether triggered by the patient or independently delivered by the ventilator, is at the preset Vt, hyperventilation is possible. This effect may be exacerbated in the obstetric patient because of the compensated respiratory alkalemia that normally accompanies pregnancy. It should be recalled that alkalemia results in a left shift of the oxyhemoglobin dissociation curve, thus making it more difficult for oxygen to be released from hemoglobin to tissues.

Intermittent Mandatory Ventilation

Intermittent mandatory ventilation (IMV) allows interspersion of spontaneous breaths by the patient with machine breaths. Spontaneous breaths are at the patient's own Vt, whereby machine breaths are delivered at the preset Vt. It was first introduced in 1971 for use with neonates with respiratory distress syndrome because conventional ventilators were unable to deliver the rapid breath rates associated with this condition. Shortly thereafter, it was proposed by Downs and colleagues (1973) as an alternative method for weaning adults from mechanical ventilation.

A schematic representation of an IMV circuit is depicted in Figure 5-2 (Marino, 1991). The patient is connected to a common source of oxygen through two parallel circuits. The first contains a volume-cycled ventilator. The other contains a reservoir bag filled with the inhaled gas mixture. A unidirectional valve in the circuit allows the patient to breathe spontaneously from the reservoir bag when a ventilator breath is not being delivered. The pattern of ventilations is such that a machine breath may be delivered at the same time the patient is spontaneously breathing. This concept, referred to as stacking of breaths, is uncomfortable for the patient and increases volume and pressure within the airway. The newer IMV system eliminates this problem by synchronizing patient and machine breaths.

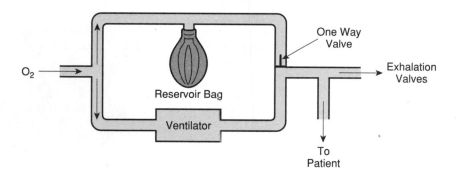

Figure 5-2. Schematic representation of an IMV (intermittent mandatory ventilation) circuit. Reproduced with permission. From "The ICU Book. Modes of Mechanical Ventilation," by P. L. Marino, 1991, Philadelphia, PA: Lea & Febiger/Williams and Wilkins.

Synchronized Intermittent Mandatory Ventilation

Synchronized intermittent mandatory ventilation (SIMV) allows spontaneous breathing between mechanically delivered ventilator breaths. This technique was introduced because of concern that a mechanical breath might be superimposed on a spontaneous breath. It prevents stacking of breaths and concomitant increases in peak inspiratory pressure, mean airway pressure, and mean intrapleural pressure. It remains the most common mode used in obstetric critical care situations.

Continuous Positive Airway Pressure

Continuous positive airway pressure (CPAP) is pressure above atmospheric, which is maintained at the airway opening throughout the respiratory cycle during spontaneous breathing. CPAP may be delivered through a special mask to patients who do not have an endotracheal or tracheostomy tube. However, the mask must fit exactly so as to prevent air leaks. This mode of ventilation was first used as positive-pressure oxygen breathing to help keep the lungs expanded in patients with crushed chest injuries and to treat infants with respiratory distress syndrome.

Gas exchange across the alveolar capillary membrane is promoted as functional residual capacity is increased. However, the patient maintains a high level of work in breathing with this mode as she is responsible for all ventilatory effort. It is more often used as a mode during weaning from mechanical ventilatory assistance.

ADJUNCTS TO MECHANICAL VENTILATION

Pressure Support Ventilation

Pressure support ventilation (PSV) augments a patient's spontaneous breaths while on mechanical ventilation. At the onset of every spontaneous breath, the negative pressure generated by the patient opens a valve that delivers the inspired gas at the desired pressure, usually 5 to 10 cm H_2O. This is designed to increase the Vt and reduce the work of breathing. In essence, the pressure boost is delivered to overcome the resistance within the endotracheal tube and ventilator circuit tubing.

Newer microprocessor-driven mechanical ventilators include pressure-support modes that operate in conjunction with their demand-flow valve systems. The principal advantages of PSV are decreased patient work of breathing and improved subjective comfort.

Positive End-Expiratory Pressure

Mechanical ventilation with positive end-expiratory pressure (PEEP) is designed for any pulmonary condition with widespread alveolar collapse. A pressure-limiting valve in the expiratory tubing prevents the pressure in the airways from returning to atmospheric pressure at the end of expiration. This positive pressure in the alveoli at end-expiration helps prevent alveolar collapse and promotes gas exchange across the alveolar-capillary interface. This ventilatory adjunct increases the functional residual capacity, the lung volume at end-expiration. In selected patients, this increases alveolar participation in gas exchange and allows the fractional concentration of inspired oxygen to be lowered.

NEWER METHODS OF MECHANICAL VENTILATION AND OXYGENATION

The primary purposes of mechanical ventilation are to achieve adequate alveolar ventilation and to improve oxygen exchange. Traditionally, volume-limited ventilation used alone or in conjunction with spontaneous breathing has been the only form of mechanical assistance commonly used in adults. In addition, enrichment of FiO_2 and the addition of positive end-expiratory pressure (PEEP) have been the principal means of improving oxygenation. Over time, newer techniques have been introduced to clinical practice. Because the majority of these newer modes are pressure-cycled, independent volume monitoring is highly desirable.

Pressure Control and Inverse I:E Ratio

It has been common practice in mechanically ventilated patients to allow at least as much time for exhalation as for inhalation. The rationale for this concept is to prevent the trapping of gas in the airways. However, gas exchange may be markedly improved when the I:E ratio is forced to values greater than 1:1. This principle is known as inverse ratio ventilation (IRV) or inverse I:E ratio ventilation. It has been applied clinically to neonates with hyaline membrane disease as well as adults with refractory acute respiratory distress syndrome and other forms of hypoxemia.

This method of ventilation may be accomplished in at least two ways. First, the rate of flow delivery during conventional volume ventilation may be decreased. More commonly, pressure-controlled ventilation is utilized. This involves maintenance of pressure at a controlled level for a fixed period of time.

The mechanism for the improvement of oxygenation with this method remains uncertain, though increased mean intrathoracic pressure and increased lung volume are most likely involved. Sustained tethering forces may recruit lung units that would otherwise remain collapsed, and units with very slow time constants may be given sufficient time to ventilate (Marini & Wheeler, 1989).

Advantages of IRV include improved oxygenation and reduced peak cycling pressures. Disadvantages of IRV include higher mean intrathoracic pressure, which may impede venous return and contribute to barotrauma. It should also be noted that patient cooperation is essential, thus adequate sedation is crucial.

High-Frequency Ventilation

High-frequency ventilation (HFV) is a collective term that refers to modes of ventilation in which tidal volumes smaller than anatomic deadspace are moved at frequencies that range from 60 to 3000 cycles per minute. **High-frequency positive pressure ventilation (HFP-PV)** is identical in concept to conventional ventilation with the exception that tidal volumes are very small and cycling frequencies are very fast. **High-frequency jet ventilation (HFJV)** works in a somewhat different way. With this method, a small-diameter injecting catheter is positioned in the central airway. This catheter then pulses gas along the axis of the lumen under high pressure at a rapid cycling rate, usually between 60 and 240 cycles per minute. HFJV is the most common type of HFV used in adult settings. Yet another type of HFV is **high frequency oscillation (HFO)**. This method works on the principle that very small volumes of gas (1–3 ml/kg) are moved back and forth by a piston at extremely high frequencies (500–3000 cycles per minute).

All forms of HFV are characterized by lower peak airway pressures than conventional ventilation. Peripheral airway pressure is generally higher than measured central airway pressure, and mean alveolar pressures may not differ greatly from those observed during conventional ventilation. With rare exception, HFV does not decrease cardiovascular side effects associated with conventional ventilation. HFV is generally utilized in carefully selected clinical situations and use during pregnancy has not been reported.

Liquid Ventilation

Liquid ventilation involves instillation of a sterile perfluorocarbon into the lungs. The substance has a low surface tension and a very high solubility for oxygen and carbon dioxide. For example, oxygen is about 20 times more soluble in fluorocarbons than in water, whereas carbon dioxide is about three times as soluble (Schaffer, Wolfson, & Clark, 1992). The first human trials of liquid ventilation were reported in 1989 and demonstrated the ability of perfluorocarbon to adequately support gas exchange in moribund infants (Greenspan, Wolfson, & Rubenstein, 1990). Since that time, investigation has continued in application to adult, pediatric, and neonatal populations.

The physiologic basis for use of liquid ventilation focuses on alteration of alveolar surface tension. The surface tension in the alveolus is a function of the air–fluid interfaces that line the alveoli. This tension can be reduced by filling the alveoli with fluid rather than gas because this eliminates the air–fluid interfaces (Fuhrman, Paczan, & DeFrancis, 1991; Tutuncu, Faithful, & Xachman, 1993; West, Dollery, Matthews, et al., 1965). Instillation of perfluorocarbon liquid may offer advantages to an injured lung for a number of reasons. Because perfluorocarbon is heavier than water, it tends to trickle down to the dependent regions of the lungs, which are usually more atelectatic (Dirkes, 1992). In addition, instillation of liquid into the lungs physically opens up and maintains the patency of dependent alveoli and provides a medium for gas exchange in areas of the lungs not previously ventilated.

Generally, there are two types of liquid ventilation. Total liquid ventilation (TLV) refers to replacement of the functional residual capacity (FRC) of the lung by instillation of a perfluorocarbon liquid. Gas exchange is accomplished by inspiration and expiration of tidal volumes of liquid (Schaffer, Wolfson, & Clark, 1992). This requires a special device to deliver and remove tidal volumes of liquid and to extracorporeally oxygenate and remove carbon dioxide from the liquid. Partial liquid ventilation (PLV) involves intratracheal instillation of perfluorocarbon liquid equal to the FRC of the lungs during conventional mechanical ventilation.

COMPLICATIONS

Initiation of mechanical ventilatory assistance is accompanied by the potential for numerous complications. A list of selected complications is summarized in Table 5-2.

Cardiovascular

One of the most significant risks associated with mechanical ventilation is decreased cardiac output. This may occur for several reasons. First, positive pressure ventilation can cause a reduction in venous return, resulting in reduced right preload. Use of PEEP, especially at high levels, may exacerbate this effect. A second factor that may contribute to decreased cardiac output is related to right ventricular afterload. Pulmonary

TABLE 5-2. Complications of Mechanical Ventilation
Cardiac
Decreased cardiac output
Dysrhythmias
Decreased blood pressure
Pulmonary
Tracheal injury
Vocal cord injury
Barotrauma
Oxygen toxicity
Hypoventilation
Hyperventilation
Atelectasis
Fluid imbalance
Infection
Gastrointestinal
Stress ulcer
Ileus

vascular resistance, the afterload that must be overcome by the right ventricle during systole, is increased as large tidal volumes and pressures are pushed into the lungs. This increase in volume and pressure stretches the intraalveolar vessels and decreases their lumen size, thus increasing resistance to blood flow. Finally, two important factors impact left ventricular compliance and may decrease cardiac output. An increase in right ventricular afterload may over time lead to increased right ventricular preload. This increased volume of blood in the right ventricle may result in a shift of the interventricular septum to the left, thus reducing left ventricular compliance. The workload required of the left ventricle is thereby increased significantly. In general, patients with normal sympathetic reflexes and normal to increased intravascular volume tolerate mechanical ventilation best from a cardiovascular standpoint.

Barotrauma

Barotrauma is a general term that refers to consequences of alveolar overdistention. Varied forms of barotrauma include interstitial emphysema, pneumomediastinum, pneumoperitoneum, subcutaneous emphysema, cyst formation, and pneumothorax. Generally, air can gain access to the pleural space in two ways. First, a disruption may occur in the visceral pleura, facilitated by obstructed airways, parenchymal inflammation, and necrosis. In addition, overdistention and rupture of individual alveoli may allow interstitial air to escape along bronchi and vessels to the mediastinum. From there, it enters soft tissues and may perforate the thin mediastinal pleura and cause a pneumothorax. If intrapleural air continues to increase within a closed intrathoracic cavity, a tension pneumothorax may result.

Individuals most at risk for barotrauma usually have underlying lung disease including acute respiratory distress syndrome or chronic obstructive pulmonary disease. In addition, the risk of barotrauma is increased in patients with high mean inspiratory pressures and who are receiving high levels of PEEP. Clinical signs and symptoms associated with pneumothorax are presented in Table 5-3. Nursing management includes notification of the patient's physician and preparation for immediate insertion of a chest tube. Urgent decompression may be accomplished with a large-bore catheter-over-needle attached to a large syringe. A chest x-ray should also be obtained if a pneumothorax is suspected.

Fluid Imbalance

Fluid retention, or development of a positive water balance, is fairly common in patients receiving mechanical ventilation. This condition occurs for a number of reasons. As increased intrathoracic pressure limits venous return, stretch receptors in the atria signal for additional antidiuretic hormone (ADH). This facilitates replenishment of intravascular volume. Compression of the atria from hyperinflated lungs may decrease atrial natriuretic factor (ANF), which in turn further increases ADH. In addition, hypotension caused

TABLE 5-3. Clinical Signs and Symptoms of Pneumothorax

Subtle
   Pleuritic pain
   Shortness of breath
   Venous distention
   Accelerated breathing
   Gradual increase in mean inspiratory pressure
   Unilateral decrease in breath sounds or chest movement
   Subcutaneous emphysema
Acute or Severe
   Bradycardia
   Shock-like appearance
   Cyanosis
   Loss of consciousness
   Tracheal and/or mediastinal shift
   Sudden rise in mean inspiratory pressure

by positive-pressure ventilation may decrease renal perfusion, redistribute renal blood flow, decrease glomerular filtration, and promote sodium retention.

The intrinsic advantage of this accumulation of fluid may be to promote cardiac output in the face of high intrathoracic pressures. However, the negative effects of central hypervolemia, including pulmonary vascular congestion and impaired gas exchange, should not be overlooked. As positive-pressure ventilation is discontinued, these fluid shifts usually reverse and may actually cause cardiac decompensation in the patient with poor hemodynamic reserve.

Infection

The three major sites for nosocomial infections in the ICU are the respiratory system (31%), the urinary tract (24%), and the bloodstream (16%) (Weinstein, 1991). Infections of the lung and upper respiratory tract are exceedingly common during mechanical ventilation. Nosocomial pneumonia most often develops in patients requiring endotracheal intubation and mechanical ventilatory support. Current estimates include a 6- to 20- fold increase in nosocomial pneumonia for patients receiving mechanical ventilation (American Thoracic Society, 1995). In addition, patients with bacterial pneumonia are also at risk for bacteremia and thus are at significant increased risk for mortality.

A number of factors associated with use of mechanical ventilation are responsible for the increased risk of infection. Endotracheal intubation prevents glottic closure, disrupts the laryngeal barrier, slows the mucociliary escalator, impedes secretion clearance, and provides an open pathway for large quantities of aspirated pharyngeal bacteria and fungi to inoculate the lung. In addition, patients exposed to respiratory therapy equipment have a higher risk for acquiring nosocomial infection because of equipment contamination. Most nosocomial bacterial pneumonia is caused by repeated aspiration of pathogens that have colonized the mucosal surfaces of the oropharynx. These organisms usually reach the lungs in a liquid bolus such as the condensate that accumulates in ventilator tubing. Intubated patients also often receive antacids through a nasogastric tube to decrease gastric acidity and prevent stress ulcers. However, as the pH of the gastric acid increases, the acid loses its bactericidal effect on gram-negative organisms. Thus, aspiration of gastrointestinal contents may initiate the colonization of bacteria, which results in pneumonia.

NURSING CARE ISSUES

Caring for the obstetric patient requiring mechanical ventilation presents unique challenges. A list of related nursing diagnoses, used to formulate a plan of patient care, is presented in Table 5-4. Guidelines for care of the obstetric patient receiving ventilatory support are presented in the last section of this book. A description of selected nursing care issues follows.

TABLE 5-4. Nursing Diagnoses Associated with Care of the Patient Requiring Mechanical Ventilation

- Anxiety related to disease process, diagnostic tests and procedures and therapy
  Sensory overload/deprivation
  Sleep deprivation
  Inability to sleep

- Breathing pattern, ineffective, related to ventilator malfunction, accidental extubation, barotrauma, pneumothorax

- Infection, potential for, related to bypass of normal filtering system
  Breach of aseptic technique for suctioning
  Repeated traumatic or intrusive suctioning or procedures

- Cardiac output, altered
  Decreased, related to increased intrathoracic pressures

- Gas exchange, impaired, related to oxygen toxicity secondary to high inspired oxygen concentrations

- Impaired fetal oxygen transport

- Injury, potential for, related to pressure sores on side of mouth, nose, tracheostomy site, hyperplasia, inflammation, scarring, and stenosis of trachea caused by trauma of endotracheal tube

Initial Settings and Goals

Following successful endotracheal intubation, the patient is connected to the ventilator. Initial ventilator settings are dependent upon the patient's disease process and the overall plan of care. However, most often, a positive-pressure volume-cycled ventilator is used for the obstetric patient. The SIMV mode is usually utilized in pregnant women. It should be recalled that because of the normal compensatory respiratory alkalemia during pregnancy, use of assist-control may precipitate respiratory alkalemia more quickly than when used in nonpregnant women. General guidelines for initial settings and goals are presented in Table 5-5 (Clark et al., 1994).

Arterial blood gases are usually obtained within 15 to 30 minutes following initiation of ventilatory support. Adjustments to the initial settings are made based on assessment data related to oxygenation and ventilation. Changes in ventilator settings are most often made by respiratory therapy personnel or by the patient's physician. However, policies within individual institutions address the issue of which professional personnel may make changes in urgent situations.

Monitoring Ventilation and Oxygenation

In the critically ill obstetric patient, an adequate oxygenation system is essential for recovery. The quality of ventilation directly impacts on the patient's oxygenation status. For these reasons, it is important to monitor both the ventilation and oxygenation status of all patients receiving ventilatory support. Common parameters used to assess these functions are presented in Table 5-6. A discussion of selected parameters follows.

It should be recalled that oxygen delivery (DO_2), the total amount of oxygen made available to tissues per minute, is dependent on cardiac output (CO), arterial oxygen content (CaO_2), saturation of hemoglobin with oxygen in the arterial system (SaO_2), and, to a small degree, the amount of oxygen dissolved under pressure in the plasma (PaO_2).

Oxygen consumption (VO_2), the total amount of oxygen consumed globally by tissues per minute, is dependent on CO, venous oxygen content (CvO_2), saturation of hemoglobin with oxygen in the venous system (SvO_2), and the amount of oxygen dissolved under pressure in venous blood (PvO_2). The relationship between VO_2 and DO_2 is expressed in the oxygen extraction ratio (O_2ER). This helps to estimate oxygen reserve in the critically ill patient. These variables are discussed fully in Chapter 4. Three additional hemodynamic parameters that are important to assess include shunt fraction, alveolar–arterial oxygen difference, and the ratio of arterial oxygen pressure to fraction of inspired oxygen.

Shunt Fraction

This variable, the percent arteriovenous shunt, expresses the extent to which arterial blood is less than maximally oxygenated as it leaves the heart. A certain percentage of venous blood bypasses

TABLE 5-5. General Guidelines for Initial Settings and Goals

Initial Settings

Mode	SIMV
Rate	12–14 breaths per minute
Tidal Volume (Vt)	12–15 ml/kg
PEEP	5 cm H_2O
FiO_2	1.0 (dependent on reason for intubation)

Goals

PaO_2	> 60 mm Hg
SaO_2	>95%
$PaCO_2$	27–32
FiO2	< 50%

SIMV = synchronized intermittent mandatory ventilation
PEEP = positive end-expiratory pressure
FiO_2 = fraction of inspired oxygen
PaO_2 = partial pressure of oxygen in arterial system
$PaCO_2$ = partial pressure of carbon dioxide in arterial system
SaO_2 = arterial oxygen saturation of hemoglobin

TABLE 5-6. Common Parameters Used to Assess Ventilation and Oxygenation Status	
Parameter	Formula
CaO_2 (ml per dl) (Arterial oxygen content)	$(1.34 \times Hgb \times SaO_2) + (PaO_2 \times 0.0031)$
CvO_2 (ml per dl) (Venous oxygen content)	$(1.34 \times Hgb \times SvO_2) + (PvO_2 \times 0.0031)$
$avDO_2$ (ml per dl) (Arteriovenous oxygen difference)	$CaO_2 - CvO_2$
DO_2 (ml per min) (Oxygen delivery)	$CaO_2 \times CO \times 10$
VO_2 (ml per min) (Oxygen consumption)	$avDO_2 \times CO \times 10$
O_2ER (percent) (Oxygen extraction ratio)	VO_2/DO_2
Qs/Qt (percent) (Shunt fraction)	$100 \times \dfrac{(1.34 \times Hgb + 0.0031) \times (PAO_2 - CaO_2)}{(1.34 \times Hgb + 0.0031) \times (PAO_2 - CvO_2)}$
$AaDO_2$ (mm Hg) (Alveolar–arterial oxygen difference)	$PAO_2 - PaO_2$

$$
\begin{aligned}
Hgb &= \text{Hemoglobin} \\
SaO_2 &= \text{Arterial oxygen saturation of hemoglobin} \\
SvO_2 &= \text{Venous oxygen saturation of hemoglobin} \\
PaO_2 &= \text{Arterial oxygen tension} \\
PvO_2 &= \text{Venous oxygen tension} \\
CO &= \text{Cardiac output} \\
PAO_2 &= \text{Alveolar oxygen tension}
\end{aligned}
$$

the pulmonary capillaries, even in healthy individuals. Some venous return from the bronchial arteries and the coronary circulation flows to the left side of the heart without being oxygenated. A shunt fraction (Qs/Qt) in a healthy individual is usually between 3% and 5%. An elevated Qs/Qt is compatible with a number of clinical conditions including those where there is inadequate alveolar participation in gas exchange.

Alveolar–Arterial Oxygen Difference

The alveolar–arterial oxygen difference ($AaDO_2$) measures the difference in partial pressure of oxygen between the alveoli and the arteries. It characterizes the efficiency of oxygen exchange between the lung alveoli and the pulmonary capillaries. Normal values of $AaDO_2$ are from 10–15 mmHg for the patient breathing room air, and from 10–65 mm Hg for the patient breath-

ing 100% oxygen. The $AaDO_2$ gradient increases approximately 5–7 mm Hg for every 10% increase in FiO_2. An abnormally large drop in oxygen partial pressure from alveoli to arteries may warn of incipient respiratory failure.

Arterial PO_2 Fraction of Inspired Oxygen Ratio

The ratio between arterial oxygen pressure and fraction of inspired oxygen (PaO_2:FiO_2 Ratio) is a simple method that has been shown to correlate with changes in Qs/Qt. When this ratio is less than 200, the Qs/Qt may be estimated at greater than 20%. Conversely, when this ratio is greater than 200, the Qs/Qt may be estimated to be less than 20% (Ahrens, Beattie, & Nienhaus, 1996).

Ventilation calculations are most meaningful under the steady state of controlled ventilation when tidal volume can be unambiguously determined. The static nature of these formulas does not allow accurate determination of ventilatory parameters under SIMV ventilation. Thus, adjustments should be taken into consideration when applying clinical meaning to these parameters when SIMV is utilized.

Minute Volume

Minute volume is a measurement of the volume of gas exchanged in the lungs per minute. It is calculated as the product of the Vt, the volume of gas inspired or expired during each respiratory cycle, and the respiratory rate. Normal ranges of minute volume are approximately 2.5–7 liters per minute, with wide variations, especially during pregnancy. Because it measures gas drawn into the lungs in a respiratory cycle, it includes both effective alveolar ventilation and the dead space ventilation. Thus it is a good index of ventilation when used in conjunction with blood gas analysis.

Minute volume increases in response to hypoxemia, hypercarbia, and acidemia. It decreases in the presence of opposite clinical conditions. One clinical condition associated with decreased minute volume is pulmonary edema.

Compliance

Compliance may be expressed as either dynamic or static. Dynamic compliance is defined as the volume increase corresponding to each unit of pressure increase in the alveoli. It is calculated as the volume change during a breath divided by the change in transpulmonary pressure from end-expiration to end-inspiration. This pressure change is the difference in the peak inspiratory pressure and the positive end-expiratory pressure. The normal range of dynamic compliance is generally between 25 and 35 ml/cm H_2O. As compliance increases, the lung is less stiff and requires less pressure to produce a given tidal volume. A sudden decrease in compliance may be indicative of an airway obstruction.

Dead Space

Physiologic dead space (Vd) refers to the volume of the lungs that is ventilated but not perfused by pulmonary capillary blood flow. This does not contribute to gas exchange and may be considered wasted ventilation. Normal Vd in healthy individuals is usually from 145 to 155 ml at rest. This is approximately 20–30% of each tidal volume. This amount may be increased in clinical conditions where blood flow is obstructed through pulmonary capillaries. It may also occur with overventilation of normally perfused alveoli.

In addition to assessment of these derived calculations, nursing care should include clinical assessment of the patient's hemodynamic and oxygenation status. These measures are outlined in the care guidelines in the last section of this book. Adjuncts useful in this assessment include pulse oximetry and end-tidal CO_2 monitoring via capnography.

Airway Care

Care of the airway of the mechanically ventilated patient includes provision of adequate humidification, measures to mobilize secretions, position changes, and suctioning. Humidification and warming of inspired gas are provided mechanically as adjuncts to the ventilator. Mobilization of secretions is most often accomplished by position change and chest physiotherapy.

Suctioning

Because it exposes the patient to risks including infection, hypoxemia, atelectasis, and aspiration, suctioning should only be performed when necessary. In general, suctioning is indicated when rhonchi are auscultated or secretions are heard during respiration. An increase in ventilator peak inspiratory pressures may indicate the presence of a mucous plug or narrowing of the airways secondary to secretions.

Various strategies have been described to decrease the risk of suction-induced hypoxemia. In a nonobstetric population, a 25–30% drop in oxygen saturation has been reported, followed by a slow rise back to baseline over a 3-minute period, during endotracheal suctioning (Stone & Turner, 1989). Recommendations based on this finding include use of intermittent suction for less than 15 seconds. Prolonged, continuous suctioning causes microatelectasis and reduction of the oxygen concentration in the tracheobronchial tree. Additional methods of reducing hypoxemia include preoxygenation, hyperoxygenation, hyperinflation, and hyperventilation. A description of each of these practices is presented in Table 5-7 (Chang, 1995).

Additional strategies for prevention of nosocomial pneumonia related to suctioning are described in Table 5-8 (Widmer, 1994).

Psychosocial Support

Use of mechanical ventilation subjects the patient to physical and emotional stress in the critical care environment. It is also a stressful time for the patient's family and support system. Factors that may contribute to emotional distress are presented in 5-9. Factors that are particularly distressing are related to the inability to speak and the pain and discomfort associated with the presence and manipulation of the endotracheal tube. Every possible effort should be made to relieve physical discomfort, minimize manipulation of the endotracheal tube, facilitate communication, and include family and support system in the provision of care.

Table 5-7. Methods of Reducing Suction-Induced Hypoxemia

Technique	Definition
Hyperinflation	Increasing the tidal volume to 1-1 1/2 times the preset ventilation volume by the use of a resuscitation bag or the sigh function of the ventilator
Preoxygenation	Administration of oxygen before suctioning
Hyperoxygenation	Administration of oxygen at a greater FiO_2 than the preset ventilator level
Hyperventilation	Increasing the respiratory/ventilator rate without changing tidal volume or oxygen concentration

TABLE 5-8. Strategies for Prevention of Nosocomial Infection During Suctioning or with Mechanical Ventilation

- Provide a clean manual resuscitation bag for each patient
- Suction oropharyngeal secretions as needed to avoid accumulation of oral secretions
- Use sterile technique when using open-suctioning techniques
- Use sterile solutions only to clear secretions from in-line suction devices
- Before deflating the cuff of the tracheal tube, suction secretions above the cuff by passing the catheter orotracheally, then provide a positive-pressure breath during deflation
- Monitor tracheal cuff pressure with a manometer, minimal seal, or minimal leak technique every 8 hours to ensure an adequate seal and avoid overpressurization
- Provide routine, meticulous mouth care
- Change ventilator circuits no more frequently than every 48 hours
- Drain accumulated condensate in ventilator tubing into a fluid trap or other collection device, particularly before repositioning the patient
- Avoid backflow of condensate into tracheal tubes or humidification devices

TABLE 5-9. Factors Contributing to Distress During Mechanical Ventilation

- Inability to speak
- Pain and discomfort from endotracheal tube
- Suctioning
- Inability to determine time of day or date
- Noise
    From other patients
    Alarms
    Water movement in ventilator tubing
    Nurses and physicians talking
    Telephone
- Concern for nearby patients
- Lack of sleep
- Bright lights
- Weaning
- Position and infrequent position change
- Pulling of ventilator tubing
- Inability to see doors or windows
- Being paralyzed while remaining alert
- Sight of unfamiliar equipment

SUMMARY

Increased use of mechanical ventilation in an obstetric setting may be anticipated with continued development of critical care capabilities in this specialty practice. Inherent advantages related to family-centered care are evident when such a level of care may be provided in an obstetric unit. When care is administered by obstetric critical care nurses confident in related patient and equipment management, timely treatment of the obstetric patient with pulmonary compromise may be facilitated.

REFERENCES

Ahrens, T. S., Beattie, S., & Nienhaus, T. (1996). Experimental therapies to support the failing lung. AACN Clinical Issues, 7(4), 507–518.

American Thoracic Society. (1995). Hospital-acquired pneumonia in adults: Diagnosis, assessment of severity, initial antimicrobial therapy and preventive strategies (consensus statement). American Respiratory Critical Care Medicine, 153, 1711–1725.

Chang, V. M. (1995). Protocol for prevention of complications of endotracheal intubation. Critical Care Nurse, 15(5), 19–27.

Clark, S. L., Cotton, D. B., Hankins, G. D. V., & Phelan, J. P. (Eds.). (1994). Adult respiratory distress syndrome. In Handbook of critical care obstetrics (pp. 179–180). Cambridge, MA: Blackwell Scientific.

Dirkes, S. (1996). Liquid ventilation: New frontiers in the treatment of ARDS. Critical Care Nurse, 16, 53–58.

Downs, J. B., Klein, E. F., Desautels, D., et al. (1973). IMV: A new approach to weaning patients from mechanical ventilators. Chest, 87, 612–618.

Dupuis, Y. G. (1986). Ventilators: Theory and clinical application (p. 126). St. Louis, MO: C. V. Mosby.

Fuhrman, B. P., Paczan, P. R., & DeFrancis, M. (1991). Perfluorocarbon-associated gas exchange. Critical Care Medicine, 19(5), 712–722.

Greenspan, J. S., Wolfson, M. R., Rubenstein, D., et al. (1990). Liquid ventilation of human preterm neonates. Journal of Pediatarics, 117(1), 106–111.

Marini, J. J., & Wheeler, A. P. (1989). Mechanical ventilation. In Critical care medicine: The essentials (pp. 65–77). Baltimore: William & Wilkins.

Marino, P. L. (1991). Modes of ventilation. In The ICU book (pp. 371–382). Malvern, PA: Lea and Febiger.

Schaffer, T. H., Wolfson, M. R., & Clark, L. C., Jr. (1992). Liquid ventilation. Pediatric Pulmonology, 14, 102–109.

Stone, K. S., & Turner, B. (1989). Endotracheal suctioning. Annual Review Nursing Research, 7, 27–47.

Troiano, N. H. & Dorman, K. (1992). Mechanical ventilation during pregnancy. Clinical

Issues in Perinatal and Women's Health Nursing, 3 (3), 399–407. Philadelphia: Lippincott.

Tutuncu, H., Faithful, S., & Lachman, B. (1993). Intratracheal perfluorocarbon administration combined with mechanical ventilation in experimental respiratory distress syndrome. Critical Care Medicine, 1(7), 962–969.

Weinstein, R. A. (1991). Epidemiology and control of nosocomial infections in adult intensive care units. American Journal of Medicine, 91(3B), 179S–184S.

West, J. B., Dollery, C. T., Matthews, C. M. E., et al. (1965). Distribution of blood and ventilation in the saline-filled lung. Journal of Applied Physiology, 20, 1107–1117.

Widmer, A. F. (1994). Infection control and prevention strategies in the ICU. Intensive Care Medicine, 20, S7–S11.

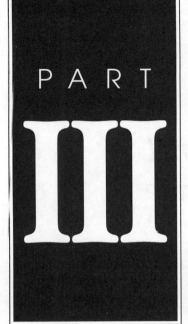

PART

III

Clinical Application

CHAPTER

6

Preterm Labor and Premature Rupture of Membranes

Kathryn Flynn

INCIDENCE AND SIGNIFICANCE

Preterm labor (PTL) is defined as labor occurring prior to the completion of 37 weeks gestation. Though the diagnosis of PTL is sometimes disputed and may be overdiagnosed, preterm delivery (PTD) represents 8–10% of all births in the United States and results in 60% of all perinatal morbidity and mortality (Berkowicz & Papierick, 1993). Despite more specific criteria for diagnosis and the availability of new treatment options, the overall incidence of preterm delivery has not decreased in the last 20 years.

Premature rupture of membranes (PROM) is the rupture of the amniotic membrane prior to the onset of labor. This event is not related to the gestational age and occurs in both term and preterm gestations. Preterm premature rupture of membranes (PPROM) refers to premature rupture prior to 37 weeks gestation. It is associated with approximately 30–50 % of preterm deliveries (Savuitz, Blackimore, & Thorp, 1991; Tucker, Goldenberg, Davis, Cooper, Winkler, & Hauth, 1991) and is the single most common event leading to the admission of a preterm infant to a neonatal intensive care unit. Widespread use of tocolytic agents to treat PTL in the last 30 years has done little to change the incidence of preterm delivery in the United States (Hugby, Xenakis, & Pauerstein, 1993). It is this unchanging pattern that has led many researchers to focus on more precise etiology of PTL, PPROM, and PTD.

In 1962, the president's panel on mental retardation began to focus on the morbidity and mortality of low-birth-weight infants. Mental retardation was originally targeted as the major risk associated with prematurity and low birth weight, but blindness and developmental problems were concerns also addressed. Neonatology developed as a specialty shortly thereafter, and studies by healthcare providers focused on the preterm infant.

Preterm labor and delivery are major unsolved problems in obstetrics. In the last several decades, research has been conducted to determine the etiology and pathogenesis of PPROM and PTL (Lockwood, 1995). Research investigating the physiology of normal term labor is being carefully studied to better understand what happens and why labor begins. It is known that rapidly increasing numbers of receptor sites for oxytocin are produced in the uterus late in pregnancy and in labor (Fuchs, Fuchs, Husslein, & Soloff, 1984). What stimulates this receptor production, however, is not very clear. It is also unclear whether the mechanisms associated with PTL are the same as those in the term pregnancy.

The lifelong effects for the child born prematurely vary both in the degree of morbidity and its effect on the family and society. Survival rates for preterm infants have steadily increased with the advancement of neonatal care. Simultaneously, the age of viability has been reduced to as low as 24 weeks gestation. For these extremely premature infants the most optimum location for delivery is in the tertiary care center with a neonatal intensive care unit. Rapid and effective infant stabilization is critical to survival. Morbidity is greatly increased with PTD. At a birth weight of less than 1500 grams or 34 weeks gestation, respiratory distress syndrome (RDS), intraventricular hemorrhage, and necrotizing enterocolitis are more likely (Levine, 1991; Main & Main, 1991). Long-term complications include bronchopulmonary dysplasia and neurologic handicaps such as cerebral palsy, developmental delays, blindness, and deafness. The more remote from term these deliveries occur, the higher the incidence of morbidity. Surfactant therapy has made it possible to enhance pulmonary function in the immediate newborn period, resulting in the reduction of time that mechanical ventilation is required, particularly at high settings. The long-term complication rate of respiratory disease seems to be declining.

Patients with PPROM are at higher risk of preterm delivery and of complications to the fetus and newborn resulting from decreased amniotic fluid volume. The most immediate risk of PPROM is preterm delivery. The latency period, or time from PROM to spontaneous delivery, decreases with advancing gestational age. At 24 weeks gestation, 40% of pregnancies with PPROM will have a latency period of more than one week. At 34 weeks gestation, this incidence falls to 20% (Hibbard, Hibbard, Ismail, & Arendt, 1993; King, 1994). When rupture occurs at very early gestations, prior to 22 weeks, pulmonary hypoplasia may occur in varying degrees due to severe oligohydramnios. Lung volume expansions may be inhibited in these fetuses due to mechanical interference as a result of compression in the intrauterine space and because amniotic fluid is not freely able to move into the lungs (Kulbride, Yeast, & Thibeault, 1989). This risk decreases as gestational age at PPROM increases. Oligohydramnios can also result in facial and limb deformities and contractures because of the inability of the fetus to move about freely.

Chorioamnionitis may be both a cause and a result of PPROM. Infection may occur in the patient with intact membranes and lead to PROM or may occur by ascending infection following rupture of membranes. Patients presenting with PROM or PTL should be carefully evaluated for signs of infection and antibiotic treatment begun when infection is evident. Numerous investigators have attempted to determine whether bacterial vaginosis (BV) is associated with PTL and PROM. More aggressive attempts at screening and treatment of BV may have some effect on changing PTL rates, though it is too early to tell if the impact will be in a significant number of women.

ETIOLOGY

The exact mechanism or event that initiates spontaneous labor remains obscure. The process appears to involve a complex series of interactions between hormones, enzymes, and cells and between fetus and mother (Figure 6-1). The appearance of certain physiologic events has been identified as occurring before or during labor. An active ripening process occurs within the cervix, which involves a breakdown of collagen by collagenase resulting in changes in cervical connective tissue. (Uldberg, Ulmsten, & Edman, 1983). Increased fibroblast activity similar to an inflammatory tissue response also occurs during this ripening process, and the cervix becomes softer and shorter (Brindley & Sokol, 1988; Liggins, 1983; Uldberg et al., 1983). In addition to cervical ripening, gap junctions and oxytocin receptors appear in the myometrium (Casey & MacDonald, 1988; Liggins, 1983).

Gap junctions are neural contacts between cells that allow the instantaneous communication necessary for rhythmic and coordinated uterine contractions (Garfield & Hayashi, 1981). The increase in number of oxytocin receptors at the time of labor increases responsiveness of the uterus to oxytocin stimuli (Brindley & Sokol, 1988; Casey & MacDonald, 1988). Serum levels do not rise appreciably before labor, but peak during the second stage (Brindley & Sokol, 1988; Casey & MacDonald, 1988). Oxytocin receptors also found in the decidua stimulate the production of prostaglandins.

The role of estrogen and progesterone in the initiation of labor remains unclear. In sheep, rising fetal cortisol levels at term activate enzymes that alter placental steroid production (Casey & MacDonald, 1988; Liggins, 1983). Estrogen is produced in greater quantities while progesterone secretion falls, resulting in increased prostaglandin synthesis. In humans, however, there is neither a demonstrable rise in fetal cortisol levels nor withdrawal of progesterone until after delivery of the placenta (Casey & MacDonald, 1988). It is possible that a change in the ratio of estrogen to progesterone may affect the initiation of labor in humans (Casey & MacDonald, 1988; Liggins, 1983).

Prostaglandins are the major hormones involved in the initiation of spontaneous labor. There is a dramatic rise in prostaglandin concentration in amniotic fluid during labor (Brindley et al., 1988). Arachidonic acid, the precursor of PGE_2 and PGF_2, is also found in increased concentration during labor. Prostaglandins not only affect cervical ripening but also promote gap junction formation and stimulate uterine contractions (Casey & MacDonald, 1988; Liggins, 1983). The mechanism of prostaglandin action on uterine contractions appears to be mediated by the enhancement of calcium transport through the plasma membrane. Calcium is a vital component in the actin and myosin coupling process necessary for smooth muscle contraction (Liggins, 1983). Prostaglandins promote both the availability of intracellular calcium for uterine smooth muscle contraction, as well as the formation of myometrial gap functions (Ulmsten, 1989). Together these two processes promote coordinated uterine contractions necessary for labor.

Prostaglandins are produced in the cervix, decidua, and myometrium. When infection or physical damage of the decidua, fetal membranes, or cervix occurs, increased prostaglandin synthesis is stimulated (Liggins, 1983). Because the decidua has many macrophage-like properties, decidual cells and macrophages both respond to infection by producing prostaglandins (Casey & MacDonald, 1988). The tissue changes that occur during cervical ripening are in fact reminiscent of an inflammatory tissue response (Casey & MacDonald, 1988; Liggins, 1983). In addition the amnion is apparently stimulated to increase production of prostaglandins through the influence of fetal urine. This effect is not noted until late in the gestation and is indicative of the possible communication occurring between mother and fetus, at least in part, via the amniotic fluid and fetal membranes (Ulmsten, 1989). The sequence of events that results in labor and parturition may be present but held in abeyance during pregnancy. It is speculated that when the fetal/placental unit somehow withdraws its sup-

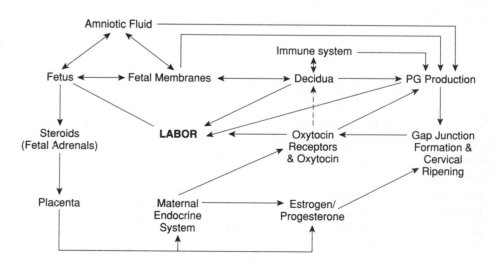

Figure 6-1. The process involved in spontaneous labor.

port of the pregnancy, the initiation of parturition begins (Hugby et al., 1993; Liggins, 1983).

RISK FACTORS

Risk factors for preterm labor are numerous, some being pregnancy-related and others related to a medical complication. Display 6-1 summarizes risk factors that have been associated with PTL. Medical conditions predating pregnancy may increase the risk for spontaneous PTL and subsequent PTD or may result in an indicated PTD. For example, a woman with hypertension and renal disease may have a compromised maternal state leading to spontaneous PTL; or the fetal state may be compromised as a result of significant maternal disease, necessitating early delivery.

Of all obstetrical risks, a history of previous preterm delivery is the most significant risk factor for PTL. The risk associated with a previous induced second-trimester abortion is actually quite low if the procedure was performed properly and without uterine or cervical damage. There is a growing body of evidence that cigarette smoking is associated with PTL and PTD. The role it plays in PROM is under investigation with mounting evidence that it has an adverse effect on placental function and oxygen exchange.

Demographic risks should be interpreted carefully. It is likely that some factors may be interrelated, such as socioeconomic status and whether or not the patient seeks early prenatal care. The patient's true risk status may be difficult to assess. Information should be evaluated in its entirety and the complete clinical picture reviewed before risk is determined.

Cervical incompetence is described as painless dilation of the cervix in the second or early third trimester of pregnancy. The etiology is unclear but may include such factors as diethylstilbestrol (DES) exposure in utero and cervical trauma from a previous medical procedure (e.g., abortion, conization). Often, there is no clear etiology. It is critical to obtain a detailed history from a patient who reports a history of an incompetent cervix (Creasy & Resnick, 1989;

DISPLAY 6-1

Summary of Risk Factors Associated with Preterm Labor and Delivery

1. **Medical Risks (preconceptual)**
   Renal disease
   Hypertension
   Previous second-trimester abortion
   Inadequate nutritional status

2. **Demographic Risks**
   Adolescence
   Advanced maternal age
   Low socioeconomic status
   Non-Caucasian
   Smoker
   Substance abuser
   Prepregnant weight less than 100 lbs.
   Psychological stress

3. **Pregnancy–Associated Risk**
   Previous preterm delivery
   Poor weight gain after 20 weeks gestation
   Poor prenatal care
   Uterine/cervical anomalies
   Multiple gestation
   Placenta previa
   Abruptio placentae
   Polyhydramnios
   Cervical incompetence
   Maternal infection
   Cervical effacement/dilation

Cunningham, MacDonald, & Gant, 1989). Careful questioning and review of medical records may reveal the patient had mild contractions, PROM or infection, which would preclude a diagnosis of incompetent cervix. Multiple factors, such as an accurate history, will contribute to the development of a management plan and deciding if cervical cerclage may be of benefit.

Multiple gestation in the current pregnancy is a significant risk factor for preterm labor and delivery. The most likely cause is uterine overdistention at an early gestational age. Distention of the uterus to full-term size despite immature gestational age may effect the length of the pregnancy. Gravitational forces and increasing pressure on the cervix may also contribute to cervical dilation, which may play a role in directly triggering PTL or may expose the amniotic membrane to bacteria, weakening the membrane and leading to PROM. Stretching of the myometrial walls caused by overdistension may stimulate the labor process.

Maternal or fetal blood loss may necessitate prompt delivery to attain the most optimal outcome to both the mother and infant. Placental abruption can be a spontaneous event, associated with PROM, related to abdominal trauma, hypertensive disease, or history of abruption in a previous pregnancy or drug use, particularly cocaine. Women with placenta previa can experience significant blood loss if cervical dilatation or manipulation have occurred. In the presence of abruptio placentae or placenta previa, preterm delivery may be indicated, though both carry significant risk to mother and fetus. A meta-analysis of patients who had chronic hypertension and abruptio placentae revealed a 10-fold increase in the likelihood of abruption when compared to the general population (Ananth, Savitz, & Williams, 1996).

There is also good evidence linking infection to preterm labor and PPROM (Romero & Mazor, 1988; Toth, Witkins, Ledger, & Thaler, 1988). Bacterial infection and endotoxin production stimulate the biosynthesis of prostaglandin at the fetal membranes and decidua. Bacterial action during the infection process releases phospholipase A_2, leading to prostaglandin prosynthesis. Prostaglandins E_2 and F_2 enhance uterine activity and dissolve and weaken collagen fibers (Bajar, Curbelo & Davis, 1981; Rayburn, 1989). Intrauterine infection most often occurs by an ascending route through the vagina, cervix, and maternal decidua. Bacteria invading the uterus are capable of crossing intact membranes and enter-

ing the intraamniotic space. The intervillous space and fetal vessels may be another possible route for infection, which when localized in the decidua and chorionic membrane can also lead to weakening of the membrane and subsequent rupture. Focal weakening of the amniotic membranes is probably due to enzymatic bacterial action, which may trigger the cascade of factors initiating labor. Changes in biochemical collagen metabolism occur in the amnion and chorion and lead to significant weakening of the membranes through collagenolysis (Vadillo-Ortega, Gonzalez–Avial, & Karchmer et al., 1990). Because of concentrations of bacteria, PPROM may be a variant of the normal process at an inappropriate time.

Systemic maternal infection, such as pyelonephritis, is also associated with preterm labor, suggesting the onset of labor in the presence of infection occurs as a protective host response controlled by either mother and/or fetus (Romero et al., 1988). Prostaglandin production, stimulated by the specific immunological response to infection, may initiate the birth process in response to a hostile maternal environment.

Certain sociological characteristics are associated with increased risk for preterm labor and delivery (Berkowicz et al., 1993). Single women, teenagers, and women over the age of 40 are at increased risk. Women of color are statistically at greater risk for preterm labor than Caucasian women, and African American women deliver babies prior to 37 weeks of gestation twice as often as do Caucasian women (Berkowicz et al., 1993; Cunningham et al., 1989). Low socioeconomic status and low educational attainment are reproducible demographic characteristics associated with an increased risk of preterm labor (Cunningham et al., 1989). There is also an association between smoking and low birth weight (Canadian Preterm Labor Investigators Group, 1992; Cunningham et al., 1989; Savitz et al., 1991).

Maternal cigarette smoking is believed to be a major contributing factor to preterm delivery in the United States (Heffner, Sherman, Speezer, & Weiss, 1993). Smoking ultimately leads to a smaller placenta with reduced oxygen available to transport to the fetus, resulting in a more aged and less optimally functioning placenta at an earlier gestational age. Substance abuse is also associated with preterm births, particularly cocaine, which is known to increase the risk of placental abruption. Many women who are substance users have multiple risk factors for preterm labor.

Low prepregnancy weight and inadequate weight gain during pregnancy put women at risk for preterm labor and delivery. Underweight women, those whose prepregnant weight is less than 90% of ideal body weight for height, are more likely to be malnourished. Nutrient transport to the fetus at early gestation may affect the earlier stages of development of the fetal–placental unit. Poor weight gain in pregnancy is often associated with poor dietary intake, further compounding the already underweight status of a women (Siega-Riz, Adair, & Hobel, 1996).

Women who are required to stand for prolonged times while working may be at risk for preterm labor. If a woman is unable to take rest breaks when feeling tired, the risk of preterm labor increases in some populations (Hickey, Cliver, Milvihill, McNeal, Hoffman, & Goldenberg, 1995). Compression of the pelvic vessels with decreased venous return and uterine blood flow have been suggested as potential causes of preterm labor when pregnancy is accompanied by prolonged standing (Hickey, Sivonen, Rukonen, Savia, & Ylikorkala, 1992).

The physiologic effects of psychologic stress during pregnancy have not been fully elucidated, although the uterus can have a variable response to catecholamine release depending on the hormonal influences operating at the time. Whereas beta-adrenergic stimulation causes vasodilation in smooth muscle, alpha-adrenergic stimulation causes vasoconstriction and increased muscle tone. Stress responses either from the maternal or fetal side stimulate corticotropin-releasing hormone (CRH). Monitoring of CRH serum levels in patients was shown to be consistently elevated in those women who delivered preterm (Bejar, Curbelo, & Davis, 1981).

It is not clear whether term parturition and the preterm birth process share similar mechanisms. The role of infection in the etiology of preterm labor is at this point in time the most clearly understood and perhaps correctable risk factor; however, infection is not responsible for or present in all cases of preterm labor. The complexity of identifiable risk factors strongly suggests multiple causes for preterm birth.

The etiology of PPROM is also poorly understood although associated factors are closely related to those of preterm labor: low socioeconomic status, smoking, poor diet, and age (Tucker et al., 1991). In addition, a history of sexually transmitted diseases has been linked to PPROM (Tucker et al., 1991). Factors that may contribute to the occurrence of PPROM include incompetent cervix, infection or inflammatory weakening of the membranes, hydramnios, trauma, multiple gestations, maternal genital tract anomalies, and abruptio placentae (Niebyl, Blake, & White et al., 1980; Tucker et al., 1991).

Women with bacterial vaginosis (BV) in the first trimester of pregnancy have an increased incidence of preterm labor, birth, and PPROM. Unfortunately, there is a high false positive rate of BV, limiting the usefulness of clinical assessment (Hickey et al., 1980).

Numerous research studies have been undertaken in an effort to better predict which women are at risk for preterm labor, and once PTL occurs, which women will have a PTD. Although patients may be screened for risk factors, identifiable risks have been found for only about half of patients who deliver prematurely. Clinical indicators that have been studied include cervical factors, uterine contractions, vaginal bleeding, fetal behavioral states, and stress (Lockwood, 1995). Cervical assessment has been studied by both manual vaginal examination and ultrasonograph. Routine manual cervical examination was shown to have little predictive value for PTD (Buekens, Alexander, & Boutsen et al., 1994). Sonographic evaluation may be more useful when the entire length of the cervix can be measured. In addition to length, endocervical funneling can be observed. This can be particularly useful in women with a shortened cervix prior to pregnancy as well as those with some symptoms of PTL (Gomez, Galasso, Romero, Mazor, Sorokin, Goncalves, & Treadwell, 1995). Changes in fetal behavioral states, specifically fetal breathing, may be highly predictive of PTD within 48 hours of delivery (Besinger, Copton, & Hayashi, 1987).

ASSESSMENT

Preterm labor is a significant complication, and thus nursing assessment of the mother and fetus begins as quickly as possible and continues throughout hospitalization. Upon admission, maternal vital signs and fetal status are evaluated concurrently with assessment of uterine activity and vaginal discharge. A careful history is taken to identify gestational age, prenatal care, and risk factors such as multiple gestation, hydramnios, history of previous preterm deliveries, uterine anomalies, and history of precipitating events.

Uterine activity and irritability are best assessed by a tocodynamometer and palpation. If the membranes are intact, cervical dilation, effacement, consistency, and position may be evaluated by gentle digital exam. If ruptured membranes are suspected, a sterile speculum exam is done to document the presence of amniotic fluid and to visualize the cervix. Cervical cultures should be obtained.

During assessment for PTL or PPROM, the patient is usually placed in the lateral recumbent position to increase blood flow to the uterus, and bed rest is prescribed. The patient is hydrated with intravenous fluids to increase blood flow to the uterus. Systematic and serial assessment continues throughout treatment and is best accomplished by continuity of care providers so as to identify subtle changes in patient status from day to day. Cervical assessment by speculum or gentle digital exam if membranes are intact to detect cervical changes may be indicated. Changes in cervical tissue consistency, cervical position, and station of the presenting part may indicate advancing labor. More precise measurement of cervical length may be done with the use of sonography. This can help to assess the full length of the cervix, measure the internal os, and decreases the number of vaginal examinations that are performed. The patient should be monitored for associated symptoms, which include the following:

1. Vaginal bleeding/spotting
2. Change in vaginal discharge color, quantity, odor, or quality
3. Low backache
4. Lower abdominal or pelvic pressure
5. Cramping
6. Diarrhea
7. Fever
8. Diminishing fetal activity

Diagnosis of preterm labor is generally accepted and confirmed when progressive cervical dilation reaches 2 cm and cervical effacement reaches 80% (Creasy & Resnick, 1989; Leveno & Cunningham, 1987). Often, treatment is begun prior to a confirmed diagnosis of PTL to stop contractions before noticeable cervical change occurs, thereby decreasing the chance of a preterm delivery. Advancement of cervical dilation beyond 4 cm is usually an indication that tocolytic therapy and other attempts to halt labor may be unsuccessful (Liu & Fairweather, 1981). Digital cervical exams should be limited to reduce stimulation of uterine irritability. In the presence of PPROM, digital exams increase the risk of infection by carrying organisms through the vagina to the endocervical canal; they are therefore avoided during management of PPROM until delivery is imminent.

Amniotic fluid examination for the lecithin-to-sphingomyelin ratio and presence or absence of phosphatidylglycerol concentration assists in the evaluation of fetal pulmonary maturity. If the specimen is retrieved through amniocentesis rather than by vaginal collection, it may also be examined for bacteria. Tests may include Gram's stain, cultures, and C-reactive protein studies as indicators of the presence of infection.

The pH of amniotic fluid is essentially neutral (6.5–7.5), whereas cervical mucus is usually slightly acidic (5.0–6.0). Urine may normally vary in pH from 4.5 to 8.0. Maternal blood near the cervix may also be near neutral (7.4) (Nagey & Saller, 1986). The overlap of these values makes nitrazine testing of a vaginal fluid specimen ineffective for the diagnosis of PROM. Examination of vaginal fluid for ferning after drying the specimen on a glass slide had proved to be a more sensitive test to confirm the presence of amniotic fluid in the vaginal vault (Reese, Chervenak, Maya, & Hobbins, 1984). Alone, none of these tests are completely reliable, but an analysis of physical findings

DISPLAY 6-2

Initial Management of Preterm Premature Rupture of Membranes[a]

The confirmation of rupture of the amniotic membranes

Determination of pathologic bacterial infection at the time of rupture

Documentation of gestational age

Determination of fetal pulmonary maturity

Early detection of developing maternal and/or fetal infections

Early detection of fetal compromise

From "Preterm Premature Rupture of the Membrane," by C. Crenshaw, 1986, Clinical Obstetrics and Gynecology, 29(4), pp. 735–738.

and history is necessary for diagnosis (see Display 6-2).

Fetal heart rate and uterine activity are monitored closely, so that any deterioration of fetal status that might require a change in the management plan of care can be recognized. Monitoring may be intermittent, continuous, or involve daily nonstress tests or biophysical profiles, depending on the patient's clinical status.

Serial ultrasounds for examination of the amount of amniotic fluid, fetal size, presentation, lower uterine segment funneling, presence of fetal breathing, and placental location all aid in improved assessment of maternal–fetal condition.

TREATMENT

Treatment of Preterm Labor

Bed rest, hydration, and sedation are conservative measures that may halt preterm contractions in up to one half of patients. Bed rest in the lateral recumbent position and intravenous hydration promote increased intravascular volume, increased uterine blood flow, and decreased pressure on the cervix (Hickey et al., 1995; Savitz et al., 1991). Failure of adequate maternal plasma

volume expansion may be a possible cause of preterm contractions and may account in part for the therapeutic success of hydration and bedrest (Hickey et al., 1995). Intravenous fluids should be limited to 400–500 ml and administered over 20–30 minutes, as excessive hydration places the patient at increased risk for pulmonary edema in the event that intravenous betamimetic or magnesium sulfate therapy become necessary (Zuckerman, Shalen, Gilad, & Katzuni, 1984). Mild sedation may be appropriate for select patients who are very anxious (Major, Lewis, Harding et al., 1994). Combined with reassurance, sedation may help decrease endogenous catecholamine production in a frightened woman.

Tocolysis refers to the pharmacological treatment of preterm contractions. Approximately one fourth to one half of women experiencing preterm contractions will not be in true preterm labor. Because success in postponing preterm birth is dependent on preventing significant cervical change, early intervention frequently precludes waiting to document cervical changes. Thus, many women may be treated with tocolytic therapy unnecessarily. Unfortunately, advances in pharmacological treatments for preterm labor have not made a significant impact on the preterm birth rate. Goals for tocolytic treatment of preterm labor are to inhibit contractions, to prevent cervical change, and to prolong fetal time in utero.

The tocolytics most frequently used to halt uterine contractions are betamimetic agents, magnesium sulfate, prostaglandin inhibitors, and calcium channel blockers. (See Display 6-3 for a summary of tocolytics.) The betamimetics used for the treatment of preterm labor include ritodrine hydrochloride and terbutaline sulfate. Isoxsuprine hydrochloride, because of its pronounced cardiovascular side effects, is rarely used today. Hexoprenaline is still in use in Europe, Africa, and at a few centers in the United States and Canada (Major et al., 1994; Kuperminc, Lessing, Yaron, & Reyer, 1993). Hexoprenaline, like ritodrine and terbutaline, is considered to have a more direct effect on myometrial relaxation. Ritodrine is the only drug currently approved by the Food and Drug Administration for tocolytic use. The Food and Drug Administration does allow for unlabeled use of medication when a stated therapy has been

DISPLAY 6-3

Summary of Medications Used for Tocolysis

Betamimetics
Commonly used
• Ritodrine hydrochloride
• Terbutaline sulfate
Infrequently used
• Hexoprenaline
• Fenoterol
• Albuterol
Magnesium Sulfate
Prostaglandin Inhibitors
• Indomethacin
Calcium Channel Blockers
• Nifedipine
Oxytocin Agonists
• Atosiban

"extensively reported in the medical literature" (FDA, 1982).

BETAMIMETICS

Betamimetic agents work by stimulating beta-adrenergic receptors. Two types of beta receptors coexist throughout the body. Beta$_1$ receptors stimulate activity in the heart, liver, pancreas, intestines, and adipose tissue. Beta$_2$ receptor stimulation causes smooth muscle relaxation in the uterus, bronchioles, and vasculature. The overlapping effects of beta$_1$ and beta$_2$ receptor activity are responsible for the adverse maternal and fetal side effects associated with these drugs, including tachycardia, hypertension, shortness of breath, and vomiting. The tocolytic effect of betamimetic drugs occurs when beta receptor stimulation activates the enzyme adenyl cyclase; this then increases cyclic adenosine monophosphate (cAMP) with-

in the uterine smooth muscle cells. The efforts of increased cAMP are a decrease in intracellular calcium, a necessary cofactor for muscle contraction, and decreased uterine smooth muscle activity. Betamimetic drugs are metabolized and inactivated by the liver and excreted in the urine (Caritis, Lin, Toig, & Wong, 1983).

The efficacy of betamimetic agents may be lost to desensitization or tachyphylaxis over time. After prolonged therapy, there is a decrease in the number of beta-adrenergic receptors resulting in a loss of efficacy. This phenomenon is known as down regulation. To avoid this, treatment may be most effective if used only until contractions have diminished and stabilized for a period of time. In the event that PTL reoccurs, betamimetic therapy may be of further benefit.

Conditions often cited as contraindications to tocolysis, or more specifically use of betamimetics, are numerous (Display 6-4). Presence of maternal cardiac disease, for example, may be readily identified as a contraindication to betamimetic therapy. However, it should be noted that previously undiagnosed cardiac disease as well as associated complications have been unmasked during tocolytic treatment with betamimetics (Caritis et al., 1983; Graber, 1989). Cerebral ischemia in patients prone to migraine headaches has been associated with the use of betamimetics (Beneditti, 1983; Caritis et al., 1983; Graber, 1989). A history of migraine headaches is particularly significant in the woman who is a candidate for tocolysis. Use of tocolytic agents in the presence of vaginal bleeding is dependent upon the reason for bleeding, maternal hemodynamic stability, fetal status, and goal of therapy.

Ritodrine can be administered intravenously or orally. When beginning therapy, the lowest possible effective dose should be given and increased at regular intervals until uterine contractions are suppressed. The usual intravenous infusion is to begin at 50–100 mcg/minute (0.05–0.1 ml/min), and with 50 mcg/minute increased every 15–20 minutes (Caritis et al., 1983). These increases should be continued until contractions stop or the maximum recommended dose of 350 mcg/minute (0.35 mg/min) is achieved. Once PTL suppression is successful, the ritodrine dose should be decreased every 20–30 minutes to 50–100 mcg/min for at least 12 hours. Oral ritodrine may be initiated 30–60 minutes before discontinuing the IV infusion. The dosage for oral therapy is 5–10 mg every 2–4 hours, with a maximum daily dose of 120 mg. Because tachyphylaxis is likely, oral therapy should be discontinued within 24–48 hours. Alternative protocols for administration, which include gradual reduction in infusion rate after effective tocolysis is achieved, have also been reported (Caritis, Darby, & Chan, 1988).

Terbutaline is also used for PTL treatment and seems to have similar effects as ritodrine. It has been used intravenously, subcutaneously, and orally. The effects are similar to those of ritodrine and the cost is significantly lower. Intravenous terbutaline is less costly than ritodrine, and its efficacy and safety appear to be comparable (Caritis et al., 1988; Moore, Briggs, & Freeman, 1988). Intravenous regimes differ slightly from center to center. Terbutaline may be given by subcutaneous injection. The usual dosage is 0.25 mg terbutaline administered subcutaneously every 1–6 hours. The frequency of administration is determined by uterine activity and maternal pulse. Terbutaline has a rapid absorption rate and a half-life of 7 minutes (Stubblefield & Heyl, 1982). Fewer and less severe side effects are seen with subcutaneous administration than with intravenous administration of any betamimetic drug (Stubblefield & Heyd, 1982).

The Canadian Preterm Investigators Group conducted a large randomized trial of ritodrine versus a placebo. The results of this study showed that perinatal mortality was not significantly affected by PTL treatment with ritodrine. It did demonstrate that delivery was delayed by 24–48 hours as compared to the placebo group. This delay was long enough to administer corticosteroids (Canadian Preterm Investigators Group, 1992).

Betamimetics are potent drugs and require vigilant maternal and fetal assessment during intravenous use. Side effects and complications of betamimetic therapy are due to stimulation of beta-adrenergic receptors distributed through-

DISPLAY 6-4

Relative and/or Absolute Contraindications to Betamimetic Therapy

Maternal
  Cardiac disease
  Cardiac arrhythmias
  Uncontrolled diabetes
  Maternal infection
  Hyperthyroidism
  Pheochromocytoma
  Preeclampsia or eclampsia
  Uncontrolled chronic hypertension
  Active vaginal bleeding
  Hypovolemia
  History of migraine headaches
  Untreated urinary tract infection
  Chronic renal or hepatic disease
  Bronchial asthma already treated with betamimetics
  Advanced labor
Fetal
  Fetal demise
  Fetal distress
  Intrauterine growth retardation
  Placental dysfunction
  Fetal anomalies incompatible with life

out the body. The occurrence of side effects may be more frequent during increases in the infusion rate than during the maintenance infusion (Caritis et al., 1983; Caritis, Toig, Heddinger, & Ashmead, 1984). It should be remembered that oral therapy does not preclude development of significant side effects and complications. The most frequent side effect of betamimetic therapy is maternal tachycardia. Maternal heart rate increases 10–20 beats per minute as a partially compensatory response to vasodilation

(Graber, 1989). Cardiac arrhythmias have been reported in association with betamimetic therapy. Associated myocardial ischemia may or may not occur (Benedetti, 1983). Widening of the pulse pressure is commonly seen without a significant reduction in mean arterial pressure. Hypotension occurs less frequently with beta$_2$ preferential drugs (i.e., ritodrine), but it is still a potential side effect.

Shortness of breath and chest pain are the most common pulmonary side effects seen with betamimetic therapy (Graber, 1989). Pulmonary edema is a serious and potentially fatal complication and, although the cause is not completely understood, it is most likely due to fluid overload and sodium retention (Benedetti, 1983; Graber, 1989). Beta-adrenergic stimulation causes sodium and water retention, and excess fluid volume may result in spite of limiting intravenous fluid intake. Iatrogenic fluid overload may also lead to pulmonary edema and should, therefore, be carefully monitored. Pulmonary edema may even occur after betamimetic infusion has been discontinued when the patient is receiving oral therapy. Risk factors for pulmonary edema include prolonged infusion (greater than 24 hours), subclinical chorioamnionitis, anemia, multiple gestation, persistent severe maternal tachycardia, and iatrogenic fluid overload (Benedetti, 1983). Glucocorticoid administration for fetal lung maturity has been implicated in the development of pulmonary edema, but its role remains controversial (Benedetti, 1983; Graber, 1989). Close assessment of fluid balance and pulmonary status should continue for at least 12 hours following cessation of intravenous therapy.

Beta-adrenergic stimulation causes glycogenolysis and hyperglycemia followed by hyperinsulinemia occurring within 4 hours of treatment (Caritis et al., 1983). Urine screening for glucose and ketones should occur at regular intervals. Ketoacidosis is a potential risk to patients with diabetes during betamimetic therapy, and a concomitant insulin infusion is often necessary. As a result of increased insulin secretion, potassium moves into the intracellular space during betamimetic administration causing decreased serum potassium (Graber,

1989). There is no change, however, in the body's total potassium because potassium excretion is not increased and serum potassium levels usually return to normal within 24 hours (Benedetti, 1983). Supplementation is rarely necessary unless serum potassium levels fall below 2.5 mg/100 ml (Benedetti, 1983; Graber, 1989). Gastrointestinal side effects of betamimetic therapy include nausea, vomiting, ileus, and diarrhea. Anxiety, apprehension, and restlessness are also common effects of betamimetic therapy.

Fetal effects of betamimetic therapy are related to placental transfer of the drug and maternal metabolic alterations. Fetal tachycardia and arrhythmias have been reported (Graber, 1989). Neonatal hypokalemia, hyperinsulinemia, and hypoglycemia may result if delivery occurs during a period of maternal metabolic changes due to betamimetic therapy (Caritis et al., 1988). Possible thickening of the intraventricular septum has been reported after prolonged exposure, but does not appear to be a permanent process and eventually normalizes (Caritis et al., 1988).

Magnesium Sulfate

Magnesium sulfate ($MgSO_4$) has become a widely used tocolytic agent and is often the first medication used for the treatment of PTL. Magnesium is a naturally occurring cation in the body and is necessary for numerous enzyme reactions in the body. As a tocolytic agent, $MgSO_4$ possibly acts to "suppress nerve transmission to uterine smooth muscle and by a direct effect on the myometrial cells" (Gordon & Iams, 1995). Studies regarding the tocolytic efficacy of $MgSO_4$ have demonstrated success rates similar to that of betamimetic agents (Hollander, Nagley, & Pupkin, 1987; Miller, Keane, & Horger, 1982; Thiagarajah, Harbert, & Bourgeois, 1985).

On an intracellular level, magnesium affects cAMP concentration and interferes with the transport of calcium extracellularly. The net effect is less calcium available for the actin myosin coupling necessary for muscle contraction. Magnesium competes with calcium, which is necessary for the conduction of nerve impulses and affects nerve impulse transmission by decreasing the availability of the neurotransmitter acetylcholine and by reducing the sensitivity of the motor end plate to acetylcholine. Because MgSO$_4$ is cleared from the body via kidneys, patients with impaired renal function are at risk for toxicity. Because of the effects of MgSO$_4$ on muscle contractility and nerve transmission, a history of myocardial infarction is a relative contraindication to the use of MgSO$_4$. The only absolute contraindication is maternal myasthenia gravis. The patient with this illness is already at high risk for serious respiratory compromise, and the effects of MgSO$_4$ on neurotransmission may result in respiratory arrest.

When MgSO$_4$ is used, a bolus of 4–6 g is usually given initially over 15–20 minutes followed by maintenance infusion administered at 2–6g/hour by infusion pump. Therapeutic maternal serum levels of magnesium range between 4 and 8 mg/dl (Givens, 1988) Magnesium sulfate has a lower rate of action than do the betamimetics and contractions may persist for some time before diminishing completely. If contractions resume, reinstitution of intravenous MgSO$_4$ therapy may be required.

The individual response to hypermagnesium is varied. Side effects of MgSO$_4$, although considerably less severe than those associated with betamimetic agents, are common. Neuromuscular blockage of striated muscle is responsible for feelings of lethargy and weakness. Visual blurring and headaches are also frequently experienced. Peripheral vasodilation frequently results in a generalized sensation of heat and complaints of nasal congestion. Transient hypotension may also occur. Gastrointestinal side effects including nausea and vomiting are common, and constipation may be troublesome (Dudley, Gagnon, & Varner, 1989). Paralytic ileus is rare but has been reported (Dudley et al., 1989). Pulmonary edema has been reported and is more likely to occur in women with an increased intravascular volume, such as those with multiple gestation or fluid overload.

Magnesium readily crosses the placenta resulting in fetal and neonatal hypermagnesemia. Reports on the fetal heart rate response to maternal MgSO$_4$ infusion have suggested either an increase or decrease in variability (Petri, 1981). Petrie suggested that increased variability may be due in part to increased placental perfusion with MgSO$_4$ therapy; however, loss of variability should not be assumed to be the result of MgSO$_4$ therapy but should be further investigated (Petri, 1981). Neonatal hypermagnesemia may result in a lower Apgar score with points lost for muscle tone. It has been suggested that infants born at less than 1500 gm following MgSO$_4$ therapy may have less incidence of cerebral palsy and of intraventricular hemorrhage (Nelson & Grether, 1995; Bottoms, Paul, & Iams, 1994).

Prostaglandin Inhibitors

Indomethacin functions as a prostaglandin inhibitor and is used as a tocolytic. Prostaglandins PGE$_2$ and PGF$_{2\alpha}$ (Zuckerman, Reiss, & Rubenstein, 1974) have been shown to be potent uterotonic substances capable of inducing labor (Ulmsten, 1989). Prostaglandins E$_2$ and F$_{2\alpha}$ are highly unstable, localized hormones, produced and synthesized rapidly with a short half-life. They have conflicting and counteracting effects, often producing a cascade of events that may result in the body's natural induction of labor. Prostaglandins act on uterine smooth muscle by increasing gap junctions, which in turn improve the coordination of uterine contractions. Prostaglandin synthetase inhibitors retard this action by suppressing cyclo-oxygenase, which prevents the synthesis of prostaglandins from arachidonic acid (Few, 1988; Morales, Smith, & Angel et al., 1989; Zuckerman, Shalev, Gilad, & Katzuni, 1984).

Indomethacin can be given orally or rectally as a tocolytic agent. Oral dosing is 50–100 mg as a loading dose, followed by 25–50 mg every 4–6 hours. The rectal dosage is 100–200 mg, then 25–50 mg every 4–6 hours. Indomethacin is metabolized in the liver, and partially excreted, unchanged in urine. As with other tocolytic agents, indomethacin has been shown to be effective in preventing delivery for 24–48 hours (Niebyl et al., 1980). One other study showed prolonged pregnancy beyond 7 days, although the diagnosis of preterm labor was less clear (Zuckerman et al., 1984).

The use of prostaglandin synthetase inhibitors is contraindicated in the presence of hypertensive disease of pregnancy, renal disease, peptic ulcers, aspirin sensitive allergy, and bleeding disorders (Abdella, 1986; Few, 1988). Maternal side effects include epigastric pain with or without nausea, vomiting, and dyspepsia. As a result of platelet function interference, these inhibitors can cause gastrointestinal bleeding. Cervical and placental site bleeding may occur during labor and the postpartum period because of the relaxation of the uterine muscle as well as platelet aggregation dysfunction. Long-term administration may be associated with headaches, dizziness, depression, and psychosis (Ulmsten, 1989). Uteroplacental circulatory effects are contradictory as vasoconstriction and placental bed dilation both occur.

Fetal physiologic effects of major concern include possible significant reduction in blood flow through the ductus arteriosus due to transient partial ductal narrowing. Doppler flow measurements have demonstrated a discernible reduction in blood flow through the ductus in about half of the fetuses studied (Moise, Huhta, Troffater, & Sharif, 1988). The reduction occurs 35–40 minutes after ingestion of indomethacin and is dose-related. These cardiovascular effects appear to resolve within a day of treatment cessation (Moise et al., 1988; Zuckerman et al., 1984). The sensitivity of the ductus arteriosus to oxygen-mediated closure may increase with gestational age. The use of prostaglandin synthetase inhibitors is generally limited to gestation of less than 34 weeks to minimize this risk (Niebyl & Witter, 1986).

Potential renal effects include reduced fetal urine output leading to a reduction in amniotic fluid production. Variable decelerations signaling umbilical cord compression may occur if severe oligohydramnios occurs. When indomethacin use is discontinued, amniotic fluid volume quickly returns to normal, usually within 24 hours.

Necrotizing enterocolitis (NEC) has been associated with indomethacin exposure in utero. If the indomethacin was given for more than 48 hours and less than 24 hours from delivery, the infant was most at risk for NEC (Major et al., 1994).

Calcium Channel Blockers

Nifedipine is the most commonly used calcium channel blocker for tocolysis. The mechanism of action is by inhibiting the uptake of extracellular calcium. The intracellular calcium level is, therefore, held more constant, inhibiting myosin activation and ultimately inhibiting smooth muscle contraction. Nifedipine is given by a sublingual or oral route and is rapidly absorbed. Recommendations for dosing vary in different studies. Most commonly, oral dosing includes an oral loading dose of 30 mg with maintenance dosing of 20 mg every 8 hours. Alternately, sublingual dosing of 10 mg up to four doses every 20 minutes, then 20 mg every 4–6 hours (Ray & Dyson, 1995).

The side effects of nifedipine are reported to be less than with ritodrine (Kuperminc, et al., 1993). Side effects include a slight elevation in maternal heart rate, transient hypotension, headache, flushing, nausea, and vomiting (Ferguson, Dyson, & Hollbrook, et al., 1989). Human studies of fetal effects resulting from calcium channel blockers have not revealed significant adverse outcomes.

Oxytocin Agonists

Increasing numbers of oxytocin receptor sites are present in the myometrium as labor proceeds. Oxytocin agonists like atosiban inactivate receptor sites, potentially inhibiting the effects of oxytocin (Zuckerman et al., 1984). Atosiban is being studied as to its effectiveness in humans. Preliminary studies were encouraging and investigation is underway to evaluate the effectiveness in patients with preterm labor (Besinger, Copton, & Hayasji, 1987). Side effects seem to be less than those seen with ritodrine and atosiban may be effective in combination with other tocolytics (Shubert, 1995).

Treatment of Preterm Premature Rupture of Membranes

It is well recognized that prematurity creates a multitude of potential problems for the neonate. Therefore, when PPROM occurs prior to 34 completed weeks, expectant management is usually recommended that attempts to prolong the pregnancy as long as the mother and fetus demonstrate signs of well-being. Eighty to ninety percent of all women will spontaneously begin the labor process within 48 hours of rupturing membranes. As gestational age decreases, the latency phase becomes longer. Because treatment for PTL involves the risks of bedrest, fluid administration, and tocolytic therapy, decision making for patients with PPROM must include evaluation for fetal and maternal risks. In the presence of chorioamnionitis, delivery is indicated. In the absence of infection, intrauterine management is usually attempted unless another complication becomes of primary concern.

The efficacy of prophylactic antibiotic therapy in prolonging pregnancy is less conclusive. Benefits from antibiotic therapy may include a longer latency period and somewhat lower maternal morbidity. However, the benefits to the neonate are less clear with some studies reporting an increase in hospital stays for the neonate born between 32 and 36 weeks gestation (Mercer, Crocker, Boe, & Sibai, 1993; Owens, Groome, & Mouth, 1993).

Preterm premature rupture of membranes resulting in oligohydramnios may then lead to umbilical cord compression and variable decelerations. Sonographic scans for fluid pockets, compromised intrauterine growth, and fetal breathing may be done serially. The absence of fetal breathing is associated with risk for infection (Hibbard et al., 1993; King, 1994). The amniotic fluid index (AFI) is also associated with the duration of the latency period, where when the AFI is normal (8.0 cm or greater), the latency period is often prolonged (MacMillan, Mann, Shmoys, & Saltzman, 1994). Amniocentesis may be done for serial assessment of fetal lung maturity and presence of bacteria. Once lung maturity is established, delivery may be indicated to avoid the risks of expectant management, which include maternal and/or fetal infection. Oligohydramnios, abruptio placentae, or fetal distress from cord entrapment or compression are also potential complications (Shubert, 1995). Antibiotic therapy is indicated when chorioamnionitis is diagnosed because of the risk for septicemia. Antibiotic therapy is necessary in the treatment of beta-hemolytic streptocci, Neisseria gonorrhoeae, and chlamydia trachomatis (Berkowicz et al., 1993).

Treatment with Glucocorticoid Therapy

The use of glucocorticoid therapy to enhance fetal lung maturation was a long-debated issue. The National Institute of Health held a consensus hearing in 1994 to address this issue. The efficacy of antenatal steroids has been demonstrated to decrease the incidence of respiratory distress syndrome (RDS) in gestational ages less than 32 weeks. Between 32 and 34 weeks the benefits are less evident, and beyond 34 weeks gestation the risk of RDS is so small that no clear benefit is seen with steroid use (Graber, 1989). When administering corticosteroids, the generally agreed upon dosage is a 12 mg intramuscular (IM) injection of betamethasone followed by a second 12 mg IM dose 24 hours later. The effects of this therapy are theorized to last approximately 7 days. Therefore, if a patient has not yet delivered at 7 days, the injections may be repeated to continue the benefit of this treatment. For patients with PPROM, steroids may not have as great an effect as in the patient with intact membranes, but the added potential benefits warrants use in most patients in the absence of chorioamnionitis (NIH, 1994).

FORMULATION OF NURSING DIAGNOSES

Nursing diagnoses are derived by reviewing the actual and potential problems of the woman experiencing PTL or PPROM. The diagnosis formulates a starting point on which the nursing plan of care is based. The more specific the nursing diagnosis, the more readily intervention can be planned. Nursing interventions are much more easily evaluated and revised throughout the woman's hospitalization when nursing diagnoses are specific and measurable.

The patient in preterm labor or with PPROM faces the potential for delivering a premature infant at risk for morbidity related to prematurity.

The anxiety the woman may experience in the face of her own hospitalization, loss of control of her body, and potential injury to her baby are assessed. Significant stress may be a deleterious factor in prolongation of the pregnancy.

Nursing diagnoses during tocolytic therapy also address prevention of severe maternal and fetal complications related to the specific drug use. For example, the potential for alteration in tissue perfusion during ritodrine infusion is related to severe maternal tachycardia, hypotension, myocardial ischemia, and an altered intravascular volume. Nursing interventions are directed toward resolving the individual's specific and immediate problems identified by the nursing diagnoses.

- Potential fetal injury related to prematurity
- Potential fetal injury related to PPROM or oligohydramnios
- Infection, potential for, related to PPROM
- Potential maternal–fetal injury related to infection
- Anxiety related to preterm labor and possible preterm delivery
- Fluid volume alteration: excess related to betamimetic tocolysis
- Potential alteration in tissue perfusion: cardiopulmonary, related to betamimetic tocolysis as evidenced by severe maternal tachycardia, chest pain, or tightness
- Potential metabolic alterations related to betamimetic tocolysis, hyperglycemia, and hypokalemia
- Potential for ineffective breathing patterns related to $MgSO_4$ tocolysis
- Alteration in comfort related to tocolytic side effects and preterm labor
- Alterations in maternal–family coping related to hospitalization during preterm labor or PPROM

NURSING CARE AND INTERVENTIONS

A patient admitted to the hospital for preterm labor or PPROM is placed in the lateral recum-bent position, and strict bed rest is prescribed. Initial assessment and interventions are carried out concurrently. During the initial observation period, intravenous hydration may be appropriate if contractions persist. Intake and output are monitored and documented immediately in the event tocolytic therapy is started.

It is possible that uterine activity can be stimulated by high levels of endogenous catecholamines produced during states of anxiety and fear (Niebyl, Caritis, Lipshitz, & Petrie, 1986; Sachs & Ringer, 1989). The anxious, frightened patient should be provided with a calm environment and frequent reassurance. It may be appropriate, at some point during the patient's hospitalization, to provide the patient with support from a psychologist or social worker. Historically, nurses have been aware that providing continuity of care promotes rapport and trust between patient and care giver, thus alleviating anxiety. Explanations concerning the plan of care, treatment, surveillance techniques, and expected outcome of the baby may need to be repeated once the patient's level of anxiety diminishes.

Family members need to be included in care planning. In this way they can participate in decision making and may address issues the patient has not identified, such as child care for other children at home. A well-thought-out system of support for the patient's partner may help to alleviate or decrease some of the stress.

Nursing care of the patient in preterm labor or with PPROM includes an ongoing assessment of uterine activity by palpation and/or electronic monitoring. Fetal well-being is assessed with continuous fetal heart rate monitoring or frequent auscultation.

During tocolytic therapy, nursing actions are directed toward monitoring and documenting the effects of tocolysis on uterine activity. If contractions continue despite tocolytic therapy, cervical changes and the station of the presenting part must be assessed and documented. Effective tocolysis is achieved when contractions become milder and less frequent. Six or more contractions in an hour should prompt physician notification and reevaluation of the method of tocolysis. In general, the frequency of digital cervical exams is determined by the clinical status of the mother. It is beneficial to limit such exams as much as possible as cervical manipulation can potentially stimulate prostaglandin production and uterine activity. In the presence of ruptured membranes, vaginal exams are limited because of the potential for infection. If possible, vaginal exams should be performed by the same examiner in order to detect any subtle changes in the cervix. Nursing management during tocolytic therapy includes prevention and recognition of serious adverse effects. Nursing management also includes minimization of the uncomfortable side effects related to drug administration.

The use of betamimetic agents requires vigilant nursing management during administration. Vital signs are taken at least hourly, with more frequent monitoring warranted in any patient with risk factors. Baseline tests prior to infusion therapy may include a maternal electrocardiogram, complete blood count, electrolyte level status, and urinalysis. Monitoring of the fetal heart rate and uterine activity should continue throughout the infusion.

The maternal fluid volume status is followed closely during therapy, with strict intake and output records maintained. If a urinary catheter is in place, intake and output can be assessed hourly, otherwise at least every 4 hours. The use of an infusion pump is mandatory for precise dosage administration. It is prudent to control the mainline by infusion pump to maintain accurate intake and to avoid fluid overload. Daily weight and serial hemograms also aid in assessing fluid status.

Cardiopulmonary complications of betamimetic therapy can be life-threatening; close monitoring of cardiopulmonary status is essential. Lung fields are auscultated for the presence of adventitious sounds. Continuous cardiac monitoring is recommended when maternal heart rate is greater than 120 beats per minute and whenever symptoms suggesting arrhythmias are present, such as an irregular heart rate. A maternal heart rate greater than 120, a systolic pressure less than 90 mm Hg or a diastolic pressure less than 40 mm Hg require immediate physician notification. The betamimetic infusion

is decreased or discontinued. Complaints of chest pain, shortness of breath, or any other abnormal reactions to the drug also require immediate physician notification and evaluation. The patient must be monitored for cardiopulmonary complications for 12–24 hours after the infusion has been discontinued. Monitoring includes strict intake and output assessment, auscultation of lung fields, and monitoring of vital signs. The patient receiving betamimetic tocolysis is usually restless and apprehensive, and nursing management should include comfort measures and provisions for periods of rest.

Prior to $MgSO_4$ tocolysis, a baseline assessment includes vital signs and deep tendon reflexes. Care providers are alerted to early signs of magnesium toxicity through assessments of the respiratory rate and deep tendon reflexes. A respiratory rate less than 12 per minute or absent deep tendon reflexes require immediate physician notification. A magnesium serum level is drawn and the infusion discontinued if magnesium toxicity is suspected. To reverse magnesium toxicity, calcium gluconate should be readily available. The recommended dose is 1 g of calcium gluconate (10 ml of 10% solution) administered intravenously over a 5- to 10-minute period. A physician should be present during calcium gluconate administration.

Fluid restriction is necessary to minimize the risks of pulmonary edema. A total hourly or daily intake should be clarified with the physician. The use of an infusion pump is mandatory to maintain precise control of the dosage administration and to control the mainline rate. Lung fields are auscultated for the presence of adventitious sounds. A urinary catheter is usually not necessary unless urinary retention is a problem or urinary output falls. The frequency, quality, duration, and patient perception of uterine contractions are monitored closely.

As with any tocolytic therapy, the patient receiving indomethacin requires careful monitoring for effectiveness of the therapy. Indomethacin is usually well tolerated by patients. Gastrointestinal side effects can be minimized by administering oral medication with food. Antacids may also help to relieve gastrointestinal discomfort. Fetal heart rate monitoring is specifically concerned with identifying variable decelerations, which may indicate cord compression due to reduction in amniotic fluid. Ultrasound evaluation to determine AFI may be indicated if indomethacin therapy continues for more than 48 hours.

Once the fetal membranes have ruptured, nursing management includes the continuing assessment of the patient for signs of infection. Fetal tachycardia is often the first sign of infection, but other clinical signs or symptoms include maternal tachycardia, rising temperature, fever, chills, uterine tenderness, foul-smelling vaginal discharge, and purulent vaginal or cervical discharge. Often, patients will report vague and nonspecific feelings of not feeling well. The nurse should pay attention to these subjective comments and look for progressive signs of labor or infection.

The optimal outcome for a woman in preterm labor or PPROM is to effectively prolong the pregnancy until 37 weeks gestation or fetal lung maturity is achieved. Unfortunately this is not always a realistic expectation. Although mothers experiencing preterm labor require reassurance from the healthcare team, they should never be offered false hopes if a preterm birth is inevitable.

The expected outcome for both mother and baby depends on the clinical status of the patient and estimated gestational age. The outcome for a woman in advanced labor with ruptured membranes and chorioamnionitis at 33–34 weeks gestation will be different than that for a woman at the same gestational age with intact membranes and a closed cervix. The expected outcome for the woman with ruptured membranes and chorioamnionitis might be vaginal delivery before significant maternal and fetal compromise occur. The goal of nursing care is to protect both mother and fetus from further harm through continuous maternal–fetal assessment and communication with the physician and other healthcare team members.

The ultimate goal in the treatment of preterm labor in the intrapartum setting is to prevent significant maternal and neonatal morbidity and mortality. The optimal outcome for the fetus/neonate is delaying birth until term or until lung maturity is attained. If cervical change continues, delaying the delivery until steroids are administered may be a more realistic goal than prevention of a preterm birth. Optimal maternal outcomes include protection from potential complications of tocolytic therapy, avoiding significant infection, especially following rupture of membranes, and a thorough understanding by the woman of the treatment and care she is receiving.

References

Aarimaa, T., Ekbald, U., Erbkola, R., et al. (1987). Effect of antepartum ritodrine on the cardiorespiratory status of the newborn after elective cesarean section. Gynecology and Obstetrics Investigations, 23, 160–166.

Abdella, T. (1986). A decision analytic approach to delivery of the very low birth-weight infant. Presentation to The Society of Perinatal Obstetricians, Sixth Annual Meeting, San Antonio, TX (Jan. 30–Feb. 1).

American College of Obstetricians and Gynecologists. (1988, April). Premature rupture of membranes. ACOG Technical Bulletin No. 115, Washington, DC: ACOG.

Ananth, C. V., Savitz, D. A., & Williams, M. A. (1996). Placental abruption and its association with hypertension and prolonged rupture of membranes: A methodologic review and meta analysis. Obstetrics and Gynecology, 88(2), 309–318.

Bejar, R., Curbelo, V., & Davis, D. (1981). Premature labor. II: Bacterial sources of phospholipase. Obstetrics and Gynecology, 57(4), 479–486.

Benedetti, T. J. (1983). Maternal complications of parenteral β-sympathomimetic therapy for premature labor. American Journal of Obstetrics and Gynecology, 145(1), 1–6.

Berkowicz, G. S., & Papierick, E. (1993). Epidemiology of preterm birth. Epidemiology Review, 15, 414–443.

Besinger, R. E., Copton, A. A., & Hayashi, R. H. (1987). The presence or absence of fetal breathing movements as a predictor of outcome in preterm labor. American Journal of Obstetrics and Gynecology, 157, 753–757.

Bottoms, S., Paul, R., Iams, J., et al. (1994). Obstetrical determinants of neonatal survival in extremely low birth weight infants. American Journal of Obstetrics and Gynecology, 170, 383.

Brindley, B. A., & Sokol, R. J. (1988). Induction and augmentation of labor: Basis and methods for current practice. Obstetrics and Gynecology Survey, 43(12), 730–743.

Buekens, P., Alexander, S., Boutsen, M., et al. (1994). Randomized controlled trial of routine cervical examinations in pregnancy. Lancet, 344, 841–844.

Canadian Preterm Labor Investigators Group. (1992). Treatment of preterm labor with the β-Adrenergic agonist ritodrine. New England Journal of Medicine, 327, 308–312.

Caritis, S., Darby, M., & Chan, L. (1988). Pharmacologic treatment of preterm labor. Clinical Obstetrics and Gynecology, 31(3), 635–651.

Caritis, S., Lin, L., Toig, G., & Wong, L. K. (1983). Pharmaco-dynamics of ritodrine in pregnant women during preterm labor. American Journal of Obstetrics and Gynecology, 147(7), 752–759.

Caritis, S. N., Toig, G., Heddinger, L., & Ashmead, G. (1984). A double blind study comparing ritodrine and terbutaline in the treatment of preterm labor. American Journal of Obstetrics and Gynecology, 150(1), 7–14.

Casey, M. I., & MacDonald, P. (1988). Biomolecular processes in the initiation of parturition: Decidual activation. Clinical Obstetrics and Gynecology, 31(3), 533–552.

Creasy, R., & Resnick, R. (1989). Maternal-fetal medicine: Principles and practice (2nd ed.). Philadelphia: W. B. Saunders.

Crenshaw, C. (1986). Preterm premature rupture of the membranes (Foreward). Clinical Obstetrics and Gynecology, 29(4), 735–738.

Cunningham, F. G., MacDonald, P. C., & Gant, N. F. (1989). Williams obstetrics (19th ed.), Norwalk, CT: Appleton and Lange.

Dudley, D., Gagnon, D., & Varner, M. W. (1989). Long-term tocolysis with magnesium sulfate. Obstetrics and Gynecology, 73, 373.

FDA. (1982). Use of approved drugs for unlabeled indications. Food and Drug Administration Drug Bill, 12, 4.

Ferguson, J. E., Dyson, D. C., Holbrook, R. H., et al. (1989). Cardiovascular and metabolic effects associated with nifedipine and ritodrine tocolysis. American Journal of Obstetrics and Gynecology, 161, 788–795.

Few, B. (1988). Indomethacin for treatment of premature labor. MCN, 13, 93.

Fuchs, A. R., Fuchs, F., Husslein, O., & Soloff, M. S. (1984). Oxytocin receptors in the human uterus during pregnancy and parturition. American Journal of Obstetrics and Gynecology, 150, 734-741.

Garfield, R. E., & Hayashi, R. H. (1981). Appearance of gap junctions in the myometrium of women during labor. American Journal of Obstetrics and Gynecology, 140(3), 254–259.

Givens, S. (1988). Update on tocolytic therapy in management of preterm labor. Journal of Perinatology and Neonatology, 21(1), 21–23.

Gomez, R., Galasso, M., Romero, R., Mazor, M., Sorokin, Y., Goncalves, L., & Treadwell, M. (1995). Ultrasonographic examination of the uterine cervix is better than cervical digital examination as a predictor of the likelihood of premature delivery in patients with preterm labor and intact membranes. American Journal of Obstetrics and Gynecology (1), 956–964.

Gordon, M. C., & Iams, J. D. (1995). Magnesium sulfate. Clinical Obstetrics and Gynecology, 38, 706–712.

Graber, E. (1989). Dilemmas in the pharmacological management of preterm labor. Obstetrics and Gynecology Survey, 44(7), 512–517.

Heffner, L. J., Sherman, C. B., Speezer, F. E., & Weiss, S. T. (1993). Clinical and environmental predictors of preterm labor. Obstetrics and Gynecology, 81(5), 750–757.

Hibbard, J. U., Hibbard, M. C., Ismail, M., & Arendt, E. (1993). Pregnancy outcomes after expectant management of premature rupture of the membranes in the second trimester. Journal of Reproductive Medicine, 38(12), 945–951.

Hickey, C. A., Cliver, S. P., Milvihill, F. X., McNeal, S. F., Hoffman, H. J., & Goldenberg, R. L. (1995). Employment related stress and preterm delivery: A contextual examination. Public Health Reports, 110(4), 410–418.

Hickey, T., Sivonen, A., Rukonen, O. V., Savia E., & Ylikorkala, O. (1992). Bacterial vaginosos in early pregnancy and pregnancy outcome. Obstetrics and Gynecology, 80(2), 173–177.

Hollander, D., Nagey, D., & Pupkin, M. (1987). Magnesium sulfate and ritrodrine hydrochloride: A randomized comparison. Obstetrics and Gynecology, 156(3), 631–637.

Hugby, K., Xenakis, E., & Pauerstein, C. (1993). Do tocolytic agents stop preterm labor? A critical and comprehensive review of efficacy and safety. American Journal of Obstetrics and Gynecology, 168, 1247–1259.

King, T., (1994). Clinical management of premature rupture of membranes. Journal of Nurse-Midwifery (Suppl. 2), 815–895.

Kulbride, H., Yeast, J., & Thibeault, D. (1989). Intrapartum and delivery room management of premature rupture of membranes complicated by oligohydramnios. Clinical Perinatology, 16(4), 863–888.

Kuperminc, M., Lessing, J. B., Yaron, Y., & Peyser, M. R. (1993). Niphedipine versus ritodrine for suppression of preterm labor. British Journal of Obstetrics and Gynecology, 100, 1090–1094.

Leveno, K. J., & Cunningham, F. G. (1987). Dilemmas in the management of preterm birth. In J. A. Pritchard, P. C. McDonald, & N. F. Gant (Eds.), Supplement to Williams' obstetrics (17th ed., Vol. 12). Norwalk, CT: Appleton and Lange.

Levine, C. D. (1991). Premature rupture of the membranes and sepsis in preterm neonates. Nursing Research, 40(1), 36–41.

Liggins, G. C. (1983). Initiation of spontaneous labor. Clinical Obstetrics and Gynecology, 26(1), 47–55.

Liu, D. T. Y., & Fairweather, D. I. V. (1981). The management of preterm labor. In M. G. Elder & C. H. Hendricks (Eds.), Obstetrics and gynecology: I. Preterm labor. London: Butterworth.

Lockwood, C. J. (1995). The diagnosis of preterm labor and prediction of preterm delivery. Clinical Obstetrics and Gynecology (pp. 675–687). MD: Lippincott–Raven.

MacMillan, W. E., Mann, S. E., Shmoys, S. M., & Saltzman, D. H. (1994). Amniotic fluid as a predictor of latency after preterm premature rupture of the membranes. American Journal of Perinatology, 11(4), 249–252.

Major, C. A., Lewis, D. F., Harding, J. A., et al. (1994). Tocolysis with indomethacin increased the incidence of necrotizing entercolitis in the low birthweight neonate. American Journal of Obstetrics and Gynecology, 170, 192–196.

Main, D. M., & Main, E. K. (1991). Preterm birth. In S. G. Gabbe, J. R. Niebyl, & J. L. Simpson (Eds.), Obstetrics: Normal and problem pregnancies (2nd ed., pp. 829–880). New York: Churchill Livingstone.

Mercer, B. M., Crocker, L. G., Boe, N. M., & Sibai, B. M. (1993). Induction versus expectant management in premature rupture of the membranes with mature amniotic fluid at 32 to 36 weeks: A randomized trial. American Journal of Obstetrics and Gynecology, 196(4), 775–782.

Miller, J., Keane, M., & Horger, R. (1982). A comparison of magnesium sulfate and terbutaline for the arrest of premature labor: A preliminary report. Journal of Reproductive Medicine, 27(6), 348–351.

Moise, K., Jr., Huhta, J., Troffater, K., & Sharif, D. (1988). Low dose aspirin therapy in the treatment of lupus anticoagulant: Effects on the human ductus arteriosus. Society of Perinatal Obstetricians Annual Meeting, 123.

Moore, B., Briggs, G., & Freeman, R. (1988). Terbutaline for tocolysis: Do advantages outweigh risks? Contemporary Obstetrics and Gynecology, 32(3), 53–65.

Morales, W. J., Smith, S., Angel, J. L., et al. (1989). Efficacy and safety of indomethacin versus ritodrine in the management of preterm labor: A randomized study. Obstetrics and Gynecology, 74(4), 567–572.

Nagey, D. A., & Saller, D. N. (1986). An analysis of the decisions in the management of premature rupture of the membranes. Clinical Obstetrics and Gynecology, 29, 826–834.

Nelson, K. B., & Grether, J. (1995). Can magnesium sulfate reduce the risk of cerebral palsy in very low birth weight infants? Pediatrics, 95, 263–269.

Niebyl, J. R., Blake, D. A., White, R. D., et al. (1980). The inhibition of premature labor with indomethacin. American Journal of Obstetrics and Gynecology, 136, 1014–1019.

Niebyl, J. R., Caritis, S., Lipshitz, J., & Petrie, R. (1986). Tocolytics: When and how to use them. Contemporary Obstetrics and Gynecology, 27, 146–162.

Niebyl, J. R., & Witter, F. R. (1986). Neonatal outcome after indomethacin treatment for preterm labor. American Journal of Obstetrics and Gynecology, 55, 747–749.

NIH. (1994). Report of the consensus development conference on the effects of corticosteroids for fetal maturation on perinatal outcomes. National Institute of Child Health and Human Development.

Owens, J., Groome, L. J., & Mouth, J. C. (1993). Randomized trial of prophylactic antibiotic therapy after preterm amnion rupture. American Journal of Obstetrics and Gynecology, 169(4), 976–981.

Petri, R. J. (1981). Tocolysis using magnesium sulfate. Seminars in Perinatology, 5(3), 226–273.

Ray, D., & Dyson, D. (1995). Calcium channel blockers. In R. Pithin & J. Scott (Eds.), Clinical Obstetrics and Gynecology, 38(4).

Rayburn, W. (1989). Prostaglandin E_2 gel for cervical ripening and induction of labor: A critical analysis. American Journal of Obstetrics and Gynecology, 160, 529–534.

Reese, E. A., Chervenak, F. A., Maya, F. R., & Hobbins, J. C. Amniotic fluid arborization: Effect of blood, meconium, and pH alterations. Obstetrics and Gynecology, 64, 248.

Romero, R., & Mazor, M. (1988). Infection and preterm labor. Clinical Obstetrics and Gynecology, 31(3), 533–582.

Sachs, R., & Ringer, S. (1989). Intrapartum and delivery room management of the very low birthweight infant. Clinical Perinatology, 16(4), 809–823.

Savitz, D. A., Blackimore, C. A., & Thorp, J. M. (1991). Epidemiologic characteristics or preterm delivery: Etiologic heterogenecity. American Journal of Obstetrics and Gynecology, 164, 467–471.

Shubert, P. J. (1995). Atosiban. Clinical Obstetrics and Gynecology, 38(4), 722–724.

Siega-Riz, A. M., Adair, I. S., & Hobel, C. J. (1996). Maternal underweight status and inadequate rate of weight gained during the third trimester of pregnancy increases the risk of preterm delivery. Journal of Nutrition, 126(1), 146–153.

Stubblefield, P., & Heyl, P., (1982). Treatment of preterm labor with subcutaneous terbutaline. Obstetrics and Gynecology, 59(4), 457–462.

Thiagarajah, S., Harbert, G. & Bourgeois, F. J. (1985). Magnesium sulfate and ritodrine hydrochloride: Systemic and uterine hemodynamic effects. American Journal of Obstetrics and Gynecology, 153(6), 666–674.

Toth, M., Wilkins, S., Ledger, W., & Tahler, H. (1988). The role of infection in the etiology of preterm birth. Obstetrics and Gynecology, 71(5), 723–726.

Tucker, J. M., Goldenberg, R. L., Davis, R. O., Copper, R. L., Winkler, C. L., & Hauth, J. C. (1991). Etiologies of preterm birth in an indigent population—Is prevention a logical explanation? Obstetrics and Gynecology, 343–347.

Uldbjerg, N., Ulmsten, U., & Edman, G. (1983). The ripening of the human uterine cervix in terms of connective tissue biochemistry. Clinical Obstetrics and Gynecology, 26(1), 14–25.

Ulmsten, U. (1989). Prostaglandins high risk obstetrics. In S. Brody & K. Ueland (Eds.), Endocrine disorders in pregnancy. Englewood Cliffs, NJ: Appleton Lange.

Vadillo-Ortega, F., Gonzalez-Avial, G., & Karchmer, S., et al. (1990). Collagen metabolism in premature rupture of amniotic membranes. Obstetrics and Gynecology, 75(1), 84–88.

Zuckerman, H., Reiss, U., & Rubenstein, I. (1974). Inhibition of human premature labor by indomethacin. Obstetrics and Gynecology, 44, 787–792.

Zuckerman, H., Shalen, E., Gilad, G., & Katzuni, E. (1984). Further study of the inhibition of premature labor by indomethacin (Pt. 1). Journal of Perinatal Medicine, 12, 19–29.

Zuckerman, H., Shalev, E., Gilad, G., & Katzuni, E. (1984). Further study of the inhibition of premature labor by indomethacin. Journal of Perinatology Medicine, 12, 19–23.

CHAPTER 7

Prolonged Pregnancy

Judy Schmidt

Establishment of an accurate due date is one of the most important activities of prenatal care. Despite diligent attention to obstetrical history, assessment of the patient, and the use of technology, only 50% of all pregnancies will deliver by the date expected. Approximately 90% will deliver within 2 more weeks (Campbell, Nochimson, & Vintzileos, 1993; Freeman & Lagrew, 1992). Once the official due date has passed and the patient has not delivered, family and friends may begin to show worry, the mother may become anxious, and medical personnel will begin to be concerned for fetal outcome.

Research studies conducted and improved technology implemented during the last 10 to 20 years have dramatically affected and improved methods of pregnancy dating through assessments such as ultrasound during the early gestation period, body temperature data combined with serum hCG (human chorionic gonadotrophin) testing, and early physical examination (Campbell et al., 1993; Freeman & Lagrew, 1992). As use of these dating techniques improve the accuracy of establishing gestational age and the estimated due date, the incidence of prolonged pregnancy appears to be decreasing, in part because of an actual decrease in falsely identified prolonged pregnancies. As falsely identified prolonged pregnancies decline, true prolonged pregnancies are identified.

Accurate dating is enhanced when prenatal care is sought early in pregnancy particularly within 5–12 weeks gestational age. Dating is most precise when an accurate last menstrual period date is known, a pelvic examination is performed, and an early ultrasound scan is obtained. When an ultrasound scan is obtained prior to 12 weeks gestation before the fetus begins to curve, the crown-rump length provides an accurate estimation of gestational age to within 3–5 days (Arulkumaran, 1997; Freeman & Lagrew, 1997). Although an ultrasound at 16–20 gestational weeks may provide a slightly less accurate due date, it does allow the important addition of screening for anomalies and is therefore overall the most cost-effective choice if only one ultrasound evaluation is to be obtained (Campbell et al., 1993). A biparietal diameter obtained during this time is accurate to within 5 days (Arulkumaran, 1997). Because of normal variation in fetal size, a third trimester ultrasound can vary between 3 to 4 weeks and this is therefore least reliable in prediction of estimated due date.

Definition and Incidence

The definition of *prolonged pregnancy* has remained consistent over the last several decades and is applied when the gestation reaches 294 days or 42 weeks from the first day of the last menstrual period in the woman with a 28-day menstrual cycle (Arulkumaran, 1997; Freeman & Lagrew, 1992), or alternatively, 280 days from the last ovulation (Campbell et al., 1993). The ovulation date is rarely known and more difficult to accurately determine, and its clinical value is therefore limited. Multiple terms have been used rather inconsistently to describe a late pregnancy such as postdate, postdatism, and prolonged pregnancy. Therefore, it is more meaningful to state the actual number of weeks and days of gestation (e.g., 40 5/7 weeks) until a true prolonged pregnancy of 42 weeks occurs.

In 1982, Rayburn noted that the incidence of prolonged pregnancy appeared to be declining with improved dating techniques and history (Campbell et al., 1993; Freeman & Lagrew, 1992). In 1986, Lagrew and Freeman noted that only 1–4% of all pregnancies actually exceed 42 weeks when improved dating is possible (Campbell et al., 1993), and other studies reported an overall incidence of 5–6% when an early ultrasound scan is performed (Arulkumaran, 1997; Boylan & McParland, 1991). The overall incidence of prolonged pregnancy is 3–10% depending upon the method used to date the pregnancy and the authority consulted (Arulkumaran, 1997; Ingemarsson & Heden, 1989). However, when the optimum dating history and assessment techniques are combined to corroborate each other, the true incidence is probably 1–2% (Wood, 1994). When a woman has a history of a previous prolonged pregnancy, the chance of her having a repeat prolonged pregnancy is 30–40% (Arulkumaran, 1997).

In addition to late or no prenatal care, other variables that complicate accurate dating include women who deviate significantly from the 28-day menstrual cycle with longer, shorter, or irregular cycles (Campbell et al., 1993). These women are more likely to be incorrectly classified as having prolonged pregnancies, especially if the gestational age derived from the last menstrual period (LMP) was not confirmed by an early physical exam or ultrasound scan. Additionally, 20–40% of all women studied cannot remember the date of their LMP or their date of conception (Ingemarsson & Heden, 1989). Because of normal cycle variation and inatten-

tion to the timing of menstrual periods, it has become important to use early ultrasound and to improve the accuracy of this technology to more precisely determine gestational age.

Maternal and Fetal Morbidity and Mortality

After reaching term gestation at 40 weeks, the overall fetal mortality rate of 1–2% begins to increase (Campbell, Nochimson, & Vintzileos, 1993). By 42 weeks the rate doubles (Freeman & Lagrew, 1997), by 43 weeks it increases fourfold, and by 44 weeks the mortality rate is 3 to 7 times higher than at term (Campbell et al., 1993). When there is evidence of placental insufficiency and the associated neonatal physical characteristics of postmaturity syndrome are present, the mortality rate leaps to 36% (Arulkumaran, 1997; Campbell et al., 1993). Morbidity also increases exponentially as gestation exceeds 40 weeks, especially in the presence of additional complications and risk factors (Arulkumaran, 1997; Freeman & Lagrew, 1997) such as placental insufficiency, macrosomia, congenital anomalies, and meconium aspiration.

Fetal morbidity and mortality is generally attributed to placental pathology, found in 20–40% of all prolonged pregnancy fetal deaths (Campbell, Nochimson, & Vintzileos, 1993). When prolonged pregnancy antepartum deaths were studied, evidence of chronic hypoxia was found in 60–70% of cases (Campbell, Nochimson, & Vintzileos, 1993). The postmature fetus experiencing chronic hypoxia from a dysmature placenta will be less able to tolerate a superimposed acute hypoxic episode without experiencing some type of morbidity. Although placental pathology due to a prolonged pregnancy can lead to problems, the placenta, which remains efficient during this time, continues to provide fetal nutrition and growth during the period following 40 weeks and may result in a macrosomic infant with the risks of traumatic labor and delivery. Hence, the consequence of experiencing a prolonged pregnancy depends upon placental function, which may take one of two pathways. Either the placenta continues to function well and may lead to *macrosomia* and the risks of birth trauma (Campbell et al., 1993), or there may be evidence of *postmaturity syndrome,* which includes a degenerating placenta, inadequate nutrition and growth retardation, oligohydramnios, inadequate fetal oxygenation, meconium staining, and fetal distress. Under either circumstance, a consequence of prolonged pregnancy may include meconium aspiration (Campbell et al., 1993), which will be discussed further in this chapter.

Common Findings

Several studies have continued the search for commonalities among women and neonates experiencing prolonged pregnancies by comparing pregnancy histories and physical findings with a control group. Most studies confer that women with prolonged pregnancies experienced a lower parity, higher maternal weight at delivery, higher blood pressure (Eden, Seifert, Wineger, & Spellacy, 1987), and were more often hypertensive and diabetic (Eden, Seifert, Wineger, & Spellacy, 1988). Their infants were heavier than the control group (Kassis, Mazor, Leiberman, Cohen, & Insler, 1991) and had more shoulder dystocia, lower apgar scores, more meconium staining and meconium aspiration syndrome (MAS), more congenital malformations, and higher mortality rates (Eden et al., 1987).

Common etiologies of prolonged pregnancy have been proposed and include estrogen secretion deficiency accompanied by a continuation of progesterone secretion and an absence of oxytocin and prostaglandins (MacMullen, Brucker, & Zwelling, 1997; Moran, McGarrigle, & Lachelin, 1992). An adrenal corticosteroid deficiency has long been associated with prolonged pregnancy, and thyroid disorders are known to change the endocrine secretion and alter the duration of pregnancy (Wood, 1994). One small study explored a connection between corticosteroid treatment and an observed increase in postmaturity syndrome (Grudev, 1990). Prolonged pregnancy can also be associated with congenital anomalies such as anencephaly, trisomy 18, or similar central nervous system malformations, which appear in 9% of cases (Ahn & Phelan, 1989). Placental sulfatase deficiency has long been associated with prolonged pregnancy. Fraidakis, Dalamanga, Mantzauvinos, Gargaropoulos, and Zourlas (1991) found that the fetal fibronectin concentration in maternal plasma was decreased in prolonged pregnancies during the third trimester, at delivery, and on day 3 postpartum. This finding provides implications for future study of fetal fibronectin as a marker for prolonged pregnancy.

Complications

One of the earliest problems associated with prolonged pregnancy may be the emotional strain that often begins with impatience when a pregnant woman's due date has come and gone and labor is not imminent. This stress may be followed by frustration, fatigue, depression, and added aggravation from the physical discomfort of pregnancy. The mother may worry about the infant's safety. As prenatal visits continue, discussions will occur between patient and care providers regarding the possible methods and outcomes of different management alternatives. These events impact in a cumulative fashion upon the mother and may at some point seem emotionally insurmountable to her (MacMullen et al., 1997; Campbell et al., 1993). Allowing the mother to express her feelings and helping her to understand they are expected and normal are very important.

Macrosomia and Shoulder Dystocia

The most frequent and often overlooked fetal and neonatal complication of prolonged pregnancy, macrosomia, arises when the placenta continues to provide adequate nutrients, thereby allowing growth of the fetus after 40 weeks. The definition of macrosomia differs from one expert to another and varies between 4.0 and 4.5 kilograms. Approximately one fourth of all prolonged pregnancies will result in fetal macrosomia (Freeman & Lagrew, 1997; MacMullen et al., 1997) compared to an incidence 4–6% in pregnancies between 38 and 40 weeks (Chervenak, Zivan, Hirsch, Girz, & Langer, 1989). Fetal macrosomia is associated with prolonged labor, shoulder dystocia, birth trauma, cephalopelvic disproportion, and cesarean delivery (Freeman & Lagrew, 1992; MacMullen et al., 1997). See Figure 7-1 for the sequence of complications related to macrosomia.

Although improvements in technology and knowledge during the past two decades have led to a decrease in the incidence of macrosomia and subsequent birth trauma, the morbidity and mortality rates for macrosomic infants of prolonged pregnancies still remain higher than for infants at term (Beckmann, 1990). A traumatic delivery of a macrosomic infant most often results from attempts to deliver the broad fetal shoulders. When shoulder dystocia occurs, the anterior shoulder lodges under the symphysis pubis. Delivery strategies employed to solve this physics problem include gentle suprapubic pressure, various types of manual rotation, and manipulation of the mother's position (e.g., McRoberts' maneuver or squatting). Shoulder dystocia and the application of maneuvers to deliver the baby may lead to brachial palsy, a fractured clavicle or humerus, and delayed delivery of the fetal body. Brachial palsies may involve a range of injuries from a temporary weakness to permanent paralysis. When delivery of the body is delayed, hemodynamics of blood flow are hindered and the lack of adequate blood flow does not permit adequate oxygen transfer during delivery. The newborn may suffer short- or long-term effects of hypoxia and possibly acidosis. Neuropsychiatric dysfunctions may result. See Display 7-1 for possible newborn sequelae of macrosomic delivery.

When prolonged pregnancy is accompanied by a large infant, there is a greater maternal risk of *prolonged labor* and *trauma* during a vaginal birth (usually associated with delivery of the fetal shoulders), including *lacerations, postpartum hemorrhage*, and *sepsis* (Arulkumaran, 1997; Freeman & Lagrew, 1997). Maternal intrapartum morbidity arises from an aftermath of localized birth trauma following an attempted and/or successful vaginal delivery. Wounds and lacerations of the birth canal vary in their extent and include cervical and vaginal lacerations and episiotomy extensions (Freeman & Lagrew, 1992). In addition, excessive pressure applied during McRoberts maneuver (in which the legs are flexed and pushed toward the mother's body with assistance) may stretch the femoral nerve and lead to a subsequent neuropathy, which interferes with motor function of the affected leg. Hemorrhage is usually related to the magnitude of birth trauma as well as the swiftness and effectiveness of treatment. An overly distended uterus may contribute to postpartum hemorrhage when the previously stretched uterine muscles become hypotonic and incapable of maintaining the uterine tone necessary for constriction of blood vessels at the placental implantation site. Maternal sepsis risks increase when tissue is traumatized and poorly perfused in a patient with already decreased compensatory responses.

Placental Insufficiency

Although macrosomia results from an adequately functioning placenta, there are complications of prolonged pregnancy that reflect placental dysfunction. These problems occur less frequently than macrosomia, but may lead to serious complications. The placenta is an organ designed to support the fetus for 40 weeks by circulating and exchanging life-sustaining nutri-

Figure 7-1.   Sequence of complications related to macrosomia.

Adequate placental function → Adequate fetal oxygenation and uteroplacental blood flow → nutritional transfer → continued fetal growth → macrosomia, 4–4.5 kg. or greater → risks of prolonged labor + newborn birth trauma + maternal birth trauma + cephalopelvic disproportion + cesarean delivery

DISPLAY 7-1

Possible Newborn Sequelae of Macrosomic Delivery

Birth Trauma

- Brachial plexus injury: temporary, permanent, partial, or complete
- Erb–Duchenne palsy—involves upper arm
- Klumpke's palsy—involves lower arm
- Facial nerve palsy
- Fractured clavicle or humerus

Hypoxic Compromise

- Mild hypoxia without permanent sequelae
- Hypoxic Ischemic Encephalopathy (HIE)
- Neuropsychiatric dysfunction, mild to severe
- Fetal demise

ents, oxygen, and other substances (MacMullen et al., 1997). At 36 weeks the placenta reaches peak function (Campbell et al., 1993), and by 38 weeks there are signs of normal deterioration. Microscopic breaks and infarcts appear in the placental villi and progress to larger placental infarcts that are clearly visible on the placenta. This inhibits not only transfer of nutrients and other substances but also prevents normal gaseous exchange between maternal and fetal

compartments. By 42 weeks the ability of the placenta to support fetal life until spontaneous labor occurs is questionable. In the presence of an aging placenta, the infant may exhibit the same physical findings of placental insufficiency (Kabler & Delmore, 1997). A small, deteriorating placenta may deprive the fetus of nutrients, causing it to use and even deplete subcutaneous fat and liver energy stores (Freeman & Lagrew, 1992). Ultrasound reports may reflect an absence of fetal growth or even a loss of fetal weight due to dwindling placental function.

Although the etiology of *oligohydramnios* is not fully understood, amniotic fluid volume decreases normally with advancing gestational age. The maximal volume of amniotic fluid occurs at 34 weeks and declines thereafter. As the placenta deteriorates, the amniotic fluid volume also diminishes and may lead to oligohydramnios. When the normal volume of amniotic fluid swallowed by the fetus is decreased, fetal urine production also falls (Trimmer, Levens, Peters, & Kelly, 1990). The decrease in amniotic fluid volume is gradual from 34–40 weeks and accelerates after 41–42 weeks. However, several cases of oligohydramnios have been documented within 24 hours of a normal amniotic fluid volume assessment in prolonged pregnancy (Clement, Schifrin, & Kates, 1987). With the decrease in amniotic fluid and thinning of the umbilical cord as its surrounding Wharton's jelly deteriorates, the risk of umbilical cord compression increases (Campbell et al., 1993). See Figure 7-2 for the sequences of physiologic changes related to placental insufficiency.

As the compression restricts blood flow to and from the fetus, the hemodynamic changes

Figure 7-2.   Sequence of physiologic changes related to placental insufficiency.

Placental deterioration ⟶ Decreased AFV ⟶ Cord compression ⟶ Fetal hypoxia ⟶ vagal reflex ⟶ meconium release ⟶ meconium staining ⟶ MAS

Placental deterioration ⟶ Inadequate maternal-fetal circulation ⟶ Nutritional deficiency ⟶ growth restriction ⟶ inadequate respiratory ability ⟶ hypoxia OR, hypoxic episodes related to uterine contractions—late decelerations ⟶ asphyxia, acidosis ⟶ neurologic sequelae of newborn

stimulate fetal baroreceptors and chemoreceptors, leading to variable decelerations of the fetal heart rate triggered by the parasympathetic nervous system. Continued placental deterioration may progress from nutritional deprivation to inadequate oxygenation of the fetus either episodically or continuously and can result in late decelerations. The continuously hypoxic fetus will not exhibit the normal interplay between the parasympathetic and sympathetic nervous systems, which appears on the fetal heart monitor as decreased fetal heart rate variability. The diminished variability may signal an acidotic fetus and may be observed in association with late decelerations, repetitive variable decelerations, or bradycardia. Tachycardia with diminished variability may signal a compensatory response to chronic hypoxia. Recognition of these observed changes and an understanding of their significance become paramount during the intrapartum period. Antepartum fetal surveillance is discussed in a later section of this chapter.

Postmaturity Syndrome

When the placenta lacks the ability to support the fetus of a prolonged pregnancy, characteristic symptoms occur. These symptoms reflect the extent and duration of placental insufficiency and are referred to as postmaturity syndrome. This syndrome appears in 2–6% of the total number of all pregnancies, 3% of term pregnancies, and 20–40% of prolonged pregnancies more than 42 weeks. Approximately 10% of infants more than 43 weeks gestation will be small for gestational age (Freeman & Lagrew, 1992). In these postmature syndrome infants, it is common to observe the characteristics of growth retardation: a loss of subcutaneous tissue mass; a body that appears long and thin; parched, dry, cracked, and loose appearing skin; thick, long hair; long nails; an alert, wide-eyed appearance; and yellow staining of the skin, umbilical cord, and placenta. See Figure 7-3. Any of the protective vernix caseosa that remains may also be stained yellow (Campbell et al., 1993; Kabler & Delmore, 1997; Freeman & Lagrew, 1997; MacMullen et al., 1997). In classic literature from the 1950s, observations reported by Clifford describe the postmaturity infant as "fragile, withered, meconium-stained with long nails" (Freeman & Lagrew, 1992). See Figure 7-4. Clifford also identified three stages of fetal dysmaturity or postmaturity syndrome, including the usual appearance of growth restriction, loss of vernix caseosa and skin maceration, long nails, and alert appearance at birth, but no meconium. In stage II there is meconium cov-

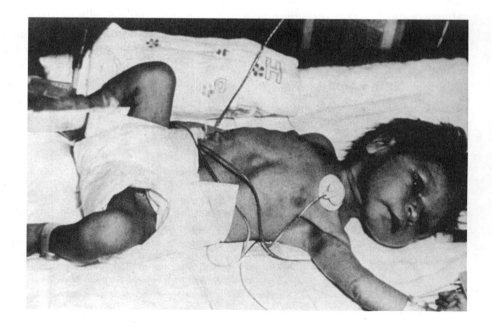

Figure 7-3. Postmature infant at two days of age showing increased alertness, decreased subcutaneous fat, and long hair.

ering the skin, placenta, and umbilical cord, which is believed to be the cause of an anoxic event. The highest mortality rate of 50% occurred in stage II, compared with an overall rate of 36%. In stage III the mortality rate drops to 15% and the nails and skin are stained yellow (Campbell et al., 1993).

Meconium-staining of amniotic fluid occurs in 25–30% of all prolonged pregnancies. This is twice the rate for term pregnancies. Meconium occurs from one of two causes: either hypoxic events or maturity of the fetus with vagal reflex (Freeman & Lagrew, 1992). Fresh meconium is more likely to be the result of acute fetal hypoxia, and when combined with oligohydramnios, may become thick and increases the risk of MAS (Beckmann, 1990). Fresh meconium occurs more frequently following umbilical cord compression, impairment of maternal–fetal blood flow, and the resulting hypoxia (Campbell et al., 1993). The timing of meconium excretion has been correlated with the degree of meconium staining. The amnion, umbilical cord, and nails take 3–6 hours to become saturated and yellow-stained, while staining of the vernix takes about 14 hours (Campbell et al., 1993). See Figure 7-5.

Although hypoglycemia, heat instability, and polycythemia are often listed as complications of the prolonged pregnancy (Freeman & Lagrew, 1992; MacMullen et al., 1997; Mannino, 1988), they may not be related to gestational age, but rather to fetal and neonatal status (Beckmann, 1990). These complications cannot be evaluated during the antepartum period but occur in the neonate.

Antepartum Fetal Surveillance

Antepartum testing is indicated when gestation exceeds 41 weeks. The intent of testing is to establish a baseline and thereby detect those few cases of compromise that will arise, and to improve morbidity and mortality outcomes (Bochner, Medearis, Davis, Oakes, Hobe, & Wade, 1987; Campbell et al., 1993; Guidetti, Divon, & Langer, 1989). Antepartum tests used in clinical practice vary from simple counting of fetal movements to more sophisticated measurements using advanced technology. Each test has its purpose, and choice of method varies with the practitioner and the clinical situation.

Fetal Movement Counts

The most basic test of counting fetal movements is accomplished in an outpatient setting by the mother. The mother is generally instructed to observe and count fetal movements or "kick counts" twice per day. Some women are able to

Figure 7-4. Postmature infant with characteristic long nails and peeling, wrinkled skin.

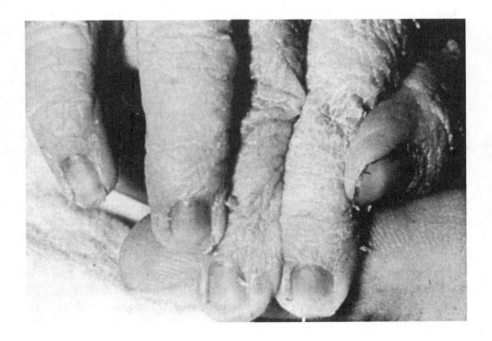

Figure 7-5. Postmature infant with meconium staining, immediately after birth.

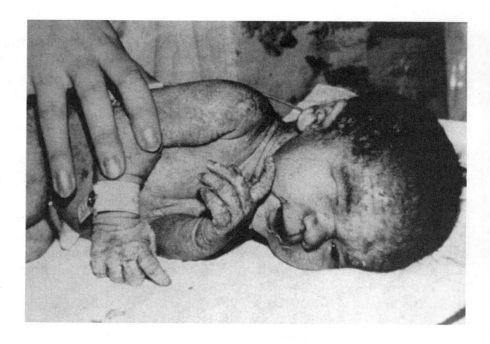

do this easily whereas others may have difficulty accurately perceiving fetal movement. The practice of counting fetal movements has not been specifically studied and validated among women with prolonged pregnancy. Its value in establishing fetal well-being is therefore questionable.

Fetal Heart Monitoring and Ultrasound Scanning

Various antepartum assessment tests and combinations of tests are preferred by care providers. Common practice includes semiweekly *nonstress testing* along with an *amniotic fluid volume (AFV) assessment* or a weekly *contraction stress test* with AFV assessment or *biophysical profile* (BPP) testing. Numerous studies have reported the significant predictive value of each testing scheme for prolonged pregnancy (Freeman & Lagrew, 1992). When variable decelerations are present that either exceed the parameters of 15 beats below the baseline with a duration of at least 15 seconds or accompany a baseline variability of less than 5 beats, the mortality rate increases to 15/1,000 (Arulkumaran, 1997; Benedetti & Easterling, 1988). Although late decelerations are the most significant fetal heart rate finding that cause concern regarding fetal well-being, they occur far less frequently than variable decelerations among patients with

prolonged pregnancy (Campbell et al., 1993; Leveno, 1986). A management dilemma occurs when variable decelerations are the only nonreassuring finding of fetal assessment.

Although testing preferences occur in clinical practice, Druzin, Karver, Wagner, Hutson, Waltner, and Kogut, (1992) found that one test does not have a significantly improved outcome over another. Studies are currently ongoing that may clarify the usefulness of one or a combination of antepartum tests for prolonged pregnancy versus others (Kabler & Delmore, 1997). Techniques coming into use may include computer analysis of the fetal heart rate, fetal pulse oximetry, ST segment analysis, magnetic resonance, and positron emission tomography scanning (Parer, 1997). As parameters are established that have reliable predictive value for prolonged pregnancies, these techniques may be increasingly used (Bartnicki, Ratanasiri, Meyenburg, & Saling, 1992).

Amniotic fluid volume changes throughout pregnancy in relationship to gestational age, peaking at 34 weeks gestation with a volume of 800–1200 ml. A gradual decline occurs between 34 weeks and term when the volume at term reaches 500–1000 ml (Schmidt, 1997). After 40 weeks AFV decreases approximately 30% per week (Eden et al., 1988). When the AFV decreases more than 50%, has a volume score less than 5 cm with vertical pockets less than 2 cm, risks for the fetus increase. *Oligohydramnios* is defined as an AFV less than 5 centimeters, whereas a 5–8 cm volume is considered borderline (Freeman & Lagrew, 1992). Eden and colleagues (1988) found that 11.5% of prolonged pregnancies have oligohydramnios compared with an incidence of less than 1% among all pregnancies (Freeman & Lagrew, 1992). Vertical pocket measurements less than 2–3 cm are predictive of fetal distress, cesarean delivery, and a higher rate of perinatal mortality (Campbell et al., 1993). (Note: Normal AFV ≥ 8 centimeters with vertical pockets ≥ 3 centimeters.) The decrease in amniotic fluid volume signals not only declining placental function but also a decrease in the liquid cushion in which the umbilical cord floats. The umbilical cord requires adequate fluid volume for protection from compression and decreased perfusion. The vagal response that often follows cord compression increases the risk of meconium release. The release of meconium into decreased amniotic fluid contents is more likely to result in thick meconium, and subsequent MAS. Vertical pocket measurement alone is rarely used to determine management and is usually used in combination with other tests to predict fetal status and need for delivery.

Doppler Flow Measurement

Various Doppler measurements provide yet another method of fetal assessment. Although its routine use is still controversial, studies have reported the value of measuring the fetal internal carotid artery pulsatility index, the descending thoracic arterial flow, the umbilical arterial flow, and umbilical arterial waveforms. Specific findings related to prolonged pregnancy include: (a) use of an umbilical arterial flow systolic/diastolic ratio cutoff of 2.4 instead of 3.0 to predict pregnancies at high risk for an abnormal outcome (Fisher, Kulhman, Depp, & Wapner, 1991); (b) combination of umbilical arterial absence of end-diastolic pressure with AFV changes to predict fetal distress in the first stage of labor (Pearce & McParland, 1991); (c) correlation of reduction in velocity of the descending thoracic

artery with oligohydramnios, meconium, nonreactive NST, and cesarean delivery (Battaglia, Larocca, Lanzani, Coukos, & Genazzani, 1991); and (d) a 20% increase in the pulsatility index of the internal carotid fetal artery in the presence of maternal hyperoxygenation is predictive of fetal distress, meconium, and lower apgars (Arduini, Rizzo, Romanini, & Mancuso, 1990).

Management Options

There is significant controversy regarding whether either the continued use of antepartum testing or induction of labor in prolonged pregnancy is advised, particularly when the cervix is unripe and no other risks are present. When the cervix is ripe and gestational age is past 41 weeks, most clinicians will opt for induction of labor (Freeman & Lagrew, 1992). A large Canadian study described morbidity and mortality among two management approaches of prolonged pregnancy: induction and serial antepartum testing. The two groups had similar outcomes except for a lower cesarean section rate (21.2%) among the induction group compared to the antepartum testing group (24.5%) (Hannah, 1990). Another similar study reported a fourfold increase in neonatal intubations among the antepartum testing group (Herabutya, Prasertsawat, Tongyai, & Isarangwin Na Ayudthya, 1992). These findings led to the recommendation that there is probably no advantage in allowing pregnancy to progress past 42–43 weeks (Campbell et al., 1993; Freeman & Lagrew, 1992; Herabutya et al., 1992). In many centers, labor is routinely induced in patients who have reached 41 gestational weeks regardless of status of cervical ripeness.

Two recent studies report success in utilizing *membrane stripping* or *sweeping* beginning near term and continuing regularly until delivery. Study groups revealed dilation upon admission exceeded 4 cm three times more often and spontaneous delivery occurred twice as often as the control group. In each study the experimental groups experienced a lower rate of infection. The group that benefitted the most from membrane stripping was the nulliparous group with a low Bishop score (el-Torkey & Grant, 1992; McColgin et al., 1990).

When the cervix remains unripe in the prolonged pregnancy, ripening agents followed by induction are generally recommended (Dyson, Miller, & Armstrong, 1987; Dyson, 1988; Papageorgiou, Tsionou, Minaretzis, Michalas, & Aravantinos, 1992). Ripening increases the success of induction of labor and reduces the incidence of complications such as fetal distress, macrosomia, postmaturity syndrome, meconium aspiration syndrome, and cesarean delivery (Freeman & Lagrew, 1992). Induction of labor in a nulliparous patient with an unripe cervix (Bishop score less than six) results in a doubled cesarean section rate compared with the general population (Arulkumaran, 1997; Freeman & Lagrew, 1992). Outpatient serial ripening (e.g., using low-dose prostaglandin in· pregnancy exceeding 41 weeks) has been used with moderate success in preparing the cervix for induction and labor (Sawai, Williams, Angel, Mastrogiannis, & Johnson, 1991).

Antepartum Care

The discomforts of pregnancy and a large uterus may become cumbersome and difficult during prolonged pregnancy. Comfort measures may help substantially and may include adding a small pillow between the knees and under the patient's abdomen to decrease pull on the hip area and round or broad ligaments while side-lying. The normal respiratory changes of pregnancy, along with enlarged uterine contents, challenge respirations. Breathing and digestion is often easier during resting when the head is elevated to a degree of comfort (Campbell et al., 1993). Digestion can also be assisted when small amounts of food are eaten frequently rather than consuming three large meals a day. For sore ligaments or joints, the application of heat should be included. While sitting or standing, dependent edema of the lower limbs in a prolonged pregnancy may be both uncomfortable and bothersome. Elevating the legs slightly to a degree of comfort will serve to aid circulation, decrease swelling, and prevent aching. The mother should be questioned about other physical discomforts and strategies applied to increase comfort, provide support, and encourage coping ability.

While awaiting labor and delivery, serial antepartum tests are likely to be employed. Teaching the pregnant woman both the purpose and technique of performing fetal movement counts while at home not only serves to enhance fetal assessment, but also provides reassurance (Campbell et al., 1993). Compliance may increase and anxiety lessen when all tests are explained before and during care, whether in an office, clinic, or a hospital. When fetal movement decreases, membranes rupture, or labor begins, the mother may be more likely to go to the hospital for close surveillance as instructed. The mother who has been taught about the early detection and treatment of symptoms of fetal compromise related to prolonged pregnancy may thereby assist in improving her outcome (Campbell et al., 1993).

Reinforcing and clarifying information given by the primary care provider is a predominant nursing function. It is helpful to know what information has been communicated to the patient either by being present during discussion or by obtaining pertinent information from the care provider or medical record. When a pregnant woman reaches term with an unripe cervix and no signs of prodromal labor, additional patient counseling is indicated, including information regarding the options of conservative management, cervical ripening, and/or induction procedures. The risks and benefits of continued surveillance or induction particular to the patient's status should be discussed. A woman with a 42-week pregnancy and an unripe cervix is unlikely to be advised to wait for spontaneous cervical ripening and labor. However, the same plan would be a reasonable choice for a woman with a 40-week pregnancy. A study of 500 pregnant women revealed that even though most women preferred conservative management before reaching term, at 41–42 weeks only one third wanted to continue with conservative management. Many women may want to deliver even though the results of antepartum testing procedures are negative for fetal risk (Roberts & Young, 1991) and the cervix is unripe, making successful induction of labor less likely.

Intrapartum Considerations

At a gestation greater than 42 weeks, 80% of pregnant women have an unripe cervix that necessitates the use of cervical ripening agents prior to or in lieu of oxytocin induction (Freeman & Lagrew, 1992). Cervical ripening agents have increased the success of induction of labor among these patients while decreasing the need for amniotomy, and decreasing post-partum sepsis and cesarean section rates (Freeman & Lagrew, 1992). When the fetus is macrosomic, the risk of labor progress becoming protracted and arrested is 22%; if the fetus is not macrosomic, the risk is 10% (Chervenak, Divon, Hirsch, Girz, & Langer, 1989). Poor uterine contractions often occur with fetopelvic disproportion (Arulkumaran, 1997), probably due to either interference with muscle coordination and effectiveness or pelvic obstruction of uterine effort. A prolonged first stage of labor and slow descent during the second stage with a fetal caput and molding is indicative of shoulder dystocia and a difficult or traumatic delivery (Arulkumaran, 1997). There is also a reported increase of uterine dysfunction in primigravid prolonged pregnancies unrelated to the size of the fetus or use of induction of labor techniques (Freeman & Lagrew, 1992; Boyd, Usher, McLean, & Kramer, 1988). In such cases, endocrine feedback mechanisms, neurological function, and actions on the cellular level of muscle cells may be problematic. One effective means to achieving a successful labor is preparation of the uterus through cervical ripening techniques.

Cervical Ripening

Prior to administering cervical ripening agents, the fetal heart rate and uterine activity should be assessed. If abnormal uterine activity or fetal heart patterns are noted, the planned ripening procedures may be curtailed. Currently available prostaglandin E_1 and E_2 ripening agents include Cervidil (dinoprostone insert), Prepidil (dinoprostone gel), Cytotec (misoprostil), and gel extemporaneously prepared in hospital pharmacies. Mechanical agents such as hygroscopic dilators are sometimes used, especially

when chemical agents such as prostaglandin are contraindicated. Serial membrane sweeping is recommended by some experts as a successful cervical ripening strategy and enhancement to labor progress.

Following administration of the ripening agent, the fetal heart and uterine activity are observed continuously for 2 hours (Freeman & Lagrew, 1992). If there are fetal heart decelerations, elevated baseline rate, poor variability, and frequent or prolonged uterine contractions, these findings are reported and suitable nursing and medical actions are taken. After 6–12 hours the cervix usually ripens adequately and the induction protocol may be initiated. If the cervix does not ripen, a second dose of cervical ripening agent may be administered before the induction is begun.

Intrapartum Surveillance and Care

Upon presentation for suspected labor, induction, or cervical ripening, the nurse does the following: carefully review the maternal antepartum and intrapartum history (Freeman & Lagrew, 1992); obtain a baseline fetal heart tracing and assess fetal status and uterine activity; maintain maternal position, such as lateral, which promotes uteroplacental perfusion; encourage comfort measures; and communicate with the patient's family regarding labor progress and fetal status (MacMullen et al., 1997). The nurses' role includes promoting a tranquil atmosphere, providing clear information and instruction to the patient and her coach, and furnishing the needed encouragement and reassurance. See Table 7-1.

During labor, close and continuous fetal surveillance and labor progress are usually recommended using a spiral electrode and intrauterine pressure catheter whenever possible (MacMullen et al., 1997); however, it is also recommended that when there are no risk factors or abnormal findings added to the prolonged pregnancy status, electronic fetal monitoring may be intermittent for 20–30 minutes every 2 hours (Arulkumaran, 1997). The methods and techniques selected for fetal surveillance should follow institutional protocols that also reflect

Table 7-1. Nursing Assessment of the Patient with Prolonged Pregnancy

Assessment of Prenatal Information

I. Reliability of gestational age
   A. Date of pregnancy documentation
      1. Accurate last menstrual period
      2. Body temperature charting plus hCG level
   B. Early prenatal exam
   C. Early ultrasound scan

II. Maternal and fetal risk factors
   A. History of prolonged pregnancy
   B. Fetal anomalies
   C. History of diabetes and macrosomia
   D. History of postmaturity syndrome

III. Antepartum surveillance
   A. Measurement trends of fundal height
   B. Maternal perception of recent fetal movements
   C. NST/CST
   D. Biophysical profile
   E. Amniotic fluid assessment: volume, vertical pockets
   F. Doppler flow

Intrapartum Assessment

Maternal Factors

I. History/events reviewed
   A. Membrane status
   B. Contraction onset
   C. Other symptoms

II. Status of cervix and station on admission

III. Uterine activity
   A. Frequency
   B. Intensity
   C. Duration
   D. Resting tone

IV. Knowledge and understanding of procedures and status
   A. Positions
   B. Surveillance
   C. Comfort
   D. Support

V. Parturition status
   A. Progress of labor descent, dilation
   B. Lacerations
   C. Blood loss

Fetal Factors

I. FHR
   A. Baseline characteristics
      1. Rate
         a. Tachycardia
         b. Bradycardia
      2. Variability
      3. Acceleration of FHR
   B. Periodic changes
      1. Late decelerations
      2. Variable and prolonged decelerations

II. Amniotic fluid
   A. Volume and vertical pockets
   B. Color, consistency, amount

III. Status during delivery
   A. Undetected meconium
   B. Fetal descent
   C. Delivery of shoulders

national standards. In addition to lateral maternal positioning, it is important to have oxygen readily available for maternal administration should nonreassuring fetal heart patterns occur (MacMullen et al., 1997). Maternal hyperoxygenation increases the maternal–fetal oxygen concentration gradient and promotes oxygen transfer within the intervilli spaces.

When caring for the patient who is undergoing induction of labor for prolonged pregnancy, the risk factors related to uterine hyperstimulation and fetal heart rate abnormalities are considered and close, competent observation becomes prerequisite. Depending upon the severity of these problems, the nurse may need to decrease or discontinue uterotonic agents such as oxytocin and possibly be prepared to administer tocolytic drugs such as terbutaline. The mother should also be assessed frequently for dehydration, infection, and exhaustion. As labor progresses it is essential to assess fetal descent and look for engagement of the vertex. Noting when these processes fail to occur improves early identification of a prolonged labor or cephalopelvic disproportion, and may help to avoid or anticipate shoulder dystocia, birth trauma, maternal exhaustion and dehydration, and other intrapartum-related complications (Freeman & Lagrew, 1992). Also, noting abnormal labor patterns will help to identify the ineffective uterine contractions of a protracted labor, especially in the uterus distended by a macrosomic fetus. In addition to protracted labor, hyperstimulation is reported to occur more frequently in the prolonged pregnancy with fetal macrosomia (Freeman & Lagrew, 1992).

Management of Meconium-Stained Amniotic Fluid

The presence of meconium-stained amniotic fluid alone presents a risk for MAS but may be more concerning when fetal heart abnormalities, maternal hypotension, or hyperstimulation are also present. To decrease the incidence and morbidity associated with variable decelerations as well as thick meconium-stained fluid, *amnioinfusion therapy* has been shown to be effective. With any combination of decreased amniotic fluid, thick meconium staining, and variable or prolonged decelerations, the nurse should anticipate enacting protocols for amnioinfusion during the intrapartum period. At the time the fetal head delivers, suctioning of the nasopharynx is implemented immediately and resuscitation protocols are employed as needed. Even though meconium may have been unobserved during the intrapartum period, it may appear at delivery, especially when oligohydramnios complicates its identification. When both meconium-stained fluid and an abnormal fetal heart rate tracing are present, the risk of MAS and neonatal hypoxia increases (Arulkumaran, 1997).

The availability of suction, resuscitation equipment, and other experts for neonatal care at delivery should be anticipated. The need for neonatal bronchial lavage following a delivery with meconium-stained amniotic fluid is utilized when indicated. It is recommended that a chest x-ray be evaluated when any symptoms of respiratory distress are noted (Kabler & Delmore, 1997).

Postdelivery Care

The appropriate postdelivery care for the mother is determined by multiple factors such as mode of delivery, complications, emotional status, teaching needs, and anticipated length of stay. A mother who experiences a vaginal delivery without complications and delivers a healthy infant may require routine postpartum care, while a mother who experiences pelvic trauma, postpartum blood loss, and prepares to care for an infant who is macrosomic or growth retarded, bruised, or hypoglycemic requires different physical care, support, and teaching. For example, if the mother experiences postpartum hemorrhage, the nurse will be called upon to provide close observation of vital functions; adequate intravenous access for fluids, drugs, and blood administration; assessment of uterine tone and massage as needed; avoidance of bladder distention; administration of oxygen therapy as needed; rapid mobilization of experts and resources; and ongoing support and information to the mother and her support persons.

Immediate newborn care involves screening for potential complications. Most premature infants will quickly stabilize, have no long-term neurological compromise, and will quickly regain lost weight (Mannino, 1988). When the infant is either large or small for gestational age, careful and extended measurement of blood glucose may be indicated and may reveal the need for additional treatment. The infant with hypoglycemia may require early feedings. Large infants and infants who have experienced difficult delivery need close examination for birth trauma including fractured clavicle or humerus, hematoma, and ecchymotic areas. Neurosensorial status is evaluated at 1–2 day intervals. At least one normal examination during the first week of life is predictive of a normal outcome and serves as a good marker of infant prognosis (Amiel-Tison, 1988).

When the mother and family are encouraged to hold and care for the infant and provide early breastfeeding as soon as possible, they will become familiar with the infant's condition and may be able to notice early changes in respiration, alertness, and color. Nevertheless, the signs of hypoglycemia and dehydration should be reviewed with the mother and her family as well as what to do.

During the early postpartum period when the infant and mother are stable, specific patient instructions in neonatal care of a postmaturity syndrome infant are given. Because these infants often have skin maceration and poor skin integrity, it is important to prevent infection and trauma by using good hand-washing technique. This can be modeled by professional staff in the hospital or during a home visit. The use of powders and most lotions should be avoided and the skin should be kept dry. The parents should be told that even though the skin of the postmature infant often appears macerated, all layers are anatomically intact, and an adequate skin barrier is present despite the multiple layers of desquamation (Kuller & Lund, 1993). For infants with long nails, the parents are instructed to trim the nails with small, blunt-ended scissors while the infant is asleep and less likely to be active (Kabler & Delmore, 1997). The nails should be cut short enough to prevent self-scratching, but not so short that there are trauma and risk of infection. Demonstrating nail cutting, then asking parents to complete the process, will ensure safety and increase parental confidence.

CONCLUSIONS

The outcomes of a prolonged pregnancy range from normal delivery of a healthy baby and mother to a life-threatening event. Early prenatal care, close observation of antepartum and intrapartum progress, and awareness of potential complications can do much to avoid or identify the problems of prolonged pregnancy. Nurses are in a position to contribute by providing knowledgeable surveillance and timely intervention, and by helping patients and families understand the importance of effective prenatal intrapartum and postpartum care.

References

Ahn, M. O., & Phelan, J. P. (1989). Epidemiologic aspects of the postdate pregnancy. Clinical Obstetrics & Gynecology, 32(2), 228–234.

Amiel-Tison, C. (1988). Cerebral handicap in full-term newborns related to late pregnancy and/or labor. European Journal of Obstetrics, Gynecology, & Reproductive Biology, 28(2), 157–163.

Arduini, D., Rizzo, G., Romanini, C., & Mancuso, S. (1990). Doppler assessment of fetal blood flow velocity waveforms during acute maternal oxygen administration as predictor of fetal outcome in post-term pregnancy. American Journal of Perinatology, 7(3), 258–262.

Arulkumaran, S. (1997). Prolonged pregnancy. In D. James, P. Steer, C. Weiner, & B. Gonik (Eds.), High risk pregnancy management options (pp. 217–228). London: W. B. Saunders.

Bartnicki, J., Ratanasiri, T., Meyenburg, M., & Saling, E. (1992). Postterm pregnancy: Computer analysis of the antepartum fetal heart rate patterns. International Journal of Gynaecology & Obstetrics, 37(4), 243–246.

Battaglia, C., Laroca, E., Lanzani, A., Coukos, G. & Genazzani, A. R. (1991). Doppler velocimetry in prolonged pregnancy. Obstetrics & Gynecology, 77(2), 213–216.

Beckmann, C. A. (1990). Postterm pregnancy: Effects on temperature and glucose regulation. Nursing Research, 39(1), 211–214.

Benedetti, T. J., & Easterling, T. (1988). Antepartum testing in postterm pregnancy. Journal of Reproductive Medicine, 33(3), 252–258.

Bochner, C. J., Medearis, A. L., Davis, J., Oakes, G. K. Hobel, C. J., & Wade, M. E. (1987). Antepartum predictors of fetal distress in postterm pregnancy. American Journal of Obstetrics & Gynecology, 157(2), 353–358.

Boyd, M. E., Usher, R. H., McLean, F. H., & Kramer, M. S. (1988). Obstetric consequences of postmaturity. American Journal of Obstetrics & Gynecology, 158(2), 334–338.

Boylan, P., & McParland, P. (1991). Fetal assessment in postterm pregnancy. [Review] [11 refs.]. Current Opinion in Obstetrics & Gynecology, 3(1), 41–44.

Campbell, W., Nochimson, D. & Vintzileos, A. (1993). Prolonged pregnancy. In R. Knuppel & J. Drukker (Eds.), High-risk pregnancy a team approach (2nd ed.). Philadelphia: W. B. Saunders.

Chervenak, J. L., Divon, M. Y., Hirsch, J., Girz, B. A., & Langer, O. (1989). Macrosomia in the postdate pregnancy: Is routine ultrasonographic screening indicated? American Journal of Obstetrics & Gynecology, 161(3), 753–756.

Clement, D., Schifrin, B. S., & Kates, R. B. (1987). Acute oligohydramnios in postdate pregnancy. American Journal of Obstetrics & Gynecology, 157(4, Pt. 1), 884–886.

Druzin, M. L., Karver, M. L., Wagner, W., Hutson, J. M., Waltner, A., & Kogut, E. (1992). Prospective evaluation of the contraction stress and nonstress tests in the management of postterm pregnancy. Surgery, Gynecology & Obstetrics, 174(6), 507–512.

Dyson, D. C. (1988). Fetal surveillance vs. labor induction at 42 weeks in postterm gestation. Journal of Reproductive Medicine, 33(3), 262–270.

Dyson, D. C., Miller, P. D., & Armstrong, M. A. (1987). Management of prolonged pregnancy: Induction of labor versus antepartum fetal testing. American Journal of Obstetrics & Gynecology, 156(4), 928–934.

Eden, R. D., Seifert, L. S., Winegar, A., & Spellacy, W. N. (1987). Perinatal characteristics of uncomplicated postdate pregnancies. Obstetrics & Gynecology, 69(3, Pt. 1), 296–299.

Eden, R. D., Seifert, L. S., Winegar, A., & Spellacy, W. N. (1988). Maternal risk status and postdate pregnancy outcome. Journal of Reproductive Medicine, 33(1), 53–57.

el-Torkey, M., & Grant, J. M. (1992). Sweeping of the membranes is an effective method of induction of labour in prolonged pregnancy: A report of a randomized trial [see comments]. British Journal of Obstetrics and Gynaecology, 99(6), 455–458.

Fisher, R., Kuhlman, K., Depp, R., & Wapner, R. (1991). Dopper evaluation of umbilical and uterine-arcua arteries in the postdates pregnancy. Obstetrics & Gynecology, 78(3, Pt. 1), 363–368.

Fraidakis, M., Dalamanga, A., Mantzavinos, T., Gargaropoulos, A., & Zourlas, P. A. (1991). Plasma and amniotic fluid concentrations of fibronectin during normal and post term pregnancy. Clinical & Experimental Obstetrics & Gynecology, 18(4), 247–250.

Freeman, R., & Lagrew, D. (1992). Prolonged pregnancy. In S. Gabbe, J. Niebyl, & J. Simpson (Eds.), Obstetrics normal and problem pregnancies (2nd ed., pp. 945–956). New York: Churchill Livingstone.

Freeman, R., & Lagrew, D. (1997). Postdate Pregnancy. In S. Gabbe, J. Niebyl, & J. Simpson (Eds.), Obstetric normal and problem pregnancies (3rd ed., pp. 887–897). New York: Churchill Livingstone.

Grudev, D. (1990). Delivery in prolonged pregnancy following preparation and induction with aprofen and prednisolone. [Bulgarian]. Akusherstvo i Ginekologiia, 29(3), 14–18.

Guidetti, D. A., Divon, M. Y., & Langer, O. (1989). Postdate fetal surveillance: Is 41 weeks too early? American Journal of Obstetrics & Gynecology, 161(1), 91–93.

Hannah, M. E. (1990). Which tests of postterm fetal well-being work? Birth: Issues in Perinatal Care & Education, 17(4), 228–229.

Herabutya, Y., Prasertsawat, P. O., Tongyai, T., & Isarangura Na Ayudthya, N. (1992). Prolonged pregnancy: The management dilemma. International Journal of Gynaecology & Obstetrics, 37(4), 253–258.

Ingemarsson, I., & Heden, L. (1989). Cervical score and onset of spontaneous labor in prolonged pregnancy dated by second-trimester ultrasonic scan. Obstetrics & Gynecology, 74(1), 102–105.

Kabler, J., & Delmore, P. (1997). Alterations in health status of newborns. In F. Nichols & E. Zwelling (Eds.), Maternal-Newborn Nursing Theory and Practice (pp. 1352–1354). Philadelphia: W. B. Saunders.

Kassis, A., Mazor, M., Leiberman, J. R., Cohen, A., & Insler, V. (1991). Management of post-date pregnancy: A case control study. Israel Journal of Medical Sciences, 27(2), 82–86.

Kuller, J., & Lund, C. (1983). Assessment and management of integumentary dysfunction. In C. Kenner, A. Brueggemeyer, & L. Gunderson (Eds.), Comprehensive neonatal nursing: A physiologic perspective (pp. 764-765). Philadelphia: W. B. Saunders.

Leveno, K. (1986). Amniotic fluid volume in prolonged pregnancy. Seminars in Perinatology, 10(2), 154–161.

Lurie, S., Matzkel, A., Weissman, A., Gotlibe, Z., & Friedman, A. (1992). Outcome of pregnancy in class A1 and A2 gestational diabetic patients delivered beyond 40 weeks' gestation. American Journal of Perinatology, 9(5–6), 484–488.

MacMullen, N. Brucker, M., & Zwelling, E. (1997). High-risk childbirth (pp. 882–883). In F. Nichols & E. Zwelling (Eds.), Maternal-Newborn Nursing Theory and Practice (pp. 1352–1354). Philadelphia: W. B. Saunders.

Mannino, F. (1988). Neonatal complications of postterm gestation. Journal of Reproductive Medicine, 33(3), 271–276.

McColgin, S. W., Hampton, H. L., McCaul, J. F., Howard, P. R., Andrew, M. E., & Morrison, J. C. (1990). Stripping membranes at term: Can it safely reduce the incidence of post-term pregnancies? Obstetrics & Gynecology, 76(4), 678–680.

Moran, D. J., McGarrigle, H. H., & Lachelin, G. C. (1992). Lack of normal increase in saliva estriol/progesterone ratio in women with labor induced at 42 weeks' gestation. American Journal of Obstetrics & Gynecology, 167(6), 1563–1564.

Papageorgiou, I., Tsionou, C., Minaretzis, D., Michalas, S., & Aravantinos, D. (1992). Labor characteristics of uncomplicated prolonged pregnancies after induction with intracervical prostaglandin E2 gel versus intravenous oxytocin. Gynelologic & Obstetric Investigation, 34(2), 92–96.

Parer, J. (1997). Electronic fetal heart rate monitoring: Research guidelines for interpretation. The National Institute of Child Health and Human Development Research Planning Workshop. Journal of Obstetric Gynecologis, and Neonatal Nursing, 26(6), 635–640.

Pearce, J. M., & McParland, P. J. (1991). A comparison of Doppler flow velocity waveforms, amniotic fluid columns, and the nonstress test as a means of monitoring post-dates pregnancies. Obstetrics & Gynecology, 77(2), 204–208.

Roberts, L. J., & Young, K. R. (1991). The management of prolonged pregnancy—An analysis of women's attitudes before and after term [see comments]. British Journal of Obstetrics & Gynaecology, 98(11), 1102–1106.

Sawai, S. K., Williams, M. C., O'Brien, WF, O. B., Angel, J. L., Mastrogiannis, D. S., & Johnson, L. (1991). Sequential outpatient application of intravaginal prostaglandin E2 gel in the management of postdates pregnancies. Obstetrics & Gynecology, 78(1), 19–23.

Schmidt, J. V. (1997). Fluid check: Intrapartum amnioinfusion. AWHONN Lifelines, 1(5), 46–51.

Trimmer, K. J., Leveno, K. J., Peters, M. T., & Kelly, M. A. (1990). Observations on the cause of oligohydramnios in prolonged pregnancy. American Journal of Obstetrics & Gynecology, 163(6, Pt. 1), 1900–1903.

Wood, C. L. (1994). Postdate pregnancy update. Journal of Nurse-Midwifery, 39(2, Suppl.), 110S–122S.

CHAPTER
8

Induction and Augmentation of Labor

Susan Pozaic

Pregnancy, in the majority of women, is a self-limiting event. Some gestations, however, require assistance in effecting parturition. Indeed, the rationale for third-trimester fetal monitoring depends upon the professional's ability to initiate a safe and timely delivery. (O'Brien, 1995). Modern obstetrics employs a number of pharmacologic and mechanical methods to ripen the cervix and to initiate or enhance the labor process. New methods to facilitate labor have been investigated and previously employed methods have been used in new ways. Oxytocin has remained the agent of choice to induce labor; however, its major deficiency is its high failure rate in women with an unripe cervix. Prostaglandins have been shown to be successful in enhancing cervical status. Interest has also been renewed in the use of various mechanical methods to enhance cervical ripening.

A common and specialized part of obstetric nursing practice is the direct care of patients who will require these labor enhancement techniques. Nursing care entails responsibility for and regulation of the pharmacologic means of stimulation of labor, specifically, prostaglandins and oxytocin; therefore, the use of these two methods are the primary focus of this chapter.

Augmentation of labor is defined as artificial stimulation of labor that began spontaneously but has progressed abnormally. Additional uterine activity is stimulated, usually by pharmacologic means, in order to bring about more progressive cervical dilation and effacement and descent of the fetal presenting part. Induction of labor is carried out when there is a medical indication to end the gestation.

PATIENT SELECTION

Though there are risks associated with pharmacologic and nonpharmacologic methods of induction and augmentation, the needs of the mother and fetus may necessitate their use. The physician must therefore consider whether labor manipulation would more likely harm or benefit both mother and fetus. Labor manipulation is indicated when the mother and/or her fetus would benefit physiologically from delivery. Factors to be considered when deciding if and when labor should be induced (Shyken & Petrie, 1995) are:

1. cervical ripeness
2. fetal pulmonary maturity
3. fetal ability to tolerate labor
4. uterine sensitivity to the proposed induction method
5. maternal condition
6. gestational age
7. fetal size and presentation

Indications for delivery are usually relative and dynamic in the sense that they change as modern obstetrical practice changes. Maternal factors may include pregnancy-induced or chronic hypertension, diabetes mellitus, antepartum bleeding including partial placenta previa or mild placental abruption, premature rupture of the membranes in a term pregnancy, chorioamnionitis, history of recurrent fetal death, renal, cardiac, hepatic, pulmonary, or malignant diseases (Musacchio, 1990; ACOG, 1995). Fetal indications include isoimmunization, intrauterine growth retardation, intrauterine fetal death, prolonged gestation, major anomalies, and fetal distress evidenced by biochemical or biophysical indicators (Musacchio, 1990; O'Brien & Cefalo, 1996).

In general, any contraindication to spontaneous vaginal delivery is a contraindication to induction of labor. Maternal contraindications to labor induction include complete placenta previa, vasa previa, classical uterine incision, extensive myomectomy, pelvic structural deformities, active or culture-proven genital herpes infection, invasive cervical carcinoma, hypertonic uterine activity, and maternal exhaustion (ACOG, 1995; Musacchio, 1990; O'Brien & Cefalo, 1996). Relative contraindications include grand multiparity, uterine overdistention as a result of hydramnios or multiple gestation, and possibly, previous cesarean section (O'Brien & Cefalo, 1996). Fetal contraindications to labor induction include abnormal presentation such as transverse lie or funic presentation, presenting part above the pelvic inlet, and the presence of fetal distress (ACOG, 1995; Musacchio, 1990).

Labor induction is initiated in the anticipation of a favorable outcome, spontaneous vaginal delivery. The likelihood of this occurring is increased when the cervix demonstrates readiness to progressively efface and dilate. Bishop (1964) developed a method by which the cervix can be clinically evaluated and scored to assist in predicting the likelihood of successful induction. The position of the cervix as it relates to the vagina, cervical consistency, dilation, and effacement, and the station of the fetal presenting part are evaluated and given a numerical value (see Table 8-1). The range of scores is 0–13 with low numbers being indicative of an unfavorable cervix and higher numbers being indicative of a more favorable cervix. In a study conducted by Friedman, Niswander, Bayonet-Riversa, & Sachtleben (1966), a cervical score of 1–4 was associated with an induction failure rate of 19.5%; a score of 5–8 with a 4.8% failure rate; and a score of 9–12 with no failures. A modified Bishop score is used by some (see Table 8-2) (Blanch, Olah, & Walkinshaw, 1996). A study conducted to evaluate factors associated with success of vaginal delivery following induced labor stated that previous delivery was most important, whereas cervical position and consistency were not important (Lyndrup, 1996). Another study suggested that only cervical dilation appears to predict the length of the latent phase of induced labor (Watson, Stevens, Welter, & Day, 1996).

Cervical assessment is also being conducted by transvaginal ultrasound. One study reported that cervical wedging defined as a triangle or "U" pattern at the area of the internal cervical os, prior to labor induction was associated with a

TABLE 8-1. Bishop's Pelvic Scoring

	0	1	2	3
Dilation	0	1–2	3–4	5–6
Effacement (%)	0–30	40–50	60–70	80
Station	–3	–2	–1 to 0	+1 to +2
Consistency	Firm	Medium	Soft	
Position	Posterior	Midposition	Anterior	

shorter latent phase and overall shorter labor (Boozarjomehri, Timor-Tritsch, & Chao, 1994).

Another factor associated with an increased likelihood of successful labor induction is the presence of fetal fibronectin in the endocervix. Fetal fibronectin is synthesized by choriodecidual cells and is released into cervical secretions early in the cervical ripening process. Its presence may reflect separation of the chorion from the decidua in the uterus (Leppert, 1995). Studies have demonstrated that the presence of fetal fibronectin in the endocervix is associated with shorter duration from induction to delivery and fewer doses of prostaglandins needed to induce labor (Ahner, Egarter, Kiss, Heinzl. Zeillinger, Schatten, Dirmeier, & Husslein, 1995; Blanch et al. 1996).

Because cervical condition plays such an important role in the induction of labor, specifically the latent phase, a variety of methods to prepare the cervix for labor have been tried. These include catheters, laminaria, breast stimulation, relaxin, oxytocin, estrogen, prostaglandin E and prostaglandin F, and antiprogestins.

Augmentation of labor is indicated when there is a lack of labor progress, that is, cervical effacement and dilation, or failure of descent of the fetal presenting part in the presence of inadequate quantities of uterine contractions. A lack of labor progress can be identified only after the woman has been in active labor, because hypotonic uterine dysfunction occurs most frequently when the cervix is dilated to 4 or more centimeters. One of the most common errors is the treatment of uterine dys-

function or hypotonus when the woman is not yet in active labor (Cunningham, MacDonald, Gant, Leveno, & Gilstrap, 1993).

An understanding of the normal labor curve developed by Friedman (1954) helps to illustrate the normal labor progress of cervical dilation and fetal descent. Labor disorders that may be treated with oxytocin include hypotonic uterine dysfunction, protraction disorders, and arrest disorders. Uterine dysfunction is frequently caused by pelvic contractures, fetal malposition, and uterine overdistention. Cervical rigidity is an uncommon cause (Cunningham et al., 1993). In hypotonic uterine dysfunction, basal tonus is normal and there is only a slight rise in pressure during a contraction that is insufficient to dilate the cervix. If indeed the patient had been in active labor as evidenced by rhythmic, uncomfortable uterine activity that has produced cervical effacement and dilatation of at least 4 centimeters, and cephalopelvic disproportion (CPD) is not present, augmentation is considered.

Protraction disorders include the following:

1. Protracted active phase dilation in which cervical dilation is less than 1.2 cm/hr in the nulliparous patient and less than 1.5 cm/hr in the multiparous patient
2. Protracted descent in which the maximum slope of descent of the fetal presenting part is less than 1 cm/hr in the nulliparous patient and less that 2 cm/hr in the multiparous patient

One third of these cases are caused by cephalopelvic disproportion (CPD) of varying degrees

TABLE 8-2. Modified Bishop Score

	0	1	2
Cervix length (cm)	2	1	0
Cervix dilation (cm)	0–1	1–2	2–3
Cervix position	Posterior	Mid	Anterior
Consistency	Firm	Medium	Soft
Station	−2	−1	0

(Cunningham et al., 1993). In the presence of CPD, cesarean section is the preferred treatment. If CPD is not present, treatment is controversial but may include augmentation.

Arrest disorders include prolonged deceleration phase, secondary arrest of dilation, arrest of descent, and failure of descent. A prolonged deceleration phase occurs when the termination of transition exceeds 3 hours in the nulliparous patient and 1 hour in the multiparous patient. Secondary arrest of dilation exists when there is no further cervical dilation for greater than two hours in the active phase. Arrest of descent is present when there is no further descent of the fetal presenting part for more than 1 hour. Failure of descent exists when there is no descent either during the deceleration phase of the first stage of labor or during the second stage of labor. If CPD is not present, augmentation of labor may be attempted.

UTERINE PHYSIOLOGY

In order to understand the mechanisms of action of methods used to prepare or "ripen" the cervix and induce or augment labor, uterine physiology as it relates to the initiation of labor must be reviewed. Cervical ripening refers to softening and effacement and is thought to represent the maturation of the reproductive system in terms of labor induction readiness. Rearrangement and realignment of the collagen, elastin, and smooth muscle cells is the most important component of cervical softening. This rearrangement occurs because of mechanical forces. Dilation occurs as a result of degradation of collagen by proteolytic enzymes. The mechanisms are not completely understood but probably involve prostaglandins, progesterone and estrogen effects, estrogen receptor down-regulation, and possibly an inflammatory reaction (Leppert, 1995).

The exact mechanism responsible for the initiation of labor has not been determined; however, a number of physiologic events are known to occur prior to or during labor. The onset of labor requires the myometrial inhibiting effect of progesterone to be diminished. Progesterone along with estrogen facilitates increased prostaglandin

synthesis. These substances play a role in the cascade of labor events: cervical ripening, gap junction formation, the increase in oxytocin receptors, and increased responsiveness of the uterus to substances that produce contractions (Schulman & Farmakides, 1987). (For a more detailed description of the underlying physiology involved in initiation of parturition, refer to Chapter 6.)

TECHNIQUES

Cervical Ripening

Cervical changes can be produced using mechanical or chemical means.

Mechanical Agents

Devices used to mechanically dilate the cervix are catheters and laminaria. The mechanism of action is simple expansion and the promotion of prostaglandin production, which in turn changes the collagen matrix of the cervix (Newton, 1987). Mechanical dilators may be indicated when pharmacologic means to ripen the cervix are contraindicated or are not feasible.

Catheters. A foley catheter inserted into the cervix and inflated, usually overnight, has been found to be an effective agent for cervical ripening (James, Peedicayil, & Seshadri, 1994; Orhue, 1995). St. Onge and Connors (1995) report the foley catheter to be as effective as prostaglandin gel for cervical ripening. A double-balloon device was reported as more effective in cervical ripening and labor induction than prostaglandin E_2 gel or oxytocin (Atad, Hallak, Auslender, Porat-Packer, Zarfati, & Abramovic, 1996). Its use has not been associated with any complications, however, infection is a potential risk.

Hygroscopic Dilators. Natural laminaria tents, and more recently, synthetic hygroscopic dilators have been tried to manually dilate the cervix prior to labor induction. The tents are placed in the cervical os and as they absorb fluid, their diameter increases. Despite their ability to enhance cervical ripeness, a recent study demonstrated no improvement in the length of labor, and no reduction in the need for cesarean section (Gilson, Russell, Izquierdo, Qualls, & Curet, 1996; Krammer, Williams, Sawai, &

O'Brien, 1995). Although cervical dilation allows for earlier amniotomy, it is unclear whether the postripening cervical state has the same predictive value for successful induction of labor as the cervical state achieved without mechanical stimulation (Krammer & O'Brien, 1995).

Chemical Agents

Chemical agents used to enhance cervical maturation include relaxin, oxytoxin, estrogen, prostaglandin E and F, and antiprogestins.

Relaxin. In many species, not including humans, serum relaxin rises 24 hours prior to labor. Elevated levels of relaxin produce softening, effacement, and dilation of the cervix by facilitating connective tissue restructuring without producing uterine contractions. Exogenous porcine relaxin has been administered by intravaginal or intracervical gel. It accelerated cervical changes and decreased the time to onset of labor without increasing uterine contractility (Weiss, 1995). No significant maternal or fetal complications are identified. The possibility of sensitization exists because relaxin is a foreign protein (Chwalisz & Garfield, 1994).

Oxytocin. Oxytocin, used by many to induce labor, may be used in various ways to induce cervical ripening. It is likely that oxytocin works to enhance cervical ripening by inducing uterine contractions, which produce biophysical and biochemical changes similar to those that occur naturally during the early latent phase of labor (Chez, Barton, Miller, & Petrie, 1988). Oxytocin is administered by slow intravenous infusion for up to 20 hours or serially over a period of days to produce the cervical change (Chez et al., 1988; Merrill & Freeman, 1986). Use of the body's natural physiologic functioning in the form of breast stimulation to cause endogenous release of oxytocin has been shown to be effective in priming the cervix (Elliott & Flaherty, 1984; Salmon, Kee, Tan, & Jen, 1986). The method of breast stimulation should be carefully evaluated for incidence of uterine hyperstimulation (Curtis, Evens, & Resnick, 1986). Gentle unilateral stimulation produces less hypertonus (Salmon et al., 1986).

Estrogen. Various estrogens have been used to induce cervical ripening. An increased estrogen-progesterone ratio is thought to enhance collagen breakdown in the cervix without producing prominent uterine contractions. It is also believed that estrogen promotes sensitivity of the cervix to prostaglandins (Uldbjerg, Ulmsten, & Ekman, 1983). Estradiol was found to be equivalent to prostaglandin E_2 and oxytocin in cervical ripening (Magann, Perry, Dockery, Bass, Chauhan, & Morrison, 1995).

Prostaglandins. Prostaglandins are hormones produced by most organs, especially the endometrium in the female. Prostaglandin E_2 (PGE_2) is the primary prostaglandin produced by the cervix and trophoblast (Schulman & Farmakides, 1987). Precursors of prostaglandins are stored as phospholipids in the cell membranes. Prostaglandins are formed just prior to their release because they are rapidly metabolized by the lungs, kidneys, and liver (Glazer & Hulme, 1987). The most important prostaglandins involved in reproduction are prostaglandin E_2 (PGE_2) and F_2 (PGF_2) formed from arachidonic acid. Exogenous sources of PGE_2 produce the same biochemical changes that occur naturally in the ripening cervix, without increasing uterine activity (Anderson, Forman, & Ulmsten, 1983; Schulman & Farmakides, 1987). PGE_2 may also alter the myometrium by changing membrane excitability, thereby preparing the uterus for parturition (Shulman, 1983). It has been postulated that prostaglandins act as a facilitator to oxytocin in the labor process (Novy & Liggins, 1980). Prostaglandin E_2 (PGE_2) is superior to prostaglandin F_2 (PGF_2) because the cervical ripening effects are greater and the incidence of systemic side effects is lower (Keirse, 1993).

It has been reported that preinduction cervical ripening with local PGE_2 increases the Bishop score, shortens the duration of labor, increases the rate of delivery within 12 hours, and increases the rate of successful induction; however, it was not shown to decrease the rate of cesarean delivery (O'Brien, 1995). In contrast, Darroca, Buttino, Miller, and Khamais (1996) reported the use of PGE_2 gel decreased the amount of oxytocin needed and decreased the cesarean section rate by 60%.

Prostaglandins used to induce labor may be given systemically; however, this is not common practice because of the side effects and risk of hyperstimulation caused by variable effective dose, narrow therapeutic range, and longer myometrial effects than are expected from the rapid degradation of prostaglandins systemically (Anderson et al., 1983).

Prostaglandins are most commonly administered locally. Prior to FDA approval of a prostaglandin E_2 gel in December 1992, a commercially prepared form of PGE_2 gel was not available and was compounded by hospital pharmacies by melting a prepared 40-milligram suppository and suspending it in a gel base. Many questions were raised as to the consistency of the drug concentration in the hospital-compounded preparation. Sanchez-Ramos, Farah, Kaunitz, Adair, Del Valle, and Fuqua (1995) compared the hospital-compounded preparation with the commercially available PGE_2 gel and reported no difference in administration of gel to delivery interval, number of doses, amount of oxytocin or adverse neonatal outcomes but noted that the cesarean section rate was significantly less in the women treated with the commercially available gel.

Murray, Buonocore, and Hawley (1995) compared PGE_2 gel with PGE_2 tablets administered vaginally in nulliparous women and found no difference in overall failed induction, cesarean section rate, assisted delivery, oxytocin need, induction to delivery interval, analgesic requirements, or neonatal condition but noted that gel was associated with an increase in fetal heart rate abnormalities requiring cesarean section, and tablets were associated with an increased need for cesarean section secondary to poor labor progress.

Prostaglandin E_2 gel is administered either vaginally or intracervically in doses ranging from 0.5 mg to 5 mg with 3 mg being the most common vaginal dose. Prostaglandin E_2 gel is available in a 2.5-cc syringe containing 0.5 mg of dinoprostone (Prepidil). A prostaglandin vaginal insert (Cervidil) containing 10 mg of dinoprostone, releases medication at a rate of 0.3 mg per hour. The insert has the advantage of being able to be removed from the vagina should hyperstimulation occur.

One study reports that the intracervical route enhances cervical ripening but is equivalent to the vaginal route in regard to other parameters (Keirse & de Koning Gans, 1995). Other studies report the vaginal route to be more efficacious for cervical ripening and labor induction (Hales, Rayburn, Turnbull, Christensen, & Patatanian, 1994). Administration as frequently as every hour appears to be safe but offers no advantage in terms of cervical ripening over the more common 6-hour dosing (Carlan, Danna, Durkee, Quinsey, & Lanaris, 1995).

Comparison studies of low-dose oxytocin for cervical ripening compared with PGE_2 demonstrated less time from beginning to delivery and increased likelihood of vaginal delivery within 24 hours in the PGE_2 group (Jackson, Sharp, & Varner, 1994; Pollnow & Broekhuizen, 1996). No other differences were detected in efficacy in another study but uterine hyperstimulation and fetal distress were seen at a rate of 4.8% in the prostaglandin group (Jackson et al., 1994). In contrast, no difference in cesarean section rate, meconium staining, hyperstimulation or Apgar scores was noted in the more recent study (Pollnow & Broekhuizen, 1996).

Recently, Misoprostol (Cytotec), a prostaglandin E_1 analog given in a dose of 25 micrograms vaginally every 2 hours for as many as 6 doses, was compared with PGE_2 given in a dose of 0.5 milligrams intracervically every 6 hours twice. Misoprostol reduced the time from drug administration to onset of three uterine contractions in a 10-minute period, time to rupture of membranes, and time to delivery. There was more uterine hypertonus with misoprostol but no related fetal morbidity (Varaklis, Gumina, & Stubblefield, 1995). In another study the same dose of misoprostol was utilized but a comparison of dosing frequency at 3- and 6-hour intervals was conducted (Wing & Paul, 1996). Patients who received doses every 6 hours had longer intervals to delivery, more frequent need of oxytocin, and more failed inductions. There was no difference in hyperstimulation, abnormal fetal heart rate patterns, meconium passage, Apgar scores less than 7, neonatal resuscitations, or admissions to neonatal intensive care. Further studies need to be conducted to determine the safety of misoprostol.

In order to keep costs down, outpatient cervical ripening and induction of labor has been studied (Sawai & O'Brien, 1995). O'Brien, Mercer, Cleary, and Sibai (1995) reported on outpatient vaginal administration of 2 milligrams of PGE$_2$ gel daily for 5 days with 10 minutes of electronic fetal monitoring before dosing and 30 minutes of electronic fetal monitoring following dosing. They found this regimen to be safe and effective in initiating labor. Sawai, O'Brien, Mastrogiannis, Krammer, Mastry, and Porter (1994) reported that outpatient PGE$_2$ suppositories self-administered daily in post-date pregnancies decreased gestational length and related cost of antepartum testing and postterm complications. Hyperstimulation is a potential problem but there are no reports of long-term adverse sequelae related to hyperstimulation with ripening agents (O'Brien, 1995). The incidence of hyperstimulation appears to be dose-related and occurs within the first hour of insertion (Bernstein, 1991).

Despite the benefits of prostaglandins, adverse effects have been reported and are primarily related to smooth muscle. These most commonly include cramping, painful uterine contractions, nausea, vomiting, diarrhea, backache, fever, chills, flushing, hot flashes, and muscular pain. Caution should be exercised in using prostaglandins in patients with asthma, hypertension, renal, hepatic, or cardiovascular disease, seizure disorders, or diabetes mellitus (Kelsey & Prevost, 1994). Oxytocin may be administered as soon as 4 hours after the last administration of prostaglandins but oxytocin is most commonly administered 6–12 hours after prostaglandins (Kelsey & Prevost, 1994).

Antiprogestins. Mifepristone (RU-486), a progesterone antagonist, has been investigated for use in induction of labor. It is believed that antiprogestins enhance myometrial responsiveness to prostaglandins and induce cervical ripening irrespective of the stage of pregnancy (Chwalisz & Garfield, 1994). Although mifepristone enhanced the rate of spontaneous labor, decreased the time to onset of labor, and decreased the total amount of oxytocin needed in patients who delivered vaginally, there was no difference in the number of women with favorable cervical scores if not delivered by day 4 and the rate of cesarean section was not improved (Frydman, Lelaidier, Baton-Saint-Mleux, Fernandez, Vial, & Bourget, 1992). The only maternal side effect was mild to moderate diarrhea. Despite the fact that mifepristone crosses the placenta, there was no increase in the incidence of fetal distress or alterations in neonatal parameters of well-being (Frydman et al., 1992). Although mifepristone is effective in inducing labor in first- and second-trimester pregnancies, its use in labor induction at term is questionable (Edwards, 1996).

Labor Induction/Augmentation

The methods described to artificially ripen the cervix may also induce labor in certain patients. Nonpharmacologic methods to induce labor will be briefly described and more detailed information will be presented regarding the pharmacologic methods of labor induction, including active management of labor, as the nurse is responsible for patient assessment and nursing management.

Nonpharmacologic Methods

Nonpharmacologic methods to induce or augment labor include amniotomy and stripping of the membranes.

Amniotomy. Amniotomy is the nonpharmacologic method most frequently used to stimulate labor. Its mechanism of action is thought to be the release of arachidonic acid and subsequent formation of the prostaglandins. These prostaglandins are thought to potentiate the action of oxytocin so myometrial activity is initiated or maintained (Husslein, Kofler, Rasmussen, 1983). In a study conducted of fetal membranes it was determined that the fetal head alone exerts more force against the cervix than the head covered with the membranes. However, before the head is directly applied to the cervix, the membranes play an important role as dilator (Manabe, Sagawa, & Mori, 1985). Amniotomy allows inspection of the amniotic fluid for meconium, placement of the fetal scalp electrode, and shortens the duration of labor (Busowski & Parsons, 1995). The main disadvantage of amniotomy to induce labor is the unpredictable interval from membrane rupture to the initiation of labor and delivery. Other associated potential hazards include maternal/fetal infection, umbilical cord prolapse (which is rare when the vertex is engaged), and umbilical cord compression producing fetal heart rate changes. After thorough consideration of the risks involved, the physician or nurse midwife may elect to rupture the membranes to augment the labor process once the presenting part is well applied to the cervix. Very often, amniotomy is used concurrently with a pharmacologic agent to further augment the labor process.

Stripping of Membranes. Stripping of the membranes is the manual separation of the chorioamniotic membranes from the lower uterine segment. Cervical stretching is often accomplished simultaneously. This procedure may initiate labor by stimulating an autonomic neural reflex, releasing endogenous oxytocin from the maternal pituitary, and by local release of prostaglandins (McKay & Mahan, 1983). A recent study reported the number of women who delivered within one week of membrane stripping at term was significantly greater than controls (Wiriyasirivaj, Vutyavanich, & Ruangsri, 1996). Additionally, among those who did not deliver in one week, women in the membrane-stripping group had cervical scores that were significantly higher, the number of days to delivery was significantly less, and the incidence of postterm pregnancy was less. Another study reported membrane stripping significantly decreased time to delivery only in women at 41 weeks gestation and beyond (Goldenberg, Dulitzky, Feldman, Zolti, & Bider, 1996). The potential risks of membrane stripping include premature rupture of the fetal membranes, maternal–fetal infection, and disruption of a low-lying placenta. Disadvantages of the procedure and variable results make the usefulness of stripping of the membranes questionable and beyond the scope of nursing practice.

Pharmacologic Methods

Oxytocin. Oxytocin increases uterine contractility by increasing free intracellular calcium. This is accomplished by increased calcium influx, mobilization of calcium stores, and inhibition of the calcium extrusion pump. Calcium is vital for the activation of smooth muscle. Sensitivity of the uterus to oxytocin depends on the concentration of myometrial oxytocin receptors. Oxytocin receptors increase throughout pregnancy with a sharp rise during parturition as a result of the increased estrogen–progesterone ratio and prostaglandin synthesis. As the oxytocin receptors increase through gestation, myometrial sensitivity to oxytocin increases and the amount of oxytocin necessary to produce uterine contractions decreases. Oxytocin probably also enhances prostaglandin production in the decidua, which in turn stimulates uterine contractions (Fuchs & Fuchs, 1996). Gap junctions in the myometrium allow rapid communication between large numbers of cells, which then are capable of producing the expulsive forces necessary for delivery. Commercially available oxytocin is a synthetic form of the hormone secreted by the hypothalamus and stored in the neurohypophysis. It is released in pulses with the frequency and/or amplitude of the pulses increasing with the progress of labor (Dawood, 1995). The only route currently approved by the FDA for the induction or augmentation of labor is by continuous intravenous infusion. Pulsatile administration of oxytocin may decrease the amount of oxytocin needed for uterine stimulation (Dawood, 1995), but it offers no other clinical advantage (Reid & Helewa, 1995; Willcourt, Pager, Wendel, & Hale, 1994). Oxytocin is removed from the plasma by the kidneys and liver and is inactivated by placental oxytocinase in the blood. Initial uterine response to intravenous oxytocin may occur almost immediately and the effect may persist for up to one hour (ASHP, 1996). The pharmacokinetic half-life of oxytocin is generally 10–15 minutes. The time to reach steady-state drug concentrations in the blood is 3 to 5 times the half-life. Earlier oxytocin induction/augmentation protocols were based on a shorter half-life and provided for an upward adjustment in dosage every 15–20 minutes. However, more recent data suggest that the pharmacokinetic half-life of oxytocin is not consistent with the time to reach maximum pharmacologic effect.

In vivo studies conducted by Seitchik and others demonstrated that the interval to reach the maximum pharmacologic effect of oxytocin was 40 minutes (Seitchik, Amico, Robinson, & Castillo, 1984; Seitchik & Castillo, 1982). Indeed, other studies have demonstrated benefits in extending the dosing interval (Gonser, 1995). These benefits include less uterine hyperstimulation, less abnormal fetal heart rate tracings, and lower maximal dose (Blakemore, Qin, Petrie, & Paine, 1990; Foster, Jacobson, & Valenzuela, 1988). Seitchik and Castillo (1983) demonstrated that 45% of patients with augmented labor will require less than 2.5 mU/min; 45% will require 2.5–5 mU/min, and 10% will require greater than 5 mU/min. Stated differently, 90% of patients will require less than 16 mU/min (ACOG, 1995).

Controversy exists regarding the optimal starting dose, incremental dose, and dose interval. Some oxytocin protocols based on the physiologic data advocate physiologic doses and others advocate pharmacologic doses (Dawood, 1990; Toaff, Hezroni, & Toaff, 1978). Advocates of the physiologic doses of oxytocin believe the normal physiologic pattern of endogenous oxytocin release is best mimicked by low doses of oxytocin, that is, 2–6 milliunits per minute. Their goal is vaginal delivery with a minimum of uterine hyperstimulation and fetal distress. Proponents of pharmacologic doses of oxytocin as well as advocates of the active management of labor have the primary goal of strong uterine contractions leading to shortened labor and vaginal delivery. They believe this leads to fewer cesarean deliveries for dystocia, fewer cases of peripartum infection, and less maternal morbidity. Dosing of oxytocin varies with parity and whether it is used for induction or augmentation of labor.

The initial starting dose and incremental rate of change were studied by Wein in 1989. Three different starting doses were used, 0.7, 1.7, and 3.3 milliunits per minute (mU/min), and were doubled every 30 minutes. Women receiving higher initial doses required higher maintenance and total doses. There was no difference in number of successful inductions or interval from induction to delivery; however, the high-dose group demonstrated a significantly greater number of infants with low 5-minute Apgar scores. The author suggests that lower dose oxytocin infusion is equally effective and may decrease untoward effects.

The starting dose as well as the magnitude of the incremental dose were studied by Satin and coworkers (Satin, Leveno, Sherman, Brewster, & Cunningham, 1992). The starting doses were 1 and 6 mU/min, which were increased by the same dose, 1 and 6 mU/min respectively, every 20 minutes. High-dose oxytocin was associated with a 3-hour shorter labor length, decreased neonatal sepsis, fewer forceps deliveries, and a 5% decrease in failed inductions. It was also associated with more hyperstimulation though not with adverse fetal effects, and more cesarean deliveries for fetal distress though the incidence of umbilical cord blood acidemia was not increased. The authors stated that labor augmentation using high-dose oxytocin is clearly superior to low dose but high dose for induction offers mixed results. The data were further analyzed for economic impact. The high-dose regimen resulted in estimated provider and consumer cost savings of $350,000 per year (Brown, Satin, & Leveno, 1994).

The magnitude of the incremental dose increase was also studied by Muller and colleagues (1992). The traditional management group was started with 0.5–1 mU/min and received increases of 1–2 mU/min every 30 minutes. The experimental group was started with 1–2 mU/min and received increases in the form of doubling the current rate every 30 minutes. The experimental group proceeded to onset of regular uterine contractions more rapidly but the overall length of labor was not decreased; the number of assisted deliveries was increased because of increased changes in the fetal heart rate. There were no differences in the rates of hyperstimulation.

Several studies address the interval for increasing the rate of oxytocin infusion. Mercer, Pilgrim, and Sabai (1991) reported that low-dose oxytocin increased at hourly intervals was superior to standard protocols involving a dosing interval of 20 minutes. Hourly dosing did not increase the time to delivery, and the rate of hyperstimulation, abnormal fetal heart rate, and cesarean delivery for fetal distress was decreased. Goni,

Sawhney, and Gopalan (1995) compared doubling the current dose of oxytocin every 20 and 60 minutes. Hourly dosing decreased the incidence of hyperstimulation, cesarean section, and assisted vaginal delivery without causing a delay in delivery.

Lazor, Philipson, Ingardia, Kobetitsch, & Carry (1993) compared 15- and 40-minute dosing protocols. Both groups were started at 1 mU/min and the incremental dose was 1 and 1.5 mU/min, respectively. The 40-minute dosing protocol had a significantly lower maximum dose of oxytocin, rate of hyperstimulation, and fetal distress in both augmented and induced patients. No differences were noted in the rate of cesarean deliveries or length of labor.

Satin, Leveno, Sherman, & McIntire (1994) compared two high-dose oxytocin protocols, both groups beginning with 6 mU/min and with incremental doses of 6 mU/min, but at 20- versus 40-minute intervals. More frequent dosing in women receiving oxytocin for augmentation was associated with decreased cesarean delivery for dystocia and no increase in hyperstimulation. In contrast, for induction, the shorter dosing interval was associated with an increase in hyperstimulation and no decrease in cesarean deliveries for dystocia. Neonatal outcomes were unaffected.

Xenakis, Langer, Piper, Conway, & Berkus (1995) studied low-dose (initial dose 1 mU/min, increased every 30 minutes by 1 mU/min) versus high-dose treatments (initial dose 4 mU/min, increased every 15 minutes by 4 mU/min) for labor augmentation. The high-dose group had a lower cesarean section rate regardless of parity, and decreased time to correct labor abnormality. There were no differences in maternal complications or neonatal outcomes.

Research supports high-dose, short-interval oxytocin dosing for labor augmentation; however, for the purpose of labor induction, low-dose, longer interval dosing is superior. Regardless of the rate of infusion and dosing interval, the dose must always be titrated to the uterine response. Factors that affect the dose response to oxytocin and increase the total dose of oxytocin are cervical dilation of 2 cm or less, nulliparity, gestation 36 weeks or less, and maternal large body surface area (Satin, Leveno, Sherman, & McIntire, 1992).

When comparing high-dose to low-dose regimens, although a shorter induction to delivery time seems to occur, there is an increase in the total amount of oxytocin required, the rate of hyperstimulation, and the potential for fetal compromise. As long as oxytocin doses are low and the dosing intervals adequate to allow the drug to reach steady-state, hyperstimulation will be avoided while ensuring adequate uterine activity (Shyken & Petrie, 1995).

Hyperstimulation of the uterus may occur as a result of either high dosage or increased patient sensitivity to oxytocin. Tetanic contractions produce excessive and extreme tension within the uterine musculature, thereby increasing the risk of uterine rupture, cervical lacerations, amniotic fluid embolus, and decreased uteroplacental perfusion with subsequent insufficiency of oxygen transfer to the fetus. Uteroplacental insufficiency causes fetal heart rate changes including late decelerations, bradycardia, tachycardia, premature ventricular contractions, and possibly death secondary to asphyxia. Another important property of oxytocin is its antidiuretic effect. When oxytocin infusions are prolonged and the infusion rate approaches 40 mU/min, there is a dramatic drop in urinary output and potential exists for water intoxication (Musacchio, 1990). Rapid intravenous infusion of oxytocin has been noted to cause severe maternal hypotension, increased heart rate, decreased venous return, and cardiac output, and electrocardiographic changes indicative of cardiac ischemia (ASHP, 1996). These cardiovascular effects may be especially hazardous to a woman receiving regional anesthesia, or with valvular heart disease, or who is hemorrhaging. However, these effects should not occur when oxytocin is properly diluted and administered by infusion pump.

Women who receive oxytocin during the intrapartum period are thought to be at higher risk for postpartum hemorrhage secondary to uterine atony. Hemorrhage may be related to oxytocin-induced thrombocytopenia, afibrinogenemia, and hypoprothrombinemia (ASHP, 1996). By carefully controlling delivery and by continuing the oxytocin infusion postpartum, this complication may be prevented.

Allergic reactions including anaphylaxis can occur and may be fatal. Injudicious use of oxytocin has resulted in maternal deaths attributed to hypertensive episodes and subarachnoid hemorrhage (ASHP, 1996).

Neonates who are delivered following oxytocin-induced labor are 1.6 times more likely to develop hyperbilirubinemia than are neonates who were not exposed to oxytocin induction or augmentation (ASHP, 1996). Hyperbilirubinemia is also more likely with very high doses of oxytocin (Beazley & Alderman, 1975). The principle fetal hazard is iatrogenic prematurity and related respiratory distress syndrome. Iatrogenic prematurity and increased cesarean sections are major problems associated with the elective induction of labor. For these reasons, elective induction or termination of pregnancy strictly for patient or physician convenience is not recommended by the Food and Drug Administration (FDA, 1978). One study found a trend toward an increased rate of cesarean section among nulliparous patients with an unfavorable cervix who were electively induced at term (Wigton & Wolk, 1994).

Active Management of Labor

The increasing incidence of cesarean deliveries in the United States has prompted an examination of the techniques of labor management. Of particular interest is the disparity in the incidence of cesarean deliveries between the United States and Ireland. With a system of labor augmentation for nulliparous women, termed active management of labor as described by O'Driscoll et al., (1969, 1973, 1984), the cesarean section rate in Ireland is 4.8%; therefore, active management is of great interest as a factor that may help decrease the cesarean section rate in this country. The basic principles of active management are presented in Display 8-1.

Active management protocols are being studied in the United States. Lopez-Zeno, Peacemen, Adaschek, and Socol (1992) reported a 26% reduction in cesarean sections in the active management group attributed to a decrease in dystocia. The length of labor in the active management group was 1.66 hours shorter, there were

DISPLAY 8-1

Principles of Active Management of Labor

1. Admission to the labor suite only if passage of blood-stained mucus, spontaneous rupture of membranes, or complete cervical effacement
2. Early amniotomy
3. Hourly cervical examinations
4. Oxytocin administration for dilattaion of less than 1 cm per hour
5. High concentrations of oxytocin in patients requiring augmentation, usually 6 mU/min, increased by 6 mU/min every 15 minutes
6. Expected duration of 12 hours from admission to delivery
7. Nurse–patient ratio of 1:1
8. Strict criteria for interpretation of fetal compromise
9. Peer review of operative deliveries

fewer infectious complications in the mothers, and there was no increase in maternal or neonatal morbidity. In contrast, Frigoletto et al. (1995) reported no difference in the cesarean section rate but noted duration of labor shortened by 2.7 hours, and a lower rate of maternal fever in the active management group.

Gerhardstein, Allswede, Sloan, and Lorenz (1995) used an active management approach to labor but reduced the dose of oxytocin to an initial dose of 2 mU/min and increased by 2 mU/min every 15 minutes. The cesarean section rate decreased by 7%. Cammu and Van Eeckhout (1996) compared routine amniotomy and early oxytocin with selective use of amniotomy and oxytocin in nulliparous women who were otherwise managed the same with supportive care provided on a 1:1 basis by a midwife. Both amniotomy and oxytocin were used more often in the active management group. The first stage of labor was decreased by 30 minutes in the active management group, while the rates of cesarean section, spontaneous vaginal delivery, and neonatal outcome were not significantly different.

Active management of labor has not been found to be associated with increased perinatal morbidity; therefore, it many offer the potential for a reduced cesarean section rate when used for labor augmentation.

Management

The decision of whether to induce or augment labor is based on physical benefit to the mother and/or fetus as previously addressed. Also, contraindications to induction or augmentation should not be present. A physician who is qualified to perform cesarean deliveries should evaluate the patient in terms of indications versus contraindications to induction/augmentation and should be readily available to manage any complications. The patient should be examined by a qualified professional prior to labor induction to determine fetal presentation, station of presenting part, and adequacy of the pelvic size. Additionally, obstetric personnel who understand oxytocin effect and are able to identify maternal and/or fetal complications should be present during the administration of oxytocin (AAP & ACOG, 1992). Proper equipment such as an infusion pump and fetal monitor must be present and available. A written protocol for the preparation and administration of oxytocin as well as nursing responsibilities should be established by the department of obstetrics in each institution. The patient should be informed of the clinical indication and procedure to be implemented and be emotionally prepared. Many patients have been informed by peers that induced labor is more painful than spontaneous labor. Oxytocin protocols that advocate low initial dose and gradual dosage increases more closely approximate spontaneous labor with gradual onset of more painful contractions as the woman adjusts to the labor process.

Immediately prior to initiation of the induction procedure, the physician or nurse must perform a vaginal exam to determine cervical status (AAP & ACOG, 1992). Leopold's maneuvers should also be employed to verify fetal position. Baseline laboratory values including complete blood count, serum electrolytes, glucose, and blood type and hold should be obtained.

Baseline maternal vital signs, uterine activity, and fetal heart rate should be evaluated prior to initiation of the labor induction procedure. Findings of the initial assessment should be documented in the clinical record.

An assessment is conducted of the patient's knowledge of the procedure including the reason for its use, possible side effects and how they will be managed, how the procedure is performed, and her anxiety related to the procedure. If the physician elects to use prostaglandin gel or tablets for the purpose of cervical ripening, the nursing role is one of support. This includes preparing the equipment and initiating maternal/fetal monitoring, as well as positioning the patient in lithotomy or dorsal position and providing emotional support. The patient may be encouraged to implement relaxation techniques. Following the procedure, fetal surveillance continues for 30 minutes to 2 hours, vital signs are reassessed, and the patient placed at rest. If the patient has no increase in uterine activity and the fetal heart rate remains reassuring, the patient may be discharged. If, however, regular uterine contractions occur, monitoring is continued and maternal signs are assessed hourly for the first 4 hours (ACOG, 1995). Documentation includes cervical examination results, drug dosage, route, side effects, and patient reaction (Glazer & Hulme, 1987). Prostaglandin gel may be followed by oxytocin for labor stimulation. Manufacturer's guidelines recommend a 6–12-hour delay. If the patient continues to have uterine activity as a result of the gel, oxytocin should be used cautiously or deferred (ACOG, 1992). A second dose of prostaglandin gel may be given 6–12 hours after the first dose if insufficient cervical change has occurred. Only Cervidil may be administered by a nurse and fetal surveillance should be maintained during the time the insert is placed (up to 12 hours). Oxytocin is administered 30 minutes after Cervidil removal.

Oxytocin is approved by the FDA for induction or augmentation of labor by the intravenous route. The oxytocin must be diluted because rapid infusion can cause maternal hypotension, dysrhythmias, cardiac ischemia, and uterine tetany. Oxytocin is commercially available as 10 units per milliliter. Oxytocin is added to a balanced salt solution such as lactated Ringer's or 0.9% sodium chloride. A balanced salt solution will not exacerbate the water-retentive properties of oxytocin. The concentration should be standardized as per institutional policy. Oxytocin dosage is measured in milliunits per minute. A common dilution is 10 units of oxytocin per 1000 ml intravenous fluid. This yields a concentration of 10 milliunits per 1 ml. An alternative dilution is 15 units of oxytocin per 250 ml intravenous solution yielding a concentration of 60 milliunits per 1 ml. This dilution is convenient for dosage administration because ml per hour are equivalent to mU/minute. See Display 8-2 for formulas which help convert milliunits of oxytocin per milliliter to an infusion rate in milliliters per hour.

Table 8-3 lists oxytocin conversions for the dilutions just listed. The oxytocin solution is labeled as to the concentration with an appropriate medication sticker. In order to administer precise dosages, an infusion pump must be utilized. The diluted oxytocin solution to be administered by pump is piggy-backed into a primary intravenous line containing electrolyte solution at the most proximal port. A primary intravenous solution is used to keep the line open should the medication need to be discontinued and/or should an intravenous fluid bolus be necessary.

Prior to initiating the infusion, baseline vital signs (temperature, pulse, respirations, and blood pressure) and fetal and uterine status should be assessed. Use of electronic fetal monitoring permits more thorough assessment of fetal heart rate responses and uterine activity. Internal or direct electronic monitoring methods permit the most accurate evaluation of fetal heart rate variability and strength of uterine activity and require cervical dilation and rupture of the membranes. As these occur, a fetal scalp electrode and an intrauterine pressure catheter may be considered.

The infusion should be initiated with a low dose because the effective dose varies greatly among women. The dose is increased by small,

DISPLAY 8-2

Formulas for Calculating Oxytocin Dosages

1. Determine mU oxytocin/ml by

$$\frac{\text{units of oxytocin}}{\text{ml of IV fluid}} \cdot 1000 = \text{milliunits per (mU/ml)}$$

2. Determine mU of oxytocin/min by

$$\frac{\text{mU/ml}}{1} \cdot \frac{\text{ml/hr}}{60 \text{ min}} = \text{milliunits per min (mU/min)}$$

3. Confirm administration rate in ml/hr by

$$\frac{\text{mU/min} \cdot 60 \text{ min/hr}}{\text{mU/ml}} = \frac{\text{ml}}{\text{hr}}$$

Example: 15 U oxytocin per 250 ml IV fluid

1. $\dfrac{15\text{ U}}{250 \text{ ml}} \cdot 1000 = 60 \text{ mU/ml}$

2. $\dfrac{60 \text{ mU}}{1} \cdot \dfrac{1 \text{ ml/hour}}{60 \text{ min}} = 1 \text{ mU/min}$

3. $\dfrac{1\text{mU/min} \cdot 60 \text{ min}}{60 \text{ mU/ml}} = 1 \text{ ml/hr}$

set increments after steady state has been achieved with the previous dosage adjustment. The American College of Obstetricians and Gynecologists (ACOG) recommends an initial dose of 0.5 to 2 mU/min with increases of 1–2 mU every 30–60 min (ACOG, 1995). This should produce a gradual onset of labor equivalent to the early latent phase of labor. It should also decrease the total dose of oxytocin and the incidence of hyperstimulation of the uterus. Three factors are continually assessed in order to determine a patient's therapeutic oxytocin dose: uterine activity, fetal response, and cervical effacement and dilatation. Uterine activity goals consist of uterine contractions with a frequency of 2–3 minutes, a duration of 40–90 seconds, and intensity of 40–90 millimeters of mercury by intrauterine monitoring (Petrie & Williams, 1993). The resting tone must be less than 20 millimeters of mercury by intrauterine monitoring. If intrauterine pressure

TABLE 8-3. Oxytocin Conversions

Rate (mU/min)	Solution Concentration	
	10 U oxytocin/1000 ml (10 mU/ml)	15 U oxytocin 250 ml (60 mU/ml)
	ml/hr	ml/hr
0.5	3	0.5
1	6	1
2	12	2
3	18	3
4	24	4
5	30	5
6	36	6
7	42	7
8	48	8
9	54	9
10	60	10
11	66	11
12	72	12
13	78	13
14	84	14
15	90	15
16	96	16
17	102	17
18	108	18
19	114	19
20	120	20

monitoring is not being used, contractions should be moderate to firm to palpation and resting tone should be adequate as identified by lack of sensation of intrauterine pressure to the examiner's hand. Should hyperstimulation occur, the infusion is decreased or discontinued.

The definitive measurement of adequate oxytocin dosage is cervical dilation. Dilation should progress by at least one centimeter per hour. The need to assess cervical change is balanced with the potential risk of infection in performing vaginal examination.

Water intoxication, a complication of prolonged high-dose oxytocin administration, is prevented by using balanced salt intravenous solutions, decreasing the total dose of oxytocin, monitoring intake and output, and observing at-risk patients for signs and symptoms, including weakness, restlessness, nausea, vomiting, diarrhea, polyuria or oliguria, and seizures.

In summary, ongoing assessment of the patient undergoing induction or augmentation of labor consists of maternal vital signs, uterine activity, fetal response, cervical dilatation, and observation for conscientious fluid management. As labor progresses to the active phase, the dose of oxytocin may need to be gradually decreased as the concentration of oxytocin receptors increases through labor making lower doses more effective.

Oxytocin is often continued in the immediate postpartum period to prevent postpartum hemorrhage.

Nursing Diagnosis

Nursing diagnosis is an essential component of the nursing process. Formulating a nursing diagnosis is the link between gathering information and developing a plan of care. It demands astute, holistic clinical judgment based on a sound knowledge base. The following are nursing diagnoses that are appropriate for patients undergoing induction or augmentation of labor.

1. *Maternal Stability*

   Alterations in cardiac output: decreased related to side effects of prostaglandins and oxytocin

   Potential fluid volume overload related to oxytocin infusion

   Potential for injury: uterine hyperstimulation

   Impaired physical mobility related to continuous monitoring

2. *Psychosocial Well-Being*

   Alterations in comfort: pain related to intense uterine activity

   Ineffective individual coping related to intense uterine activity

   Fear related to unknown methods: effects of induction/augmentation techniques

   Fear related to self and fetal well-being

   Knowledge deficit related to unknown methods: effects of induction/augmentation techniques

   Disturbance of self-concept: role performance related to altered birth plan

3. *Fetal Well-Being*

   Potential for injury: fetal compromise related to decreased oxygenation

   Potential for injury: fetal compromise related to infectious process

Expected Outcomes

Maternal Stability

The patient will

1. Maintain vital signs within normal ranges
2. Maintain adequate urinary output
3. Avoid vena caval compression and hypotension by maintaining a lateral position
4. Achieve adequate uterine activity
5. Avoid uterine hyperstimulation and subsequent injury

Psychosocial Well-Being

The patient will

1. Verbalize understanding of procedures including risks
2. Verbalize understanding of the monitoring process
3. Verbalize decreased fear of procedure and unknown
4. Demonstrate ability to relax during uterine activity
5. Verbalize feelings related to role performance
6. Demonstrate normal maternal/infant bonding

Fetal Well-Being

The fetus will

1. Maintain fetal heart rate between 110–160 beats per minute
2. Maintain a reassuring fetal heart rate pattern on the electronic fetal heart rate monitor as evidenced by
   a. minimum or greater fetal heart rate variability
   b. presence of long-term variability
   c. absence of fetal heart rate decelerations
   d. presence of accelerations
3. Exhibit intrauterine activity

REFERENCES

American College of Obstetricians and Gynecologists (1995). Induction of labor. (Technical Bulletin 217) Washington, DC: Author.

Ahner, R., Egarter, C., Kiss, H., Heinzl, K., Zeillinger, R., Schatten, C., Dormeier, A., & Husslein, P. (1995). Fetal fibronectin as a selection criterion for induction of term labor. American Journal of Obstetrics and Gynecology, 173(5), 1513–1517.

American Academy of Pediatrics and the American College of Obstetricians and

Gynecologists. (1996). Guildelines for perinatal care (4th ed.). Elk Grove Village, IL: Author.

American Society of Hospital Pharmacists. (1996). AHFS Drug Information 1996. Bethesda, MD: Author.

Andersson, K. E., Forman, A., & Ulmsten, U. (1983). Pharmacology of labor. Clinical Obstetrics and Gynecology, 26(1), 56–77.

Atad, J., Hallak, M., Auslender, R., Porat-Packer, T., Zarfati, D., & Abramovici, H. (1996). A randomized comparison of prostaglandin E_2, oxytocin, and the double-balloon device in inducing labor. Obstetrics and Gynecology, 87(2), 223–227.

Beazley, J. M., & Alderman, B. (1975). Neonatal hyperbilirubinemia following the use of oxytocin in labor. British Journal of Obstetrics & Gynaecology, 82, 265–271.

Bernstein, P. (1991). Prostaglandin E_2 gel for cervical ripening and labour induction: A multicentre placebo-controlled trial. Canadian Medical Association Journal, 145, 1249–1254.

Bishop, E. H. (1964). Pelvic scoring for elective induction. Obstetrics and Gynecology, 24(2), 266–268.

Blakemore, K. J., Qin, N. G., Petrie, R. H., & Paine, L. L. (1990). A prospective comparison of hourly and quarter-hourly oxytocin dose increase intervals for the induction of labor at term. Obstetrics and Gynecology, 75(5), 757–761.

Blanch, G., Olah, K. S. J., & Walkinshaw, S. (1996). The presence of fetal fibronectin in the cervicovaginal secretions of women at term—Its role in the assessment of women before labor induction and in the investigation of the physiologic mechanisms of labor. American Journal of Obstetrics and Gynecology, 174(1, Pt. 1), 262–266.

Boozarjomehri, F., Timor-Tritsch, I., & Chao, C. R. (1994). Transvaginal ultrasonographic evaluation of the cervix before labor: Presence of cervical wedging is associated with shorter duration of induced labor. American Journal of Obstetrics and Gynecology, 171(4), 1081–1087.

Brown, C. E. L., Satin, A. J., & Leveno, K. J. (1994). The economic advantages of measured change in health care: An example from obstetrics. Obstetrics and Gynecology, 84(5), 893–895.

Busowski, J. D., & Parsons, M. T. (1995). Amniotomy to induce labor. Clinical Obstetrics and Gynecology, 38(2), 246–258.

Cammu, H., & Van Eeckhout, E. (1996). A randomized controlled trial of early versus delayed use of amniotomy and oxytocin infusion in nulliparous labour. British Journal of Obstetrics & Gynaecology, 103, 313–318.

Carlan, S. J., Danna, P., Durkee, D., Quinsey, C., & Lanaris, B. (1995). Randomized study of pre-induction cervical ripening with sequential use of intravaginal prostaglandin E_2 gel. Obstetrics and Gynecology, 85, 608–613.

Chez, R. A., Barton, D. M., Miller, F. C., & Petrie, R. H. (1988). When and how to induce labor. Contemporary Obstetrics and Gynecology, 32, 145–153.

Chwalisz, K., & Garfield, R. E. (1994). Antiprogestins in the induction of labor. Annals of the New York Academy of Sciences, 734, 387–413.

Cunningham, F. G., MacDonald, P. C., Gant, N. F., Leveno, K. J., & Gilstrap, L. C. (1993). Williams' obstetrics (19th ed.). East Norwalk, CT: Appleton and Lange.

Curtis, P., Evens, S., Resnick, J., et al. (1986). Uterine responses to three techniques of breast stimulation. Obstetrics and Gynecology, 67(1), 25–28.

Darroca, R. J., Buttino, L., Jr., Miller, J., & Khamais, H. J. (1996). Prostaglandin E_2 gel for cervical ripening in patients with an indication for delivery. Obstetrics and Gynecology, 87(2), 228–230.

Dawood, M. Y. (1990). Uterine stimulation with oxytocin. In R. E. Garfield (Ed.), Uterine contractility. Serono Symposia, Norwell, MA.

Dawood, M. Y. (1995). New approach to oxytocin induction-augmentation of labor. Application of oxytocin physiology during pregnancy [Review]. Advances in Experimental Medicine and Biology, 395, 585–594.

Edwards, M. S. (1996). Mifepristone: Cervical ripening and induction of labor. Clinical Obstetrics and Gynecology, 39(2), 469–473.

Elliott, J. P., & Flaherty, J. F. (1984). The use of breast stimulation to prevent postdate pregnancy. American Journal of Obstetrics and Gynecology, 149(6), 628–632.

Food and Drug Administration. (1978). New restrictions on oxytocin use. FDA Drug Bulletin, 8(5), 30. Washington, DC.

Foster, T. C. S., Jacobson, J. D., & Valenzuela, G. J. (1988). Oxytocin augmentation of labor: A comparison of 15- and 30-minute dose increment intervals. Obstetrics and Gynecology, 71(2), 147–149.

Friedman, E. A. (1954). The graphic analysis of labor. American Journal of Obstetrics and Gynecology, 68(6), 1568–1575.

Friedman, E. A., Niswander, K. R., Bayonet-Rivera, N. P., & Sachtleben, M. R. (1966). Relation of prelabor evaluation to inducibility and the course of labor. Obstetrics and Gynecology, 28(4), 495–501.

Frigoletto, F. D., Lieberman, E., Lang, J. M., Cohen, A., Barss, V., Ringer, S., & Datta, S. (1995). A clinical trial of active management of labor. New England Journal of Medicine, 333(12), 745–750.

Frydman, R., Lelaidier, C., Baton-Saint-Mleux, C., Fernandez, H., Vial, M., & Bourget, P. (1992). Labor induction in women at term with mifepristone (RU 486): A double-blind, randomized, placebo-controlled study. Obstetrics and Gynecology, 80(6), 972–975.

Fuchs, A. R., & Fuchs, F. (1996). Physiology and endocrinology of parturition. In S. G Gabbe, J. R. Niebyl, & J. L. Simpson (Eds.), Obstetrics: Normal and problem pregnancies (3rd ed.). New York: Churchill Livingstone.

Gerhardstein, L. P., Allswede, M. T., Sloan, C. T., & Lorenz, R. P. (1995). Reduction in the rate of cesarean birth with active management of labor and intermediate-dose oxytocin. Journal of Reproductive Medicine, 40(1), 4–8.

Gilson, G. J., Russell, D. J., Izquierdo, L. A., Qualls, C. R., & Curet, L. B. (1996). A prospective randomized evaluation of a hygroscopic cervical dilator, Dilapan, in the preinduction ripening of patients undergoing induction of labor. American Journal of Obstetrics and Gynecology, 175(1), 145–149.

Glazer, G., & Hulme, M. A. (1987). Prostaglandin gel for cervical ripening. Maternal Child Nursing, 12(1), 28–31.

Goldenberg, M., Dulitzky, M., Feldman, B., Zolti, M., & Bider, D. (1996). Stretching of the cervix and stripping of the membranes at term: A randomized controlled study. European Journal of Obstetrics Gynecology & Reproductive Biology, 66(2), 129–132.

Goni, S., Sawhney, H., & Gopalan, S. (1995). Oxytocin induction of labor: A comparison of 20- and 60-minute dose increment levels. International Journal of Obstetrics and Gynecology, 48, 31–36.

Gonser, M. (1995). Labor induction and augmentation with oxytocin: Pharmacokinetic considerations. Archives of Gynecology & Obstetrics, 256, 63–66.

Hales, K. A., Rayburn, W. F., Turnbull, G. L., Christensen, H. D., & Patatanian, E. (1994). Double-blind comparison of intracervical and intravaginal prostaglandin E_2 for cervical ripening and induction of labor. American Journal of Obstetrics and Gynecology, 171(4), 1087–1091.

Husslein, P., Kofler, E., Rasmussen, A. B., et al. (1983). Oxytocin and the initiation of human parturition: IV: Plasma concentrations of oxytocin and 13, 14-dihydro-15-ketoprostaglandin $F_{2\alpha}$ during induction of labor by artificial rupture of the membranes. American Journal of Obstetrics and Gynecology, 147(5), 503–507.

Jackson, G. M., Sharp, H. T., & Varner, M. W. (1994). Cervical ripening before induction of labor: A randomized trial of prostaglandin E_2 gel versus low-dose oxytocin. American Journal of Obstetrics and Gynecology, 171(4), 1092–1096.

James, C., Peedicayil, A., & Seshadri, L. (1994). Use of the foley catheter as a cervical ripening agent prior to the induction of labor. International Journal of Gynaecology & Obstetrics, 47(3), 229–232.

Keirse, M. J. (1993). Prostaglandins in preinduction cervical ripening: Meta-analysis of worldwide clinical experience. Journal of Reproductive Medicine, 38, 89–100.

Keirse, M. J. N. C., & de Koning Gans, H. J. (1995). Randomized comparison of the effects of endocervical and vaginal prostaglandin E_2 gel in women with various degrees of cervical ripeness. American Journal of Obstetrics and Gynecology, 173(6), 1859–1864.

Kelsey, J. J., & Prevost, R. R. (1994). Drug therapy during labor and delivery. American Journal Hosp Pharm, 51(19), 2394–2402.

Krammer, J., & O'Brien, W. F. (1995). Mechanical methods of cervical ripening. Clinical Obstetrics and Gynecology, 38(2), 280–286.

Krammer, J., Williams, M. C., Sawai, S. K., & O'Brien, W. F. (1995). Pre-induction cervical ripening: A randomized comparison of two methods. Obstetrics and Gynecology, 85(4), 614–618.

Lazor, L. Z., Philipson, E. H., Ingardia, C. J., Kobetitsch, E. S., & Curry, S. L. (1993). A randomized comparison of 15- and 40-minute dosing protocols for labor augmentation and induction. Obstetrics and Gynecology, 82(6), 1009–1012.

Leppert, P. C. (1995). Anatomy and physiology of cervical ripening. Clinical Obstetrics and Gynecology, 38(2), 267–269.

Lopez-Zeno, J. A., Peacemen, A. M., Adaschek, J. A., & Socol, M. L. (1992). A controlled trial of a program for the active management of labor. New England Journal of Medicine, 326, 450–454.

Lyndrup, J. (1996). Induction of labor by PGE$_2$ and other local methods: Physiology, methods and guidelines for patient selection. Acta Obstetrica Gynaecoligica Scandinavica, 75, 86–97.

Magann, E. F., Perry, K. G., Dockery, J. R., Bass, J. D., Chauhan, S. P., & Morrison, J. C. (1995). Cervical ripening before medical induction of labor: A comparison of prostaglandin E$_2$, estradiol, and oxytocin. American Journal of Obstetrics and Gynecology, 172(6), 1702–1708.

Manabe, Y., Sagawa, N., & Mori, T. (1985). Experimental evidence for the progress of labor with the increase in the force of cervical dilatation after rupture of the membranes. American Journal of Obstetrics and Gynecology, 152(6), 696–704.

McKay, S., & Mahan, C. S. (1983). How worthwhile are membrane stripping and amniotomy? Contemporary Obstetrics and Gynecology, 184, 173–181.

Mercer, B., Pilgrim, P., & Sibai, B. (1991). Labor induction with continuous low-dose oxytocin infusion: A randomized trial. Obstetrics and Gynecology, 77(5), 659–663.

Merrill, P. A., & Freeman, R. K. (1986). Serial induction of labor. Contemporary Obstetrics and Gynecology, 27, 51–54.

Muller, P. R., Stubbs, T. M., & Laurent, S. L. (1992). A prospective randomized clinical trial comparing two oxytocin induction protocols. American Journal of Obstetrics and Gynecology, 167(2), 373–381.

Murray, H. G., Buonocore, A., & Hawley, J. (1995). A randomized trial of two preparations of vaginal prostaglandin for pre-induction cervical ripening. Obstetrics and Gynecology, 86(6), 880–885.

Musacchio, M. J. (1990). Oxytocins for augmentation and induction of labor. New York: March of Dimes.

Newton, E. R. (1987). Using mechanical dilators for cervical ripening. Contemporary Obstetrics and Gynecology, 30, 47–64.

Novy, M. J., & Liggins, G. C. (1980). Role of prostaglandins, prostacyclin, and thromboxanes in the physiologic control of the uterus and in parturition. Seminars in Perinatology, 4, 45–65.

O'Brien, W. F. (1995a). Cervical ripening and labor induction: Progress and challenges. Clinical Obstetrics and Gynecology, 38(2), 221–223.

O'Brien, W. F. (1995b). The role of prostaglandins in labor and delivery. Clinics in Perinatology, 22(4), 973–984.

O'Brien, W. F., & Cefalo, R. C. (1996). Labor and delivery. In S. G. Gabbe, J. R. Niebyl, & J. L. Simpson (Eds.), Obstetrics: Normal and problem pregnancies. New York: Church Livingston.

O'Brien, J. M., Mercer, B. M., Cleary, N. T., & Sibai, B. M. (1995). Efficacy of outpatient induction with low-dose intravaginal prostaglandin E$_2$: A randomized, double-blind, placebo-controlled trial. American Journal of Obstetrics and Gynecology, 173(6), 1855–1859.

O'Driscoll, K., Foley, M., & MacDonald, D. (1984). Active management of labour as an alternative to cesarean section for dystocia. Obstetrics and Gynecology, 63(4), 485–490.

O'Driscoll, K., Jackson, R. J. A., & Gallagher, J. T. (1969). Prevention of prolonged labour. British Medical Journal, 2, 477–480.

O'Driscoll, K., Stronge, J. M., & Minogue, M. (1973). Active management of labour. British Medical Journal, 3, 135–137.

Orhue, A. A. (1995). Induction of labour at term in primigravidae with low Bishop's score:

A comparison of 3 methods. European Journal of Obstetrics, Gynecology & Reproctive Biology, 58(2), 119–125.

Petrie, R. H., & Williams, A. M. (1993). Induction of labor. In R. A. Knuppel & J. E. Drukker (Eds.), High-risk pregnancy: A team approach (2nd ed.). Philadelphia: Saunders.

Pollnow, D. M., & Broekhuizen, F. F. (1996). Randomized, double-blind trial of prostaglandin E$_2$ intravaginal gel versus low-dose oxytocin for cervical ripening before induction of labor. American Journal of Obstetrics and Gynecology, 174(6), 1910–1916.

Reid, G. J., & Helewa, M. E. (1995). A trial of pulsatile versus continuous oxytocin administration for the induction of labor. Journal of Perinatology, 15(5), 364–366.

Salmon, Y. M., Kee, W. H., Tan, S. L., & Jen, S. W. (1986). Cervical ripening by breast stimulation. Obstetrics and Gynecology, 67(1), 21–24.

Sanchez-Ramos, L., Farah, L. A., Kaunitz, A. M., Adair, C. D., Del Valle, G. O., & Fuqua, P. (1995). Preinduction cervical ripening with commercially available prostaglandin E$_2$ gel: A randomized, double-blind comparison with a hospital-compounded preparation American Journal of Obstetrics and Gynecology, 173(4), 1079–1084.

Satin, A. J., Leveno, K. J., Sherman, M. L., Brewster, D. S., & Cunningham, F. G. (1992). High- versus low-dose oxytocin for labor stimulation. Obstetrics and Gynecology, 80(1), 111–116.

Satin, A. J., Leveno, K. J., Sherman, M. L., & McIntire, D. D. (1992). Factors affecting the dose response to oxytocin for labor stimulation. American Journal of Obstetrics and Gynecology, 166, 1260–1261.

Satin, A. J., Leveno, K. J., Sherman, M. L., & McIntire, D. D. (1994). High-dose oxytocin: 20- versus 40-minute dosage interval. Obstetrics and Gynecology, 83(2), 234–238.

Sawai, S. K., & O'Brien, W. F. (1995). Outpatient cervical ripening. Clinical Obstetrics and Gynecology, 38(2), 301–309

Sawai, S. K., O'Brien, W. F., Mastrogiannis, D. S., Krammer, J., Mastry, M. G., & Porter, G. W. (1994). Patient-administered outpatient intravaginal prostaglandin E$_2$ suppositories in post-date pregnancies: A double-blind, randomized, placebo-controlled study. Obstetrics and Gynecology, 84(5), 807–810.

Schulman, H. (1983). Prostaglandins. In F. Fuchs & A. Klopper (Eds.), Endocrinology of pregnancy (3rd ed.). New York: Harper & Row.

Schulman, H., & Farmakides, G. (1987). Role of the unfavorable cervix in the induction of labor. Clinical Obstetrics and Gynecology, 30(1), 50–55.

Seitchik, J., & Castillo, M. (1982). Oxytocin augmenetation of dysfunctional labor. I: Clinical data. American Journal of Obstetrics and Gynecology, 144(8), 899–905.

Seitchik, J., & Castillo, M. (1983). Oxytocin augmentation of dysfunctional labor. III: Multiparous patients. American Journal of Obstetrics and Gynecology, 145(7), 777–780.

Seitchik, J., Amico, J., Robinson, A. G., & Castillo, M. (1984). Oxytocin augmentation of labor. IV: Oxytocin pharmacokinetics. American Journal of Obstetrics and Gynecology, 150(3), 225–228.

Shyken, J. M., & Petrie R. H. (1995). The use of oxytocin. Clinics in Perinatology, 22(4), 907–931.

St. Onge, R. D., & Connors, G. T. (1995). Preinduction cervical ripening: A comparison of intracervical gel versus the foley catheter. American Journal of Obstetrics and Gynecology, 172(2, Pt. 1), 687–690.

Toaff, M. E., Hezroni, J., & Toaff, R. (1978). Induction of labour by pharmacological and physiological doses of intravenous oxytocin. British Journal of Obstetrics & Gynaecology, 85, 101–108.

Uldbjerg, N., Ulmsten, U., & Ekman, G. (1983). The ripening of the human cervix in terms of connective biochemistry. Clinical Obstetrics and Gynecology, 67(1), 14–26.

Varaklis, K., Gumina, R., & Stubblefield, P. G. (1995). Randomized controlled trial of vaginal misoprostol and intracervical prostaglandin E$_2$ gel for induction of labor at term. Obstetrics and Gynecology, 86, 541–544.

Watson, W. J., Stevens, D., Welter, S., & Day, D. (1996). Factors predicting succesful labor induction. Obstetrics and Gynecology, 88(6), 990–992.

Wein, P. (1989). Efficacy of different starting doses of oxytocin for induction of labor. Obstetrics and Gynecology, 74, 863–868.

Weiss, G. (1995). Relaxin used to produce the cervical ripening of labor. Clinical Obstetrics and Gynecology, 38(2), 293–300.

Wigton, T. R., & Wolk, B. M. (1994). Elective and routine induction of labor. A retrospective analysis of 274 cases. Journal of Reproductive Medicine, 39(1), 21–26.

Willcourt, R. J., Pager, D., Wendel, J., & Hale, R. W. (1994). Induction of labor with pulsatile oxytocin by a computer-controlled pump. American Journal of Obstetrics and Gynecology, 170(2), 603–608.

Wing, D. A., & Paul, R. H. (1996). A comparison of differing dosing regimens of vaginally administered misoprostol for pre-induction cervical ripening and labor induction. American Journal of Obstetrics and Gynecology, 175, 158–164.

Wiriyasirivaj, B., Vutyavanich, T., & Ruangsri, R. A. (1996). A randomized controlled trial of membrane stripping at term to promote labor. Obstetrics and Gynecology, 87(5), 767–770.

Xenakis, E. M. J., Langer, O., Piper, J. M., Conway, D., & Berkus, M. D. (1995). Low-dose versus high-dose oxytocin augmentation of labor–A randomized trial. American Journal of Obstetrics and Gynecology, 173(6), 1874–1878.

CHAPTER

9

Hypertensive Disorders in Pregnancy

Terry G. Leicht and Carol J. Harvey

Pregnancy-induced hypertension (PIH) is a significant cause of maternal and fetal/neonatal morbidity and mortality. fifty thousand women die worldwide each year from eclampsia (Duley, 1992). Hypertensive complications are the second leading cause of maternal death in the United States, second only to embolic events (Koonin, Atrash, Rochat, & Smith, 1989). In a recent retrospective review of 1,840 maternal deaths occurring between 1987 and 1990, 18% were attributable to complications of PIH (Berg, Atrash, Koonin, & Tucker, 1996). PIH complicates 6–8% of all pregnancies in the United States and presents a clinical challenge to the perinatal healthcare team.

Although several theories have been proposed, the etiology of PIH remains unclear. Scientific research has provided clinicians with information regarding risk factors for the disease, pathophysiologic effects, and proposed methods of clinical management.

The purpose of this chapter is to provide information to the clinician regarding the pathophysiology of PIH, evaluation and management of the hypertensive obstetric patient, and current theories under investigation regarding the etiology and possible prevention of the disease.

CLASSIFICATION OF DISEASE

Various nomenclature systems exist in the literature that attempt to classify the subsets of hyper-

tension in pregnancy. The systems reflect the evolution of the body of knowledge about this disease process and some individual authors' viewpoints. This chapter describes the classification system developed by the National Institutes of Health Working Group on High Blood Pressure in Pregnancy (1990) (see Display 9-1). A brief description of this system follows.

Chronic Hypertension/Coincidental Hypertension

Chronic hypertension is defined as hypertension present prior to pregnancy or diagnosed before the 20th week of pregnancy. Hypertension that persists after the 42nd postpartum day is also classified as chronic.

Pregnancy-Induced Hypertension

Three distinct clinical groups are included in this classification. The first describes patients presenting with hypertension without proteinuria or edema.

The second, preeclampsia, includes patients with hypertension accompanied by proteinuria, edema, or both. The incidence of preeclampsia in the general obstetric population is approximately 5–7%. Women at increased risk for preeclampsia include those having their first baby; women less than 17 years of age; women with diabetes mellitus, chronic hypertension, or preexisting vascular disease; and women with

DISPLAY 9-1

Classification of Hypertensive States in Pregnancy

I. Pregnancy-Induced Hypertension
  A. Hypertension without proteinuria and/or edema
  B. Preeclampsia: hypertension with proteinuria and/or edema
    1. mild
    2. severe
  C. Eclampsia

II. Chronic Hypertension/Coincidental Hypertension

III. Preeclampsia/Eclampsia Superimposed on Chronic Hypertension

IV. Transient Hypertension

Source: Developed by the National Institutes of Health Working Group on High Blood Pressure in Pregnancy (1990).

multiple gestation. In a recent large prospective study (Sibai, 1995), 2,947 nulliparous women were evaluated for clinical characteristics predictive of the development of preeclampsia. Preeclampsia developed in 5.3% of the study participants. Four characteristics predicted the development of preeclampsia: systolic blood pressure ($p < .001$), prepregnancy weight ($p < .01$), smoking history ($p < .01$), and gravidity ($p < .05$). It is interesting to note that systolic blood pressure was a better predictor of preeclampsia when compared to diastolic blood pressure or mean arterial blood pressure. Also, the higher the participant's systolic pressure at entry into the study (13–27 weeks gestation) and the higher the participant's prepregnancy weight, the greater the risk for the development of preeclampsia. Contrary to previous reports, this study found that being African American was not a risk factor for the development of PIH.

Preeclampsia can be further categorized as mild or severe, reflecting the extent of end-organ derangement or damage. Display 9-2 lists the clinical manifestations of severe preeclampsia.

The third clinical group includes eclampsia, and those patients presenting with hypertension and seizures and/or coma. The incidence of eclampsia in patients who have pregnancy-induced hypertension has decreased over the past several decades and has recently been estimated at 1:2,000–1:2,500 deliveries (Cunningham et al., 1997; Douglas & Redman, 1994). Maternal mortality for patients with eclampsia has also decreased in the past 50 years primarily because of improved surveillance in the perinatal period and improved access to perinatal care. Currently, mortality rates for eclampsia are difficult to extrapolate because of underreporting. In a recent study (Eclampsia Trial Collaborative Group, 1995) maternal mortality was estimated to be between 3 and 5% depending on the type of therapy prescribed for the seizure activity. Reported perinatal mortality in this study ranged from 130 to 300 per 1,000.

Eclampsia is a consequence of severe preeclampsia; however, it is not always preceded by hypertension, significant proteinuria, or edema. In two published series (Chesley, 1978; Diekman, 1952) 20% of eclamptic women had systolic blood pressures of less than 140 mm/Hg.

Preeclampsia/Eclampsia Superimposed on Chronic Hypertension

Women with preexisting hypertension have a greatly increased risk for the development of PIH when compared to the overall population. Up to 20% of patients with preexisting hypertensive disorders may develop this disease. Older gravidas have an increased incidence of developing preeclampsia most likely related to their overall increased incidence of chronic hypertensive disease. The morbidity for both mother and fetus in this group of patients is also higher than for patients with chronic hypertension or preeclampsia alone, with an increased incidence of abruptio placenta, intrauterine

DISPLAY 9-2

Clinical Criteria for Severe Preeclampsia

The presence of one or more of these parameters in a patient with pregnancy-induced hypertension is classified as severe preeclampsia:

- Blood pressure >160 mmHg systolic or >110 diastolic, on two occasions 6 hours apart with the patient at bed rest
- Proteinuria >5 grams in 24 hours or 3+ to 4+ on qualitative assessment
- Oliguria <400 ml of urine in 24 hours
- Cerebral or visual disturbances
- Epigastric or right-upper-quadrant pain
- Pulmonary edema or cyanosis
- Impaired liver function of unclear etiology
- Thrombocytopenia

growth retardation (IUGR), and intrauterine fetal death (IUFD).

Transient Hypertension

Transient hypertension is defined as the development of mildly elevated blood pressure during pregnancy or in the first 24 hours postpartum with no other signs of chronic disease or preeclampsia. The hypertension usually resolves following delivery but may recur with future pregnancies. Because the identification of hypertension in the pregnant woman may be a precursor to pregnancy-induced hypertension, continued assessment for other symptoms of PIH throughout pregnancy should be performed. Thus, the diagnosis of transient hypertension can only be made after the postpartum period is complete.

PREGNANCY-INDUCED HYPERTENSION

Historically, PIH has been diagnosed following the onset of the classic triad of clinical signs: hypertension, proteinuria, and edema. However, these symptoms can be attributed to a variety of common pregnancy conditions, frequently making a definitive diagnosis difficult.

The diagnosis of hypertension in the obstetric population is controversial. Average blood pressure for young women (age <30 years) is 120/60. Thus, the use of measurements of 140 systolic and 90 diastolic to define hypertension in this group may not accurately capture all pregnant women with elevated blood pressure. Therefore, some clinicians have used an increase in blood pressure of 30 mm Hg systolic or 15 mm Hg diastolic to identify patients possibly at risk for developing PIH. However, increased blood pressure in pregnancy may be a normal physiologic change. Villar and Sibai (1989) reported a prospective study to determine the predictive value of a threshold increase of 15 mm Hg diastolic and/or a 30 mm Hg increase in systolic blood pressure, and the subsequent development of PIH. They reported that a threshold elevation of diastolic blood pressure had a positive predictive value of less than 35%. An elevation in systolic blood pressure had a similar poor predictive value of less than 33%. Additionally, elevation in calculated mean arterial blood pressure was also weakly predictive of subsequent development of PIH. The authors concluded that neither threshold elevations of systolic and/or diastolic blood pressure nor mean arterial pressure were significantly predictive of the development of PIH.

Blood pressure elevations during the second half of pregnancy warrant increased surveillance for the development of other signs of PIH. Because normal physiologic events may incrementally increase maternal blood pressure over time, it is reasonable for clinicians to use an increase in systolic and/or diastolic blood pressure to 140 mm Hg and 90 mm Hg, respectively, for the diagnosis of hypertension in pregnancy.

Proteinuria is defined as the presence of 300 mg or greater of protein in a 24-hour period or 100 mg/dl in two random urine samples 6 hours apart. The degree of protein can vary in 24 hours, making a single random sample insufficient. Although the presence of proteinuria is considered a sign of worsening disease process, in some patients it is a late developing sign. Eclampsia has occurred in the absence of proteinuria. In a review of 298 eclamptic patients 41% did not have proteinuria (Naidoo & Moodley, 1980). In another series of 199 patients, 13% had negative or trace proteinuria prior to seizure (Chesley, 1978).

Edema is a common finding in many pregnant women and as an isolated finding is not diagnostic of PIH. Edema of the hands and face that persists throughout the day is considered to be more significant than the finding of dependent edema. However, 10–15% of pregnant women whose blood pressure remains normal throughout pregnancy develop edema of the hands and face (Thomson, Hytten, & Billewicz, 1967). The edema associated with PIH is thought to be related to endothelial damage and subsequent leakage of fluid into the extravascular space.

Pathophysiology

Vasospasm and endothelial damage are the underlying pathophysiologic events in PIH. The concept of vascular changes that could be described as vasospastic in nature was first described in 1918 (Volhand, 1918). Vasospasm may cause elevation in arterial blood pressure and resistance to blood flow. It is unclear whether vasospasm produces damage to the vessels or if damage to the vessels produces vasospasm. Regardless, the restriction of blood flow is associated with endothelial cell damage, which in turn stimulates platelet and fibrinogen utilization. The vascular changes alter blood flow and result in hypoxic damage to vulnerable organ systems.

In addition to endothelial damage and vasospasm, women with PIH have exaggerated responses to angiotensin II. Angiotensin II is made by the renin–aldosterone pathway in the kidney when enzymes are released to convert angiotensin I to angiotensin II. Angiotensin II is a

potent vasoconstrictor and can produce arterial hypertension. Normal pregnancy decreases or blunts a patient's response to angiotensin II. In women with PIH, however, this normal "blunting" does not occur. This finding was the physiologic premise behind attempts to identify the patient who may ultimately develop PIH by using the "roll-over" test. The roll-over test, like other antepartum screening tests for PIH, has low specificity and has been abandoned in clinical practice.

Patients with PIH have been found to have an imbalance between prostacyclin and thromboxane. Prostacyclin has a direct effect on the tone of the arterial smooth muscles and works as a vasodilating agent; conversely, thromboxane is a potent vasoconstrictor. The exact mechanism that causes this imbalance remains unclear. However, in patients with PIH, placental production of prostacyclin has been found to be significantly decreased and thromboxane A_2 is significantly increased (Walsh, 1985).

The vascular effects of PIH ultimately may compromise individual organ systems by decreased blood flow, increased microvascular obstruction, and cellular hypoxia.

Complications
Cardiovascular

In the normal pregnancy, circulating blood volume is increased from 40–50%. In the severe preeclamptic patient, because of vasoconstriction and increased vascular permeability, there is a significant decrease in plasma volume resulting in decreased perfusion to end organs. The intravascular compartment of the patient with severe preeclampsia generally remains contracted until sometime during the postpartum period. Increased membrane permeability and the autotransfusion immediately following delivery place these patients at risk for the development of pulmonary edema.

Hemodynamic changes in patients with PIH are difficult to predict based on noninvasive assessments. Additionally, researchers disagree on the hemodynamic findings of patients with PIH.

For example, though elevation of blood pressure is a diagnostic clinical finding in PIH, it may be the result of either increased systemic vascular resistance or an increase in cardiac output. The extreme hypertension that may occur with this disease process can cause significant organ damage and must be controlled to prevent serious morbidity and mortality for the patient and fetus.

Renal

Decreased renal blood flow in some preeclamptic patients leads to a decrease in glomerular filtration rate (GFR), decreased clearance of uric acid, and sodium retention. Plasma creatinine levels may be above normal values for those of the nonpregnant woman. Glomerular damage causing increased permeability of the membrane results in the diagnostic finding of proteinuria. Patients in the clinical setting may have variation in the degree of proteinuria. This is theorized to be related to the degree of renal vasospastic activity. As the disease worsens and further damage to the glomerulus occurs, the size of protein molecule that can cross the membrane increases and proteinuria increases.

In severe preeclampsia, renal damage can occur from severe vasospasm. Creatinine levels may be as much as 2–3 times higher than in the nonpregnant patient. There is usually complete recovery of renal function after delivery.

Hematologic

The vasospastic activity in PIH may contribute to endothelial damage in the blood vessels. Platelet aggregation at the site of the injury and destruction of platelets and red blood cells as they pass through the narrowed vessel lumens then occurs. Thrombocytopenia, defined as a platelet count less than 100,000, and hemolysis are laboratory markers for this phenomenon in patients with severe PIH. Transfusion of platelets is not usually recommended, except for prophylaxis in the stable patient with a platelet count of <10,000–20,000 or in the preoperative patient with a count of under 50,000 (FDA Drug Bulletin, 1989). If platelet transfusion is indicated because of surgical or invasive procedures, patients should be transfused immediately prior to the procedure. This is because of the ongoing pathology of PIH, which rapidly destroys circulating platelets. Hemolysis occurring from PIH is rarely significant enough to cause anemia warranting the transfusion of blood. However, organ damage may be worsened by a decrease in the oxygen-carrying capacity of the blood. The transfusion of packed red blood cells may be utilized as a means of improving oxygen delivery. Other clotting abnormalities do not usually occur in this disease process.

Hepatic

The vasospasm and ischemia that are associated with PIH cause hepatocellular damage. Continued and profound vasospasm can lead to life-threatening complications such as hepatic hemorrhage, rupture, and necrosis. Elevation of serum glutamic-oxaloatic transaminase (SGOT) is a laboratory marker in the patient with hepatic dysfunction.

Clinical signs and symptoms of epigastric or right-upper-quadrant pain, nausea, or vomiting with or without accompanying hypertension should cause a high index of suspicion for hepatic involvement and warrant further evaluation.

Neurologic

Visual disturbance is a common neurologic finding in the patient with severe preeclampsia. Vasospasm of the retinal artery is the most likely cause of this symptom. Amourosis, the temporary blindness that occurs in approximately 1–3% of patients with severe PIH, and retinal detachment are much less common neurologic complications that can occur in this disease. The retinal detachment is usually unilateral and temporary. Surgical intervention is rarely required and vision is usually restored within about 1 week.

Serious, life-threatening neurologic complications may occur in severe preeclampsia. The presence of seizure activity in the patient with PIH is the diagnostic criteria for the classification of eclampsia. Eclampsia most frequently occurs in the third trimester of pregnancy. The onset of eclamptic seizures is associated with greater morbidity and mortality to both the mother and fetus. The patient with eclamptic seizures may lapse into a coma for varying lengths of time. Hypoxia, cerebral hemorrhage, and death are sequelae associated with eclampsia.

HELLP Syndrome

The constellation of symptoms that make up the HELLP syndrome (Display 9-3), hemolysis, elevated liver enzymes, and low platelets, are evidence of the impact of severe preeclampsia on end organs. Researchers (Crosby, 1991; Sibai et al., 1993) have found evidence of this syndrome in 15–20% of patients with severe preeclampsia or eclampsia.

One proposed theory for the etiology of these complications focuses on the vasospastic activity associated with preeclampsia (Rolfes & Ishak, 1986). Endothelial cells in the liver are damaged by the vasospastic activity that occurs in preeclampsia leading to platelet aggregation, adherence, and fibrin deposition. The resultant increase in intraluminal pressure may induce hemorrhage and rupture in the hepatic vessels. Hemorrhagic necrosis is the likely cause of elevated liver enzymes found in these patients. Serious complications of HELLP include hepatic infarction and hepatic rupture. Hepatic infarction may occur following gross ischemia and obstruction to blood flow from fibrin deposits. Bleeding from these areas of infarction and necrosis may cause subcapsular hematoma or hepatic rupture, a life-threatening event. The onset of symptoms associated with liver rupture is usually sudden upper abdominal or right-upper-quadrant pain, shoulder pain, nausea, and vomiting. Liver enzymes are grossly elevated and prothrombin time is prolonged. Urgent surgical intervention is most often required. Maternity morbidity and mortality following liver rupture is high. Smith and associates (1991) reviewed 35 cases of hepatic rupture that were associated with preeclampsia and reported a mortality rate of 30%.

Management of the patient with HELLP syndrome includes bed rest, frequent assessment of blood pressure, control of hypertension, laboratory evaluation of liver function, blood glucose, and coagulation status, and intensive fetal surveillance.

Fetal Implications

The pathophysiologic effects of PIH predispose the fetus to IUGR, fetal hypoxia, and death. Chronic hypoxia and acute placental abruption have both been cited as causative factors in fetal

DISPLAY 9-3

The HELLP Syndrome

H = Hemolysis
EL = Elevated Liver Enzymes
LP = Low Platelets

The HELLP Syndrome is diagnosed when patients with preeclampsia have measurable physiologic changes from the vasospasm and the endothelial damage associated with the disease.

---

demise. Patients diagnosed with PIH require ongoing antepartum surveillance to assess for fetal well-being. In the intrapartum period continuous electronic fetal monitoring is usually employed. These fetuses are at increased risk for uteroplacental insufficiency and the additional stress of uterine contractions may result in hypoxia, manifested by a variety of fetal heart rate changes. Consideration should be given to the fetal status prior to the initiation of procedures that may further compromise uteroplacental perfusion, such as epidural anesthesia or augmentation of labor. Interventions to maximize perfusion may include judicious administration of an intravenous fluid bolus and maternal repositioning. Other interventions are dependent on maternal assessment findings.

Clinical Management

The goals of treatment for the patient with severe pregnancy-induced hypertension include delivery of the fetus, control of hypertension, prevention of seizure activity, and close observation for complications.

Delivery of the Fetus

The only "cure" for PIH begins with delivery of both the fetus and the placenta. Delivery of the placenta is essential in resolving the disease process. PIH has been diagnosed in patients with a hydatidiform molar pregnancy in which no fetus develops.

Mode of delivery is patient-specific and depends on gestational age, fetal presentation, and maternal condition. Because PIH may occur remote from term, the administration of steroids to accelerate fetal lung maturity is often prescribed for preterm pregnancies. Patients who present with severe PIH at previable or borderline viable gestational age present a unique challenge to the healthcare team. There is little agreement in the scientific literature on the best course of management. Historically, immediate delivery of the extremely preterm infant has been done to avoid further physiologic insult to the mother and to offer the fetus a theoretically less hostile environment in a neonatal intensive care unit.

Recent studies, however, have shown that there may be some benefit to delay of delivery for as many days as possible to allow for improved fetal lung maturity. Sibai and co-workers (1994) randomly assigned a group of 95 pregnant women at 28 to 32 weeks of gestation to either an aggressive management protocol group or an expectant management protocol group. Aggressive management patients were prepared for delivery, either by cesarean section or induction of labor, after 48 hours of glucocorticoids were administered for fetal lung maturity. Patients in the expectant management group were prescribed bed rest and oral antihypertensives, and received daily antenatal fetal testing. There was no eclampsia in either group and the two groups had similar incidences of abruptio placenta (4.1% vs. 4.3%). The expectant management group reached a significantly higher gestational age than the aggressive management group (32.9 weeks vs. 30.8 weeks). The expectant management group also had higher neonatal birth weights, lower incidence of admission to the neonatal intensive care unit, lower mean days of hospitalization in the neonatal intensive care unit, and lower incidence of neonatal complications. The authors concluded that expectant management of patients with severe PIH may be an option for these women; however, intensive daily assessment of both the mother and fetus were paramount to ensure patient safety. Patients with severe PIH who are managed expectantly may be referred to a tertiary care center with both obstetric and neonatal critical care capabilities.

Seizure Prophylaxis

In the United States magnesium sulfate is the drug of choice for the prevention and abatement of seizure activity in the patient with PIH. The exact mechanism of action remains controversial, but its use results in a decreased incidence of eclampsia and improved perinatal outcome (Sibai, 1990.)

Magnesium sulfate can be administered intravenously or intramuscularly to the patient with PIH. Once administered, it circulates primarily unbound to protein, and is excreted in the urine by functioning nephrons. The excretion of magnesium is filtration dependent; thus, the patient with decreased glomerular filtration is at risk for increased serum magnesium levels.

Magnesium slows or blocks neuromuscular conduction, potentially depressing central nervous system irritability and, in theory, increases seizure threshold. Side effects of magnesium therapy are most commonly the result of neuromuscular blockade on the respiratory and cardiovascular systems. The effects of serum magnesium levels on physiologic findings are presented in Display 9-4.

Administration of magnesium sulfate is typically accomplished by one of two methods. The first is a combination of intravenous and intramuscular techniques (IV/IM). In the IV/IM protocol, an initial dose of 2–4 G of magnesium sulfate is administered intravenously over 2–4

DISPLAY 9-4

Physiologic Effects of Increased Serum Magnesium

Effect	Serum Magnesium Level (mg/dL)
Therapeutic	4–8
Loss of deep tendon reflexes	9–12
Respiratory arrest	>15
Cardiac arrest	>25–30

minutes, and 10 G of magnesium sulfate is administered intramuscularly at the same time. Additional doses of 5 G magnesium sulfate are administered IM every 4 hours until therapy is discontinued.

Because intramuscular injections must be repeated in the patient on magnesium seizure prophylaxis and serum level cannot be controlled over a short period of time, many clinicians elect to administer magnesium sulfate via continuous intravenous (IV) infusion. Using the IV protocol, patients are given an intravenous loading dose of 4–6 G of magnesium sulfate over 15–30 minutes, followed by a continuous infusion of magnesium sulfate at 1, 2, or 3 grams per hour.

Therapeutic levels of serum magnesium can only be assessed by standardized laboratory analysis of the patient's serum. Lower infusion rates of magnesium may be required if glomerular filtration and urine output are decreased. Deep tendon reflexes do not correlate with serum magnesium levels, unless they become absent over the course of therapy. Thus, decisions about increases and decreases in the magnesium dosage should be based on analysis of serum blood chemistry.

Magnesium toxicity is rare in the patient with normal renal function. To prevent toxicity, patients receiving magnesium therapy should be frequently assessed for adequate urine output, presence of DTRs, and respiratory rate and effort. If toxicity occurs, 10 cc of 10% calcium gluconate is administered intravenously slowly over 1–3 minutes until signs and symptoms are reversed.

Eclamptic seizures are rare, and are generally grand mal in nature. Seizure activity can occur in patients in the antepartum, intrapartum, and postpartum periods. Eclamptic seizures have been documented in the first trimester and in postpartum patients several weeks after delivery. If seizure activity should occur, the clinician caring for the patient should establish an airway as soon as possible, turn the patient to her side, protect the patient from injury, apply oxygen therapy, have suction available, and evaluate the maternal and fetal response. The clinician at the bedside should avoid restraining the patient during or after seizure activity, and should avoid ambitious attempts to insert a tongue blade or oral airway if the patient's teeth are clenched. If the eclamptic patient is already receiving magnesium sulfate therapy, an additional 2 grams of magnesium sulfate is administered intravenously over 3–5 minutes. If the patient has not received any magnesium sulfate, a loading dose of 4 grams is administered intravenously over 5 minutes. If the seizure continues, an additional 2 grams of magnesium sulfate can be administered over 3–5 minutes. If, after the administration of 4–6 grams of magnesium sulfate, the seizure activity continues, a paralytic agent can be administered, followed by endotracheal intubation and mechanical ventilation.

In many centers outside the United States, benzodiazepines continue to be the major anticonvulsant agent utilized for the patient with preeclampsia (Roberts, 1994). The Eclampsia Trial Collaborative Group (1995) conducted a randomized trial of anticonvulsant therapy in 1,687 women with preeclampsia. Outcome measurements included recurrence of convulsions, maternal and fetal morbidity, and maternal and fetal mortality. One group of 453 patients on magnesium sulfate were compared to a group of 452 patients receiving diazepam. There were 50% fewer seizures in the magnesium group and maternal deaths were significantly lower (3.8% vs. 5.1%). There were no differences reported in perinatal or maternal morbidity and no differences in the number of inductions of labor or cesarean sections. Cree, Meyer, and Hailey (1973) found that the use of diazepam resulted in hypothermia, hypotonia, and respiratory depression in a high number of neonates.

A second study compared a group of 388 patients receiving magnesium sulfate versus a group of 387 patients on phenytoin. The magnesium group had 67% fewer recurrent seizures and maternal mortality was 50% less in the magnesium sulfate group than in the phenytoin group (2.6% vs. 5.2%). Other findings of this study included that the women in the magnesium sulfate group were less likely to require ventilator support, to develop pneumonia, and to be admitted to the intensive care unit than those in the phenytoin group. The neonates of women in the magnesium sulfate group were also less likely to require intubation at delivery or to be admitted to the neonatal ICU than those whose mothers were on phenytoin.

Lorazepam, a benzodiazepine derivative, had even more severe side effects. Whitelaw and associates (1981) evaluated 53 neonates born to mothers who received lorazepam. They reported that lorazepam was conjugated slowly by the neonates and remained detectable in the urine for 7 days. Full-term neonates whose mothers received oral lorazepam had a slight delay in establishing feeding. The neonates whose mothers had received intravenous lorazepam had significantly lower Apgar scores, need for ventilation, hypothermia, and poor sucking. Preterm neonates whose mothers received lorazepam by either route had a high incidence of low Apgar scores, need for ventilation, hypothermia, and poor sucking. Although lorazepam was found to be an effective sedative and anxiolytic and there were no seizures in women treated with this agent, researchers suggest that the use of lorazepam by oral route prior to 37 weeks, and intravenous use at any gestational age, should be restricted to hospitals with facilities for neonatal intensive care.

Antihypertensive Agents

The physics of arterial blood pressure are complex and include the forces of flow and resistance. Hypertension may be the result of a high flow state (increased cardiac output), an elevated systemic vascular resistance (increased resistance), or both. Antihypertensive therapy may thus be directed toward reduction of cardiac output, vascular resistance, or both.

The administration of antihypertensive medications is, in general, limited to patients at risk for hypertensive crisis. Hypertensive crisis is defined as a sustained elevation of blood pressure greater than 200 mm Hg systolic and/or 120 mm Hg diastolic. At these pressures, rapid vascular damage can occur in flow-sensitive organs and the incidence of cerebral hemorrhage is increased. The use of antihypertensive agents in PIH is generally indicated when diastolic blood pressures reach or exceed 110 mm Hg. The goal

of therapy is to reduce the risk of cerebral vascular accident, while maintaining uteroplacental perfusion. Thus, management is directed at reducing the diastolic blood pressure to a value less than 110 mm Hg, but greater than 95–100 mm Hg.

Blood pressure control in the PIH patient is challenging, as these patients may be volume depleted, volume adequate, or volume overloaded at the time of hypertensive crisis. Thus, no one agent or protocol for intervention will be successful in treating all patients. Therefore, a second-line pharmacologic therapy may be necessary for this group of patients.

The classification of currently available antihypertensive agents is listed in Display 9-5.

Diuretics are not recommended in the acute management of PIH in the absence of invasive hemodynamic findings indicating central hypervolemia. Because diuretics decrease preload and thus cardiac output, serious maternal and fetal compromise may occur if administered to a patient who is volume depleted.

Centrally acting agents (sympatholytics) such as alpha-methyldopa have been used in the long-term treatment of hypertension during pregnancy with good results. In the acute care setting, however, the delayed onset of these agents limit their clinical utility during hypertensive emergencies.

DISPLAY 9-5

Classification System of Currently Available Antihypertensive Pharmacologic Agents

- Diuretics
- Centrally Acting Agents
- A and B Adrenergic Blockers
- Vasodilators
- Calcium Channel Blockers
- Angiotensin-Converting Enzyme Inhibitors

Vasodilators are the most common category of antihypertensive agents used in the treatment of hypertensive emergencies in pregnancy. This class of agents includes hydralazine and sodium nitroprusside. Hydralazine is a direct vasodilator and has an onset of action of 10–20 minutes after IV administration. Hydralazine reduces systemic vascular resistance (SVR), increases heart rate, and increases cardiac output. It is usually administered via IV bolus in dosages of 5–10 mg. Intravenous dosage may be repeated at 20-minute intervals until a desired response is seen. Hydralazine "failure" is considered when a total of 40 mg has been administered without a satisfactory reduction in blood pressure. Hydralazine is rarely administered in a continuous drip because of the prolonged half-life of the drug.

Labetalol is a nonselective (mixed) alpha- and beta-adrenergic antagonist. Its onset of action, 1–2 minutes, is more rapid compared to hydralazine with a peak action obtained at 10 minutes after infusion. Labetalol decreases maternal heart rate, but does not significantly decrease cardiac output. It may be given as an IV bolus or as a titrated drip. When given intravenously, 10 mg is initially administered over 2 minutes and incremental doses of 20–50 mg are given every 10 minutes as necessary to a maximum of 300 mg. Continuous intravenous infusion is administered at 0.5–1.0 mg/minute via a volume-controlled pump, and titrated to the desired blood pressure. The maximum rate is 2 mg per minute.

Sodium nitroprusside is a potent vasodilating agent that is reserved for the patient in whom antihypertensive therapy with first- and second-line agents has failed, and in the patient who presents with life-threatening hypertension. The onset of action is 15–30 seconds with a peak action at 1–2 minutes following intravenous administration. It is administered as a titrated drip via a volume-controlled infusion device. Because the half-life of the drug is so brief, intraarterial blood pressure monitoring is recommended to safely titrate medication.

Sodium nitroprusside is metabolized in the liver and produces cyanide as a byproduct. Prolonged usage should be avoided in the antepartum period, as the drug crosses the placenta and will depend on the fetal liver for metabolism. The risk of fetal cyanide toxicity exists, particularly in the immature fetus. Therapy with this agent may be undertaken for a brief period of time in the acutely hypertensive patient who is to be delivered immediately. The patient with PIH and impaired hepatic function is at increased risk for maternal cyanide toxicity as well. Patients requiring nitroprusside administration for greater than 24–48 hours should be assessed for elevated maternal serum cyanide levels.

Calcium channel blockers reduce blood pressure by blocking the intracellular pathways of calcium movement, resulting in smooth muscle relaxation and subsequent vasodilation. Nifedipine, a calcium channel blocker, has been used in pregnant patients for over a decade with good results. More recently, calcium channel blockers have been under increased scrutiny following reports that there may be a relationship between these agents used in hypertensive emergencies and resultant myocardial ischemia and infarction. At this time, the use of Nifedipine in pregnancy has not been clearly associated with maternal ECG changes, cardiac enzyme elevation, and/or myocardial infarction. However, the use of any calcium channel blocker in the acute management of hypertensive emergencies should be undertaken with close observation for evidence of myocardial ischemia.

Angiotensin-converting enzyme (ACE) inhibitors reduce blood pressure by blocking the conversion of angiotensin I to angiotensin II in the renin–aldosterone–angiotensin system. The use of ACE inhibitors in pregnancy has been abandoned after association with fetal anomalies and immune system dysfunction were discovered.

Invasive Monitoring in PIH

The use of invasive hemodynamic monitoring may be of benefit in women with severe preeclampsia when one or more of the complications shown in Display 9-6 are present.

There is no one hemodynamic profile that is characteristic of patients with PIH; rather, PIH produces a hemodynamic continuum from high cardiac output with decreased SVR to low cardiac output, depressed left ventricular function, and high SVR. Common hemodynamic findings reported at the time of pulmonary artery catheter placement in the patient with PIH are increased cardiac output, normal SVR, normal PCWP, low central venous pressure (CVP), and elevated left ventricular stroke work index (Benedetti et al., 1980; Benedetti, Kates, & Williams, 1985; Clark, et al., 1989). However, low cardiac output, abnormal SVR, PCWP and left ventricular failure may also be evident (Fox, Troiano, & Graves, 1996).

Clark and colleagues (1986) described three hemodynamic subsets of patients with PIH who underwent invasive hemodynamic monitoring due to oliguria unresponsive to administration of a fluid challenge. The first group of patients had low filling pressures, normal to low normal cardiac output, and normal systemic vascular resistance. In this group, the oliguria was hypothesized to be the result of inadequate renal perfusion from the low intracardiac filling pressures and cardiac output. The second subset included patients who had normal filling pressures, normal cardiac output, and normal afterload. In this group, renal arterial vasospasm out of proportion to systemic arterial vasospasm was thought to be responsible for the oliguria. In the third group, patients were found to have elevated filling pressures, low cardiac output, and elevated systemic vascular resistance. In this final group, oliguria was believed to be the result of decreased renal perfusion from elevated left ventricular afterload and low cardiac output.

Of interest is the finding that in patients with PIH, the CVP does not correlate with PCWP and may provide misleading estimates of left ventricular filling (Cotton et al., 1985). Therefore, when filling pressures and intravascular volume determination is needed for clinical management, the use of a pulmonary artery catheter is superior to the use of a central venous catheter.

Oxygen Transport Observations

Adding support to the theory that preeclampsia has an immunologic basis are the recently reported oxygen transport findings of patients with severe preeclampsia. Oxygen delivery in PIH patients was described as normal or above

DISPLAY 9-6

Indications for Invasive Hemodynamic Monitoring

Clinical indications for arterial line and/or pulmonary artery catheter placement in patients with severe PIH are as follows:

- Oliguria unresponsive to fluid challenge
- Pulmonary edema
- Hypertensive crisis refractory to conventional therapy
- Cerebral edema
- Disseminated intravascular coagulation
- Multisystem organ failure

normal, dependent upon the degree of hyperdynamic left ventricular function or cardiac output. Oxygen consumption, however, was remarkably "fixed," or constant in patients with severe manifestations of the disease. The fixed consumption pattern implies that these patients remain oxygen delivery dependent at high output states, and are similar to nonpregnant patients with Systemic Inflammatory Response Syndrome (SIRS), which has been strongly correlated with the degree of inflammatory mediator production.

Prevention

Various drugs and management protocols have been recommended for the prevention of preeclampsia. In prospective studies however, no benefit has been found for dietary salt restriction, diuretic therapy, or high protein diets. (Steegers et al., 1991). Calcium supplementation, aspirin therapy, and magnesium therapy have also been investigated.

Calcium Supplementation

Studies have shown that populations who have a higher intake of dietary calcium also report lower maternal blood pressure (Belizan & Villar,

1980). Also, recent reports from a large meta-analysis and a review of clinical trials have supported the hypothesis that calcium supplementation during pregnancy decreased the mean arterial blood pressure of study subjects (Bucher et al., 1996; Carroli, Duley, Bellizan, & Villar, 1994). The recent CPEP (Calcium for Preeclampsia Prevention) trial, a prospective, double-blind, placebo-controlled trial in normal healthy primigravidas, evaluated the effect of calcium supplementation on blood pressure, incidence and severity of preeclampsia, and pregnancy outcome. Approximately 4,500 women participated and received either calcium supplementation or placebo beginning at 13–21 weeks of gestation until the end of pregnancy. The results showed that calcium had no protective effect from preeclampsia. Measured systolic and diastolic blood pressures, incidence and severity of preeclampsia, gestational age at onset of preeclampsia, and neonatal outcomes were the same in both groups (Levine et al., 1997).

Aspirin Therapy

Aspirin is a prostaglandin synthesis inhibitor. When administered during pregnancy, it decreases platelet aggregation and increases vasodilation. Because platelet aggregation and an imbalance of thromboxane and prostacyclin are known as pathophysiologic events in PIH, the administration of aspirin to prevent the disease was studied.

Hauth and colleagues (1993) reported results of a prospective randomized study that evaluated the effect of aspirin therapy on the incidence of preeclampsia and IUGR in a low-risk population. Approximately 600 healthy nulliparous women were randomized to aspirin therapy or placebo at 24 weeks gestation. The incidence of preeclampsia was significantly lower in the aspirin group than in the placebo group. However, the incidence of preterm births related to severe preeclampsia, neonatal complications, and maternal complications were identical in both groups.

In 1993, the NIH Maternal–Fetal Medicine Network reported on a multicenter, randomized trial of aspirin therapy. Approximately 3,000 nul-

liparous women were enrolled in the study and received either aspirin or placebo. Overall, the results demonstrated a significant reduction in the incidence of preeclampsia in the aspirin group. However, there was no difference in gestational age at delivery, birth weight, or neonatal complications between the two groups. Additionally, of concern was the finding that women in the aspirin group had significantly higher rates of abruptio placenta than in the placebo group (Sibai et al., 1993).

To date, studies have detected no agent or dietary supplement that prevents preeclampsia. Research continues regarding biochemical supplements that may prove beneficial in the worldwide challenge of preeclampsia prevention.

SUMMARY

PIH is a complex multisystem disease that results in impaired oxygen transport to vital organs. Resultant hypoxic changes within affected organ systems produce the characteristic diagnostic criteria and clinical signs and symptoms. Such symptoms are indicative of the extent of the disease pathology and may include life-threatening complications. The goals of clinical management are prompt diagnosis, blood pressure control, prevention of seizures, optimization of oxygen transport to the patient and the fetus, and delivery of the fetus.

The nurse caring for the patient with PIH should be knowledgeable of pathophysiologic principles related to the disease, associated complications, and the framework for maternal–fetal clinical management.

REFERENCES

Belizan, J. M., & Villar, J. (1980). The relationship between calcium intake and edema, proteinuria, and hypertension-gestosis. An hypothesis. American Journal of Clinical Nutrition, 33, 2202–2210.

Benedetti, T. J., Cotton, D. B., Read, J. C., et al. (1980). Hemodynamic observations in severe pre-eclampsia with a flow-directed pulmonary artery catheter. American Journal of Obstetrics & Gynecology, 136, 330–334.

Benedetti, T. J., Kates, R., & Williams, V. (1985). Hemodynamic observations in severe preeclampsia complicated by pulmonary edema. American Journal of Obstetrics & Gynecology, 152, 465–470.

Berg, C. J., Atrash, H. K., Koonin, L. M., & Tucker, M. (1996). Pregnancy-related mortality in the United States 1987–1990. Obstetrics and Gynecology, 88, 161.

Bucher, H. C., Guyatt, G. H., Cook, R. J., Hatala, R., et al. (1996). Effect of calcium supplementation on pregnancy-induced hypertension and preeclampsia. A meta-analysis of randomized controlled trials. Journal of the American Medical Association, 275, 1113–1117.

Carroli, G., Duley, L., Belizan, J. M., & Villar, J. (1994). Calcium supplementation during pregnancy: A systematic review of randomized controlled trials. British Journal of Obstetrics & Gynaecology, 101, 753–758.

Chesley, L. C., (1978). Hypertensive disorders of pregnancy. New York: Appleton–Century-Crofts.

Chesley, L. C., (1985). Diagnosis of preeclampsia. Obstetrics and Gynecology, 65, 423.

Clark, S. L., Cotton, D. B., Wesley, L., et al. (1989). Central hemodynamic assessment of normal term pregnancy. American Journal of Obstetrics & Gynecology, 161, 1439–1442.

Clark, S. L., Greenspoon, J. S., Aldahl, D., et al. (1986). Severe preeclampsia with persistent oliguria: Management of hemodynamic subsets. American Journal of Obstetrics & Gynecology, 154, 490–494.

Cotton, D. B., Gonik, B., Dorman, K., et al. (1985). Cardiovascular alterations in severe pregnancy-induced hypertension: Relationship of central venous pressure to pulmonary capillary wedge pressure. American Journal of Obstetrics & Gynecology, 151, 762–764.

Cree, J. E., Meyer, J., & Hailey, D. M. (1973). Diazepam in labor: Its metabolism and effect on the clinical condition and thermogenesis of the newborn. British Medical Journal, 282, 1106.

Crosby, E. T. (1991). Obstetrical anesthesia for patients with the syndrome of haemolysis, elevated liver enzymes, and low platelets. Canadian Journal of Anaesthesia, 38, 227.

Cunningham, F. G., MacDonald, P. C., Gant, N. F., Leveno, K. J., Gilstrap, L. C., Hankins, G. D. V., & Clark, S. L. (Eds.). (1997). Williams Obstetrics (20th ed., pp. 693–744). Stamford, CT: Appleton and Lange.

Diekman, W. L. (1952). The toxemias of pregnancy (2nd ed.). St. Louis, MO: Mosby.

Douglas, K. A., & Redman, C. W. G. (1994). Eclampsia in the United Kingdom. British Medical Journal, 309, 1395.

Duley, L. (1992). Maternal morbidity associated with hypertensive disorders of pregnancy in Africa, Asia, Latin America and the Caribbean. British Journal of Obstetrics and Gynaecology, 99, 547.

Eclampsia Trial Collaborative Group. (1995). Which anticonvulsant for women with eclampsia? Evidence from the collaborative eclampsia trial. Lancet, 345, 1455.

Food and Drug Administration. (1989). FDA Drug Bulletin, 19, 14.

Fox, D. B., Troiano, N. H., Graves, C. R. (1996). Use of the pulmonary artery catheter in severe preeclampsia: A review. Obstetrical and Gynecological Survey, 51(11), 684–695.

Hauth, J. C., Goldenberg, R. L., Parker, C. R., Jr., Phillips, J. B., III, Cooper, R. L., DuBard, M. B., & Cutter, G. R. (1993). Low-dose aspirin therapy to prevent preeclampsia. American Journal of Obstetrics & Gynecology, 168, 1083.

Koonin, L. M., Atrash, H. K., Rochat, R. W., & Smith, J. C. (1989). Maternal mortality surveillance, United States, 1980–1985. Maternal Mortality World Review, 37, 19.

Levine, R. L., Hauth, J. C., Curet, L. B., Sibai, B. M., Catalano, P. M., Morris, C. L., DerSimonian, R., Esterlitz, J. R., Raymond, E. G., Bild, D. E., Clemens, J. D., & Cutler, J. A. (1997). Trial of calcium to prevent preeclampsia. New England Journal of Medicine, 337(2), 69–76.

MacGillivary, I., Rose, G. A., & Rowe, D. (1969). Blood pressure survey in pregnancy. Clinical Science, 37, 395.

Naidoo, D. M., & Moodley, J. (1980). A survey of hypertension at the King Edward VIII Hospital, Durban. S Afr Med. J, 58, 556.

Roberts, J. M. (1994). Pregnancy-related hypertension. In R. K. Creasy & R. Resnik (Eds.), Maternal–fetal medicine: Principles and practice (3rd ed., pp. 804–843). Philadelphia: W. B. Saunders.

Rolfes, D. B., & Ishak, K. G. (1986). Liver disease in pregnancy. Histopathology, 10, 555.

Sibai, B. M. (1990). Magnesium sulfate is the ideal anticonvulsant in preeclampsia-eclampsia. American Journal of Obstetrics & Gynecology, 162, 1141–1145.

Sibai, B. M., Caritis, S. N., Thom, E., et al. (1993). Prevention of preeclampsia with low-dose aspirin in healthy nulliparous pregnant women. New England Journal of Medicine, 329, 1213–1218.

Sibai, B. M., Gordon, T., Thom, E., Caritis, S. N., Klebanofff, M., McNellis, D., & Paul, R. H. (1995). Risk factors for preeclampsia in healthy nulliparous women: A prospective multicenter study. The National Institute of Child Health and Human Development Network of Maternal–Fetal Medicine Units. American Journal of Obstetrics & Gynecology, 172(2, Pt. 1), 642–648.

Sibai, B. M., Mercer, B. M., Schiff, E., & Friedman, S. (1994). Aggressive versus expectant management of severe preeclampsia at 28 to 32 weeks' gestation: A randomized controlled trial. American Journal of Obstetrics & Gynecology, 171(3), 818–822.

Sibai, B. M., Ramadan, M. K., Usta, I., Salama, M., Mercer, B. M., & Friedman, S. A. (1993). Maternal morbidity and mortality in 442 pregnancies with hemolysis, elevated liver enzymes and low platelets (HELLP syndrome). American Journal of Obstetrics & Gynecology, 169, 1000.

Smith, L. G., Moise, K. G., Dildy, G. A., et al. (1991). Spontaneous rupture of the liver during pregnancy: Current therapy. Obstetrics and Gynecology, 77, 171.

Steegers, E. A., van Lakwijk, H. P., Jougsma, H. W., et al. (1991). Physiological implications of chronic dietary sodium restriction during pregnancy: A longitudinal prospective randomized study. British Journal of Obstetrics and Gynaecology, 98, 980–987.

Thomson, A. M., Hytten, F. E., & Billewicz, W. Z. (1967). The epidemiology of oedema during pregnancy. Journal of Obstetrics and Gynaecology of the British Commonwealth, 74, 1.

Villar, M. A., & Sibai, B. M. (1989). Clinical significance of elevated mean arterial blood pressure in second trimester and threshold increase in systolic or diastolic blood pressure during third trimester. American Journal of Obstetrics & Gynecology, 160(2), 419–423.

Volhand, F. (1918). Die doppelseitigen haematogenen Nierenerkrankunger. Berlin: Springer.

Walsh, S. W. (1985). Preeclampsia: An imbalance in placental prostacyclin and thomboxane production. American Journal of Obstetrics & Gynecology, 152, 335.

Whitelaw, A. G. L., Cummings, A., & McFadyen, I. R. (1981). Effect of maternal lorazepam on the neonate. British Medical Journal, 282, 1106.

Working Group on High Blood Pressure in Pregnancy National Institutes of Health. (1990). National high blood pressure education program working group report on high blood pressure in pregnancy. American Journal of Obstetrics & Gynecology, 163, 1689–1712.

CHAPTER 10

Cardiac Disorders During Pregnancy

Susan B. Drummond and Nan H. Troiano

During pregnancy, profound alterations in the maternal cardiovascular system occur. These physiologic changes have been described thoroughly in Chapter 1. The pregnant woman with normal cardiac function usually adapts to these changes without difficulty. The woman with a cardiac disorder, however, may be at significant risk for morbidity or mortality when faced with these changes.

Cardiac disorders occur in approximately 1% of all pregnancies and represent one of the most important nonobstetric causes of maternal death (Cunningham, et al., 1993; Oakley, 1989). It is the most common indirect cause of maternal mortality, and following hypertension, hemorrhage, and infection, the fourth most common direct cause (Gilstrap, 1989). This chapter describes specific cardiac lesions and how they impact the woman during pregnancy, with an emphasis on intrapartum management.

CLASSIFICATION

The risk of perinatal morbidity and mortality for the pregnant woman with preexisting cardiac disease is dependent on three factors: (1) the specific cardiac lesion, (2) the functional abnormality produced by the lesion, and (3) development of pregnancy-related complications, such as hemorrhage, infection, and pregnancy-induced hypertension (Gianopoulos, 1989). A classification system describing risk of mortality associated with specific cardiac lesions during pregnancy has been described by Clark (1991) as shown in Table 10-1. It is preferable that women be counseled preconceptually so that they thoroughly understand their risk for morbidity and mortality if they become pregnant. However, for those who become aware of their unique risk following conception, this system may be used to aid the patient in deciding whether or not to continue the pregnancy.

Functional ability also influences pregnancy outcome. The New York Heart Association (NYHA) system classifies cardiac disease according to the patient's functional ability. This system is often utilized as part of a thorough assessment of the pregnant cardiac patient. A description of the NYHA system is found in Table 10-2. (NYHA, 1979). Patients classified as NYHA I or II prior to pregnancy generally do well during pregnancy. Those with class III or IV disease have a significantly increased risk of morbidity and mortality with pregnancy. Although this system is useful in caring for the pregnant cardiac patient, as many as 40% of women who develop congestive heart failure and pulmonary edema during pregnancy are functional class I prior to pregnancy (Clark, 1991). Therefore it is imperative to assess the patient at each prenatal visit and reclassify her according to any signs of deteriorating status.

TABLE 10-1. Mortality Risk Associated with Pregnancy

Group I: Mortality <1%
  Atrial septal defect
  Ventricular septal defect (uncomplicated)
  Patent ductus arteriosus
  Pulmonic and tricuspid disease
  Corrected tetralogy of Fallot
  Biosynthetic valve prosthesis (porcine and human allograft)
  Mitral stenosis, NYHA class I and II

Group II: Mortality 5–15%
  Mitral stenosis with atrial fibrillation
  Mechanical valve prosthesis
  Mitral stenosis, NYHA class III or IV
  Aortic stenosis
  Coarctation of the aorta (uncomplicated)
  Uncorrected tetralogy of Fallot
  Previous myocardial infarction
  Marfan syndrome with normal aorta

Group III: Mortality 25–50%
  Pulmonary hypertension
  Coarctation of the aorta (complicated)
  Marfan syndrome with aortic involvement

Cardiac disease during pregnancy may generally be categorized as congenital, acquired, or ischemic in nature. Selected lesions within each of these categories are described.

CONGENITAL CARDIAC DISORDERS

Incidence

The incidence of congenital heart disease is approximately 1 per 100 liveborn infants (Hoffman, 1995). The frequency of congenital as opposed to acquired cardiac disease has increased (Szekely, Twener, & Snaith, 1973). Two factors have contributed to this increased incidence. First, more patients with congenital cardiac disease are surviving to reproductive age due to tremendous progress in medical technology. Second, the incidence of rheumatic fever in the United States has decreased significantly over the years. The ratio of rheumat-

ic cardiac disease to congenital cardiac disease seen during pregnancy was approximately 20:1 in the early 1950s; decreased to 3:1 by the late 1970s, and has now approached unity in some populations (Ullery, 1954; Ueland, 1978; Shime et al., 1990).

Etiology

Congenital cardiac lesions are thought to be multifactorial in 90% of cases, whereby effects of a number of genes coupled with an environmental catalyst result in genetic predisposition (Ramen, Maberry, & Gilstrap, 1989). Such lesions may also be associated with maternal disease, viral infection, and drug or alcohol ingestion. In addition, cardiac disease may represent a component of other genetic syndromes such as trisomy 21.

Maternal diseases that increase the risk of fetal cardiac disorders include diabetes mellitus, lupus erythematosus, and phenylketonuria. For example, infants of insulin-dependent diabetic mothers have a 3–5% risk of congenital cardiac defects including ventricular septal defects, coarctation of the aorta, and transposition of the great vessels (Nora, Nora, & Wexler, 1981). Maternal systemic lupus erythematosus is associated with fetal cardiac abnormalities, most commonly complete heart block. Infants of mothers with phenylketonuria are at a 25–50% risk of cardiac lesions including ventricular and atrial septal defects and tetralogy of Fallot (Nora, Nora, & Wexler, 1981). Infants exposed to rubella in utero have approximately a 35% incidence of cardiac defects, including ventricular and atrial septal defects as well as patent ductus arteriosus (Ramen, Maberry, & Gilstrap, 1989). It has also been reported that mothers who use alcohol during pregnancy have a 25–50% risk of fetal cardiac anomalies such as septal defects and patent ductus arteriosus (Nora, Nora, & Wexler, 1981). The following specific congenital cardiac disorders are presented focusing on those aspects that are unique to pregnancy.

Atrial Septal Defect

Atrial septal defect (ASD) is one of the most common congenital cardiac lesions found during pregnancy. Two important potential com-

TABLE 10-2. New York Heart Association—Functional Classification System

Class	Description
I	Asymptomatic No limitation of physical activity
II	Asymptomatic at rest Symptomatic with heavy physical activity Slight limitation of physical activity
III	Asymptomatic at rest Symptomatic with minimal physical activity Considerable limitation of physical activity
IV	Symptomatic with any physical activity May be symptomatic at rest Severe limitation of physical activity

plications seen with ASD are dysrhythmias and heart failure. The onset of atrial dysrythmias generally occurs after the fourth decade of life and therefore is unlikely to be encountered in the pregnant patient (Clark, 1991). Hypervolemia associated with pregnancy results in an increased left-to-right shunt through the ASD that inflicts a significant burden on the right ventricle (Clark, 1991). Though this additional right preload is tolerated well by most patients, congestive heart failure and death have been reported (Hibbard, 1975). An additional risk of fluid overload is a potential for shunt reversal. ASD is characterized by normal to low pulmonary artery pressures. Therefore, the development of pulmonary hypertension is uncommon. The majority of patients with ASD tolerate pregnancy, labor, and delivery without complications.

Ventricular Septal Defect

Ventricular septal defect (VSD) may occur as a single lesion or in combination with other con-

genital cardiac anomalies, such as tetralogy of Fallot or transposition of the great vessels. Many VSDs are diagnosed by ultrasound in utero and corrected soon after birth. The majority of VSDs are diagnosed and repaired before the patient reaches childbearing age. In patients with uncorrected lesions, the size of the defect is the most important determinant to the development of complications during pregnancy. Risk is associated primarily with fluid overload. In patients with small defects, labor, delivery, and postpartum are usually tolerated without difficulty. Larger defects are associated more commonly with congestive heart failure or the development of pulmonary hypertension as fluid pressures increase on the right side of the heart. A large VSD may also be associated with aortic regurgitation, which can add to the risk of congestive heart failure (Clark, 1991).

Patent Ductus Arteriosus

Although a common congenital cardiac anomaly, patent ductus arteriosus (PDA) is generally detected and closed during the newborn period. Therefore it is an unusual finding during pregnancy. Patients who do present with a PDA during pregnancy usually tolerate the hemodynamic stress of pregnancy, labor, and delivery without difficulty. However, the high-pressure, high-flow, left-to-right shunt associated with a large uncorrected PDA can result in the development of pulmonary hypertension (Clark, 1991).

Tetralogy of Fallot

Tetralogy of Fallot refers to the complex of four lesions: ventricular septal defect, overriding aorta, pulmonary stenosis, and right ventricular hypertrophy. The major physiologic risk posed by tetralogy of Fallot is the potential shunting of blood past the lungs without being oxygenated. As much as 75% of the venous blood returning to the heart may pass directly from the right ventricle into the aorta without becoming oxygenated. Most cases are successfully surgically corrected in early childhood. The procedure involves opening the pulmonary stenosis, closing the septal defect, and reconstructing the flow pathway into the aorta. The majority of patients with corrected tetralogy of Fallot experience good outcomes in pregnancy (Meyer et al., 1964; Loh & Tan, 1975). Patients with an uncorrected VSD can experience worsening of the right-to-left shunt related to the decrease in SVR that accompanies pregnancy. A poor prognosis has been associated with patients having a prepregnancy hematocrit > 65%, history of syncopal episodes, oxygen saturation < 80%, high right ventricular pressures, or cardiomegaly (Jacoby, 1964).

Coarctation of the Aorta

The most common site of coarctation is the origin of the left subclavian artery (Clark, 1991). This condition may be associated with a bicuspid aortic valve, aortic stenosis or regurgitation, thoracic aortopathy, aneurysm of the circle of Willis, and the cardiac and systemic results of long-standing arterial hypertension (Wooley & Sparks, 1992). Untreated patients with coarctation are at risk for the development of arterial hypertension, congestive heart failure, infectious aortitis or endocarditis, myocardial infarction, cerebrovascular accidents, aortic aneurysms, and dissection or rupture complicating aortopathy (Wooley & Sparks, 1992).

Historically, pregnancy in women with coarctation of the aorta was discouraged. In a review of 200 pregnant women with coarctation of the aorta before 1940, Mendelson (1940) reported 14 maternal deaths, concluded that pregnancy, labor, and delivery posed significant risk to patients with this disorder, and suggested contraception, therapeutic abortion, cesarean section, and sterilization as therapeutic and prophylactic measures. He followed with similar recommendations in 1960. More recently, Deal and Wooley (1973) presented 28 women with unoperated coarctation of the aorta who had 83 pregnancies. All were classified as NYHA class I or II prior to pregnancy. In this group of women, no maternal deaths or permanent cardiovascular complications occurred. In contrast, patients with known aortic aneurysm or aneurysm in the circle of Willis may have a mortality risk of as high as 15%; therefore, pregnancy termination should be considered (Clark, 1991).

Eisenmenger Syndrome

Eisenmenger syndrome develops when progressive pulmonary hypertension leads to a shunt reversal in the presence of a congenital left-to-right shunt. The syndrome is more likely to occur with a VSD or a PDA because of the high pressure and high flow associated with these defects. Decreased SVR normally associated with pregnancy increases the occurrence of right-to-left shunting, resulting in decreased pulmonary perfusion and hypoxemia for the mother and the fetus. Continued pulmonary hypertension leads to systemic hypotension and decreased right heart pressures that may be inadequate to perfuse the pulmonary arterial bed. This insufficiency may result in sudden severe hypoxemia and death.

Women with Eisenmenger's syndrome should be counseled with respect to the significant risks that accompany pregnancy. Maternal mortality associated with this syndrome is reported between 30% and 50% (Mendelson, 1960). Termination of pregnancy is usually recommended. However, one report (Gleicher et al., 1979) describes 13 pregnancies in 12 women with this syndrome who decided to continue their pregnancies despite recommendations for therapeutic abortion. Three maternal deaths occurred, and eight infants were born alive. In this group of women, successful outcomes were attributed to prolonged bed rest and the use of heparin and oxygen therapy.

ACQUIRED CARDIAC DISORDERS

Mitral Stenosis

Mitral stenosis is the most common rheumatic lesion of pregnancy. Rheumatic fever is caused by group A streptococci and occurs most often after infections such as scarlet fever, middle ear infections, or sore throat. Antibodies formed in response to the infection may also react against the body's own tissues, specifically the mitral valve, causing immunologic or inflammatory damage. Scar tissue forms over the valve leaflets and chordae tendineae resulting in valvular stenosis. The valve orifice becomes progressively narrowed and immobile, impeding forward flow of blood through the heart. If the orifice is reduced to less than one half of normal, blood can flow to the left ventricle only with abnormally elevated atrial-to-ventricular pressure gradients. Adequate time for left ventricular filling is essential to maintain cardiac output.

Labor, delivery, and the immediate postpartum period pose significant stress for these patients. The normal high-output/low-resistance state of pregnancy, as well as marked fluctuations in cardiac output during labor and delivery (Table 10-3), fluid shifts, and peripartum blood loss may not be tolerated well by patients with mitral stenosis (Kennedy, 1995). The autotransfusion from the utero-placental circulation that occurs at the time of delivery may produce acute pulmonary edema. Pulmonary artery catheterization is utilized in patients with NYHA class III or IV disease as well as other selected patients. Because of the need to avoid central volume overload yet maintain adequate volume to support cardiac output, it is especially important to assess fluid status. It is important to note, however, that in patients with mitral stenosis, PCWP is not an adequate appraisal of left ventricular diastolic filling pressure. Frequent assessment of cardiac output is indicated to evaluate left ventricular function, especially if the patient has received diuretics for volume reduction (Clark, 1986; Clark et al., 1985).

Atrial fibrillation is often associated with mitral stenosis and may have serious implications. The stenotic valve does not allow complete emptying of blood from the left atrium into the left ventricle, therefore pooling of blood occurs around the valve. As pregnancy is a hypercoagulable state, thrombi can rapidly form here. Fibrillation can dislodge the thrombi and cause arterial embolism.

Aortic Stenosis

Aortic stenosis, though occasionally congenital in nature, is most commonly of rheumatic origin. It generally does not become hemodynamically significant until the orifice has diminished to one third or less of normal. The major difficulty associated with this lesion is maintenance of cardiac output. Because of the increased plasma volume, most patients tolerate early pregnancy well and have an improved cardiac output. However, patients may experience a relatively fixed cardiac output, which during exertion may be insufficient to sustain cardiac or cerebral perfusion.

The time of greatest risk for patients with aortic stenosis is intrapartum or pregnancy termination (Arias & Pineda, 1978). The maintenance of cardiac output is vital. Continuous evaluation with invasive hemodynamic monitoring permits thorough evaluation of all aspects of hemodynamic function. Because hypovolemia is a much greater risk than pulmonary edema, the PCWP should be maintained at a slightly higher than normal level to provide a margin of safety against unexpected blood loss during delivery or immediately postpartum (Clark, 1991).

Peripartum Cardiomyopathy

Peripartum cardiomyopathy is defined as cardiomyopathy developing in the last month of pregnancy or in the first six months postpartum in a patient with no previous history of cardiac disease and after elimination of all other causes of cardiac failure (Demakis & Rahimtoola, 1971). The incidence in the United States is reported between 1 in 1,300 and 1 in 15,000 pregnancies (Pierce, Price, & Joyce, 1963; Woolford, 1952; Cunningham et al., 1986). The majority of affected American patients are of African descent and tend to reside in the southern region of the United States at time of diagnosis (Veille, 1984). Other suggested risk factors

TABLE 10-3. Cardiac Output During Normal Labor and Delivery

Stage of Labor	Cardiac Output (%)
Early first*	↑ 15
Late first*	↑ 30
Second*	↑ 45
Postpartum—5 minutes	↑ 65
Postpartum—60 minutes	↑ 40

*An additional 15% increase accompanies each uterine contraction.

include twin pregnancy (Fillmore & Parry, 1977), pregnancy-induced hypertension (Homans, 1985) and more recently reported, long-term oral tocolytic therapy (Lampert et al., 1993). The exact etiology is unknown; however, speculation includes nutrition deficiency, small coronary vessel abnormalities, intimal thickening of itramural coronary arteries and hormonal autoimmune response to fetal antigens (Homans, 1985).

The patient presents with dyspnea, fatigue, and peripheral or pulmonary edema. Cardiomegaly and pulmonary edema are noted on chest radiograph. These patients are best managed with sodium and fluid restriction, decreased physical activity, inotropic support, and diuretic therapy. Over 60% of patients will recover and return to normal cardiac function; however, a notable feature of peripartum cardiomyopathy is its tendency to recur with subsequent pregnancies (Clark, 1991; Gianopoulos, 1989). Therefore, future pregnancy is generally not advisable.

Marfan Syndrome

Marfan syndrome is an autosomal dominant disorder characterized by generalized weakness of connective tissue resulting in skeletal, ocular, and cardiovascular abnormalities. It has an estimated prevalence of 4 to 6 cases per 10,000 persons with no difference in prevalence related to sex, race, or ethnicity (Pyeritz & McKusik, 1979). Women with Marfan syndrome who become pregnant assume two risks: a potentially fatal acute aortic dissection and the risk of having a child who has inherited the syndrome. In a review of the literature published up to 1980, Pyeritz (1981) reported 32 women with Marfan syndrome who had experienced at least one pregnancy. Acute aortic dissection was diagnosed in 20 of these women. Sixteen women died during or shortly after pregnancy, and four died later in the postpartum period because of aortic rupture or regurgitation. Preexisting cardiovascular abnormalities among the patients included aortic dilation, coarctation of the aorta, aortic regurgitation, patent ductus arteriosus, hypertension, and cardiomegaly.

Women with Marfan syndrome should receive preconceptual counseling regarding the risk for potential pregnancy-related complications and the risk for transmitting the syndrome to the baby. For the pregnant patient who has a substantial dilation of the aorta and does not choose therapeutic abortion, surgical intervention or treatment with beta-blocking agents has been suggested (Ginz, 1970).

Ischemic Cardiac Disease

Coronary artery disease and myocardial infarction in pregnancy are rare. However, ischemic cardiac disease is the leading cause of death in the United States, and, with the trend toward childbearing later in life, it is reasonable to predict such complications may increase in incidence. It has been estimated that myocardial infarction occurs in 1 out of every 10,000 pregnancies (Hankins et al., 1985). Fewer than 100 cases of myocardial infarction during pregnancy have been reported. In a review by Hankins and colleagues, 70 well-documented cases in the world literature were analyzed (Hankins, 1985). Of those patients, only 13% had known coronary artery disease antedating their pregnancy. Two thirds had an infarct in the third trimester with a mortality rate of 45%. When delivery occurred within 14 days of infarction, mortality was greatly increased. Thus, hemodynamic demands associated with pregnancy may serve as a stress to the coronary circulation, thereby producing ischemia in patients with previously asymptomatic disease. Typically invasive hemodynamic monitoring is utilized to guide control of preload and afterload during labor and delivery.

MANAGEMENT

Initial clinical assessment of the patient with cardiac disease begins with a thorough history. The patient's chief complaint should be determined and documented. History of her present cardiac disease should be elicited and include review of the specific lesion or disorder, functional classification, and current medications. The patient should be questioned regarding presence of symptoms such as chest pain, dyspnea, cyanosis, fatigue, palpitations, or skin changes. Complaints of pain require further evaluation including onset, duration, character, location, radiation, alleviating factors, aggravating factors, and accompanying signs or symptoms. Past medical history should also be reviewed including previous illnesses, surgical procedures, or hospitalizations. Family history should be evaluated including hereditary, familial diseases that pertain to the cardiovascular system. Assessment of social history includes use of alcohol or tobacco, chemical dependence, occupation, educational level, and support system.

General physical assessment involves use of inspection, palpation, percussion, and auscultation to determine the presence or absence of signs and symptoms associated with cardiac disease. Additional noninvasive assessment parameters include level of consciousness, blood pressure, oxygen saturation, electrocardiographic findings, and urinary output.

Cardiac output, the amount of blood ejected from the left ventricle, is determined by four variables: preload, afterload, contractility, and heart rate. Cardiac output may be adjusted by manipulating any one of these four variables. Preload, determined primarily by the volume of blood in the ventricles at end-diastole, is significantly affected by venous return to the heart. If the amount of blood entering the heart during diastole is increased, then the end-diastole volume will be increased and the heart muscle will stretch to accommodate the volume. The normal heart responds with increased velocity of contraction and therefore increased cardiac output. Factors affecting preload (Elkayam, Ostrzega, Shotan, & Mehra, 1995) are as follows.

Increase in Preload	Decrease in Preload
Mitral insufficiency	Mitral stenosis
Left ventricular damage	Decreased circulating fluids
Increased circulatory fluids	Conduction anesthesia
Vasoconstricting agents	Vasodilating agents
Patient position	Patient position

A high afterload results in increased left ventricular stroke work, leading to increased myocardial oxygen consumption, which can result in left ventricular failure. The following are factors affecting afterload (DeAngelis, 1985).

Increase in Afterload	Decrease in Afterload
Aortic valvular stenosis	Vasodilating agents
Peripheral arterial vasoconstriction	Hemorrhage
Hypertension	Conduction anesthesia
Polycythemia	Patient position
Vasoconstricting agents	
Patient position	

Contractility of the heart muscle may be manipulated by various pharmacological agents, which are shown in the following list (DeAngelis, 1985).

Positive Effect	Negative Effect
Digitalis	Quinidine
Isoproterenol	Barbiturates
Calcium	Propranolol
Catecholamines	
Norepinephrine	
Epinephrine	
Dopamine	
Dobutamine	

Cardiac output is also impacted by heart rate. Sustained tachycardia can lead to heart failure due to decreased filling time and shortened ejection times. Conversely, cardiac output may also be compromised if the heart rate is too slow, as with heart block. Additional strategies include prevention of thromboembolism, infection, and anemia.

HEMODYNAMIC STATUS

The intense cardiovascular demands of pregnancy actuate a challenge in the management of the cardiac patient. Labor, delivery, and the immediate postpartum period provide a time of increased risk due to the rapid volume changes that occur. For the patient with valvular disease, during the intrapartum period the major management considerations are preload reduction, control of heart rate, alterations in afterload, and prevention of hypotension or other events resulting in fluid imbalance (Austin & Davis, 1991).

Invasive hemodynamic monitoring may be indicated for certain patients to evaluate more accurately hemodynamic function and adequacy of cardiac output. It is recommended that all patients with cardiac disease classified as NYHA III or IV have central hemodynamic monitoring during the intrapartum period. Accurate hemodynamic measurements can reinforce or dispute clinical impressions and give continuous information of hemodynamic changes. Invasive monitoring is most often accomplished through the use of a pulmonary arterial catheter. Fiberoptic pulmonary arterial catheters permit the additional assessment of oxygen dynamics, of particular interest in the patient with cardiac compromise. Normal hemodynamic values are presented in Table 10-4 (Clark et al., 1989).

Epidural anesthesia is appropriate for most patients with cardiac disease during labor. By eliminating pain, associated changes in heart rate and cardiac output may be avoided. Epidural anesthesia also decreases preload secondary to peripheral vasodilation. Hypotension, a common side effect of epidural anesthesia, should be avoided, however. Keeping the patient in the lateral recumbent position, as well as careful administration of intravenous fluids, will promote the maintenance of blood pressure.

Vaginal delivery is advisable for most patients with cardiac disease, with cesarean section retained for obstetric indications, such as fetal distress, cephalopelvic disproportion, and failure to progress. Continuous invasive monitoring is advantageous because of the autotransfusion that occurs at delivery. It is then possible to carefully evaluate rapid changes in heart rate, cardiac output, and PCWPs. Changes in cardiac output during labor and delivery are noted in Table 10-3.

Antiobiotic prophylaxis is indicated for selected patients with cardiac disease becasue of their predisposition to developing endocarditis during invasive procedures. Bacteremia may be more frequent following cesarean section depending on circumstances and indications of operative delivery. Despite the American Heart Association's opinion that prophylaxis is not necessary for patients with valvular heart disease undergoing vaginal delivery, many physicians prefer to order prophylaxis in light of the risk–benefit ratio. Current recommendations for prophylaxis are presented in Table 10-5 (ACOG, 1992).

Specific recommendations for intrapartum nursing care of patients with selected cardiac lesions are reviewed in Table 10-6 (see p. 182). Additional nursing issues may be identified when providing care for intrapartum patients with cardiac disease. These include the following:

- Single room care if possible
- Sufficient space to accommodate specialized procedures and equipment
- Proper positioning of patient to optimize cardiac output
- Administration of drugs as ordered to optimize hemodynamic function
- Regulation of all intravenous fluids with infusion pump

TABLE 10-4. Normal Hemodynamic Values in Pregnancy

Parameter	Value and Standard Deviation
Cardiac output (liter/minute)	6.2 ± 1.0
Systemic vascular resistance (dyne/sec/cm^{-5})	1210 ± 266
Pulmonary vascular resistance (dyne/sec/cm^{-5})	78 ± 22
Mean pulmonary artery pressure (mm Hg)	13 ± 2
Pulmonary capillary wedge pressure (mm Hg)	7.5 ± 1.8
Central venous pressure (mm Hg)	3.6 ± 2.5
Left ventricular stroke work index (g/m/m^{-2})	48 ± 6

- Frequent assessments of intake and output
- Avoidance of hypotension
- Investigation of cause of tachycardia
- Anticipation of autotransfusion following delivery
- Avoidance of the lithotomy position during the second stage of labor

As with any obstetric patient, the nurse also is responsible for continuous fetal surveillance. A less than optimal cardiac output in the mother will be reflected in the fetal heart rate tracing. Proper maternal positioning and maintenance of hemodynamic values within normal limits will contribute to adequate placental perfusion and therefore provide proper oxygenation to the fetus.

NURSING DIAGNOSES

The use of nursing diagnoses can expedite the plan of care for the pregnant patient with cardiac disease. Examples include the following:

1. Alteration in comfort: pain related to uterine contractions
2. Anxiety
3. Potential for impaired gas exchange related to pulmonary edema
4. Potential for infection related to: pulmonary congestion, invasive hemodynamic monitoring, or valvular disease

5. Potential for decreased cardiac output related to structural defects, congestive heart failure, or pulmonary edema
6. Potenital for injury: fetal, related to decreased uteroplacental blood flow secondary to decreased cardiac output
7. Potential for activity intolerance related to decreased cardiac output
8. Potential for thromboembolism related to: valvular defects, decreased venous return, or hypercoagulability of pregnancy

Expected Outcomes

During the intrapartum period, the patient with cardiac disease will do the following:

1. Maintain adequate cardiac output to meet maternal demand
2. Maintain optimal hemodynamic parameters
3. Maintain adequate gas exchange and tissue perfusion
4. Exhibit normal electrocardiographic findings
5. Exhibit no signs or symptoms of thromboembolism
6. Exhibit no signs or symptoms of infection
7. Maintain reassuring fetal heart rate responses

SUMMARY

Care of the pregnant patient with known cardiac disease presents a unique challenge to the critical care nurse. Knowledge of the disease process as well as astute assessment of hemodynamic function during pregnancy are essential. Nursing care should focus on assessment, early detection of problems, treatment, and prevention. When these women are cared for outside a tertiary care center with capabilities for obstetric critical care, collaboration between critical care nurses and obstetric nurses is strongly advised.

REFERENCES

American College of Obstetrians and Gynecologists. (1992). Cardiac disease in pregnancy. ACOG Technical Bulletin 168, Washington, DC: ACOG.

Arias, F., & Pineda, J. (1978). Aortic stenosis and pregnancy. Journal of Reproductive Medicine, 20, 229.

TABLE 10-5. Recommendations for Bacterial Endocarditis Prophylaxis

Ampicillin 2 g intravenously and Gentamicin 1.5 mg/kg/ intravenously OR	30 minutes prior to delivery
Vancomycin 1 g intravenously and Gentamicin 1.5 mg/kg/intravenously	30 minutes to 1 hour prior to delivery
	Every 8 hours for 3 dosages

TABLE 10-6. Intrapartum Management of Selected Cardiac Lesions

Mitral Stenosis	Aortic Stenosis	Pulmonary Hypertension
Left atrial outflow obstruction with decreased left ventricular diastolic filling rate and a "fixed" cardiac output.	Left ventricular outflow obstruction with "fixed" cardiac output and left ventricular hypertrophy.	Often the result of an uncorrected congenital left-to-right shunt (PDA, ASD, VSD) and ultimately leading to reversal of the shunt.
• SBE prophylaxis • Continuous pulse oximetry • Maintain PCWP = 12–14 mm Hg • Maintain HR < 100 bpm • may use propranolol to treat tachycardia • Epidural anesthesia—avoid hypotension • Vaginal delivery preferred—decrease PCWP prior to delivery • Anticoagulation with atrial fibrillation	• SBE prophylaxis • Continuous pulse oximetry • Maintain PCWP = 16–18 mm Hg • Avoid hypotension • Avoid tachycardia • Treat blood loss promptly • Epidural anesthesia • Vaginal delivery preferred	• SBE prophylaxis • Continuous pulse oximetry • Anticoagulation • Maintain PCWP = 16–18 mm Hg • Epidural with caution—avoid hypotension—must maintain adequate right preload • Oxygen administration—helps to keep pulmonary vasculature maximally dilated • Vaginal delivery preferred

Austin, D. A., & Davis, P. A. (1991). Valvular disease in pregnancy. Journal of Perinatal Neonatal Nursing, 5, 2.

Avila, W. S., Grinberg, M., Snitcowsky, R., et al. (1995). Maternal and fetal outcome in pregnant women with Eisenmenger's syndrome. European Heart Journal, 16, 460–464.

Clark, S. L. (1986). How labor and delivery influence mitral stenosis. Contemporary Obstetrics and Gynecology, 27, 127.

Clark, S. L. (1991). Structural cardiac disease in pregnancy. In S. L. Clark, G. D. V. Hankins, D. B. Cotton, & J. P. Phelan (Eds.), Critical care obstetrics (2nd ed.). Boston: Blackwell.

Clark, S. L., Cotton, D. B., Lee, W., et al. (1989). Central hemodynamic assessment of normal term pregnancy. American Journal of Obstetrics and Gynecology, 161, 1439.

Clark, S. L., Phelan, J. P., Greenspoon, J., et al. (1985). Labor and delivery in the presence of mitral stenosis: Central hemodynamic observations. American Journal of Obstetrics and Gynecology, 152, 986.

Criteria Committee of the New York Heart Association. (1979). Nomenclature and criteria for diagnosis of diseases of the heart and great vessels (8th ed.). New York: New York Heart Association.

Cunningham, E. G., Pritchard, J. A., Hankins, G. D. V., et al. (1986). Peripartum heart failure: Idiopathic cardiomyopathy or compounding cardiovascular events? Obstetrics and Gynecology, 67, 157–168.

Cunningham, F. G., MacDonald, P. C., Gant, N. F., et al. (1993). Williams obstetrics (19th ed.). Stamford, CT: Appleton & Lange.

Deal, K., & Wooley, C. F. (1973). Coarctation of the aorta and pregnancy. Annals of Internal Medicine, 78, 706–710.

DeAngelis, R. (1985). The cardiovascular system. In J. G. Alspach & S. M. Williams (Eds.),

Core curriculum for critical care nursing (3rd ed., pp. 101–118). Philadelphia: Saunders.

Demakis, J. G., & Rahimtoola, S. H. (1971). Peripartum cardiomyopathy. Circulation, 44, 964–968.

Elkayam, U., Ostrzega, E., Shotan, A., & Mehra, A. (1995). Cardiovascular problems in pregnant women with the Marfan syndrome. American College of Physicians, 123, 2.

Fillmore, S. J., & Parry, E. O. (1977). The evolution of peripartal heart failure in Zaria. Circulation, 56, 1058–1061.

Gianopoulos, J. G. (1989). Cardiac disease in pregnancy. Medical Clinics of North America 73, 3.

Gilstrap, L. C. (1989). Heart disease during pregnancy. Clinical Obstetrics and Gynecology, 32, 1.

Ginz, B. (1970). Myocardial infarction in pregnancy. Journal of Obstetrics and Gynaecology British Commonwealth, 77, 610.

Gleicher, N., Midwall, J., Hochberger, D., et al. (1979). Eisenmenger's syndrome and pregnancy. Obstetrics and Gynecology Survey, 34, 721.

Hankins, G. D. V., Wendel, G. D., Leveno, K. J., et al. (1985). Myocardial infarction in pregnancy: A review. Obstetrics and Gynecology, 65, 139.

Hibbard, L. T. (1975). Maternal mortality due to cardiac disease. Clinical Obstetrics and Gynecology, 18, 27.

Hoffman, J. I. (1995). Incidence of congenital heart disease: II Perinatal incidence. Pediatric Cardiology, 16(4), 155–165.

Homans, D. C. (1985). Peripartum cardiomyopathy. New England Journal of Medicine, 312, 1432–1437.

Jacoby, W., Jr. (1964). Pregnancy with tetralogy and pentalogy of Fallot. American Journal of Cardiology, 14, 866.

Kennedy, B. B. (1995). Mitral stenosis: Implications for critical care nursing. JOGNN, 24(5), 406–412.

Lampert, M. B., Hibbard, J., Weinert, L., et al. (1993). Peripartum heart failure associated with prolonged tocolytic therapy. American Journal of Obstetrics and Gynecology, 168, 493–495.

Loh, T. F., & Tan, N. C. (1975). Fallot's tetralogy and pregnancy: A report of a successful pregnancy after complete correction. Medical Journal of Australia, 2, 141.

Mendelson, C. L. (1940). Pregnancy and coarctation of the aorta. American Journal of Obstetrics and Gynecology, 39, 1014–1021.

Mendelson, C. L. (1960). Cardiac disease in pregnancy: Medical care, cardiovascular surgery and obstetric management as related to maternal and fetal welfare. In C. E. Heaton (Ed.), Obstetrics and gynecology monographs (pp. 124–132). Philadelphia: Davis.

Meyer, E. C., Tulsky, A. S., Sigman, P., et al. (1964). Pregnancy in the presence of tetralogy of Fallot. American Journal of Cardiology, 14, 874.

Nolan, T. E., & Hankins, G. D. V. (1989). Myocardial infarction in pregnancy. Clinical Obstetrics and Gynecology, 32, 68.

Nora, J. J., Nora, A., & Wexler, P. (1981). Hereditary and environmental aspects as they affect the fetus and newborn. Clinical Obstetrics and Gynecology, 24, 851.

Oakely, C. M. (1989). Pregnancy and heart disease: Pre-existing heart disease. Cardiovascular Clinics, 19, 57.

Pierce, J. A., Price, B. O., & Joyce, J. W. (1963). Familiar occurrence of postpartal heart failure. Archives of Internal Medicine, 111, 651–655.

Pyeritz, R. E. (1981). Maternal and fetal complications of pregnancy in the Marfan syndrome. American Journal of Medicine, 71, 784–790.

Pyeritz, R. E., & McKusik, V. A. (1979). The Marfan syndrome: Diagnosis and management. New England Journal of Medicine, 300, 772–777.

Ramen, S. M., Maberry, M. C., & Gilstrap, L. C. (1989). Congenital heart disease. Clinical Obstetrics and Gynecology, 32, 41.

Shime, J., Mocarski, E. J. M., Hastings, D., et al. (1990). Congenital heart disease and pregnancy. In U. Elkayam & N. Gleicher (Eds.), Cardiac problems in pregnancy: Diagnosis and management of maternal and fetal disease (2nd ed., p. 73). New York: Alan Liss.

Szekely, P., Turner, R., & Snaith, L. (1973). Pregnancy and the changing pattern of rheumatic heart disease. British Heart Journal, 35, 1293.

Ueland, K. (1978). Cardiovascular diseases complicating pregnancy. Clinical Obstetrics and Gynecology, 21, 429.

Ullery, J. C. (1954). Management of pregnancy complicated by heart disease. <u>American Journal of Obstetrics and Gynecology</u>, <u>67</u>, 834.

Veille, J. C. (1984). Peripartum cardiomyopathies: A review. <u>American Journal of Obstetrics and Gynecology</u>, <u>148</u>, 805–818.

Wooley, C. F., & Sparks, E. H. (1992). Congenital heart disease, heritable cardiovascular disease and pregnancy. <u>Progress in Cardiovascular Diseases</u>, <u>35</u>(1), 41–60.

Woolford, R. M. (1952). Postpartum myocardiosis. <u>Ohio State Medicine</u>, <u>48</u>, 924–930.

CHAPTER 11

Pulmonary Disorders in Pregnancy

Karen Dorman

Asthma is common among women of childbearing age, but the incidence of most primary pulmonary disorders in the pregnant population is rare. More commonly, they occur as a consequence of other disease processes and include disorders such as pulmonary edema, pulmonary emboli, and acute respiratory distress syndrome (ARDS). Pneumonia of viral or bacterial etiology or as a result of gastric aspiration may also occur during pregnancy. However, it is difficult to accurately ascertain the incidence of each of these disorders as they often represent varying degrees of the same ongoing process. For example, amniotic fluid embolism often results in the development of pulmonary edema, which may progress to ARDS. In addition, many pulmonary disorders have similar symptoms and may require invasive testing to confirm the diagnosis. Therefore, misdiagnosis and unconfirmed diagnosis also contribute to an underestimation of the true incidence. Although relatively uncommon, pulmonary disorders during pregnancy may result in significant maternal morbidity and mortality. Thus, a thorough understanding of normal pulmonary physiology and the precipitating factors of these disorders, and careful attention to pulmonary assessment, are paramount to caring for patients with pulmonary compromise.

PULMONARY PHYSIOLOGY

Planning and provision of nursing care require an understanding first of normal respiratory function. *Ventilation* refers to the actual movement of air in and out of the lungs. *External respiration* refers to the oxygen exchange at the alveolar level, and *internal respiration* refers to the gas exchange at the cellular level. Although technically three separate entities, in reality it is difficult to separate these processes. The lungs have approximately 300 million alveoli that are composed of 90% type I alveolar epithelial cells and 10% type II alveolar epithelial cells (West, 1985). Type I cells are involved with the transfer of gas across the capillary membrane, are easily destroyed by injury, and do not regenerate. By contrast, type II alveolar cells produce and store surfactant, a phospholipid that prevents the collapse of the alveoli at end expiration and maintains elasticity of the lung. They can also regenerate and even become type I alveolar cells if there is a need. When surfactant is diminished, atelectasis occurs and diffusion is impaired. Sighing helps expand alveoli and spread surfactant into the distal areas of the lung not well ventilated with every breath. Each alveolus is completely surrounded by a dense network of capillaries, each of which allows one red blood cell to pass at a time. As a red blood cell passes through the capillaries, it is exposed

185

to approximately three alveoli in three fourths of a second. During this time, the oxygen saturation increases from 75% (normal mixed venous blood) to greater than 97% saturation (normal arterial blood). This saturation can occur in one fourth of a second in cases of tachycardia (West, 1985). Oxygen and carbon dioxide diffuse easily across the alveolar capillary membrane; however, diffusion is decreased when the membrane is thickened as in ARDS and cardiogenic pulmonary edema.

Exchange of oxygen and carbon dioxide occurs by a process of diffusion, defined as movement from an area of high concentration to an area of low concentration to reach an equilibrium. The majority is carried by the hemoglobin molecules (measured as oxygen saturation) with approximately 1–2% dissolved in plasma (measured as PaO_2) (Thelan, Davie, & Urden, 1990). As oxygen molecules dissolved in plasma diffuse into the tissue cells, more oxygen is released from hemoglobin molecules to be dissolved into plasma. Hemoglobin has a rather constant affinity for oxygen, though at a lower PaO_2 oxygen is more quickly released from hemoglobin to the tissues. At higher levels of PaO_2 the saturation of the hemoglobin molecules remains essentially constant. In conditions such as fever, increased $PaCO_2$ (hypercarbia), and acidosis, hemoglobin dissociation is enhanced, which allows more oxygen to be released for use by the tissues. The opposite is true in conditions such as hypothermia, alkalemia, and hypocarbia. Oxygen delivery to the tissues is also affected by cardiac output and hemoglobin.

Another important aspect in ventilation is the movement of gas into and out of the alveoli. The diaphragm does approximately 80% of the work of ventilation during normal inhalation. Exhalation is a passive process. As the diaphragm contracts, the pleural cavity enlarges, creating a negative pressure that allows air to rush in. The pulmonary circuit is the largest vasculature of the body and generates a systolic and diastolic pressure far lower than those of the systemic circulation. The increase in plasma volume seen in pregnancy does not affect pulmonary pressure. Changes in intrathoracic

pressure caused by maternal hyperventilation or positive pressure ventilation cause a profound variation in pulmonary pressure. This effect should be considered if invasive monitoring is to be used.

The pulmonary circuit is so intricate that hypoxemia can result from many different causes. The three most common categories are shunt, alveolar hypoventilation, and ventilation and perfusion inequality. The term *shunt* refers to a condition in which blood enters the arterial system without passing through ventilated parts of the lungs (Thelan, Davie, & Urden, 1990). Shunts can be caused by congenital cardiac defects or arteriovenous fistulas. However, shunting can also be caused by hypoventilation of a portion of the lung as occurs in atelectasis with alveolar collapse, pneumonia causing alveolar consolidation, and/or excessive mucous production as in chronic bronchitis. Hypoxemic patients with true shunts are not able to increase the PaO_2 to normal limits even with the administration of 100% oxygen. When the amount of oxygen available in the alveoli is less than required by the metabolic processes in the tissues, alveolar hypoventilation is the cause. In most cases this is also associated with an elevated $PaCO_2$. Causes include reduced chest expansion, depressed central nervous system function, and lung expansion restriction. Oxygen therapy will benefit this condition; however, mechanical ventilation is often required.

Ventilation/perfusion (V/Q) inequality occurs when the alveoli are underventilated or underperfused. Common causes of V/Q mismatch are chronic obstructive lung disease, asthma, pneumonia, and pulmonary thromboembolism. Administration of oxygen is beneficial in these patients (West, 1985). Many of the shunts described here reflect impairment of gas exchange. The most common is fluid in the lungs as in cardiogenic and noncardiogenic pulmonary edema. Another problem with gas exchange occurs in ARDS when the interstitial membrane thickens and prevents the diffusion process from occurring. With these patients, perfusion is normal but ventilation is impaired. Thus, shunt also refers to the portion of the lung that is not able to oxygenate the blood.

Significant maternal hypoxemia places the fetus at increased risk for morbidity or mortality. The placenta serves as the organ of respiration for the fetus with the exchange of oxygen and carbon dioxide occurring as a passive process. The oxygen supply available to the fetus is dependent on adequate maternal arterial oxygen content (PaO_2), placental perfusion, and fetal saturation of hemoglobin. Removal of carbon dioxide is dependent on fetal blood flow to the placenta, subsequent diffusion of carbon dioxide, and uptake by the maternal circulation. Normal umbilical cord blood gases are listed in Table 11-1. Several mechanisms exist that facilitate fetal adaptation to brief periods of maternal hypoxemia. First, diffusion of oxygen to the fetus is enhanced because of elevation of maternal PaO_2 and reduction of arterial carbon dioxide concentration ($PaCO_2$) associated with pregnancy. In addition, fetal hemoglobin has a stronger affinity for oxygen than does maternal hemoglobin and fetal hematocrit levels are higher than adult hematocrit levels. Finally, the fetus exhibits a compensatory mechanism that shunts blood flow to the brain and heart in the presence of hypoxic stress (Morin & Weiss, 1992). Chronic maternal hypoxemia, however, may result in failure of these compensatory responses and can lead to fetal hypoxemia, acidemia, or death. Other complications include polycythemia and intrauterine growth retardation. Fetal hypoxia often results in the passage of meconium from the gastrointestinal tract, which if aspirated by the fetus during labor or delivery may cause respiratory distress syndrome.

PULMONARY DISORDERS

Although the etiologies of the various pulmonary disorders differ, signs of pulmonary compromise are similar. Thus, it is extremely important for the care provider to understand the etiologies and predisposing factors of these complications to correctly diagnose and treat the patient accordingly. Early detection and resolution of the disease process is crucial to successful therapy.

Pulmonary Edema

Pulmonary edema is defined as an abnormal accumulation of water, more than may be drained by the lymphatic system, in the extravascular portions of the lung. This may involve both the interstitial and alveolar spaces (Hatjis & Swain, 1988). Although not always

TABLE 11-1. Normal Umbilical Blood Gases Reported as Average, Standard Deviation, and Ranges

	Umbilical Venous	Umbilical Arterial
pH	7.35 ± 0.05	7.28 ± 0.05
	(7.24–7.49)	(7.15–7.43)
PCO_2 (mm Hg)	38.2 ± 5.6	49.2 ± 8.4
	(23.2–49.2)	(31.1–74.3)
PO_2 (mm Hg)	29.2 ± 5.9	18.0 ± 6.2
	(15.4–48.2)	(3.8–33.8)
HCO_3 (mEq/liter)	20.4 ± 2.1	22.3 ± 2.5
	(15.9–24.7)	(13.3–27.5)

Source: From "Assessment of fetal and newborn acid-base status," by the American College of Obstetricians and Gynecologists, April 1989, ACOG Technical Bulletin, 127.

TABLE 11-2. Estimate of Delivered Oxygen Concentrations with Low-Flow Oxygen Devices

O₂ Flow Rate(liter/minute)	FiO₂
Nasal Cannula	
1	0.24
2	0.28
3	0.32
4	0.36
5	0.40
6	0.44
O₂ Mask	
5–6	0.40
6–7	0.50
7–8	0.60
Mask with reservoir bag	
6	0.60
7	0.70
8	0.80
9	0.80+
10	0.80+

Note: Normal ventilatory patterns are assumed.
Source: From Clinical Application of Respiratory Care, by B. A. Shapiro, R. A. Harrison, R. A. Kacmarek, and R. D. Cane, 1985, Chicago: Year Book Medical Publishers.

clinically obvious until moderate in severity, it is frequently an early finding in the progression of many other disease processes. The overall incidence of pulmonary edema in pregnancy is unclear. However, it has been reported that patients receiving intravenous betamimetic therapy for preterm labor have a 5% incidence of cardiogenic pulmonary edema related to sodium and water retention (Katz, Robertson, & Creasy, 1981). The incidence is as high as 50% for pregnancies of twins treated with betamimetics. This risk may be increased as hydration is frequently the first therapy used to

halt preterm contractions, although a definitive answer regarding efficacy has not been reported (Freda & DeVore, 1996). It is interesting to note that this complication associated with betamimetic therapy is unique to pregnancy and is not seen in other patients treated with much higher doses of these same agents (Pisani & Rosenow, 1995). The symptoms usually occur 24–48 hours after initial intravenous therapy and have been reported to occur with oral or subcutaneous administration as well (Deblieux & Summer, 1996).

Normally the pulmonary capillaries are permeable to fluid, and there is constant movement of fluid across the capillary membrane into the interstitial spaces and back into the capillaries. The flow of fluid is regulated by the balance of two opposing forces. Pulmonary capillary hydrostatic pressure forces fluid out of the vessels, and plasma oncotic pressure pulls fluid into the vessels by the attraction of fluid to protein molecules in the blood. Pulmonary hydrostatic pressure is greater in the arterioles, and plasma oncotic pressure is greater in the venules. These two forces are usually balanced. The lymphatic system is also available to absorb any excess fluid that may accumulate in the interstitial space. This balanced system may be altered primarily by two mechanisms. An increase in capillary hydrostatic pressure results in cardiogenic pulmonary edema, and an increase in the permeability of the capillary membrane results in noncardiogenic pulmonary edema. Both mechanisms cause excess fluid accumulation in the extravascular compartment, the interstitial spaces, and the alveoli. Although the end result is the same, therapy is directed toward the causative factor. If the underlying cause is inappropriately identified, treatment may actually be detrimental to the patient.

Cardiogenic Pulmonary Edema

Cardiogenic, or hydrostatic, pulmonary edema, as the name implies, occurs as a result of heart dysfunction. The causes of ventricular failure in obstetrics include elevated preload, most frequently related to iatrogenic fluid overload; decreased contractility, secondary to myocardial infarction or cardiomyopathy; and elevated afterload, related to aortic stenosis or severe hypertension (Benedetti, Kates, & Williams, 1985; Keefer, Strauss, Civetta, & Burke, 1981). Regardless of the cause of left ventricular failure, the left ventricle becomes unable to empty efficiently, fluid accumulates, and results in an elevated pressure. As the ventricular failure continues, the left atrial pressure rises, which increases capillary hydrostatic pressure forcing excessive fluid into the extravascular spaces. The condition worsens as alveoli fill with fluid, preventing gas exchange across the membrane.

Noncardiogenic Pulmonary Edema

In contrast, noncardiogenic, or non-hydrostatic, pulmonary edema is caused by increased pulmonary capillary permeability and does not involve heart dysfunction. It occurs as a result of physical or chemical damage of the pulmonary vascular membrane, which allows fluid as well as protein molecules to escape into the extravascular spaces. The causes of noncardiogenic pulmonary edema in obstetrics include aspiration of gastric contents, sepsis, blood transfusion reactions, disseminated intravascular coagulation, and amniotic fluid embolism (Pritchard, McDonald, & Gant, 1985). The increased protein content in the extravascular spaces attracts additional fluid, which increases the pulmonary edema. This process results in a clinical picture similar to cardiogenic pulmonary edema. Signs and symptoms include tachypnea, tachycardia, basilar crackles, chest discomfort, and/or dyspnea on exertion. An increased incidence as well as morbidity from noncardiogenic pulmonary edema is noted when preterm labor is associated with maternal infection.

In patients with cardiogenic or hydrostatic pulmonary edema, insertion of a pulmonary artery catheter reveals an elevated pulmonary capillary wedge pressure, indicative of left ventricular failure, as well as increased pulmonary arterial pressures. The focus of treatment is improvement of left ventricular function and reduction of hydrostatic pressure with diuretics, inotropic medications, and afterload reduction with antihypertensives or possibly in combination, dependent on the primary problem. Patients with noncardiogenic pulmonary edema experience increased pulmonary capillary permeability. In contrast, insertion of a pulmonary artery catheter reveals a normal-to-low pulmonary capillary wedge pressure. Because the permeability of the membrane cannot be manipulated, treatment is usually supportive in nature until membrane stabilization occurs. When detected early, cardiogenic pulmonary edema can be easily reversed. However, when pulmonary edema is caused by cardiac failure or occurs in the presence of other complicating factors, reversal is much more difficult.

Pneumonia

Pneumonia in pregnancy may result from aspiration of gastric contents as well as viral or bacterial pathogens. In general, pneumonia is not tolerated as well by pregnant women as it is by nonpregnant women. Pneumonia is a relatively common entity that carries moderately low morbidity and mortality since the introduction of antibiotics (Benedetti, Valle, & Ledger, 1982). The clinical course of women in labor with pneumonia is dependent on many factors, such as the organism involved, the resistance of the host, prompt diagnosis, and treatment.

Bacterial pneumonia is rarely seen in patients with intact immune systems (0.04–1%) (Maccato, 1990). The incidence increases if defense mechanisms are altered, by a decrease in mechanical barriers from intubation, by decreased clearance of organisms related to poor cilial function as a result of smoking or certain viral infections, and by decreased immune response caused by immunosuppressive drugs or chronic anemia (Maccato, 1990). The most common causative organism is *Streptococcus pneumonae*, but other pathogens include *Haemophilus influenzae, Staphylococcus aureus,* and *Klebsiella pneumoniae. Mycoplasma pneumoniae* produces a slow-onset pneumonia, which is accompanied by low-grade fever that frequently abates without treatment. Antibiotics specific for that pathogen are preferred; however, broad-spectrum antibiotic coverage pending sputum culture results and oxygen therapy are the mainstays of treatment for bacterial pneumonia. Recently, there has been a rise in the number of patients with drug-resistant strains of bacteria in whom other drug therapy was required.

Although pregnant women are not at great risk for contracting influenza, there is evidence that women in the third trimester are at increased risk for developing secondary viral pneumonia following exposure to influenza, varicella, and measles (Kort, Cefalo, & Baker, 1986). For high-risk patients such as those with cardiac or respiratory disease or a compromised immune system, vaccination is advisable as such infection may occasionally be fatal during pregnancy. Pneumonia generally occurs 2–3 days after infection with influenza and is treated with ribavirin. Patients are then carefully assessed for secondary bacterial infection. There is a 20% reported incidence of lung involvement in adults with varicella and in pregnant women this is associated with significant mortality (Luby, 1987). Symptoms include dyspnea, cough, chest pain, and bloody sputum within 3–6 days of vesicular eruption. Acyclovir is the drug of choice for treatment of varicella pneumonia. The increase in the number of pregnant women with the AIDS virus has also led to an increase in secondary pneumonia with the organism *Pneumocystis carinii*. The drugs of choice are trimethoprim/sulfamethoxasole (TMX/SMX). Although these drugs have not been fully tested in pregnancy, the potential mortality from *Pneumocystis carinii* far outweigh the potential problems with the treatment (Riley, 1997).

Gastric aspiration occurs most commonly during intubation for general anesthesia but may also occur during eclamptic seizures. Pregnant women are at increased risk for aspiration caused by relaxation of the gastroesophogeal sphincter and displacement of the stomach by the uterus to a horizontal angle. In addition, there is an increase in gastric acid secretion and a decrease in gastric motility. Sedatives used in labor may decrease normal reflexes, thereby further increasing risk. Gastric aspiration during intubation for general anesthesia may be prevented by the use of cricoid pressure during intubation (Selick's maneuver) (Selick, 1974).

The complications that arise as a result of gastric aspiration are directly related to the amount and acidity of the gastric contents. The greater the amount and the greater the acidity, the more damage done. The clinical course may be apparent within minutes or may evolve over several hours. Noncardiogenic pulmonary edema, bronchospasm, atelectasis, decreased airway compliance, and even hypotension may occur (Pritchard, McDonald, & Gant, 1985). Prior to general anesthesia, it is common to administer metoclopramide hydrochloride (Reglan), which empties the stomach. Ranitidine hydrochloride (Zantac), a histamine 2 blocker, is also given to stop production of gastric acid. Both of these medications require 30–45 minutes for maximal effect. Thus, administration of sodium citrate neutralizes any gastric acid still present (Lahiri, Thomas, & Hodgson, 1973).

Once aspiration has occurred, treatment includes prompt suctioning and possibly bronchoscopy if large particulate matter is involved. In the past, saline lavage was used but is contraindicated as it may actually spread aspirate throughout the lung. Though controversial, steroids and antibiotics are frequently given to stabilize the cellular membrane and prevent secondary bacterial infection. Prompt initiation of respiratory support including oxygen is imperative and, when necessary, mechanical ventilation is initiated.

Pulmonary Embolism

Pulmonary embolism refers to the condition where a plug composed of a detached clot, bacteria, or other foreign body occludes a blood vessel in the pulmonary circulation. Deep vein thrombosis is the most common predisposing condition for pulmonary embolism and pregnant women are at high risk for deep vein thrombosis because of increased venous stasis as well as the hypercoagulable state of pregnancy. The incidence in the antepartum period is the same as in nonpregnant patients (Villasanta & Granados, 1983). However, the incidence in the postpartum period increases by 3 to 8 times. Patients with documented deep venous thrombosis require heparin therapy until after delivery with brief interruption of therapy around the delivery. Pulmonary thromboembolism results when a portion of a clot is dislodged from the venous circulation and migrates into the pulmonary vasculature where it occludes a pulmonary arteriole, preventing blood flow and infarcting the area beyond the clot (Roberts, 1987). The severity of symptoms correlates with the size and location of the embolus. The most common symptoms of pulmonary embolism are tachypnea, dyspnea, chest discomfort, and apprehension. Because these symptoms are rather vague and indicative of many disease states, the presence of pulmonary embolism should be documented prior to instituting anti-coagulant therapy. Diagnosis may be made with a V/Q scan, which reveals interruption of blood flow. If inconclusive, pulmonary angiography may be required. Treatment for pulmonary embolism includes heparin administration and supportive oxygen therapy. In cases of a very large pulmonary embolus, some studies have reported successful treatment with intravenous urokinase to dissolve the clot, administered under fluoroscopy (Kramer, Belfort, Saade, Surani, & Moise, 1995).

Amniotic Fluid Embolism

Though the exact mechanism remains unclear, amniotic fluid embolism results from escape of amniotic fluid into the maternal venous circulation. The incidence of amniotic fluid embolism is reported to be 1:8000–80,000 deliveries (Killam 1985). Because the incidence is so rare, Clark and coworkers established a national registry to gather data on patients with amniotic fluid embolism. Forty-six charts were reviewed for multiple variables. Maternal mortality (most within 5 hours of the event) was determined to be 61%, but only 15% of women who survived were neurologically intact. Fetal survival was found to be 39%. The majority of patients (70%) were antepartum and of those whose first symptoms were postpartum, 69% did so within 8 minutes of delivery. The most common symptoms were seizures, dyspnea, fetal bradycardia, hypotension, and cyanosis. Forty patients (87%) had a cardiac arrest while four others had a serious dysrhythmia. If the patient survived the initial insult, disseminated intravascular coagulation occurs to some extent in up to 100% of patients with amniotic fluid embolism (Killam, 1985; Courtney, 1974). Pulmonary edema also occurs in a large percentage of these patients. Several factors have been reported to be common to the majority of reported cases of amniotic fluid embolism. These include average maternal age of 32 years, multiparity, strong uterine contractions, significant amount of particulate matter in the amniotic fluid, larger than average fetus, stillbirths, and premature placental separation (Morgan, 1979). However, the analysis of these 46 cases yields no factors specific to these patients when compared to the general population. Detection of fetal squamous cells, hair, lanugo, and mucin in maternal blood has been the cornerstone for diagnosis, with many cases diagnosed at autopsy. Several clinicians have reported finding fetal squamous cells in blood aspirated from the pulmonary artery in patients without symptoms (Kuhlman, Hidvegi, & Tamma, 1985; Lee, Ginsburg, Cotton, & Kaufman, 1986). Many have suggested the primary finding is severe pulmonary arterial vasospasm as a result of amniotic fluid entering the lungs, followed by severe noncardiogenic pulmonary edema (Courtney, 1974; Morgan, 1979; Clark, Montz, & Phelan, 1986). From analysis of the data from the registry as well as Clark's earlier work, he states that the name amniotic fluid embolism should be discarded and the syndrome of acute peripartum hypoxia, hemodynamic collapse, and coagulopathy should be known as "anaphalactoid syndrome of pregnancy." Initial treatment is aimed at restoring and maintaining cardiovascular and respiratory function and includes fluid, oxygen therapy, possibly mechanical ventilation, and administration of inotropic and vasoactive drugs.

Acute Respiratory Distress Syndrome

Previously referred to as shock lung, hemorrhagic pulmonary edema, and pump lung, acute respiratory distress syndrome was first described in 1967 (Ashbaugh, et al., 1967). Acute respiratory distress syndrome occurs in a small number of pregnant women. However, its exact incidence is difficult to determine because it is not a primary process and actually represents the end point of many different pulmonary disorders. Diagnosis is made in patients with moderate-to-severe hypoxemia, bilateral diffuse infiltrates, no history of primary pulmonary disease, presence of a predisposing disease, and no increase in left atrial pressure. Other symptoms include cyanosis and decreased pulmonary compliance. Onset of the disease process becomes obvious several hours to several days following the initial insult. Predisposing factors include severe pulmonary edema, aspiration pneumonia, sepsis, pulmonary trauma, multiple transfusions, and pulmonary embolism (Ashbaugh et al., 1967; Bernard & Bradley, 1986; Hankins, 1991). Acute respiratory distress syndrome is characterized by severe pulmonary edema, pulmonary hemorrhage, formation of hyaline membranes, hyperplasia, and interstitial fibrosis (Hankins, 1991). Treatment is mainly supportive and includes mechanical ventilation, oxygen therapy with inspired oxygen concentration of 60% or less, and the use of positive end expiratory pressure to force fluid in the extravascular spaces back into the vessels and open collapsed alveoli (Craig, Pierson, & Carrico, 1985).

Asthma

Asthma is a complex chronic disorder with an unknown etiology, which affects an estimated 9–12 million people in the United States, with approximately 7% of those being women of childbearing age (National Institutes of Health, 1992). The disease is characterized by a hyperresponsive airway, with acute exacerbations of severe bronchospasm in response to many physical, chemical, and pharmacologic agents. The Report of the Working Group on Asthma and Pregnancy reported that during pregnancy, asthma improved in approximately one third of the population, worsened in one third, and one third were unchanged (Stenius-Aarniala, Piirila, & Teramo, 1988). Other studies show improvement in 6–69% of patients, the variety related to the population studied and the method used to study the patients (Juniper et al., 1989; Hudak,

Gallo, & Lohr, 1986). Noncompliance with medicine regimens and upper respiratory infections are associated with a worse pregnancy course. Maternal complications include preeclampsia, hyperemesis gravidarum, increased tendency for hemorrhage following delivery, and difficult labor. Fetal complications, which correspond to the severity of disease, include increased risk of intrauterine death, intrauterine growth retardation, preterm birth, low birth weight, and neonatal hypoxia. Successful treatment includes a combination of medications including beta-agonists, beclomethasone, sodium cromoglycate, oral theophylline, and often systemic corticosteroids. Avoidance and/or prompt treatment of upper airway infections is also advisable. Although there is no evidence that these medications cause harm to the fetus, there is a tendency for both the patient and her primary physician to want to decrease her medication use during pregnancy. Patient education regarding prompt treatment of symptoms directly relates to decreasing the severity of exacerbations.

PULMONARY ASSESSMENT

Physical assessment of the patient with pulmonary complications should begin with a complete history. Symptoms such as shortness of breath, dyspnea, and chest pain, as well as explicit explanations of the severity and duration of these symptoms, should be included. During an acute incident, the history remains important though relevant information should be gathered as quickly as possible from the patient or from another reliable source. While gathering the patient's history, attention should be directed to general appearance, noting skin condition, ventilatory pattern, respiratory effort, and symmetry of chest wall movement. Central cyanosis, if present, is a fairly late sign of hypoxia as it represents desaturation of greater than 5 gm/dl of blood in the capillaries (Shapiro, Harrison, Kacmarek, & Cane, 1985). This must be differentiated from peripheral cyanosis, which represents localized hypoxia.

Chest wall palpation may reveal tender areas and lumps. Assessment of the chest position is important as deviation may signify a large pleural effusion, pneumothorax, or severe atelectasis. Presence of tactile fremitus, elicited via use of the palmar surface of the examiner's hands to evaluate vibrations caused by the patient's speech, may reveal pleural effusions or consolidation represented by increased and decreased vibrations, respectively. Respiratory excursion may be better evaluated using the examiner's hands placed on the patient's back to evaluate symmetry of movement. Pneumonia, pneumothorax, and splinting often cause asymmetrical movement.

Chest wall percussion is used to differentiate organ densities. The air-filled lung sounds resonant, whereas the stomach sounds tympanic, and muscle sounds flat. Percussion should be performed especially on initial assessment, and abnormalities should be further investigated. Auscultation of breath sounds is an important part of every physical examination. The quality and phases of respiration change throughout the lung fields as air moves from the trachea to the alveoli. The pattern of respiration as well as the presence or absence of adventitious sounds should be noted. The names of adventitious sounds have been simplified and are now referred to as crackles, wheezes, and pleural friction rubs. Crackles, previously referred to as rales, are caused by different pressures throughout the lung fields and opening of collapsed alveoli. They are only heard during inspiration. Wheezes are indicative of airway constriction and are heard throughout the respiratory cycle. Pleural friction rubs are caused by irritated surfaces rubbing together causing a grating sound during inhalation and exhalation. Consolidation can best be detected by listening to the patient say *"e,e,e"* or *"ninety-nine,"* while listening to the posterior chest wall with a stethoscope. The sounds heard from a normal lung should be *"e,e,e"* and *"nin, nin."* If consolidation is present, the examiner would hear *"a,a,a"* or *"ninety-nine,"* clearly.

Evaluation of arterial blood gases is also an important step in the assessment of pulmonary disease. When interpreted correctly they are helpful in determining the origin, chronicity, and severity of pulmonary dysfunction, as well as the patient's response to treatment. They should be obtained prior to initiation of therapy in order to establish a baseline. Patients requiring multiple arterial blood gases may benefit from an indwelling arterial catheter to reduce the risk of traumatic injury to the artery from repeated punctures. The values in this section represent the normal values for the pregnant patient. The PaO_2 value refers to the amount of oxygen dissolved in arterial blood. The normal range for adults on room air is 104–108 mm Hg. The PaO_2 should be assessed first because, if it is low, oxygen supplementation is instituted immediately while the remainder of the values are assessed. The normal range of blood pH is 7.40–7.45. If less than 7.40, the patient is acidemic; if greater than 7.45, the patient is alkalemic. The next value examined is $PaCO_2$ to determine respiratory acidemia, respiratory alkalemia, or normalcy. This value reflects the adequacy of ventilation; the normal range is 27–32 mm Hg. The normal range for bicarbonate is 18–22 mEq/liter. A low bicarbonate level represents metabolic acidosis and a high level is indicative of metabolic alkalosis. The blood gas values of the pregnant woman differ from those of a nonpregnant woman because of the normal change of hyperventilation of pregnancy; thus, gases reflect a mild compensated respiratory alkalemia. A thorough review of the alterations in the pulmonary system is presented in Chapter 1.

An adjunct to the intermittent monitoring of arterial blood gases is continuous pulse oximetry. Hemoglobin saturated with oxygen absorbs more light than does unsaturated hemoglobin. Thus, pulse oximetry introduces a beam of light into the capillary bed and measures the amount that is absorbed by the hemoglobin. The absorbed amount is indicative of the oxygen saturation of hemoglobin in the body. This value is not a substitute for arterial blood gases but can be used as additional information obtained on a continuous basis to monitor trends in the patient's condition.

Because many pulmonary disorders have vague or similar symptoms, additional tests are often required to differentiate the diagnosis. For the patient with pneumonia, sputum must be obtained for Gram stain and culture, as well as a blood culture. Chest x-ray is one of the most commonly used tests, is easily performed, and can be done at the patient's bedside if necessary. X-rays make it possible to differentiate structures of different densities within the chest with bone being the most dense and air the least dense. Thus, bone and muscle appear white; blood and fluid, gray; and air, black. The presence and location of additional radiopaque items such as an endotracheal tube, pulmonary artery catheter, and chest tubes can be documented with chest x-ray. The best view of the chest is the postero-anterior view with the patient standing and lungs fully expanded. This view is usually only available when the x-ray is taken in the radiology department. Portable film shows the anteroposterior view with patients either upright or supine, and frequently not able to expand their lungs adequately. Thus the quality of film and clarity of structures are less than optimal and often inconclusive.

Ventilation/perfusion scans are most often used to diagnose pulmonary emboli. Hypothetically in patients with normal pulmonary function, the ratio between ventilation and perfusion should be 1:1. However, because of normal physiological and anatomical shunting, there is always a mild mismatch. Patients with problems in either ventilation or perfusion have a greater mismatch. The test is performed in two stages, first perfusion and then ventilation. Radioactive dye is injected into the patient's vein, and the flow of dye through the pulmonary vasculature is reported through a cathode-ray tube, and photographs are taken. Obstructions to blood flow are usually representative of pulmonary embolism although tumors, pulmonary hypertension, arteriovenous fistulas, and vasculitis may also impede blood flow. Next the patient inhales a radioactive gas, and the distribution is carefully monitored. Ventilation abnormalities are suggestive of chronic obstructive pulmonary disease, pneumonia, severe pulmonary edema, cystic fibrosis, and airway obstruction. Portable V/Q scans are now available for critically ill patients. Pulmonary function tests are used to quantify respiratory function, by actually measuring lung volume during normal and maximal

ventilation. These tests are usually conducted on patients with known pulmonary disease or those who complain of dyspnea for baseline evaluation of lung mechanics to follow changes in respiratory function caused by a chronic disease process. They are also performed for preoperative evaluation prior to surgery in patients with known pulmonary disease. The values routinely obtained are tidal volume, inspiratory reserve, inspiratory capacity, expiratory reserve volume, vital capacity, residual volume, functional reserve capacity, and total lung capacity. Patient understanding and cooperation are essential for measurement of many of these parameters.

DIAGNOSES

Pulmonary Edema (Cardiogenic)

Ventilation and perfusion ratios, altered, related to excessive accumulation of fluid in alveoli

Cardiac rhythm, altered, related to hypoxia, hypokalemia, medications or anxiety and concomitant disease

Anxiety (acute), related to pain and discomfort, fear of suffocation

Cardiac output, altered, related to left ventricular dysfunction

Fluid and electrolyte imbalance, altered, related to diuretic therapy

Acute Respiratory Failure (Related to Amniotic Fluid Embolism, Pulmonary Embolism, Acute Respiratory Distress Syndrome)

Anxiety related to dyspnea and fear of dying

Airway clearance, ineffective, related to secretions, bronchial edema, bronchospasm, fibrosis, and parenchymal destruction

Infection, related to retained secretions, use of respiratory equipment, impaired pulmonary defense system

Impaired gas exchange, related to alveolar hypoventilation

Tissue perfusion, altered, cardiopulmonary (decreased) related to embolism

Gastrointestinal function, altered, related to ulcers and gastritis

Mechanical Ventilation

Anxiety related to disease process, diagnostic tests and procedures, therapy
>   Sensory deprivation (overload)
>   Sleep deprivation
>   Disorientation
>   Inability to talk

Breathing pattern, ineffective, related to ventilator malfunction, accidental extubation, barotrauma, pneumothorax

Infection, potential for, related to bypass of normal filtering system

Breach of aseptic technique for suctioning through tracheal tube; repeated traumatic or intrusive suctioning procedures

Breathing pattern, ineffective, related to hyperventilation or hypoventilation

Cardiac output, altered decreased, related to increased intrathoracic pressures associated with mechanical ventilation (and, if used, positive end-expiratory pressure)

Gas exchange, impaired, related to oxygen toxicity secondary to high inspired oxygen concentrations

Injury, potential for, related to pressure sores on side of mouth, nose, tracheostomy site, hyperplasia and inflammation, scarring and stenosis of trachea caused by trauma of endotracheal tube

THERAPY AND NURSING CARE

In addition to oxygen therapy, pharmacologic support may be administered to restore normal respiratory function. The drugs used in the treatment of pulmonary disorders vary according to the underlying problem. However, use of small amounts of sedation may be beneficial in most types of respiratory distress to quell the anxiety-triggered hyperventilation associated with air hunger. Morphine sulfate in small increments not only calms patients but also has a relaxant effect on the pulmonary vasculature and slightly decreases venous return, which may be beneficial in disease states such as cardiogenic pulmonary edema. Care must be taken to monitor the effects as even mild overdosage could depress the respiratory center of the central nervous system, thus decreasing the stimulus to breathe.

Another frequently used class of medication is steroids. Although use is often controversial, they are frequently used in the treatment of aspiration pneumonia, amniotic fluid embolism, and for many of the other precipitating causes of noncardiogenic pulmonary edema. The rationale for use of steroids is to decrease the local inflammatory response and stabilize the cellular membrane. They are usually instituted immediately after the initial insult and continued for several days afterward. Antibiotic therapy is not routinely indicated for all pulmonary disorders. Many carry increased risk of infection either from the actual disease process as in bacterial or aspiration pneumonia or from manipulation of the airways permitting introduction of bacteria. In many pulmonary disorders, fluid and sputum accumulate in the alveoli, creating a facilitative medium for bacterial growth.

Care of the woman in labor with pulmonary compromise is especially challenging as both mother and fetus are at risk for hypoxia. Adequate maternal oxygenation is important; however, adequate cardiac output and placental perfusion are equally essential for fetal oxygenation. Oxygen is the most frequently used and misused drug for patients with a pulmonary disorder, and it has both positive and detrimental effects. The goal of oxygen therapy is to achieve a PaO_2 of 70–100 mm Hg with a hemoglobin saturation of at least 90% at the lowest therapeutic amount. The concentration required to treat patients is dependent on the total clinical picture including cardiac output and the amount and quality of hemoglobin. The patient's respiratory status must be frequently assessed including rate, effort, skin color, and oxygen saturation via pulse oximetry. Arterial blood gases should be monitored if there is a change in respiratory status or therapy. Auscultation of breath sounds is required at least every 8 hours, more often if the patient's status changes. The fetus should be monitored closely for evidence of hypoxia, as reflected by abnormal fetal heart rate responses.

The method selected for oxygen delivery is dependent on the amount of oxygen required as well as patient comfort. It must be emphasized that the inspired concentration of oxygen is based on normal tidal volume and respiratory rate. Nasal cannulas are frequently used to deliver low concentrations of oxygen (i.e., 1–5 liters/minute) or an FiO_2 of 0.24–0.44. Cannulas are advantageous in that they are inexpensive, easy to use, and comfortable to wear. Higher flow rates should be avoided because of drying of the nasal mucosa. There have been concerns regarding the effectiveness of a nasal cannula with patients who predominantly breathe through their mouth, and studies have reported conflicting results (Spearman, 1982; Domigan-Wenta, 1985). In general, masks are less comfortable and many patients report a claustrophobic feeling. Simple masks are most commonly used for short-term oxygen therapy. They can deliver up to 0.60 FiO_2; however, actual concentration can be greater or more dilute as a result of the oxygen concentration of the exhaled air and rate of breathing. The mask may also be used for delivery of humidification or aerosol treatments.

The nonrebreathing mask has a reservoir and a one-way valve that prevent exhaled air from entering the reservoir bag. This mask requires a higher rate of flow (at least 8 liters/minute) to keep the reservoir bag inflated. A tightly fitting nonrebreathing mask can deliver an FiO_2 of 0.90–1.00. However, because of loosely fitting masks and rapid respiratory rates, the concentration delivered is usually approximately 0.63 FiO_2 (Domigan-Wenta, 1985). High-flow systems deliver all the air required by the patient, in addition to the proper concentration of oxygen from a FiO_2 of 0.24–1.00. An advantage of this system is that respiratory rate and breathing pattern have no effect on the inspired oxygen concentration. The Venturi mask is the most reliable mask for delivering exact oxygen concentrations, regardless of the patient's respiratory pattern. The mask delivers 100% oxygen at high velocity through an orifice the size of which can be adjusted to deliver different oxygen concentrations. The inspired oxygen concentration with various delivery devices are shown in Table 11-2. Humidification of inspired air is necessary when the upper airway is

bypassed as with intubation or when supplemental oxygen is required. It is important to prevent drying and irritation of the respiratory system, minimize fluid loss, and liquefy secretions so they may be expectorated. Patients who already require ventilation are at greater risk for these complications. Humidification can be accomplished with warm or cold humidifiers, although cold humidifiers are only 50% effective.

Patients who have refractory hypoxemia or tissue hypoxia with supplemental oxygen therapy and are therefore unable to ventilate sufficiently require intubation and mechanical ventilation. The most commonly used ventilators are positive pressure ventilators of which there are three types: volume cycled, pressure cycled, and time cycled. A detailed explanation of ventilators and care of the patient requiring mechanical ventilation can be found in Chapter 5.

Adding positive end-expiratory pressure may be required in patients with decreased compliance or fluid-filled alveoli. This keeps the alveoli open during the expiratory phase and can force pulmonary fluid out of the alveoli toward the vasculature. Continuous positive airway pressure works on the same principle but is used when patients are not receiving intermittent positive pressure with a ventilator. Continuous positive airway pressure can be delivered by a tight-fitting mask, though an endotracheal tube is most often used (Domigan-Wenta, 1985). Positive end-expiratory pressure and continuous positive airway pressure must be carefully monitored, especially if the patient is hemodynamically unstable. Venous return and thus cardiac output are decreased with increased intrathoracic pressure. When high levels of positive end-expiratory pressure are required, inotropic drugs or fluid therapy may be required to maintain cardiac output (Gallagher, Civetta, & Kirby, 1978). Use of positive end-expiratory pressure in conjunction with mechanical ventilation may allow a reduction of FiO_2 to less toxic levels below 0.50.

Evaluation of other mechanisms to improve oxygenation are currently being investigated. They include extracorporeal carbon dioxide removal (ECCO$_2$R) and extracorporeal membrane oxygenation (ECMO) (Dirkes, 1996). There are multiple disadvantages to these therapies including bleeding, and excessive requirements of resources such as trained personnel and vast blood bank services. Additionally, although ECMO has been successful in the treatment of neonatal RDS, more research is required to determine the effects in adults. Liquid ventilation therapy, which involves instillation of a liquid perfluorocarbon, is another mode of therapy being tested. Early studies show substantial improvements in gas exchange, increase in lung compliance, and a reduction in intraalveolar hemorrhage, pulmonary vascular congestion, and infiltrates (Hirschl, Tooley, Parent, Johnson, & Bartlett, 1996). The liquid perfluorocarbons are heavier than water, causing them to settle into dependent portions of the lung, opening collapsed alveoli and providing a medium for gas exhange using a liquid with a high solubility for oxygen and carbon dioxide. More research is needed prior to clinical applications of these procedures.

ACUTE RESPIRATORY COMPROMISE

In the event of acute respiratory failure, priorities include attainment of a secure airway, ventilation with 100% oxygen if possible, and assessment and support of circulatory function. These must be maintained until further assistance is available. If the patient is breathing but experiencing difficulty, a mask delivering a high concentration of oxygen should be placed on the patient and a quick assessment performed to determine the cause of respiratory failure. If the patient has aspirated, rapid suctioning should be done prior to ventilation to prevent the gastric contents from being forced farther into the lungs. During the acute phase of respiratory failure, attention should be directed toward stabilization of the mother. Only after the mother has been stabilized should attention be directed toward the fetus. An important caveat to remember is if the mother is hypoxic, the fetus is also hypoxic and the outcome will often be improved with in utero resuscitation. However, if the mother's condition includes absence of

cortical activity or no chance of survival, cesarean section may be performed depending on fetal gestational age and condition.

It should be remembered that maternal hypoxia often triggers labor as a protective mechanism caused in part by decreased uteroplacental perfusion. Thus, the woman in labor with pulmonary complications should be assessed for uterine activity and rupture of membranes that may result from uterine contractions. If the patient is found to be in preterm labor and tocolytics are ordered, decisions regarding tocolysis require careful thought. For example, betamimetics may be indicated as they also cause bronchodilation. However, cardiovascular side effects could be devastating in the patient who is critically ill.

Nursing care of the patient requiring mechanical ventilation presents additional challenges. Though a lifesaving measure, mechanical ventilation can be quite frightening and introduces another set of possible complications to the already compromised patient. Care must be taken to assure that the ventilator is working properly prior to connection to the patient and that it continues to function for the duration of therapy. A qualified respiratory therapist must be readily available to troubleshoot ventilator problems. The nurse at the bedside must also be familiar with the ventilatory settings and alarms, must know how to detect common problems, and must be able to appropriately ventilate the patient with an Ambu bag until any problem is solved. All procedures and equipment should be explained thoroughly as this is the most effective way to allay fear and enhance patient cooperation. The patient must be able to communicate by writing on a pad or chalkboard, because speech is impossible and lip reading is difficult when the patient is orally intubated. Ventilatory settings must be validated according to hospital standards, and a complete patient assessment including breath sounds should be done at appropriate intervals. Suctioning is also an important therapy when the patient is being mechanically ventilated, because she can no longer cough to clear secretions. Not a benign procedure, suctioning should be done only when necessary to clear the airway. Hyperoxygenation should be accomplished before and after suctioning. Suctioning should be rapid, using only intermittent suction during withdrawal of the catheter. If the patient requires positive end-expiratory pressure, a special valve is available so that the positive pressure can be maintained if open suctioning is performed.

REFERENCES

Ashbaugh, D. G., Bigelow, D. R., Petty, T. L., et al. (1967). Acute respiratory distress in adults. Lancet, 2, 319.

Benedetti, T. J., Kates, R., & Williams, V. (1985). Hemodynamic observations in severe preeclampsia complicated by pulmonary edema. American Journal of Obstetrics and Gynecology, 152, 330.

Benedetti, T, L., Valle, R., & Ledger, W. J. (1982). Antepartum pneumonia in pregnancy. American Journal of Obstetrics and Gynecology, 144, 413.

Bernard, G. R., & Bradley, R. B. (1986). Adult respiratory distress syndrome: Diagnosis and management. Heart Lung, 15, 250.

Clark, S. L., Hankins, G. D. V., Dudley, D. A., Dildy, G. A., & Porter, T. F. (1995). Amniotic fluid embolism: Analysis of the national registry. American Journal of Obstetrics and Gynecology, 172, 1158.

Clark, S. L., Montz, F. J., & Phelan, J. P. (1986). Hemodynamic alterations associated with amniotic fluid embolism: A reappraisal. American Journal of Obstetrics and Gynecology, 151, 617.

Courtney, L. D. (1974). Amniotic fluid embolus. Obstetrics and Gynecology Survey, 29, 169.

Craig, K. C., Pierson, D. J., & Carrico, C. (1985). The clinical application of positive end-expiratory pressure (PEEP) in the adult respiratory distress syndrome (ARDS). Respiratory Care, 30, 184.

Deblieux, P., & Summer, W. R. (1996). Acute respiratory failure in pregnancy. Clinical Obstetrics and Gynecology, 39(1), 143.

Deirkes, S. (1996). Liquid ventilation: New frontiers in the treatment of ARDS. Critical Care Nurse, 16, 53.

Domigan-Wenta, J. (1995). CPAP mask. American Journal of Nursing, 85, 813.

Freda, M. C., & DeVore, N. (1996). Should intravenous hydration be the first line of defense with threatened preterm labor? A critical review of the literature. Journal of Perinatology, 16(5), 385.

Gallagher, T. J., Civetta, J. M., & Kirby, R. R. (1978). Terminology update: Optimal PEEP. Critical Care Medicine, 6, 323.

Greenberger, P. A., & Patterson, R. (1988). The outcome of pregnancy complicated by severe asthma. Allergy Proceedings, 9(5), 539.

Hankins, G. D. V. (1991). Adult respiratory distress syndrome. In S. L. Clark, G. D. V. Hankins, D. B. Cotton, & J. P. Phelan (Eds.), Critical care obstetrics (2nd ed.). Boston: Blackwell.

Hatis, C. G., & Swain, M. (1988). Systemic tocolysis for premature labor is associated with an increased incidence of pulmonary edema in the presence of maternal infection. American Journal of Obstetrics and Gynecology, 159, 723.

Hirschl, R. B., Tooley, R., Parent, A., Johnson, K., & Bartlett, R. H. (1996). Evaluation of pulmonary function, pulmonary compliance and lung injury during total and partial liquid ventilation in acute respiratory distress syndrome. Critical Care Medicine, 24(6), 1001.

Hudak, C. M., Gallo, B. M., & Lohr, T. (1986). Critical care nursing—A holistic approach. Philadelphia: Lippincott.

Juniper, E. F., Daniel, E. E., Roberts, R. S., et al. (1989). Improvement in airway responsiveness and asthma severity during pregnancy. American Review of Respiratory Disease, 140, 924–931.

Katz, M., Robertson, P. A., & Creasy, R. K. (1981). Cardiovascular complications associated with terbutaline treatment for preterm labor. American Journal of Obstetrics and Gynecology, 139, 605.

Keefer, J. R., Strauss, R. G., Civetta, J. M., & Burke, T. (1981). Noncardiogenic pulmonary edema and invasive cardiovascular monitoring. Obstetrics and Gynecology, 58, 47.

Killam, A. (1985). Amniotic fluid embolus. Clinical Obstetrics and Gynecology, 28, 32.

Kort, B. A., Cefalo, R. X., & Baker, V. V., (1986). Fatal influenza A pneumonia in pregnancy. American Journal of Perinatology, 3, 179.

Kramer, W. B., Belfort, M., Saade, G. R., Surani, S., & Moise, K. J. (1995). Successful urokinase treatment of massive pulmonary embolism in pregnancy. Obstetrics and Gynecology, 86, 660.

Kuhlman, K., Hidvegi, D., & Tamma, R. (1985). Is amniotic fluid material in the central circulation of peripartum patients pathologic? American Journal of Perinatology, 2, 295.

Lahiri, S. K., Thomas, T. A., & Hodgson, R. M. H. (1973). Single-dose antacid therapy in the prevention of Mendelson's syndrome. British Journal of Anaesthesia, 45, 354.

Lee, W., Ginsburg, K. A., Cotton, D. B., & Kaufman, R. E. (1986). Squamous and trophoblastic cells in the maternal pulmonary circulation identified by invasive hemodynamic monitoring during the peripartum period. American Journal of Obstetrics and Gynecology, 55, 999.

Luby, J. P. (1987). Southwestern Internal Medicine Conference: Pneumonia in adults due to mycoplasma, chlamydia, and viruses. American Journal of Medical Science, 294, 45.

Maccato, J. (1990). Pneumonia in pregnancy. In L. C. Gilstrap & S. Faro (Eds.), Infections in pregnancy. New York: Alan R. Liss.

Morgan, M. (1979). Amniotic fluid embolism. Anesthesia, 34, 20.

Morin, F. C., & Weiss, K. I. (1992). Response of fetal circulation to stress. In R. A. Polin & W. M. Fox (Eds.), Fetal and Neonatal Physiology, Philadelphia: W. B. Saunders.

National Institutes of Health. (1992, October). Report of the working group on asthma and pregnancy: Management of asthma during pregnancy. (NIH Publications No. 93-3279A).

Pisani, R. J., & Rosenow, E. C. (1995). Pulmonary edema associated with tocolytic therapy. Annals of Pharmacotherapy, 29, 521.

Pritchard, J. A., McDonald, P. C., & Gant, N. F. (1985). Williams obstetrics (17th ed.). Norwalk, CT: Appleton Century-Crofts.

Riley, L. (1997). Pneumonia and tuberculosis in pregnancy. Infectious Disease Clinics of North America, 11(1), 119.

Roberts, R. B., & Shirley, M. A. (1974). Reducing the risks of acid aspiration during cesarean section. Anesthesia and Analgesia, 53, 589.

Roberts, S. L. (1987). Pulmonary tissue perfusion altered: Emboli. Heart Lung, 16, 128.

Selick, B. A. (1961). Cricoid pressure to control regurgitation of stomach contents during induction of anesthesia. Lancet, 2, 204.

Shapiro, B. A., Harrison, R. A., Kacmarek, R. M., & Cane, R. D. (1985). Clinical application of respiratory care. Chicago: Year Book Medical.

Spearman, C., & Sheldon, R. (1982). Egans fundamentals of respiratory therapy (4th ed.). St. Louis, MO: Mosby.

Stenius-Aarniala, R. Piirila, P., & Teramo, K. (1988). Asthma and pregnancy: A prospective study of 198 pregnancies. Thorax, 43, 12.

Thelan, L. A., Davie, J. K., & Urden, L. D. (1990). Textbook of critical care nursing: Diagnosis and management. St. Louis, MO: Mosby.

Villasanta, U., & Granados, J. L. (1983). Deep vein thrombophlebitis during pregnancy. In F. P. Zuspan & C. D. Christian (Eds.), Controversies in obstetrics and gynecology. Philadelphia: Saunders.

West, J. B. (1985). Respiratory physiology: The essentials (3rd ed.). Baltimore: Williams & Wilkins.

CHAPTER 12

Sepsis and Systemic Inflammatory Response Syndrome: Critical Complications During Pregnancy

Julie M. R. Arafeh

Infection resulting in septic shock is a leading cause of death in adult intensive care units (Ackerman, 1994). This statistic remains true despite the use and continued advances in antimicrobial therapy in the last decade. The search for new therapies and determination of the physiologic events that lead to septic shock have been the subjects of much research in the critical care arena. This information is useful in understanding the pathophysiology of sepsis and in planning care for the infected obstetric patient.

Although maternal death from sepsis is estimated to be between 3 and 8%, the low incidence of maternal death in general makes sepsis a major cause of mortality (Gonik, 1991; Simpson, 1995). When sepsis is identified in the obstetric patient it is most often related to endometritis after delivery, with cesarean section being the delivery route mentioned most often (Gonik, 1991). As far as reported bacterial infections, urinary tract infections are the most common, with *Escherichia coli* being the isolate identified most frequently (Savoia, 1995). Other infections linked with sepsis are pyelonephritis and chorioamnionitis (Gonik, 1991).

Other avenues for the introduction of organisms are invasive procedures. It is well known that the common procedure of intravenous cannulation has increased the risk of infection after the catheter has been in place for 72 hours (Nichols, 1992). Electron microscopy has identified coagulase-negative staphylococci adherent to catheters as soon as 30 minutes after insertion (Norwood, 1995). Although central venous catheters are associated with a 6.9–11.5% risk of infection, use of the internal jugular site is associated with greater risk possibly related to increased movement and proximity near the mouth and nose (Norwood, 1995). The risk of infection increases 5–10% per day each day an indwelling urinary catheter is in place (Nichols, 1992). After 24 hours endotracheal tubes are typically colonized with gram negative bacteria (Taylor, 1992).

DEFINITIONS

Regardless of the etiology of the infection it is important to be consistent in the use of terminology. Inconsistent use of terms like sepsis and septic shock make dissemination of information and collaborative research projects among institutions difficult. An attempt to standardize terminology resulted in a 1992 joint publication of definitions by the American College of Chest Physicians and the Society of Critical Care Medicine (American College of Chest Physicians et al., 1992). The terms defined for use were infection, bacteremia, systemic inflammatory response syndrome (SIRS), sepsis, severe sepsis, septic shock, hypotension, and multiple organ dysfunction syndrome. These terms include physiologic parameters that can be equated to clinical assessments and laboratory results. There are several distinctions made in describing sepsis. Sepsis is defined as the response to infection, and severe sepsis occurs when the infected patient demonstrates organ dysfunction or hypotension. Septic shock implies that this condition persists despite fluid resuscitation. See Display 12-1 for definitions and physiologic parameters (American College of Chest Physicians et al., 1992). Of all of the terms, SIRS is the most unfamiliar and will be discussed in further detail.

SYSTEMIC INFLAMMATORY RESPONSE SYNDROME (SIRS)

The role of the immune system is to defend the body from invading organisms. The series of events that occurs in response to invasion is known as inflammation. Inflammation allows fluid and cells from the blood stream into the affected area through the processes of vasodilation and increased vasopermeability. With the cells from the immune system in the area, the infectious agent is surrounded and destroyed (Sell, 1987). Under these controlled circumstances inflammation is protective, destroying foreign and dead cells and removing debris to promote return to normal tissue function. However, when this response is not controlled or occurs systemically, tremendous damage to healthy tissue and cells can occur. This phenomenon is known as SIRS. Widespread vasodilation and vasopermeability result in low intravascular volume, generalized edema, and tissue damage (Sell, 1987). In order to understand the pathophysiology leading to SIRS, the role of the endothelium, selected immune cells, and mediators or signaling molecules that initiate and maintain the inflammatory response will be reviewed.

THE ROLE OF THE ENDOTHELIUM

The innermost cellular lining of the vascular bed is known as the endothelium. The endothelium has many functions, the most recognized of which is related to the smooth lining, which discourages clot formation and enhances blood flow through the vessel. Other functions include diffusion and filtration of substances between the intravascular and extravascular spaces and formation and release of mediators such as prostaglandins and thromboxanes. Release of mediators contributes to the size of the vessel and hemostasis. For example, the prostaglandin prostacyclin causes vasodilation and inhibits platelet aggregation, whereas thromboxane causes vasoconstriction and platelet aggregation. The endothelium plays a critical role in the inflammatory process by the formation of adhesion molecules on its surface that will attract and bind with cells such as neutrophils. When the endothelium and neutrophils are stimulated during the inflammatory process, adhesion molecules appear on both the neutrophils and the endothelium, which cause the neutrophils to roll along the side of the vessel, become attached, and move through the vessel into the tissue (Huddleston, 1992; Guyton & Hall, 1996; Vedder & Harlan, 1995).

When the endothelium is damaged or becomes over-stimulated by substances such as endotoxin, it turns into a secretory organ releasing mediators resulting in vasodilation, vasopermeability, and increased formation of adhesion molecules. As neutrophils become stimulated and bind with the endothelium, release of their strong enzymes can occur, causing damage to the lining and releasing even more procoagulant factors such as tissue factor. The formation of blood clots and clumps of aggregated neutrophils decrease blood flow by occluding the vessel (Huddleston, 1992; Vedder & Harlan, 1995).

COMPONENTS OF THE IMMUNE SYSTEM

The role of the immune system is not fully understood and is the subject of much research. Whereas the function of immune cells is fairly well understood, the communication pattern between these cells and how other cells are

DISPLAY 12-1

Consensus Conference Definitions of Sepsis

Infection: Microbial phenomenon characterized by an inflammatory response to the presence of microorganisms or the invasion of normally sterile host tissue by those organisms.

Bacteremia: The presence of viable bacteria in the blood.

Systemic Inflammatory Response Syndrome: The systemic inflammatory response to a variety of severe clinical insults. The response is manifested by two or more of the following conditions:

> Temperature >38°C or <36°C
> Heart rate >90 beats/min
> Respiratory rate >20 breaths/min or $PaCO_2$ <32 torr (<4.3 kPa)
> WBC >12,000 cells mm³, <4000 cells/mm³, or >10% immature (band) forms

Sepsis: The systemic response to infection. This systemic response is manifested by two or more of the following conditions as a result of infection:

> Temperature >38°C or <36°C
> Heart rate >90 beats/min
> Respiratory rate >20 breaths/min or $PaCO_2$ <32 torr (<4.3 kPa)
> WBC >12,000 cells/ mm³, <4000 cells/mm³, or >10% immature (band) forms

Severe Sepsis: Sepsis associated with organ dysfunction, hypoperfusion, or hypotension. Hypoperfusion and perfusion abnormalities may include, but are not limited to, lactic acidosis, oliguria, or an acute alteration in mental status.

Septic Shock: Sepsis with hypotension, despite adequate fluid resuscitation, along with the presence of perfusion abnormalities that may include, but are not limited to, lactic acidosis, oliguria, or an acute alteration in mental status. Patients who are on inotropic or vasopressor agents may not be hypotensive at the time that perfusion abnormalities are measured.

Hypotension: A systolic BP of <90 mm Hg or a reduction of >40 mm Hg from baseline in the absence of other causes for hypotension.

Multiple Organ Dysfunction Syndrome: Presence of altered organ function in an acutely ill patient such that homeostasis cannot be maintained without intervention.

---

made to respond during inflammation is being discovered. It is known that many cells, not just immune cells, release substances called mediators. These mediators are signaling molecules that can stimulate or limit the action of white blood cells, endothelial cells, and smooth muscle (Sell, 1987). Some of the mediators have a local effect whereas others affect cells distant from where they were released. The molecular weight and size of the mediator in part determines how far the mediator can travel to influence cells. Mediators that are very small tend to have a local effect whereas the larger mediators can travel further distances (Stroud et al., 1990). Selected cells of the immune system and mediators will be reviewed.

SELECTED CELLS IN THE IMMUNE SYSTEM

Mast Cells

Mast cells are located near vessels and submucosal tissue and are responsible for initiating and controlling the inflammatory response. They have the ability to release many mediators such as arachadonic acid metabolites, histamine, and proteases resulting in the contraction of endothelial cells and vasodilation. This allows increased blood flow to the area and encourages movement of cells into tissue (Sell, 1987; Huddleston, 1992).

Macrophages

Macrophages are large phagocytic cells or scavenger cells that can be found in tissues and in the blood stream (Sell, 1987). Their role includes detection and destruction of invading organisms by phagocytosis, initiation of inflammation, and destruction of aging cells and necrotic tissue. Because they reside in noninflamed tissue, macrophages are key in initiating the inflammatory process in response to bacteria or invading organisms. They do this in several ways. First, they can destroy the invading organisms by phagocytosis. In this process the macrophage binds to the organism and ingests it. Once inside the macrophage the organism is exposed to several destructive substances that result in the death of the organism in ideal circumstances. In this way healthy tissue is protected from the destructive forces the macrophage utilizes. In addition to phagocytosis of foreign cells, macrophages also destroy necrotic tissue, which clears the site of acute inflammation to allow for healing and regeneration of tissue (Sell, 1987; Ganz, 1995). In initiating the inflammatory response, macrophages can release chemotaxic factors, which attract other cells of the immune system or other macrophages to the area. Macrophages also release mediators such as tumor necrosis factor (TNF), Interleukin-1 (IL-1), Interleukin-6 (IL-6) and Interleukin-8 (IL-8) (Ganz, 1995). These mediators will be discussed in more detail later.

Neutrophils

Neutrophils compose 50–90% of the peripheral white blood cell count (Sell, 1987). They are very mobile and are the first cells to respond to invading organisms. Neutrophils contain granular tissue that releases strong enzymes capable of destroying cells. Chemotaxis is required to move neutrophils to the area being invaded. When neutrophils are activated they develop adhesion molecules that bind with adhesion molecules on the endothelial lining. The process of neutrophil alignment along the endothelial lining is known as margination. After attaching to the lining of the vessel, they squeeze through into the tissues (Secor, 1994).

Lymphocytes

Lymphocytes compose approximately 30% of the white blood cell count and have a well recognized role in inflammation (Sell, 1987). They are activated by antigens and are responsible for immunity displayed against certain infections such as measles or chickenpox (Guyton & Hall, 1996). Lymphocytes can be divided into three groups; B cells, T cells and large granular cells called natural killer cells. They are divided into these groups dependent upon where they generally reside after maturation (Sell, 1987). Precursor cells to all lymphocytes originate in the bone marrow, then T cells migrate to the thymus and eventually reside in lymph nodes and the spleen, whereas B cells differentiate in several different areas with mature cells found mainly in the plasma. Although immunity is the role most associated with lymphocytes, they also play a role in the inflammatory process. Natural killer cells act directly to destroy other cells under the influence of mediators released by lymphocytes (Seller & Owen, 1993). Substances like endotoxin stimulate lymphocytes and cause the release of mediators such as IL-1 and IL-2.

MEDIATORS

Cytokines

Cytokines are chemical messengers that are released by cells such as macrophages, lymphocytes, neutrophils, and endothelial cells. There are at least 30 known cytokines such as Interleukin-1 (IL-1), Interleukin-6 (IL-6), Interleukin-8 (IL-8), Interleukin-10 (IL-10), and tumor necrosis factor (TNF). The terminology involving cytokines can be confusing. In many instances these mediators were named based on the effect they had on cells or the cells from which their release was first identified. A very small amount of these mediators, picomolar or less, can cause diverse biologic responses such as activation of white cells and the endothelium, depression of the myocardium, anorexia, fever, hypotension, and hypercoagulability. Gram-negative sepsis and the role cytokines play in the process have been studied in the animal and human model. The release of endotoxin, found in the outer membrane of gram-negative bacteria, stimulates TNF and after a short period of time IL-1. The combined effect of these two cytokines is worse than the effect of one alone as shown in animal studies where one or the other cytokine was blocked with decreased mortality noted. Furthermore, cytokines can be divided according to the effect they have on inflammation. Cytokines associated with a proinflammatory effect are IL-1, IL-8, and TNF. Those associated with an anti-inflammatory effect are IL-10 and IL-6. It is believed that cytokines are released in a cascading fashion. One cytokine will result in the release of another, which then results in the release of another cytokine, and so on. The release of anti-inflammatory cytokines would imply an attempt to modulate or control the effects of the proinflammatory cytokines and has prompted new therapies to attempt to boost these mediators in syndromes such as SIRS. In the animal model total blockage of IL-1 resulted in increased mortality of the animal, therefore it is believed that cytokines are important in controlled amounts (Shapiro & Gelfand, 1995; Christman, 1995). Research continues with discovery of new cytokines and additional biologic actions of known cytokines occurring on a regular basis.

Free Oxygen Radicals

A free oxygen radical is an oxygen molecule with an unpaired electron. Radicals are unstable and can destroy cells, denature proteins, and increase capillary permeability (Huddleston, 1992). Oxygen radicals are a large part of the considerable arsenal neutrophils use to destroy cells (McCord, 1995). In combination with other elements, oxygen radicals can form hydroxyl radicals, which are even more destructive than oxygen radicals. Free oxygen radicals are produced in small amounts when oxygen is used in metabolism (Huddleston, 1992). Normally antioxidants balance the production of oxygen radicals but in sepsis there appears to be an imbalance allowing increased levels of oxygen radicals (Stroud et al., 1990).

Proteases

Proteases are proteolytic enzymes that break down proteins in plasma and tissue. They are released from mast cells, neutrophils, and macrophages to destroy foreign cells and damaged tissue. When overstimulated, proteases break down collagen and elastin in healthy tissue, destroying vessels and even organ parenchyma. Free oxygen radicals can exacerbate the damage done by proteases by breaking down enzymes that control them (Huddleston, 1992; Stroud et al., 1990).

Platelet-Activating Factor

As with most of the mediators, platelet-activating factor (PAF) can be released by many different cells. PAF causes platelets to activate and aggregate as the name suggests. It also stimulates neutrophils to marginate along the endothelium and to release enzymes (Sell, 1987; Huddleston, 1992; Vedder & Harlan, 1995).

Arachadonic Acid Metabolites

Arachadonic acid is a precursor cell found in the membranes of all cells except red blood cells. When stimulated, arachadonic acid is released and can then follow one of three pathways that result in the release of eicosanoids. Leukotrienes, prostaglandins, and thromboxanes are eicosanoids. These metabolites influence the size of vessels, vasopermeability, and aggregation of platelets, and can stimulate other cells in the inflammatory response (Sell, 1987; Huddleston, 1992; Halushka et al., 1995).

Inflammation

Inflammation is comprised of a complex series of events. A summary of these events is depicted in Figure 12-1. The first event of inflammation is temporary vasoconstriction, which is felt to be under the control of the sympathetic nervous system. This vasoconstriction lasts only a short period of time and is not well understood (Sell, 1987). Acute vascular response occurs next. Initiation of this response may occur from mast cells or macrophages, which identify invading organisms, and release mediators resulting in endothelial cell contraction and vasodilation. Through these processes of vasodilation and vasopermeability, fluid and cells leave the blood vessel, which results in the classic signs of inflammation; edema, redness, heat, and pain (Sell, 1987). Neutrophils drawn to the area by chemotaxis marginate or bind with the endothelial lining. As the endothelial cells contract, neutrophils move into the tissues to destroy the organisms. Platelets and fibrinogen in the tissue result in coagulation, which provides a "scaffolding" for new tissue growth (Sell, 1987). If the infection or injury is limited, the acute phase of the inflammatory response is all that is required

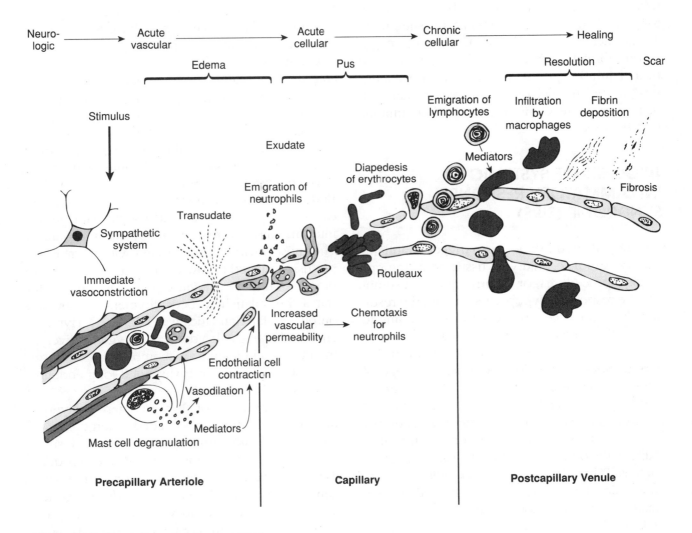

Figure 12-1. The inflammatory response.

to return the tissue to normal function. However, cells such as macrophages are often necessary to remove debris from the area for normal tissue function to be restored (Sell, 1987).

As stated earlier, this protective response can turn very destructive if inflammation is not well controlled. Widespread vasodilation lowers systemic vascular resistance. When combined with widespread vasopermeability, intravascular volume moves into the tissues or the "third space," making adequate perfusion difficult. Tissue edema interferes with organ function. The release of mediators can result in some vessels dilating and others constricting, which can result in the shunting of blood from underperfused tissues. Stimulation of neutrophils leading to margination and enzyme release can cause extensive damage to the endothelial lining of vessels and tissues. Damaged endothelium becomes secretory, releasing prostaglandins and tissue factor. Tissue factor is a powerful stimulant of coagulation. Formation of clots in the vascular space further inhibits perfusion. As perfusion continues to decline because of these events, cell death occurs, resulting in even further stimulus for SIRS (Secor, 1994).

TRIGGERS OF SYSTEMIC INFLAMMATORY RESPONSE SYNDROME (SIRS)

A variety of circumstances can trigger an inflammatory response. Injury to tissue from trauma, surgical procedures, or a burn injury can stimulate the response. Hypoperfusion with the resultant drop in oxygen delivery to cells leading to cell death and tissue damage can also stimulate SIRS. However, one of the most recognized triggers of SIRS is infection (American College of Chest Physicians et al., 1992; Huddleston, 1992). Infection resulting from gram-negative bacteria results in the release of endotoxin. Endotoxin is a well-studied exogenous mediator of SIRS. It is found in the outer membrane of all gram-negative bacteria. When the bacteria either multiply or die, endotoxin is released (Secor, 1994). Extremely small amounts of endotoxin (nanograms/kg) can initiate SIRS. Endotoxin also stimulates macrophages to release tumor necrosis factor and IL-1.

Both of these mediators have proinflammatory properties leading to activation of neutrophils, myocardial depression, and stimulation of the endothelium. The cascading effect of cytokine release can be seen with endotoxin stimulation. Even though endotoxin does not remain in the bloodstream for long periods of time, the stimulation of tumor necrosis factor will continue the destructive action of endotoxin. TNF will stimulate the release of IL-1 and the cascade continues to propagate the initial action of endotoxin (Secor, 1994; Kellum & Decker, 1996). It is known that women develop sepsis less frequently than men. In the animal model, high levels of HDL and LDL cholesterol are associated with increased survival. It is believed that the high cholesterol levels bind to and neutralize endotoxin. The hormone prolactin is believed to have a similar effect (Zellweger, 1997). Elevated cholesterol and prolactin levels in pregnancy may have a beneficial effect in the event of endotoxin release.

Gram-negative bacteria are located in the intestinal tract and are contained by a healthy epithelial lining in the gut, components of the immune system, and other intestinal flora. If any of these protective devices fail, gram-negative bacteria can attach to the intestinal wall and "translocate" or pass through the intestinal lining into other tissues and compartments in the body. Endotoxin may also translocate (Fink, 1991). In cases of trauma, sepsis, and shock, damage to intestinal mucosa may occur by several routes. The most obvious insult occurs with decreased perfusion related to low cardiac output or when blood is shunted to vital organs. During shock states the splanchnic bed allotment of cardiac output can fall dramatically (Fink, 1991). Hypoxemia and anemia also decrease oxygen delivery. In critically ill patients any combination of these three states can occur. If sustained long enough this results in cell death.

During periods of low oxygen delivery, mucosal cells produce needed energy in an anaerobic fashion causing a build up of substances that, when combined with oxygen during reperfusion, cause the formation of free oxygen radicals. When free oxygen radical production is increased beyond what the normal protective devices can contain, cellular damage occurs. In addition, accumulations of neutrophils have been noted in the gut during low perfusion states. The reason for the accumulation is not known but when stimulated the neutrophils can cause considerable damage. Malnutrition, particularly a lack of the amino acid glutamine, has been linked with increased translocation in the animal model. It is believed that a lack of important amino acids and fatty acids contributes to translocation in humans particularly in times of stress by depriving mucosal cells of important nutrients, which makes them more susceptible to damage during low perfusion states (Fink, 1991; Bower, 1993). So, whether or not the critically ill patient has a primary diagnosis of infection, gram-negative bacteria or endotoxin may gain access to body tissues to initiate SIRS (Fink, 1991).

Other bacteria besides gram-negative can release harmful exogenous mediators. Certain strains of the gram-positive bacteria *Staphlococcus aureus* have been shown to release toxic shock syndrome toxin-1 (TSST-1), which can result in the disease for which it was named (Creehan, 1995). Exotoxins from gram-positive bacteria have been linked with increased capillary permeability, damage to both white and red blood cells, and platelet aggregation (Kellum & Decker, 1996). Other substances that have been linked with initiation of SIRS are antigens from parasites, enterotoxins, and fungal infections (Kellum & Decker, 1996).

SEPSIS

As reviewed in the introduction, colonization through invasive procedures is a well-documented phenomenon. There is an estimated 24% increase in nosocomial infection in the ICU versus non-ICU patient population and infection can be a deadly complication for the critically ill patient (Ringer & Darovic, 1995). Prevention of the introduction of organisms to patients in the ICU through strict aseptic technique, rigorous compliance to protocols concerning invasive procedures, and thorough handwashing are important preventive care measures. Nurses, as around-the-clock care providers, are responsible for the majority of care provided to the patient, particularly concerning invasive techniques and maintenance of invasive lines including intra-

venous catheters and central venous lines. In this light they have the opportunity to decrease the number of organisms introduced to the patient by following proper techniques and protocols.

The first step in reducing nosocomial infection is proper handwashing using friction for at least 10 seconds before handling any invasive device. Gloves also reduce the transmission of bacteria from the hands as well as provide protection to the provider from pathogens in blood and body fluids. Correlation exists between organisms on the skin at insertion sites and later development of infection. Cleansing insertion sites with antiseptic soap and water followed by 70% alcohol or 10% povidone–iodine solution helps to reduce the number of organisms on the skin (Ringer & Darovic, 1995). Insertion sites for central lines have differing infection rates. Although the internal jugular site is preferred for central line insertion in the obstetric patient, it is associated with a higher infection rate than the subclavian site (Norwood, 1995). Observation for signs of infection at the insertion site and systemic infection should be done routinely. Signs of infection at the insertion site include induration, redness, purulent discharge, or pain (Ringer & Darovic, 1995). Established protocols or standards for line assessment and replacement, dressing change, and catheter replacement should be strictly followed (Kellum & Decker 1996; Ringer & Darovic, 1995).

CLINICAL PRESENTATION OF INFECTION

The clinical presentation of sepsis can be subtle, requiring close observation of vital signs and organ function for trends. Detection of trends coupled with laboratory findings assist in finalizing the diagnosis. Regular review of organ systems with attention to specific physiologic parameters is a crucial part of nursing care.

Cardiovascular

The processes of vasodilation and vasopermeability associated with SIRS and sepsis result in loss of intravascular volume and a decrease in systemic vascular resistance (SVR). Initially the sympathetic nervous system will compensate by increasing heart rate. Tachycardia and a bounding pulse are noted at this time. The pulse pressure widens and blood pressure begins to fall. One study looking for characteristics of survivors of septic shock examined clinical parameters of 48 septic patients. Those with a heart rate less than 106 beats per minute (bpm) in the early stage of sepsis, characterized by a hyperdynamic state, had higher survival rates. Twenty-four hours into treatment the heart rate of the survivors had decreased to less than 95 bpm (Porembka, 1993). However, if volume continued to be depleted and was not adequately replaced, tachycardia continued but the character of the pulse became weak and thready. Also, peripheral circulation was impaired with poor capillary refill in nail beds and the skin became cool and clammy with a mottled appearance. The combination of low intravascular volume and mediator-related vasodilation decreases the vessel's ability to respond to catacholamines attempting to correct the vasodilation, resulting in hypotension. Persistent hypotension despite fluid resuscitation is associated with higher mortality rates (Parker et al., 1993).

Pulmonary

Respiratory rate increases because of hypoxemia. Damage to pulmonary capillaries results in atelectasis and increased secretions. Thus, as sepsis continues, breath sounds are diminished bilaterally with crackles and wheezes present. Use of pulse oximetry to determine the saturation of oxygen in arterial hemoglobin (SaO_2) is a convenient, noninvasive parameter to assess arterial oxygen content. Normal pregnancy SaO_2 level is 96% or greater but in critically ill patients maintaining a SaO_2 of at least 90% correlates with a PaO_2 of 60 mm Hg, which is associated with adequate oxygenation (Dorman, 1992). SaO_2 levels initially remain stable but if damage to lung tissue is severe, acute respiratory distress syndrome (ARDS) can occur, which is associated with declining SaO_2 levels that fall despite oxygen therapy. Another noninvasive measurement that is gaining popularity in the adult ICU is transcutaneous oxygen and carbon dioxide monitoring.

This measurement is accomplished by placing an electrode on the skin, which heats the area under the electrode and affects the lipoproteins in the skin. These lipoproteins change states, allowing gases to diffuse from subcutaneous tissues to the electrode for measurement. This measurement is felt to be more reflective of perfusion and oxygenation in the tissues than are PaO_2 or oxygen delivery values (Shoemaker & Parsa, 1995).

Renal

Renal damage during sepsis can occur by several routes. Decreased blood flow to the kidney, the effects of inflammatory mediators, and toxicity of drugs used to treat infection can separately or in combination cause renal damage. If circulating volume is not or cannot be adequately replaced, signs of acute renal failure occur. Irreversible damage can occur in 60–90 minutes if ischemia is not corrected (Lancaster, 1992). The most obvious sign of renal failure is oliguria, however nonoliguric renal failure should be considered if the patient has adequate or increased urine output with other signs of renal failure. These signs include elevated serum creatinine (normally <1.0 mg/dL) and blood urea nitrogen (BUN) levels, electrolyte abnormalities, and acid-base abnormalities (Lancaster, 1992). Commonly used medications that can cause renal toxicity include gentamicin, lasix, corticosteroids, cephalothin, sulfonamides, and nonsteroidal anti-inflammatory agents such as indomethacin (Lancaster, 1992). Although administration of these medications is often necessary in septic patients, close attention to dosage for body size, administration routes and times, as well as being observant for signs of renal failure are important nursing assessments.

Central Nervous System (CNS)

The exact mechanism of CNS injury in sepsis is unknown, however, it is believed to be related to decreased perfusion and the effect of circulating mediators. Changes in level of consciousness are noted as the CNS fails. Early symptoms include malaise, a general sense of not feeling well, and restlessness with increasing CNS dysfunction evidenced by confusion, stupor, and coma (Dasch, 1992).

Body Temperature

Under the influence of mediator stimulation to the hypothalmus and increased metabolic rate, body temperature rises. In later stages of sepsis, body temperature falls and may even be subnormal related to hypothalmus dysfunction and decreased metabolism (Secor, 1994; Robins, 1992; Franklin, Darovic, & Dan, 1995).

Central Hemodynamic Monitoring

In the American College of Obstetricians' (ACOG) Technical Bulletin No. 121 on invasive hemodynamic monitoring, shock is listed as a condition that may benefit from use of invasive hemodynamic monitoring (ACOG, 1992). As with other potentially critical illnesses, the decision to use invasive monitoring is based on the patient condition and initial response to supportive therapy.

Hemodynamic Parameters

Systemic Vascular Resistance (SVR)

SVR is decreased in sepsis. Mediator-induced vasodilation coupled with tissue hypoxia are responsible for the low SVR (Robins, 1992).

Cardiac Output (CO)

CO increases because of several compensatory mechanisms. The sympathetic nervous system increases venous return, heart rate, and myocardial contractility. Uncontrolled mediator release causes disturbance in blood flow and can contribute to shunting of blood in the vasculature. Ventricular dilation in sepsis is well documented and, combined with low left afterload, increases CO in an attempt to increase delivery to tissues. Research has correlated this ventricular dilation with higher survival rates and normal ventricular size with low survival rates (Porembka, 1993). Volume resuscitation is necessary to maintain adequate CO as fluid begins to leak into the third space. If volume resuscitation is not sufficient, CO may decline and thus, tissue oxygenation.

Pulmonary Capillary Wedge Pressure (PCWP)

The PCWP and pulmonary artery pressure (PAP) are variable in the patient with sepsis. A study using human volunteers for infusion of endotoxin to study hemodynamic changes revealed no significant change in PCWP after infusion with adequate volume replacement (Porembka, 1993). However, if intravascular volume is low, PCWP may also be low.

Left Ventricular Stroke Work Index (LVSWI)

LVSWI is usually depressed during sepsis. The decrease in left ventricular function is attributed to myocardial depressant factor (Parker et al., 1994; Suffredini et al., 1989). Further studies have shown that increase in LVSWI with adequate volume replacement was predictive of survival (Porembka, 1993).

Oxygenation Parameters

Arterial Blood Gases (ABG)

In the nonpregnant adult population an initial respiratory alkalosis is reported with sepsis. However, with the state of compensated respiratory alkalemia that is normal in pregnancy, this change may not be significant. As hypoxemia develops, metabolic acidosis and increased lactate are noted. It can be assumed that the obstetric population would develop metabolic acidosis at a more rapid rate because of the compensated state with less base available to buffer acids.

Oxygen Delivery (DO_2)

Oxygen delivery increases during septic shock largely because of the increased CO. Survivors of septic shock consistently demonstrate elevated DO_2 levels. Although there is controversy, improved survival rates have been reported in patients with severe sepsis that had DO_2 levels increased to supranormal values, defined as approximately 600 mL/min/m² in the non-obstetric patient population (Shoemaker & Parsa, 1995; Mims, 1992). However, elevation of oxygen delivery does not mean the cells are able to utilize or are receiving oxygen. Trends in the delivery of oxygen and the use or consumption of that oxygen by the body are important to review together.

Oxygen Consumption (VO₂)

VO_2 is a measurement of the use of oxygen by the body. Under normal oxygen delivery states the cells will consume a set amount of oxygen in a steady state. When cells do not consume a baseline level of oxygen because of low oxygen delivery, this is referred to as a supply dependent or delivery dependent state. Low VO_2 indicates that cells are not being well oxygenated and if this state continues will die. In sepsis VO_2 is initially decreased but survivors demonstrate a gradual increase in VO_2. Again, higher survival rates have been reported in patients with adequate volume resuscitation and adequate DO_2 and subsequently more available oxygen for consumption (Shoemaker & Parsa, 1995; Mims, 1992).

Laboratory Studies

Many laboratory tests are generally evaluated during the course of treatment for sepsis and depend on the particular organ system demonstrating evidence of dysfunction or failure. The diagnosis of sepsis and SIRS are suggested by changes in the white blood cell (WBC) count. These changes include either elevation of the WBC greater than 12,000 cells/mm³ or less than 4000 cells/mm³ (American College of Chest Physicians et al., 1992). Because the WBC count increases during pregnancy, particularly during labor, it may be more helpful to look at immature forms of white cells or bands that are greater than 10% in sepsis and SIRS (American College of Chest Physicians et al., 1992). Evaluation of trends in WBC counts is generally more predictive than a single value. Because an infectious organism is the cause of sepsis, cultures and appropriate treatment are important components of patient care.

TREATMENT

The major treatment goals for the patient with sepsis include identification and treatment of the infection, support of cardiac output and oxygen transport, nutritional support, and identification and support of failing organ systems (Huddleston, 1992).

Treating Infection

Identification of the source of infection and initiation of treatment for infection are early treatment goals that coincide with early support of cardiac output and oxygen delivery. All body fluids and cavities that could be infected should be cultured. In pregnancy this includes amniotic fluid and, if delivery of the fetus has occurred, the uterine cavity secondary to the potential for endometritis. Once cultures are obtained, broad spectrum antibiotic therapy can be instituted until a specific organism is isolated. However, the patient may have clinical symptoms of sepsis and appropriate laboratory changes but no organism isolated. Approximately 50% of patients with septic shock or severe sepsis will not have positive blood cultures and approximately 33% will not have positive cultures from any source (Stroud et al., 1990). In these cases the patient may have been exposed to endotoxin or other products of bacterial lysis such as in translocation (Stroud et al., 1990). In these situations, broad spectrum antibiotics may be continued in case an error in laboratory technique occurred or the organism simply was not obtained.

SUPPORTIVE CARE

Hemodynamic support includes measures to maintain an optimum cardiac output. Evaluation of preload status and subsequent volume replacement when indicated are considered integral components of therapy. However, as ventricular function is often abnormal in sepsis, the ventricle may not respond as expected to inotropic support. Maintenance of PCWP readings between 12 and 18 have been proposed by several authors with the caution to follow other hemodynamic patterns and evaluate all patients individually (Porembka, 1993; Shoemaker & Parsa, 1995). Use of SVR is not reflective of actual perfusion pressure because the patient is in a form of distributive shock. In this situation, use of mean arterial pressure (MAP) is more indicative of perfusion and is used to guide therapy. MAP of at least 60 mm Hg is the goal (Porembka, 1993). If vasopressors are used to maintain MAP, the agent should be evaluated for patient and fetal response.

Support of oxygen delivery is accomplished to a large extent by augmenting cardiac output. However, optimizing CO without significant increases in DO_2 may require blood transfusion to impact oxygen delivery. Studies have reported that supranormal DO_2 levels have decreased hospital days in septic patients. Supranormal DO_2 levels are greater than 600 mL/min/m² in the nonobstetric patient population. Following VO_2 values can help determine delivery dependent states. VO_2 of greater than 170 mL/min/m² is considered supranormal values, again in the nonobstetric patient population. If the patient consistently uses this amount of oxygen, most cells have oxygen accessible. Typically when VO_2 drops the patient is in a delivery-dependent state that responds to increasing DO_2. However, in sepsis cells may not be able to use oxygen if damaged, and despite adequate DO_2, VO_2 does not increase (Porembka, 1993; Parker et al., 1994).

Nutrition Support

Nutritional status of the patient should be addressed as soon as possible. Consulting with nutrition services is important to ensure all nutrients are given in the correct amounts and by the appropriate routes. The two routes utilized most frequently in critically ill patients are enteral and parenteral. The advantage of using total parenteral nutrition (TPN) is that nutrients can be delivered regardless of atony in the gut. The main disadvantage is the higher infection rate in patients receiving TPN over those receiving enteral feedings. In a study comparing the two methods, patients receiving solely TPN had a higher incidence of pneumonia and abdominal abscess over those receiving enteral support. The major disadvantage of enteral feeding is build up of volume in the gut related to atony. This may eliminate this form of feeding in some

patients unless a tube can be placed further in the intestinal tract. Another consideration currently under research is the composition of the feeding. Studies have compared standard feedings currently in use with feedings augmented with proteins and fats. Patients receiving the special formula had significantly fewer infections and fewer days in the hospital. More research is being done to determine the correct blend of nutrients for critically ill patients and the most advantageous routes of administration (Krenitsky, 1996).

In addition to the obvious assessments of the gastrointestinal tract—presence and character of bowel sounds, abdominal distention, diarrhea, and blood in the stool—measurement of gastric mucosal pH has been correlated with patient outcome. The pH is measured by gastric tonometry. A low pH is associated with tissue hypoxia and increased mortality (O'Neill, 1992).

FUTURE THERAPIES

Because antimicrobial therapy alone has not been successful in treating sepsis, researchers have turned their attention to modulating the mediators released in the septic cascade. The mediator initially studied was endotoxin. This choice was based on the fact that most infections are gram-negative. In addition, all gram-negative bacteria release the same endotoxin. Through the process of translocation both gram-negative bacteria and endotoxin can slip from the intestinal tract into the circulation. Subsequently, several antibodies to endotoxin were developed that were very encouraging in animal studies.

The administration of an antibody to bind with and neutralize endotoxin looked promising but failed to show significant results when used in septic patients. It is believed that the timing of such a medication is crucial. Endotoxin may be released in very small amounts and is only present for a short time in the bloodstream (Hazinski, 1994). The effect of endotoxin on the mediators TNF and IL-1 was examined next. Antibodies were developed against these mediators as well as receptor antagonists to block their ability to interface with receptor sites. Again, promising animal studies failed to yield the same results in clinical trials. Because these mediators occur naturally in the body and their effect in physiologic amounts is not well known, blockage of these mediators may be harmful (Hazinski, 1994).

Another treatment that has been studied is decontamination of the gut to prevent translocation of bacteria and endotoxin. However, this has not been associated with decreased mortality (Hazinski, 1994). Another treatment that is currently in clinical trials is the medication ibuprofen. This medication, as well as other nonsteroidal anti-inflammatory agents, blocks one of the pathways of arachadonic acid and therefore reduces the production of thromaboxane A2 and certain prostaglandins (Hazinski, 1994). Although research continues, there is currently no medication that is known to consistently reduce mortality in the septic patient.

SUMMARY

Sepsis remains a formidible foe in the critically ill patient. Until definitive therapy can be discovered, supportive care attentive to clinical parameters and maintenance of adequate perfusion remain the keys to improving survival. As research continues to unravel the role of inflammatory mediators under physiologic and pathologic circumstances, sepsis and other syndromes associated with uncontrolled mediators may be detected and treated more effectively.

REFERENCES

Ackerman, M. H. (1994). The systemic inflammatory response, sepsis, and multiple organ dysfunction. Critical Care Nursing Clinics of North America, 6, 243–250.

ACOG. (1992). Invasive hemodynamic monitoring in obstetrics and gynecology. ACOG Technical Bulletin, 121.

American College of Chest Physicians/Society of Critical Care Medicine Consensus Conference. (1992). Definitions for sepsis and organ failure and guidelines for the use of innovative therapies in sepsis. Critical Care Medicine, 20, 864–874.

Bower, R. H. (1993). Nutrition during critical illness and sepsis. New Horizons, 1(2), 348–352.

Christman, J. W. (1995). Pulmonary host defense and inflammatory lung disease. In S. M. Ayres, A. Grenvik, P. R. Holbrook, & W. C. Shoemaker (Eds.), Textbook of critical care. Philadelphia: Saunders.

Creehan, P. A. (1995). Toxic shock syndrome: An opportunity for nursing intervention. JOGNN, 24(6), 557–561.

Dasch, V. (1992). The central nervous system: Dysfunction and exhaustion. In V. B. Huddleston (Ed.), Multisystem organ failure. St. Louis, MO: Mosby.

Dormar, K. (1992). Pulmonary disorders in pregnancy. In L. K. Mandeville & N. H. Trioano (Eds.), High-risk intrapartum nursing. Philadelphia: Lippincott.

Fink, M. P. (1991). Gastrointestinal mucosal injury in experimental models of shock, trauma, and sepsis. Critical Care Medicine, 19(5), 627–641.

Franklin, C. M., Darovic, G. O., & Dan, B. B. (1995). Monitoring the patient in shock. In G. O. Darovic (Ed.), Hemodynamic monitoring: Invasive and noninvasive clinical application. Philadelphia: Saunders.

Ganz, T. (1995). Macrophage function. In S. M. Ayres, A. Grenvik, P. R. Holbrook, & W. C. Shoemaker (Eds.), Textbook of critical care. Philadelphia: Saunders.

Gonik, B. (1991). Septic shock in obstetrics. In S. L. Clark, D. B. Cotton, G. D. V. Hankins, & J. P. Phelan, (Eds.), Critical care obstetrics. Boston: Blackwell Scientific.

Guyton, A. C., & Hall, J. E. (1996). Textbook of medical physiology. Philadelphia: Saunders.

Halushka, P. V., Geisel, J., Reines, H. D., & Cook, J. A. (1995). Prostaglandins, thromboxanes, leukotrienes, and other products of arachadonic acid. In S. M. Ayres, A. Grenvik, P. R. Holbrook, & W. C. Shoemaker (Eds.), Textbook of critical care. Philadelphia: Saunders.

Hazinski, M. F. (1994). Mediator-specific therapies for the systemic inflammatory response syndrome, sepsis, severe sepsis, and septic shock: Present and future approaches. Critical Care

Nursing Clinics of North America, 6(2), 309–319.

Huddleston, V. B. (1992). Multisystem organ failure. St. Louis, MO: Mosby.

Kellum, J. A., & Decker, J. M. (1996). The immune system: Relation to sepsis and multiple organ failure. AACN Clinical Issues, 7(3), 339–350.

Krenitsky, J. (1996). Nutrition and the immune system. AACN Clinical Issues, 7(3), 359–369.

Lancaster, L. E. (1992). Acute renal failure. In V. B. Huddleston (Ed.), Mulitsystem organ failure. St. Louis, MO: Mosby.

McCord, J. M. (1995). Oxygen-derived free radicals. In S. M. Ayres, A. Grenvik, P. R. Holbrook, & W. C. Shoemaker (Eds.), Textbook of critical care. Philadelphia: Saunders.

Mims, B. C. (1992). Imbalance of oxygen supply and demand. In V. B. Huddleston (Ed.), Multisystem organ failure. St. Louis, MO: Mosby.

Nichols, R. L. (1992). Bacterial infectious disease considerations in the surgical patient. In J. M. Civetta, R. W. Taylor, & R. R. Kirby (Eds.), Critical care. Philadelphia: Lippincott.

Norwood, S. (1995). Catheter related infections and associated bacteremia. In S. M. Ayres, A. Grenvik, P. R. Holbrook, & W. C. Shoemaker (Eds.), Textbook of critical care. Philadelphia: Saunders.

O'Neill, P. L. (1992). Gastrointestinal system: Target organ and source. In V. B. Huddleston (Ed.), Multisystem organ failure. St. Louis, MO: Mosby.

Parker, M. M., Ognibene, F. P., & Parrillo, J. E. (1994). Peak systolic pressure/end-systolic volume ratio, a load-independent measure of ventricular function, is reversibly decreased in human septic shock. Critical Care Medicine, 22(12), 1955–1959.

Porembka, D. T. (1993). Cardiovascular abnormalities in sepsis. New Horizons, 1(2), 324–341.

Ringer, M., & Darovic, G. O. (1995). Infusion-related sepsis. In G. O. Darovic (Ed.), Hemodynamic monitoring: Invasive and noninvasive clinical application. Philadelphia: Saunders.

Robins, E. V. (1992). Maldistribution of circulating volume. In V. B. Huddleston (Ed.), Multisystem organ failure. St. Louis, MO: Mosby.

Savoia, M. C. (1995). Bacterial, fungal, and parasitic disease during pregnancy. In G. N. Burrow & T. F. Ferris (Eds.), Medical complications during pregnancy. Philadelphia: Saunders.

Secor, V. H. (1994). The inflammatory immune response in critical illness. Critical Care Nursing Clinics of North America, 6(2), 251–264.

Sell, S. (1987). Basic immunology. New York: Elsevier.

Seller, M. C., & Owen, D. (1993). Physiologic response to infection. In J. M. Clochesy, C. Breu, S. Cardin, E. B. Rudy, & A. A. Whittaker (Eds.), Critical care nursing. Philadelphia: Saunders.

Shapiro, L., & Gelfand, J. A. (1995). Cytokines. In S. M. Ayres, A. Grenvik, P. R. Holbrook, & W. C. Shoemaker (Eds.), Textbook of critical care. Philadelphia: Saunders.

Shoemaker, W. C., & Parsa, M. H. (1995). Invasive and noninvasive physiologic monitoring, diagnosis and treatment of the shock syndromes. In S. M. Ayres, A. Grenvik, P. R. Holbrook, & W. C. Shoemaker (Eds.), Textbook of Critical Care. Philadelphia: Saunders.

Simpson, K. R. (1995). Sepsis during pregnancy. JOGNN, 24, 550–556.

Stroud, M., Swindell, B., & Bernard, G. (1990). Cellular and humoral mediators of sepsis syndrome. Critical Care Nursing Clinics of North America, 2(2), 151–160.

Suffredini, A. F., Fromm, R. E., Parker, M. M., Brenner, M., Kovacs, J. A., Wesley, R. A., & Parrillo, J. E. (1989). The cardiovascular response of normal humans to the administration of endotoxin. New England Journal of Medicine, 321(5), 280–287.

Taylor, R. W. (1992). Sepsis, sepsis syndrome and septic shock. In J. M. Civetta, R. W. Taylor, & R. R. Kirby (Eds.), Critical care. Philadelphia: Lippincott.

Vedder, N. B., & Harlan, J. M. (1995). Neutrophil-endothelial cell interactions. In S. M. Ayres, A. Grenvik, P. R. Holbrook, & W. C. Shoemaker (Eds.), Textbook of critical care. Philadelphia: Saunders.

Zellweger, R., Wichmann, M. W., Ayala, A., Stein, S., DeMaso, C. M., & Chaudry, I. H. (1997). Females in proestrus state maintain splenic immune functions and tolerate sepsis better than males. Critical Care Medicine, 25(1), 106–110.

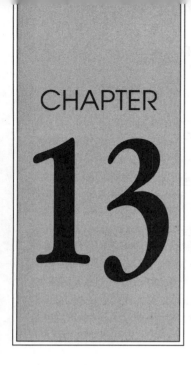

CHAPTER 13

Disseminated Intravascular Coagulation

Melissa C. Sisson and Donna Ruth

INCIDENCE

Disseminated intravascular coagulation (DIC) has been described since the 1950s, most notably in obstetrical literature, presumably because of its propensity to accompany certain obstetrical conditions. DIC is not a separate clinical entity, rather it is an intermediary of other diseases. It represents a derangement of the balance between the procoagulant and fibrinolytic systems that occurs when normal regulatory mechanisms fail. As Weiner (1986) suggests, DIC is probably best viewed on a continuum along which clinical presentation and course may vary widely depending on the inciting mechanism.

A consequence of this tendency toward clinical variation is difficulty in ascertaining the incidence of DIC in pregnancy. In the case of abruptio placenta accompanied by intrauterine fetal demise (IUFD), the occurrence of DIC may be as high as 100% (Sher & Statland, 1985). In contrast, DIC associated with IUFD without abruption is quite rare except when products of conception are retained beyond 5 weeks. An insidious consumptive coagulopathy is more common in the obstetric patient than an acute, fulminating DIC (Finley, 1989). More imperative than defining actual incidence is the recognition that pregnant women may be predisposed to DIC, particularly when besieged by obstetrical complications (Weiner, 1986).

Though acute coagulopathy during pregnancy is a rare event, it can have profound consequences for maternal–fetal well-being. Obstetric complications in isolation may carry significant risk for mother and fetus, but when compounded by disseminated coagulopathy, morbidity and mortality increase considerably. It is therefore incumbent upon all practitioners caring for pregnant women to be knowledgeable about DIC, thereby facilitating both early detection and improved outcome.

NORMAL COAGULATION

Central to any discussion of DIC is an understanding of normal coagulation. Hemostasis is the process by which blood is maintained in a liquid state within vessels, with loss of blood from damaged vessels prevented. Contributors to this process include the vascular endothelium, platelets, and circulating blood proteins. Disruption of the endothelium as a result of vascular damage sets into motion the first phase of hemostasis, which is formation of a temporary platelet plug. Exposure of subendothelial collagen results in platelet activation and adhesion. Release of histamine and serotonin promote local vasconstriction, platelet cohesion occurs, and a temporary plug is formed.

The second phase of hemostasis involves the local activation of the coagulation cascade resulting in thrombin production and eventual formation of a fibrin clot. Circulating blood proteins, the third component of hemostasis, include those of the coagulation system, the fibrinolytic system, the kinin system, and the complement system. These systems participate by providing a system of checks and balances that regulate clot formation.

The blood proteins in the coagulation system, traditionally referred to as clotting factors, can be functionally divided into enzymes and cofactors (Brandt, 1985). The enzymes (serine proteases) are activated clotting factors, and cofactors are substances that accelerate the rate of substrate activation by enzymes. The coagulation system is a series of self-amplifying substrate to enzyme interactions, activated by three types of injuries: trauma to tissue, trauma to vascular endothelium, and trauma to red blood cells or platelets.

When one or more of these intiating injuries occurs, thrombin is generated via the intrinsic pathway (contact system) or via the extrinsic pathway (tissue factor). The intrinsic pathway is activated when factor XII or Hageman factor is exposed to collagen, phospholipid, kallikrein, or in a condition such as sepsis (Finley, 1989). The extrinsic pathway is activated by tissue thromboplastin. The final stages of clot formation begin with the activation of factor X, the first step in a converging pathway that brings the intrinsic and extrinsic pathways together. (See Figure 13-1.)

The activation of factor X begins the final common pathway and leads to the conversion of circulating prothrombin to thrombin. Thrombin acts as a proteolytic enzyme cleaving fibrinopeptides A and B from fibrinogen, a large circulating plasma protein. Fibrin monomers are formed as a result of this cleavage, then are polymerized or joined by activated factor XIII and a stable clot is produced (Finley, 1989).

Three major regulatory mechanisms control coagulation: the fibrinolytic system, antithrombin III, and protein C. These systems, aided by rapid blood flow and removal of activated clotting factor by the reticuloendothelial system, serve to localize clot formation and to maintain the liquid state of blood.

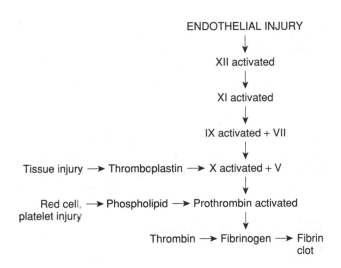

Figure 13-1. Summary of Clotting Sequence.

The fibrinolytic system begins the breakdown of fibrin when the clot is formed. (See Figure 13-2.) Plasminogen is incorporated into the fibrin clot and when activated is converted to plasmin, which systematically lyses fibrin. Four major fragments called fibrin degradation products (FDP) or fibrin split products (FSP) are liberated: X, Y, D, and E. The fibrin-split products have anticoagulant properties including disruption of fibrin polymerization, coating of platelets, and formation of soluble fibrin monomer complexes (SFMC) (Finley, 1989). FDPs exert their anticoagulant effect when they cannot be adequately cleared because of excess fibrin formation.

Antithrombin III (AT III) is the central physiologic antagonist to coagulation. It is a glycoprotein that binds to activated factors XII, XI, IX, and X and slowly inactivates thrombin. AT III inactivates thrombin by forming a 1:1 molecular complex with it and the presence of these

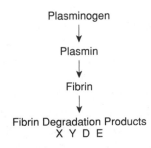

Figure 13-2. Summary of Fibrinolysis.

thrombin-antithrombin complexes (TAT) denotes activation of the coagulation system (Sen, Madazh, Davuzlu, Ocak, & Tolun, 1994). When AT III combines with heparin, thrombin inactivation is accelerated and occurs rapidly. Protein C is a vitamin K-dependent proenzyme that is found in plasma. When activated by thrombin, protein C degrades activated cofactors V and VIII. Protein C then exerts an anticoagulant effect by inhibiting a portion of the coagulation cascade.

COAGULATION DURING PREGNANCY

Pregnancy has been referred to as a hypercoagulable state (see Display 13-1). There are elevations of all coagulation factors with the exception of factors XIII and XI, which are believed to decrease (Finley, 1989). In addition, fibrinolytic activity appears to be decreased during pregnancy, with a speculated increase in plasminogen activator inhibitor. Levels of protein C are reduced to 88% of prepregnancy values, while levels of AT III remain unchanged (Finley, 1989). Protein S, which potentiates the action of protein C, is also decreased (Finley, 1989). Alterations in the hemostatic mechanism occur in order to maintain the pregnancy and to protect from blood loss at delivery.

PATHOPHYSIOLOGY OF DIC

DIC represents a failure of the normal regulatory mechanisms so that fibrin generation is no longer confined to the area of the injury. As a consequence of one or more precipitating events, there is massive consumption of the circulating clotting factors and activation of the fibrinolytic system. The result is: (1) hemorrhage, (2) systemic production of fibrin monomers/polymers with fibrin thrombi producing end-organ ischemia/necrosis, (3) activation of the kinin system with resultant vascular permeability and hypotension, and (4) activation of the complement system with systemic manifestation (Finley, 1989). The process is self-perpetuating and the clinical picture is one of excessive thrombosis, depletion of circulating blood proteins necessary for normal coagulation, and lysis of existing fibrin, all resulting in hemorrhage and shock.

DISPLAY 13-1

Hemostatic Alterations in Pregnancy

- Increase in factors V, VII, VIII, IX, X, XII, prothrombin
- Increased fibrinogen 2–4 Gms/L to 4–6 Gm/L
- Decrease in factors IX and XIII
- Decreased protein C
- Decreased fibrinolysis

PREDISPOSING OBSTETRICAL CONDITIONS

DIC is an intermediary of many primary disease processes, a number of them specific to the practice of obstetrics. (See Display 13-2.) In normal pregnancy, the coagulation and fibrinolytic systems appear to be in a hyperdynamic state with both increased production and turnover of many procoagulants (Hewitt & Davies, 1983). It has therefore been suggested that pregnancy may represent a primed state in which there is an increased susceptibility to DIC. The intrapartum activation of coagulation, as evidenced by increases in fibrinopeptide A (FPA), activated Hageman factor, and SFMCs, and activation of fibrinolysis indicated by increased FDPs, implies that normal parturition may actually represent a low-grade DIC (Finley, 1989). Hypothetically then, a pregnant woman exposed to an appropriate stimulus, such as release of tissue thromboplastin during placental abruption, may be at far greater risk for overt coagulopathy than her nonpregnant counterpart. The obstetrical conditions more commonly associated with DIC and related coagulation abnormalities are described next.

Placental abruption, occurring in 1:250 deliveries, is considered the most common obstetric cause of DIC (Weiner, 1991). Up to 20% of patients with a clinically significant abruption

DISPLAY 13-2

Predisposing Conditions

General	Obstetric
Sepsis	Abruptio Placenta
Metastatic Carcinoma	Preeclampsia-Eclampsia
Transfusion Reactions	Retained IUFD
Hemolytic Conditions	Saline Abortion
Malignant Hypertension	Amniotic Fluid Embolus
Trauma	
Snake Bite	

may have a gross clotting defect, and 25% of these will experience postpartum hemorrhage (Weiner, 1991). Severe coagulation defects occur most often when the abruption results in fetal demise (Finley, 1989). The average blood loss associated with an intrauterine fetal demise secondary to abruption is 2500ml (Weiner, 1991). When the abruption is severe, the coagulopathy is related to systemic consumption of clotting factors and activation of fibrinolysis, rather than local consumption of clotting factors during retroplacental clot formation (Gilabert, Estelles, Aznan, & Galbis, 1985). The trophoblast contains the highest concentration of tissue thromboplastin, and its continued release into the systemic circulation results in disseminated consumption of clotting factors and secondary fibrinolysis (Gilabert, Estelles, Aznan, & Galbis, 1985). In their series of 19 patients, Gilabert and coworkers (1985) found that thrombocytopenia, hypofibrinogenemia, and increased FDPs were the most frequently occurring laboratory abnormalities when the abruption was severe. Postpartum hemorrhage is the most common cause of maternal morbidity secondary to placental abruption and may occur in up to 2.5% of cases (Finley, 1989).

Preeclampsia-eclampsia is rarely associated with an overt coagulopathy and thrombocytopenia will be present first (Ledue et al., 1992).

Of women with severe preelampsia-eclampsia, 10% develop thrombocytopenia (Weiner, 1991), which is likely due to increased platelet consumption (Orlikowski & Rocke, 1992). Some authors contend that preeclampsia-eclampsia represents a chronic low-grade DIC (Kobayashi & Terao, 1987). This conclusion is based primarily on the observation of decreased AT III in preeclampsia and superimposed preeclampsia (Weiner, 1988). AT III is unaltered in the normal pregnancy and in the pregnancy complicated by chronic hypertension (Sen, Madazh, Davuzlu, Ocak, & Tolun, 1994). Weiner (1988) recommends that patients at high risk for preeclampsia have an early pregnancy baseline AT III level. Other coagulation changes include increased factor VIII consumption and increased FPA concentration (Sen, Madazh, Davuzlu, Ocak, & Tolun, 1994).

Van Dam and colleagues (1989) reported DIC in 10 of 19 patients with hemolysis, elevated liver enzymes, and low platelet (HELLP syndrome) and found these patients most likely to develop life-threatening complications at delivery. Though many patients with preeclampsia-eclampsia demonstrate a subclinical coagulopathy, those experiencing compounding complications such as placental abruption or the HELLP syndrome are at significantly greater risk for mortality.

Amniotic fluid embolus (AFE) is associated with a maternal mortality of 80%. Should the initial cardiorespiratory insults associated with AFE be survived, 45% will develop DIC within 4 hours (Finley, 1989). The etiology of the coagulopathy is controversial. Though amniotic fluid is known to have a procoagulant effect, its role in the syndrome remains inconclusive (Weiner, 1991). Laboratory abnormalities suggest excess fibrinolytic activity with decreased plasminogen, increased plasmin activator, and elevated FDPs (Weiner, 1991). Hypofibrinogenemia is also reported in most cases (Weiner, 1991). The cornerstone of the management of patients surviving AFE is blood component replacement. Prophylactic administration of heparin has been advocated by a number of authors, though its benefit remains unproven (Finley, 1989).

Maternal and perinatal outcomes reflect the severity of the precipitating event and the ease with which it is eliminated. Fortunately, most cases of obstetrical DIC are amenable to correction of the underlying process and respond favorably to termination of pregnancy.

DIAGNOSIS OF THE PATIENT WITH DIC

As outlined previously, the patient with DIC may present with a diverse clinical picture. Signs and symptoms may be as innocuous as epistaxis or as disastrous as multiportal hemorrhage. Acute, fulminant DIC is most often associated with severe placental abruption and amniotic fluid embolism. Chronic low-grade DIC is the more typical obstetrical presentation as is associated with preeclampsia-eclampsia and retained IUFD. However, patients with a chronic DIC clinical presentation are at increased risk for the development of fulminant DIC.

Though hemorrhage is the initial sign of coagulopathy, it is always preceded by thrombosis, the signs of which vary with the organ affected. Seven percent of patients have clinical signs of thrombosis, which may include peripheral cyanosis, gangrene, renal impairment, drowsiness, confusion, coma, and cardiorespiratory failure (Hewitt

TABLE 13-1. Laboratory Abnormalities in DIC	
Platelet count	Decreased
Fibrinogen	Decreased
Prothrombin time	Prolonged
Partial thromboplastin time	Prolonged
Antithrombin III	Decreased activity
FSPs/FDP	Greater than 40
SFMCs	Increased
D-Dimer	Increased

& Davies, 1983). Oozing may occur from venipunctures and other sites of trauma. Epistaxis, ecchymosis, purpura, petechaie, and other disruptions of the skin are common. Red cell lysis secondary to activation of the complement system is a potential occurrence (Finley, 1989). Hypotension due to hemorrhage or activation of the kinin system almost always accompanies DIC.

In the patient presenting with massive hemorrhage, the collection of laboratory data may prove academic, due to the obvious need for expedience. However, as a screening tool and guide for therapy, laboratory evaluation is essential. A barrage of laboratory tests are available and presented in Table 13-1.

AT III levels are the most sensitive determinants of DIC, showing a decline in activity due to increased consumption (Weiner, 1986). FDP/FSPs are nonspecific unless exceeding 40 mg and can be increased with the breakdown of old clot. D-dimer is a unique fibrin degradation fragment (DD), which is liberated when plasmin lyses cross-linked fibrin clot (Carr, McKinney, & McDonagh, 1989). D-dimer suggests clot synthesis because fibrin becomes cross-linked only after the thrombin-mediated activation of factor XIII (Carr, McKinney, & McDonagh, 1989). In contrast, fragments X, Y, D, and E are generated by lysis of fibrinogen and non-cross-linked fibrin. D-dimer then affords the advantage of reflecting both clot synthesis and breakdown. Carr and associates (1989) recommend screening with FDPs and confirming with D-dimer to maximize sensitivity and specificity. Because FPA has a half-life of 3 minutes, it indicates excessive fibrin production and more accurately reflects current coagulation status (Finley, 1989). FPA is the first strand cleaved from fibrinogen during fibrin formation. The presence of SFMCs is also indicative of recent thrombin activity (Finley, 1989).

The more common and most available tests for coagulation assessment include serum fibrinogen, prothrombin time (PT), partial thromboplastin time (PTT), and platelet count. The PT, which reflects extrinsic coagulation, is prolonged in DIC as is PTT, which measures intrinsic coagulation. Generally, these tests are far less specific, but in the asymptomatic patient may be useful for screening. Fifty percent of patients with DIC have a normal PT and PTT, while most have a decreased fibrinogen, and 90% have thrombocytopenia (Weiner, 1986). Additional lab work should include hemoglobin, hematocrit, and a peripheral smear.

Recently, Orlikowski and Rocke (1992) have advocated thromboelastography (TEG) for global assessment of hemostatic function. TEG can provide bedside measurement of all aspects of coagulation within 20–30 minutes, and in 60 minutes can provide information about clot stability and fibrinolysis (Orlikowski & Rocke, 1992). The machine generates a waveform as fibrin strands form and their elasticity is measured. The authors have suggested that TEG may be more useful than D-dimer because of the ease with which fibrinolysis is diagnosed (Orlikowski & Rocke, 1992).

MANAGEMENT OF DIC

Therapy for DIC is predicated on the degree to which the underlying mechanism can be eliminated. Generally, removal of the products of conception results in arrest of the process. Of equal importance is the management of the systemic manifestations of DIC with volume replacement, blood component therapy, and cardiovascular and respiratory support.

A chronic subclinical DIC can be successfully treated by removing the underlying cause, often accomplished by pregnancy termination. Once the stimulus for coagulopathy is eliminated, serial monitoring of clotting studies, volume replacement as necessary, and periodic clinical evaluation are sufficient.

An acute, fulminant DIC mandates a more aggressive approach. Acute hemorrhage accompanied by hypovolemic shock can rapidly result in reduction in blood flow and oxygen delivery to the capillaries and tissues with ultimate progression to cell injury and death. Blood component administration is the cornerstone of therapy (see Table 13-2). In the actively bleeding patient with hypovolemic shock, it is essential to transfuse red blood cells (RBCs). This will restore oxygen-carrying capacity and increase oxygen delivery to the tissues. The restoration of tissue perfusion and oxygenation are critical to the resolution of the shock state.

Platelet transfusion is generally not recommended except as prophylaxis in the patient with a count of less than 10,000–20,000 or in the preoperative patient with a count of under 50,000 (ACOG, 1994). Platelet transfusion is not indicated for prophylaxis with massive blood transfusion. Transfusion of fresh frozen plasma (FFP) strictly for volume replacement is not recommended; however, it is advocated in patients with a demonstrated clotting factor deficiency (ACOG, 1994). Cryoprecipitate provides an alternative to FFP for the volume-restricted patient, but poses a disadvantage because it does not contain AT III. Correction of specific clotting factor deficiencies and thrombocytopenia during massive blood replacement will minimize further transfusion requirements (Weiner, 1991).

AT III concentrate is available and is effective in the treatment of obstetrical causes of DIC; however, it is also contained in FFP. In a multicenter trial, Maki and associates (1987) compared AT III concentrate to a synthetic protease inhibitor and found it to be clinically superior in the control of symptoms of DIC. However, there

TABLE 13-2. Blood Component Therapy

Component	Content	Volume	Goal
Pack red blood cells	Red cells 1 unit increases hematocrit 3%	200–225 ml	Hematocrit 30%

FFP	Clotting factors
	1 unit increases
	  Fibrinogen 10mg/dL,
	  Factors, 2–3%
		180–200 ml	Replace clotting factors
			Fibrinogen greater than
			  100 mg/dL

Cryoprecipitate	Clotting factors
	1 unit increases
	  Fibrinogen 10mg/dL
		15–20 ml	Replace clotting factors
			Fibrinogen greater than
			  100 mg/dL

Platelet concentration	Platelets
	1 unit increases
	  count 50,000/
	  microliter
		50 ml	Platelet count 50,000/
			  microliter or greater

is no consensus that transfusion of AT III concentrate is superior to conventional blood component therapy (Finley, 1989).

Heparin does not seem to be generally accepted as useful therapy for obstetrical causes of DIC. Heparin acts to neutralize thrombin by accelerating the activity of AT III. However, if AT III levels are depleted, as occurs in fulminant DIC, heparin therapy would not seem efficacious. Maki and colleagues (1987) concluded that single-agent therapy with AT III is effective and safer than combination therapy with heparin. Finley suggests limited low-dose heparin administration only in those patients with intact vascular systems, no evidence of bleeding diathesis, and those with a prolonged triggering mechanism (Finley, 1989).

Fluid volume therapy is crucial to the successful management of the bleeding patient with DIC. The challenge inherent in fluid replacement is to promote prompt restoration of circulatory volume without compromising ventilation by fluid overload. Isotonic crystalloid solutions are recognized universally as the primary fluid for acute intrasvascular volume expansion (Gould, Lensing, Sehgal, & Moss, 1992). For most patients, the use of crystalloids with the addition of blood products is adequate for volume resuscitation (Griffen & Kaufmann, 1993).

FORMULATION OF NURSING DIAGNOSES

The formulation of nursing diagnoses provides a framework from which a plan of care is derived. A number of nursing diagnoses pertain to the parturient with DIC (Doenges, Kenty, & Moorhouse, 1988). These include:

Alteration in hemostatis
Fluid volume deficit, actual or potential
Gas exchange, impaired, fetal
Alteration in health maintenance secondary to
  Impaired cardiovascular function, actual or
    potential
  Impaired renal function, actual or potential
  Impaired liver function, actual or potential
  Impaired pulmonary function, actual or
    potential
  Impaired central nervous system function,
    actual or potential
Anxiety
Alteration in family process

THEORETICAL BASIS OF NURSING CARE/INTERVENTION

The demands of caring for the patient with potential or manifest DIC vary from astute surveillance to active intervention. Initially, impact on the severity of the process can be maximized if the risk is recognized and coagulopathy is detected early. Assessment is also of paramount importance, and the attentive perinatal nurse who detects the subtle signs of DIC may avert catastrophe.

The detection of an alteration in hemostasis, secondary to abnormal coagulation, requires assessment of both clinical and laboratory data. Laboratory screening includes a baseline hemoglobin, hematocrit, serum fibrinogen, platelet count, PT, PTT, FSPs and/or D-dimer. The frequency of collection of further laboratory data is determined by abnormalities that are detected. Spurious results may be obtained if coagulation studies are drawn from an arterial line (Hewitt & Davies, 1983). Physical assessment should be thorough and systematic with particular attention paid to discovery of petechiae, ecchymoses, hematoma formation, vaginal bleeding, gingival bleeding, hematuria, and hemorrhages in the conjunctiva. Trauma such as venipuncture or intramuscular injection should be avoided.

In the actively bleeding patient, blood loss should be quantitated when possible. Blood component replacement is often necessary and has been described previously. The risks of blood administration include transfusion reaction, transmission of infectious disease, and circulatory overload (ACOG, 1994). Currently the risk of contracting hepatitis B is 1:50,000, hepatitis C 1:3,300, and HIV 1:1,000,000 (ACOG, 1994). The risk of fatal transfusion reaction is 1:100,000 (ACOG, 1994). The onset of transfusion reaction is characteristically rapid and signs and symptoms may include: fever, chills, chest and flank pain, cardiovascular collapse, and DIC (Brandt, 1985). If an adverse reaction occurs the transfusion should be stopped immediately, the intravenous tubing flushed with normal saline, and the patient managed empirically. Rigid adherence to procedure for proper identification of blood components is critical.

Rapid administration of blood products may be hampered by their viscosity. Fifty to 100 ml of normal saline can be added to a unit of RBCs, which may triple the flow rate (Moucha & Rosenthal, 1993). Warming of blood not only protects the patient from hypothermia but will increase the flow rate up to 2½ times (Moucha & Rosenthal, 1993). Blood filters add resistance but this can be minimized by replacing them after every 3–4 units of blood, or by using microaggregate filters when multiple transfusions are anticipated.

Fluid volume deficit accompanies hemorrhage and is responsible for significant morbidity in cases of DIC. The need for fluid replacement may be assessed by measurement of urine specific gravity, hematocrit, central venous pressure and pulmonary artery, wedge pressure, and intake and output.

Many factors influence the effectiveness of fluid administration including the size of the catheter and tubing, the viscosity of the fluid, and infusion techniques. As large a catheter as possible should be placed because flow rate is a function of the radius of the catheter and the length of the tubing. It has been observed that multilumen catheters sacrifice flow, and should not be used in fluid resuscitation (Marino, 1991). For the same reason, extension sets, y-connectors, and piggyback devices should also be avoided (Falk, O'Brien, & Kerr, 1993). Pressure bags increase the flow rate by 2–3 times baseline gravity flow (Marino, 1991). Rapid volume infusion systems are also available, and patients resuscitated with them experience fewer complications and require less fluid volume (Dunham, 1991).

The amount and rate of fluid replacement therapy required will vary depending on the severity of the deficit. The best indication that fluid therapy is successful will be the resolution of the clinical signs and symptoms of shock and the return to normal oxygen consumption.

Impaired fetal gas exchange may occur as a consequence of decreased uteroplacental perfusion due to maternal hemorrhage and shock. Continuous electronic fetal monitoring during the intrapartum period is beneficial for assessment of fetal well-being. Late decelerations, tachycardia, and loss of variability may be ominous, and depending on maternal condition, may dictate expedient delivery. Additional interventions include lateral maternal positioning and administration of oxygen.

The systemic nature of DIC can precipitate impairment of cardiovascular, renal, liver, central nervous system, and pulmonary function, particularly when blood loss is great. Nursing care centers on obtaining and analyzing the patient's clinical condition and laboratory data in order to ascertain compromise of major organ systems.

Blood pressure, pulse, and peripheral perfusion are monitored frequently with particular attention to the development of hypotension and tachycardia. Inotropic support may be necessary to maintain perfusion. Urine output should be measured hourly and specific gravity checked. An output of greater than 25 ml/h generally coincides with adequate perfusion of the kidneys. Serum creatinine and blood urea nitrogen (BUN) are monitored closely for elevations consistent with renal involvement. Liver function tests are monitored serially with attention to elevation of SGOT, SGPT, and bilirubin. Nausea, vomiting, and right upper quandrant or shoulder pain suggest liver involvement. Continuous assessment of mental status is imperative because any alteration may be an early expression of cerebral hemorrhage. Pulmonary involvement may represent an iatrogenic complication resulting from fluid overload. Observation for dyspnea, tachypnea, cyanosis, and frequent auscultation of breath sounds assist in determining the presence of pulmonary edema. Pulse oximetry and measurement of arterial blood gases may also prove useful.

Emotional support is crucial in the patient and family reeling from a life-threatening complication such as DIC. Anxiety is common, as is disruption in family process. Interventions include encouraging verbalization, establishing trust, and offering explanations of procedures and equipment. The family should be encouraged to visit, and if possible, maternal–infant bonding is facilitated by the perinatal nurse.

In summary, intensive surveillance is mandated in the intrapartum patient at risk for DIC. If the patient is acutely affected, many aspects of supportive care fall within the realm of nursing practice. The degree to which the patient responds to supportive measures, once the precipitating event is eliminated, determines outcome.

EXPECTED OUTCOMES

If the initiating cause of DIC is successfully removed and the response to supportive therapy is positive, the following outcomes are possible.

1. Maintenance of hemostasis
2. Maintenance of adequate cardiac output and tissue perfusion
3. Prevention of fetal distress
4. Prevention of permanent renal dysfunction
5. Prevention of permanent liver dysfunction
6. Prevention of permanent pulmonary dysfunction
7. Prevention of permanent CNS dysfunction
8. Alleviation of anxiety
9. Diminished disruption of family process

REFERENCES

American College of Obstetricians and Gynecologists (ACOG). (1994). Blood component therapy. Technical Bulletin 199.

Brandt, J. T. (1985). Current concepts in coagulation. Clinical Obstetrics and Gynecology, 28, 3.

Carr, J. M., McKinney, M., & McDonagh, J. (1989). Diagnosis of disseminated intravascular coagulation. Journal of Clinical Pharmacology, 91, 3.

Doenges, M. E., Kenty, J. R., & Moorhouse, M. (1988). Maternal newborn care plans guidelines for client care. Philadelphia: F. A. Davis.

Dunham, C. M., Belzberg, H., Lyles, R., Weireter, L., Skurdal, D., Sullivan, G., Esposito, T., & Namini, M. The rapid infusion system: a superior method for the resuscitation of hypovolemic trauma patients. Resuscitation 21(2–3); 207–227, April 1991.

Falk, J., O'Brien, J., & Kerr, R. (1993). Fluid resuscitation in traumatic hemorrhagic shock. Critical Care Clinics, 8(2), 333–339.

Finley, B. E. (1989). Acute coagulopathy in pregnancy. Medical Clinics of North America, 73, 723.

Gilabert, J., Estelles, A., Aznan, J., & Galbis, M. (1985). Abruptio placenta and disseminated intravascular coagulation. Acta Obstetrica Gynaecoligica Scandinavica, 64, 35.

Gould, J. F., Lensing, R., Sehgal, H. L., & Moss, G. S. (1992). Hypovolemic shock. Critical Care Clinics, 9(2), 235–245.

Griffe, M., & Kaufman, B. S. (1993). Pharmacology of crystalloids and colloids. Critical Care Clinics, 9(2), 235–245.

Hewitt, P., & Davies, S. (1983). The current state of DIC. Intensive Care Medicine, 9, 249.

Kobayashi, T., & Terao, T. (1987). Preeclampsia as chronic disseminated intravascular coagulation. Gynecology and Obstetric Investigation, 24, 170.

Ledue, L., Wheeler, J. M., Kirshon, B., et al. (1992). Coagulation profile in severe preeclampsia. Obstetrics and Gynecology, 79, 14.

Maki, M., Terao, T., Ikenoue, T., Takemura, T., Sekiba, K., Shirakawa, K., & Soma, H. (1987). Clinical elevation of antithrombin III concentrate for disseminated intravascular coagulation. Gynecology and Obstetric Investigation, 23, 230.

Marino, P. L. (1991). Colloid and crystalloid resuscitation. The ICU Book. Philadelphia: Lea & Febiger.

Mouchanar, A., & Rosenthal, M. (1993). A pathophysiological approach to the patient in shock. International Anesthesiology, 31(d), 1–20.

Orlikowski, C. E. P., & Rocke, D. A. (1992). Coagulation monitoring in the OB patient. International Anesthesiology Clinics, 32(2), 173–191.

Sen, C., Madazh, R., Davuzlu, C., Ocak, V., & Tolun, N. (1994). The value of antithrombin III and fibronectin in hypertensive disorders of pregnancy. Journals of Perinatal Medicine, 22, 20.

Sher, G., & Statland, B. E. (1985). Abruptio placenta with coagulopathy: A rational basis for management. Clinical Obstetrics and Gynecology, 28, 15.

Vam Dam, P. A., Reinier, M., Backlandt, M., Buyaert, P., & Uyttenbroeck, F. (1989). Disseminated intravascular coagulation and the syndrome of hemolysis, elevated liver enzymes and low platelets in severe preeclampsia. Obstetrics and Gynecology, 73, 97.

Weiner, C. P. (1986). The obstetric patient and disseminated intravascular coagulopathy. Clinics in Perinatology, 13, 705.

Weiner, C. P. (1988). The mechanism of reduced antithrombin III activity in women with preeclampsia. Obstetrics and Gynecology, 72, 847.

Weiner, C. P. (1991). Disseminated intravascular coagulopathy associated with pregnancy. In Clark, et al. (Eds.), Critical Care Obstetrics. Boston: Blackwell Scientific.

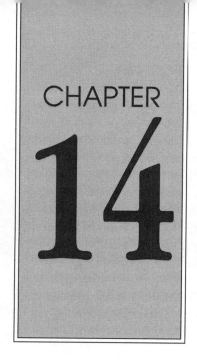

CHAPTER 14

Diabetes Mellitus in Pregnancy

Jo M. Kendrick

INCIDENCE AND CLASSIFICATION

Approximately 4% of all pregnancies are complicated by diabetes, accounting for more than 150,000 pregnancies annually in the United States (Engelgau, Herman, Smith, German, & Aubert, 1995). Diabetes mellitus is generally classified into three categories. Pregestational diabetes consists of women with Type 1 or insulin-dependent diabetes mellitus (IDDM) and Type 2, noninsulin diabetes (NIDDM). The American Diabetes Association (ADA), the National Institute of Diabetes and Digestive and Kidney Diseases, and the Centers for Disease Control and Prevention, Division of Diabetes Translation now recommend the elimination of the terms IDDM and NIDDM exclusively using the terms Type 1 and Type 2 using arabic numerals (ADA, 1997). The majority (90%) of diabetic gravidas are gestational diabetics defined as onset or recognition of abnormal carbohydrate metabolism during pregnancy. Type 1 diabetes is characterized by pancreatic beta cell dysfunction with a resultant lack of insulin production requiring exogenous insulin therapy as a mainstay of treatment as well as dietary management. The average age of diagnosis for Type 1 is less than 30. Type 2 diabetes is usually diagnosed at greater than 40 years of age, so this type of dia-

betes is not encountered as frequently in pregnancy, although it is by far the most prevalent type of diabetes nationwide. This type of diabetes results from defects in secretion and action of insulin and does not always require insulin or oral hypoglycemic agents for treatment but often can be managed by appropriate diet, exercise, and weight management. Type 1 diabetics tend to be lean, whereas 60% of Type 2 diabetics are obese (Neiger & Kendrick, 1994). Weight loss in the obese Type 2 diabetic very often results in an improvement in glucose control, decreasing or eliminating the need for oral hypoglycemic agents or insulin and achieving euglycemia with diet only.

Priscilla White developed a classification system in 1949 for diabetes in pregnancy with associated risks for predicting prognosis for perinatal outcome based on the presence and degree of microvascular disease (White, 1949). Gestational diabetes (class A) was not added to this classification until later to designate whether the diabetes is controlled by diet (A-1) or by insulin administration in addition to diet (A-2) (Table 14-1) (Hagay & Reece, 1992). Although White's classification is still widely used for descriptive purposes, pregnancy outcome for all diabetics has improved based on advanced obstetric and neonatal care. Degree of metabolic control prior to and during preg-

TABLE 14-1. Classification of Diabetes in Pregnancy

Pregestational Diabetes

Class	Age of Onset (Year)	Duration (Year)	Vascular Disease	Therapy
A	any	any	no	diet only
B	>20	<10	no	insulin
C	10–19	10–19	no	insulin
D	<10	>20	benign retinopathy	insulin
F	any	any	nephropathy	insulin
R	any	any	proliferative retinopathy	insulin
H	any	any	heart disease	insulin

Gestational Diabetes

Class	Fasting Glucose Level	Postprandial Glucose Level
A-1	<105 mg/dL and	<120 mg/dL
A-2	>105 mg/dL and/or	>120 mg/dL

Reproduced with permission from Hagay Z. J., & Reece, E. A. (1992).

nancy and presence or absence of maternal vasculopathy are factors greatly influencing perinatal outcome.

SIGNIFICANCE

The risk for adverse pregnancy outcome in women with diabetes has improved considerably over the last two decades due to improved obstetric care and tighter glycemic control, but the incidence of complications remains higher than in the general population. As the duration of diabetes increases, so does the risk for poor perinatal outcome. Gestational diabetes, if well-controlled, has no greater risk for adverse outcome than for the nondiabetic population.

In spite of advances in the care of pregnancies complicated by diabetes, fetal and neonatal mortality remains at 2–4% (Matheson & Efantis, 1989). The major cause of perinatal mortality with diabetes can be attributed to con-

genital malformations and unexplained fetal death. Congenital malformations account for approximately 40% of perinatal deaths in diabetes with no specific associated malformation (Reece, Gabrielli, & Abdalla, 1988). The congenital malformations associated with diabetes are usually multiple, more severe, and more often fatal than birth defects found in offspring of nondiabetic women. It has long been known that early maternal hyperglycemia is associated with a higher incidence of congenital malformations. The incidence of babies with birth defects born to mothers with diabetes improves significantly with preconception control as evidenced by lower glycosylated hemoglobin levels at the time of organogenesis.

Infants of diabetic mothers are at significant risk for neonatal hypoglycemia during the first 24 hours of life with a reported incidence of 25%–40% (Reece & Homko, 1994). Poor glycemic control antenatally and elevated maternal glucose during the intrapartum period place the infant at risk for hypoglycemia in the immediate neonatal period. Fetal blood glucose levels are normally approximately 70%–80% of maternal levels. With maternal hyperglycemia, the fetus responds by releasing increased insulin, resulting in hyperinsulinemia. Chronic fetal hyperinsulinemia also depresses the counter-regulatory response of glucagon, which stimulates glycogen release from the liver, therefore inhibiting a normal physiologic protective response to hypoglycemia. The combined effects of increased insulin and decreased glycogen result in neonatal hypoglycemia once the cord is cut at delivery and transplacental glucose is halted. Insulin levels may remain elevated for 24 hours, requiring frequent neonatal glucose assessment to prevent severe hypoglycemia and the neurologic sequelae associated with it.

Hypocalcemia and hypomagnesemia are two other neonatal metabolic derangements that are significantly increased among Type 1 offspring. The etiology of hypocalcemia may be due to diffusion from intracellular to extracellular fluid during periods of acidosis (Reece & Homko, 1994). Hypomagnesemia develops as a result of greater renal loss of magnesium associated with polyuria in response to hyperglycemia. One third of infants will exhibit neonatal polycythemia due to chronic intrauterine hypoxia that leads to increased red blood cell production. Polycythemia and birth trauma increase the risk for neonatal hyperbilirubinemia.

Fetal hyperinsulinemia also may delay fetal lung maturation by inhibiting the development of enzymatic precursors to surfactant production (Bourbon & Farrell, 1985). In the past, the risk for infants of diabetic mothers to develop respiratory distress syndrome (RDS) was five- to six-fold greater than infants of the same gestational age born to nondiabetic women. Stringent metabolic control has decreased that risk in recent years. Yet despite tight control, elective preterm delivery for fetal or maternal compromise and an increased incidence of cesarean births continue to contribute to the development of RDS in infants delivered to diabetic women.

Fetal growth aberrations are also a common complication associated with diabetes. Macro-

somia, defined as a fetal weight ≥ 4000 grams, occurs in approximately 26% of infants born to diabetic mothers compared to 8% in nondiabetic women (Cordero & Landon, 1993). These large infants increase the risk for birth trauma, particularly shoulder dystocia and the need for cesarean birth. Intrauterine growth retardation occurs in 20% of diabetic pregnancies as a result of maternal vascular disease (classes D–F) and is an associated factor with some malformations (Cordero & Landon, 1993). Uteroplacental insufficiency is believed to be the underlying mechanism in growth retardation when the pregnancy is complicated by maternal vascular disease. Disturbances in maternal fuels such as amino acids during organogenesis have also been suggested as another cause of growth retardation in diabetic offspring. (Cordero & Landon, 1993).

Hypoglycemia is the most common maternal complication (6–41%) of insulin-controlled diabetes and is an expected result of tighter glycemic control (Reece, Homko, & Hagay, 1995). Hypoglycemia has not been found to pose a risk for the fetus so concern is primarily focused on maternal well-being. Morning sickness, reduced food intake, and increased insulin sensitivity contribute to the development of hypoglycemia in the first trimester. Nocturnal hypoglycemia can be life-threatening when the mother does not awaken with early symptoms.

Although rare among gestational diabetics, a more serious complication of diabetes in pregnancy is the development of diabetic ketoacidosis (DKA). DKA develops at lower blood glucose levels and more rapidly in pregnancy due to lowered buffering capacity in pregnancy and the accelerated conversion to fat metabolism. The use of beta sympathomimetics and corticosteroids in women with Type 1 diabetes may induce DKA in pregnancy. Maternal mortality with DKA is low but fetal mortality has been reported to range from 30–90% (Hagay, 1994; Rodgers & Rodgers, 1991). Due to the high perinatal mortality, prompt recognition of risk factors for development of ketoacidosis such as infection or stress and early detection of ketosis are important management strategies for prevention.

Women with diabetes of longer durations (10–20 years) or with histories of poor glycemic control may have chronic complications that require intensive management in pregnancy for a successful outcome. Retinopathy, a microvascular complication, has an incidence of 20–27% in reproductive age women with Type 1 diabetes (Reece, Homko, & Hagay, 1996). The classification of this progressive disorder includes background, preproliferative, or proliferative. Background retinopathy is usually asymptomatic and does not pose a threat to vision. Microaneurysms, exudates, and small hemorrhages characterize background retinopathy (Reece, Homko, & Hagay, 1996). Preproliferative retinopathy is considered to be a transitional stage associated with cotton-wool spots and intraretinal microvascular abnormalities (Reece, Homko, & Hagay, 1996). Neovascularization occurs with proliferative retinopathy, which may cause retinal detachment as a result of distortion and contraction of the vitrous gel representing a serious threat to vision. Pregnancy accelerates the progression of retinopathy although a significant number of women experience regression after delivery (Klein, Moss, & Klein, 1990) Photocoagulation therapy and ophthalmic surveillance are therefore indicated in the pregnant woman with proliferative retinopathy. Because retinopathy is caused by poor metabolic control leading to vascular disease, it is associated with poorer perinatal outcomes than in patients who do not yet have vascular complications of diabetes.

Nephropathy, also a microvascular complication, poses a more serious threat to successful pregnancy outcome. Diabetic nephropathy has been associated with congenital malformations, intrauterine growth retardation, intrauterine fetal death, and preterm delivery. The mother is at risk for renal failure during or after pregnancy, hypertension, superimposed preeclampsia, and edema. Differentiation between preeclampsia and worsening of hypertension can be very difficult but is an important distinction to make, because delivery may be indicated in preeclampsia for improvement whereas early delivery may not be necessary with hypertension.

METABOLIC ALTERATIONS OF PREGNANCY

Providing care for pregnant women with diabetes mellitus or gestational diabetes requires a knowledge of the normal metabolic adaptations to pregnancy. This will ensure a better understanding of the impact that diabetes has on pregnancy. The metabolic alterations associated with pregnancy allow for the availability of glucose and other nutrients for the growth and development of the fetus even with maternal fasting and intermittent feeding. The beta cells of the pancreas become hypertrophied in early pregnancy as a result of stimulation by increased circulating levels of estrogen and progesterone. This results in an increased response (hyperinsulinemia) to glucose, which allows increased tissue storage of glycogen and peripheral glucose utilization. Increased fat synthesis, fat cell hypertrophy, and inhibition of lipolysis result in increased fat storage or anabolism in early pregnancy (Boden, 1996). This prepares the mother for the increased demands of the fetus for amino acids and glucose in the latter half of pregnancy.

Fasting blood glucose levels are 10–15 mg/dL lower in gravid women compared to nongravid (Buchanan, Metzger, & Freinkel, 1990). Restraint of maternal hepatic glucose production and fetal siphoning of glucose are thought to be two processes that contribute to fasting hypoglycemia in early pregnancy (Buchanan & Kitzmiller, 1994). Fasting hypoglycemia in late pregnancy may result from the increased volume of glucose distribution as the mass of the fetus increases and as maternal gluconeogenesis decreases (Buchanan & Kitzmiller, 1994).

The fetal demand for glucose in the late third trimester is met during maternal fasting by hepatic glucose production, which increases 15–30% by late third trimester (Catalano et al., 1993). The liver begins to supply glucose within 6 hours of the last meal when absorption of nutrients from the intestinal tract ceases (Boden, 1996). Depletion of glycogen stores results from this accelerated hepatic glucose production.

Pregnancy has been characterized as a "diabetogenic state" due to persistent hyperglycemia in the presence of hyperinsulinemia. Post-prandial glucose levels are significantly elevated in pregnancy, which allows placental transfer of glucose to the fetus readily by passive diffusion (Lesser & Carpenter, 1994). Hyperglycemia persists after feeding due to decreased sensitivity to insulin in both the liver and in post-receptor cell membranes in the peripheral tissues. The beta cells of the pancreas respond to this decreasing sensitivity to insulin by producing progressively more insulin. Increased insulin production parallels the rise of maternal and placental hormone production of human chorionic somatomammotropin (HCS), estrogen, progesterone, prolactin, and cortisol, all of which are considered insulin antagonists (Buchanan & Kitzmiller, 1994). Lower fasting values offset the postprandial elevations resulting in 24-hour mean glucose values similar to nongravid women (Cousins, Rigg, & Hollingsworth, 1980).

Late pregnancy has also been characterized as a catabolic phase or a period of accelerated starvation, which consists of an earlier switch from carbohydrate to fat metabolism (lipolysis) with fasting (Carpenter, 1993). This metabolic response to fasting develops in 14–18 hours in pregnant individuals and in 2–3 days in non-pregnancy (Buchanan & Kitzmiller, 1994). This assures a continuous supply of glucose and nutrients to the fetus while the mother uses lipids as an energy source; however, it increases maternal ketone production increasing the risk for the development of ketoacidosis in Type 1 diabetics and ketosis in Type 2 and gestational diabetics. Ketonemia may have detrimental effects on fetal brain development (Rizzo, Metzger, Burns, & Burns, 1991).

PRECONCEPTION ASSESSMENT AND COUNSELING

Ideally women with preexisting diabetes mellitus, Type 1 or Type 2, should have planned pregnancies allowing for preconceptual assessment, counseling, and management. However, only 20% of diabetic women seek prepregnan-

cy care (Landon, Gabbe, & Sachs, 1990). This is not unusual considering that approximately 60% of all pregnancies are unintended (Adams, Bruce, Shulman, Kendrick, & Brogan, 1993). The primary goal of preconception care is to improve the metabolic profile before conception and throughout the early weeks of pregnancy to decrease the risk of first trimester spontaneous abortion and major congenital anomalies (Miller, 1994). Preconception programs with the goal of normalization of blood glucose levels in the preconception period have significantly decreased the incidence of congenital anomalies among infants of insulin-dependent diabetics (Greene, 1993; Kitzmiller et al., 1991; Miller et al., 1981; Steele, Johnstone, & Hepburn, 1990; Willhite et al., 1993).

The preconception assessment should include a thorough history of diabetes type, age at diagnosis, presence of acute and chronic complications such as hypoglycemia, diabetic ketoacidosis (DKA), retinopathy, nephropathy, hypertension, neuropathy, diabetic regimen, and current glucose control. Particular emphasis should be placed on episodes of hypoglycemia and DKA because this provides an overall indication of glucose control and possibly compliance.

The history should also include an assessment of knowledge deficits that would determine educational needs. Many Type 1 diabetics were diagnosed as children and may not have received recent intensive diabetic education. They may be very adept at techniques for glucose monitoring and self-administration of insulin but may have very little understanding of the pathophysiology of the disease and long-term outcomes. The goal of education is to empower the woman to take control of her disease. Due to the overwhelming amount of information the woman with diabetes needs, education may need to be provided in several scheduled sessions. Education should be individualized and be provided in a variety of formats. Written materials that emphasize the material covered will allow the woman to review at her own pace.

Registered dieticians should be part of the diabetic mangement team and be included in this initial assessment and on an ongoing basis. Dietary manipulations may be necessary and should be individualized to the patient's lifestyle and activity level. Supplementation with folic acid and prenatal vitamins during the preconception period and first trimester may decrease the risk of neural tube defects (Czeizel & Dudas, 1992).

A psychosocial assessment is another important component of preconception care. This can be done by the perinatal nurse or by a social worker if one is part of the diabetic team. When presented with the diagnosis of diabetes, most individuals will experience a grief reaction that usually resolves within the first year (Speelman-Rhiley, 1993). The adjustment to diabetes is a continuous process that requires adaptation and reevaluation at each stage of life. The desire to become pregnant or pregnancy itself requires the woman with diabetes to reevaluate how her life will be affected. The woman, her partner, and her family need to know the impact that pregnancy may have on diabetes including potential maternal, fetal, and neonatal complications. They should be provided a thorough explanation of the plan of care with cost implications. They should be informed of their Hgb A1c level and provided an explanation of risks for delivering an infant with congenital anomalies or of spontaneous abortion if elevated. They also must understand that lowering the Hgb A1c to an acceptable value may take 6 weeks to 6 months depending on the difficulty in achieving near euglycemia. Commitment to pregnancy and intensive self-management should be determined prior to pregnancy. Past and current history of stress and coping methods needs to be determined. Available support systems should be explored. Symptoms of depression require referral to an appropriate provider for evaluation. A plan for meeting needs including appropriate referrals should be devised jointly with the patient with the realization that psychosocial assessment should be continuous throughout the preconception and perinatal period and adapted as needed.

The physical examination of a woman with diabetes should be thorough with special attention to signs of vascular disease. An ophthalmologic exam is indicated annually for women with diabetes. The woman should be screened for proliferative retinopathy, which, if present, requires laser treatment prior to conception because neovascularization worsens with pregnancy (ADA, 1996). The cardiac examination of women who have had diabetes for >10 years or who have signs and symptoms of coronary artery disease should include an electrocardiogram (ECG) and an exercise treadmill. Other cardiovascular studies should be ordered as indicated. Coronary artery disease is associated with a high mortality rate in pregnancy and women with this diagnosis are usually advised to avoid pregnancy (ADA, 1996). Women with hypertensive disease may need adjustment of their medications. Angiotensin-converting enzyme (ACE) inhibitors, beta-adrenergic blocking agents, or diuretics are contraindicated in pregnancy. Other hypertensive agents that are safe to use during pregnancy should be prescribed. Women need to know that hypertension may worsen during pregnancy and that pregnancy-induced hypertension is a potential risk. Women with renal insufficiency as evidenced by creatinine clearance of <50 ml/min, serum creatinine of >2 mg/dL or >2 grams/24 hour proteinuria should be counseled to avoid pregnancy until after stabilization from renal transplantation (ADA, 1996). Women with evidence of less serious nephropathy should be counseled on the high risk of developing hypertension and/or intrauterine growth retardation, warranting total bedrest and the potential for early delivery by cesarean section. This may be too difficult for women with small children who do not have family support. The woman should be evaluated for orthostatic hypotension, which may be evidence of autonomic neuropathy. This is a serious complication of diabetes that is a relative contraindication to pregnancy (ADA, 1996). Autonomic neuropathy may affect the cardiovascular system or the viscera. Gastropathy or gastroparesis with symptoms of nausea, vomiting, abdominal pain, or early satiety are serious neuropathic complications because of the inability to maintain adequate nutrition

(Hare, 1994). Evidence of peripheral neuropathy such as decreased sensation in the feet to heat and pain or absence of the ankle jerk reflex may require referral to a neurologist for specialized testing. Lower extremity examination focuses on assessment of evidence of vascular disease, neuropathy, deformity, or infection. Special attention should be given to the skin assessment noting any bruising or hypertrophic areas at insulin injection sites. Skin and foot care should be reinforced at this time.

Initial laboratory evaluation should include:

CBC, electrolytes
Hgb A1c
Urinalysis
Urine culture
24-hour urine for creatinine clearance and total protein
Thyroid profile—include antithyroid antibodies for Type 1 diabetes
Lipid profile

Effective contraceptive options should be recommended to allow the woman to achieve metabolic control prior to conception. The choice should be made jointly by the woman and her healthcare provider taking into consideration her disease and lifestyle. Barrier methods such as condoms, cervical caps, or diaphragms when used with spermicidal jellies provide safe, effective contraception if used appropriately. Parous, monogamous diabetic women may use an intrauterine device (IUD) as the incidence of pelvic inflammatory disease, discontinuation rates, and accidental pregnancy rates with IUD use is comparable in diabetic and nondiabetic women (Mestman & Schmidt-Sarosi, 1993). The use of hormonal contraception in women with diabetes is controversial due to possible adverse risks on carbohydrate and lipid metabolism. Although studies of the use of combined oral contraceptives have not conclusively revealed adverse effects on these parameters, most clinicians prefer to use progestin-only oral contraceptives that are deemed relatively safe for women with diabetes. Progestin implants and long-acting injectable progestins have not been studied in women with diabetes.

SCREENING AND DIAGNOSIS OF GESTATIONAL DIABETES MELLITUS (GDM)

Controversy exists worldwide on whether all women should be screened for GDM or only select populations based on age, incidence, or history. It is known that GDM is rare in women <20 years of age and that certain populations such as the Pima Indians have a very high prevalence of GDM. The taking of a medical history has been studied for its screening value revealing only a 50% detection rate for GDM (Marquette, Klein, & Niebyl, 1985). In the United States, 75% of obstetricians and 90% of perinatologists universally screen for GDM (Landon, Gabbe, & Sachs, 1990). Universal screening at 24–28 weeks gestation has been advocated by the American Diabetes Association until July 1997 when their position was changed to selective screening (ADA, 1997). ADA now recommends the avoidance of screening in women who are considered low risk: less than 25 years of age, normal body weight, no family history of diabetes, and not a member of an ethnic/racial group at high risk for diabetes (Hispanic, African American, Native American, Asian) (ADA, 1997). The American College of Obstetricians and Gynecologists (ACOG) changed their 1986 position recommending selective screening for women <30 years of age with risk factors and universal screening for all women aged 30 or older (ACOG, 1986). ACOG now recommends selective screening in low-risk populations such as adolescent prenatal clinics and universal screening in higher prevalence groups (ACOG, 1994).

Screening for GDM is usually obtained between 24 and 28 weeks gestation by administering a 50-gram oral glucose challenge regardless of timing of the last meal. Venous blood should be drawn fasting and 1 hour after glucose ingestion. Women should be advised not to eat, drink, or smoke until after their blood has been drawn. Capillary blood and the use of reflectance meters is not recommended due to their 15% margin for error (Carr, Coustan, Martelly, Broscoe, & Rotondo, 1989).

Screening earlier in pregnancy should be considered in women with risk factors (see Display 14-1). Regardless of when screening is performed, an abnormal result should be followed by administrations of the 3-hour oral glucose tolerance test (OGTT), which is considered to be the diagnostic "gold standard" for gestational diabetes. Women with an abnormal 3-hour OGTT who are less than 20 weeks gestation are probably previously undiagnosed Type 1 or Type 2 diabetics. The diagnosis of preexisting diabetes mellitus can only be made definitively after delivery.

A result of 140 mg/dL from the 1-hour glucose challenge is considered a positive screening test requiring diagnostic testing. The threshold of 140 mg/dL is accepted by the American Diabetes Association (ADA) (ADA, 1995) and the National Diabetes Data Group (NDDG) (NDDG, 1979). The American College of Obstetricians and Gynecolgists recognizes a positive threshold between 130 mg/dL and 140 mg/dL (ACOG, 1994). With a value of 140 mg/dL, 14% of women will be positive and require further testing (ACOG, 1994). However, 10% of women with GDM will be missed by using 140 mg/dL as the threshold (ACOG, 1994). Because of this, many practitioners use 130 mg/dL as a cutoff, which results in approximately 25% of women screened who will require diagnostic testing (ACOG, 1994). A blood glucose of 200 mg/dL or greater from the screening glucola is considered diagnostic for GDM and requires no further testing.

The criteria for diagnosis of gestational diabetes are based on the work of O'Sullivan and Mahan (1964). These criteria were based on whole blood and were used for approximately 15 years, after which laboratory methods for detecting glucose changed from whole blood to venous plasma. The National Diabetes Data Group converted O'Sullivan's criteria by adding 14% to the original whole blood values (NDDG, 1979). These criteria listed in Table 14-2 are accepted by the American Diabetes Association (ADA, 1995) and the American College of Obstetricians and Gynecologists (ACOG, 1994) ACOG also recognizes Carpenter and Coustan's conversion of O'Sullivan's original criteria to venous plasma, which are based on the hexaki-

DISPLAY 14-1

Criteria for Screening for GDM <24 Weeks Gestation

first degree relative with diabetes

persistent glycosuria

previous glucose intolerance

polyhydramnios

obesity (>150% ideal body weight)

history of unexplained fetal death or stillborn

multiple spontaneous abortions

previous infant with congenital anomalies

history of infant weighing >4000 grams

oral betamimetic therapy

corticosteroid therapy

Note. If early testing yields a negative result, screening should be repeated at 24–28 weeks gestation.

nase method of glucose determination (see Table 14-2) (ACOG, 1994). Regardless of the criteria used, two values must be met or exceeded for a diagnosis of GDM. A fasting blood glucose value of >120 mg/dL is diagnostic for GDM without the need for administration of the 3-hour OGTT.

One abnormal value on the 3-hour OGTT has been associated with an increased incidence of macrosomia and various other adverse pregnancy outcomes (Langer et al., 1989). One third of women with one abnormal value will demonstrate two abnormal values on a repeat test 1 month later, consistent with a diagnosis of GDM (Neiger & Coustan, 1991). There is no consistent approach recognized when one value is elevated. Management of patients with one abnormal value can include repeating the test 1 month later as pregnancy affects increase, diet therapy, and blood glucose monitoring or continued observation.

TABLE 14-2. Diagnostic Criteria for Gestational Diabetes

100 g Oral Glucose Tolerance Test	Whole Blood (O'Sullivan)	Venous Plasma (NDDG)	Carpenter Conversion
Fasting	90	105	95
1 hour	170	190	180
2 hours	145	165	155
3 hours	125	145	140

Note. Diagnostic for GDM with two abnormal values.

Written and verbal instructions for women scheduled for the 3-hour oral glucose tolerance test should include the following:

- explanation for the necessity of the test and possible impact on pregnancy outcome if undiagnosed or untreated
- carbohydrate loading diet for the 3 days preceding the test
- nothing by mouth after midnight except water
- no smoking for 12 hours prior to test
- procedure and interval for venous sampling
- nausea and/or vomiting may result from ingestion of glucose solution
- no smoking, eating, or drinking during test
- inform when woman can expect results

METABOLIC MANAGEMENT FOR THE PREPREGNANT AND PREGNANT DIABETIC

Diet Therapy

The cornerstone for diabetes management is diet therapy with the goal of attainment and maintenance of euglycemia and adequate weight gain during pregnancy avoiding hypoglycemia and ketosis. Caloric intake for pregnant women as recommended by ACOG (1994) for women with a current weight of less than 80% ideal body weight are 35-40 kcal/kg daily; for those 80–120%, 30 kcal/kg; for those 120–150%, 24 kcal/kg; and for those >150%, 12–15 kcal/kg (ACOG, 1994). This represents a caloric restricted diet (1080–1350 calories per day) for obese women, who comprise the majority of Type 2 and gestational diabetics. Hypocaloric diets have been studied for dietary management of obese pregnant women with small sample sizes with inconclusive recommendations (Knopp, Magee, Raisys, Benedetti, & Bonet, 1991; Magee, Knopp, & Benedetti, 1990). Therefore, hypocaloric diets are not recommended, nor would obese women be apt to follow such a strict regimen.

Jovanovic and Peterson (1993) recommend daily calorie intake based on prepregnancy body weight. Women whose prepregnancy weight is at the desired level are encouraged to gain 25–35 pounds and consume 30 kcal/kg/day. Overweight women who are >120% desirable prepregnancy weight should consume 24 kcal/kg/day and gain 15–25 pounds. Underweight women (<90% desirable prepregnancy weight) should consume 36–40 kcal/kg/day and gain 28–40 pounds (Jovanovic & Peterson, 1993). The diet for pregnancy should be comprised of 40–50% carbohydrates (CHO), preferably high in fiber, 20% protein, and 30–40% fat (Kitzmiller et al., 1991). These calories should be eaten preferably in three meals and four snacks to decrease postprandial hyperglycemia and the risk of between-meal hypoglycemia (Miller, 1994). Aspartame has been determined to be safe as a nonnutritive sweetener in pregnancy except in women with phenylketonuria (American Dietetic Association, 1993). Saccharin does cross into placental circulation but there is no evidence of harmful fetal effects (American Dietetic Association, 1993).

Prepregnancy diets for Type 1 and Type 2 diabetics should consist of 55–60% CHO, 12–20% protein, and <30% fat (Jovanovic & Peterson, 1993). Active women in prepregnancy programs require 30 kcal/kg per day, whereas sedentary or obese women need only 20 kcal/kg per day.

Assessment and reevaluation of dietary needs by a registered dietician should occur ideally prior to conception, and then on an ongoing basis thereafter, and finally in the postpartum period. Dietary adjustments at the minimum will be needed with each trimester. Weight gain or loss should be monitored closely and diet and insulin therapy should be adjusted as indicated. Special considerations and written instructions for emesis or "sick day" management in pregnancy should be provided. (See Display 14-2.) Counseling for dietary management of diabetes in pregnancy should be individualized to incorporate the woman's personal preferences, cultural beliefs, financial limitations, lifestyle, and activity level.

Exercise

The role of exercise for pregnant women with diabetes has been gaining acceptance, but still remains controversial. Exercise involving cardiovascular conditioning facilitates glucose utilization by increasing insulin binding and affinity for its receptor (Artal, Wiswell, & Romem, 1985). Exercise during pregnancy in women with diabetes should be discontinued if uterine activity results. Women with diabetes who are already involved in an exercise program should be allowed to continue during their pregnancy but should be counseled that a decrease in exercise may be required as pregnancy progresses. They also should be instructed to check their blood glucose before and after exercise with the understanding that in an insulin-deficient state, glucose levels will rise. Exercise during euglycemia may cause hypoglycemia during the exercise or hours later (Plovie, 1991). Other measures to improve safety of exercise in pregnancy include exercising postprandially at the same time of day, every day (Plovie, 1991). Pregnant women should not exercise alone and should always have a carbohydrate snack available (Plovie, 1991). Mild exercise programs such as walking can safely be encouraged in Type 1, Type 2, and gestational diabetes. Pregnant women with diabetes who have not achieved metabolic control should not exercise nor should those with complications of diabetes such as vasculopathy, hypertension, proliferative retinopathy, and severe neuropathy of the lower extremities. Hopefully, future research will determine the safety and efficacy of exercise in pregnancy providing appropriate guidelines for intensity level and monitoring methods.

Education and Self-Management

The diagnosis of gestational diabetes mellitus (GDM) requires extensive, individualized education for the pregnant woman and significant others. A sample of a diabetic education checklist can be found in Display 14-3. The woman needs an explanation of the abnormal values on her 3-hour oral glucose tolerance test and reassurance that she did not cause her diabetes. A discussion of glucose transport, the role of insulin in providing energy for bodily functions, and the growth and development of the fetus provides the foundation for understanding gestational diabetes. A brief overview of the role of placental hormones and the development of glucose intolerance in the susceptible woman should be provided. The role of diet therapy and self-monitoring of blood glucose and the necessity for controlling diabetes in pregnancy are also discussed. Possible fetal and neonatal complications should be discussed so the woman understands the importance of compliance with the diabetic regimen. The use of a reflectance meter including quality control, cleaning, and the technique for blood glucose testing with return demonstration is vital to the success of self-management. Glucose testing in the gestational diabetic who is not on insulin is generally required fasting and 2 hours postprandially or 4 times daily. The woman should be instructed on documentation of blood glucose values and any unusual reactions on a log. Recording the foods ingested allows the dietician or diabetes nurse to determine whether carbohydrate intake

DISPLAY 14-2

Diabetes and Pregnancy Sick Day Guidelines**

These guidelines should be followed only for short-term illness such as nausea, vomiting, or diarrhea when the regularly prescribed diet cannot be tolerated. In the case of severe vomiting, contact your healthcare provider.

1. Take your insulin at the usual time. Do not discontinue insulin, even if you are vomiting and unable to tolerate your prescribed diet. Infectious illnesses increase the need for insulin and can raise your blood sugar level.

2. Check your urine for ketones when you first get up in the morning and anytime your blood glucose value is greater than 180 mg/dL. If you are vomiting, check your urine ketones every 4–6 hours and notify your healthcare provider of positive results at the moderate level.

3. If you are vomiting excessively, check you blood sugars every 2 hours. Notify your healthcare provider at levels of 200 mg/dL.

4. If you are unable to eat solid foods, replace the carbohydrates or carbohydrate exchanges you normally would eat with soft foods or liquids if your blood sugar is below 100 mg/dL (see the list below). Replacing the calories from meats (protein) and fats is not of prime importance.

5. Drinking plenty of liquids is very important during illness to prevent the development of dehydration that could lead to ketoacidosis. If your blood sugar is above 120 mg/dL, drink sugar-free beverages.

15 Grams Carbohydrates

any bread exchange	1 cup cream soup
1 slice toast/bread	1/2 cup custard
1/2 cup regular gelatin	1/2 cup orange juice
1/2 cup cooked cereal	1/3 cup grape juice
1/2 cup ice cream	2 1/2 tsp. sugar
1/2 cup sherbet	1 cup citrus Gatorade
6 saltines	1 cup tomato juice
1/2 cup cooked macaroni	1/2 regular twin popsicle
1 small baked potato	1/2 cup regular coke, sprite, or pepsi

**Adapted from the Diabetes Center Guidelines at the University of Tennessee Medical Center.

is appropriate. This becomes especially important when attempting to establish euglycemia. Euglycemia is defined as blood glucose values <105 mg/dL fasting and <120 mg/dL postprandially. Blood glucose determinations should be obtained 4 times daily for the first week to determine the success of diet therapy. If values are in the normal range, then home glucose testing may be decreased to 2 days weekly (usually a weekday and weekend day) as long as the patient understands that diet therapy must continue until delivery to prevent or minimize fetal

TABLE 14-3. Glycemic Goals for Diabetes in Pregnancy (ACOG, 1994)				
Diabetic Type	Fasting	Premeal	Postmeal	2–6 A.M.
Type 1, Type 2	60–90 mg/dL	60–105 mg/dL	1hr, <140 mg/dL 2 hrs, <120 mg/dL	60–90 mg/dL
GDM	105 mg/dL		1 hr, <140 mg/dL 2 hrs, <120 mg/dL	

or neonatal complications. Daily testing can be resumed if reported values reveal elevations. Random testing should be obtained at office visits. Weekly contact to report blood glucose values to the diabetes nurse educator who can consult with the woman's healthcare provider comprises comprehensive management.

Compliance with diet therapy in gestational diabetes may be improved if the nutritional education by the registered dietician is provided after the educational session on GDM. Guidelines for diet therapy in pregnancy are discussed in the previous section. Keeping a diet diary the first week after instruction for the dietician to review will identify possible problems, lack of understanding, or need for adjustment. Lack of adequate weight gain or weight loss with or without ketosis warrants investigation by the dietician. If diet therapy fails to provide metabolic control, insulin therapy is instituted that will require further dietary adjustments.

Self-care practices should be explored during preconception or early pregnancy and individualized education provided. Technique of insulin adminstration and glucose monitoring should be observed and documented and any deficiencies corrected. Knowledge of insulin action, timing of injection, storage, mixing, and site selection and rotation should be assessed and reviewed with the woman. Oral hypoglycemics should be changed to insulin during the preconception period due to the theoretic risk of teratogenicity and fetal/neonatal hypoglycemia (Neiger & Kendrick, 1994). Insulin adjustment algorithms should be reviewed and euglycemic goals defined with the woman. Preprandial levels of 70–100 mg/dL and postprandial values of <140 mg/dL at 1 hour and <120 mg/dL at 2 hours are accepted by the American Diabetes Association (ADA, 1996). These goals may be unrealistic in women with hypoglycemia unawareness and may need reevaluation and adjustment. The reflectance meter should be calibrated for accuracy and the diabetic should know when and how to perform quality control on the meter according to the manufacturer's recommendations.

Self-monitoring in pregnant women with Type 1 and Type 2 diabetes consists of more intensive surveillance than is required in gestational diabetes. Diagnosis of pregnancy in women with pregestational diabetes who have not been enrolled in a preconception program may require hospitalization for institution of intensive therapy if they are in or near the period of organogenesis (gestation 5–8 weeks). If they are very well controlled with an acceptable Hgb A1c value, outpatient treatment may be acceptable. Women who have Type 2 diabetes who are being controlled by oral hypoglycemics will need to be instructed on insulin administration. The schedule of office visits and frequency of fetal testing should be explained. Glycemic goals for diabetic pregnancy are listed in Table 14-3. To achieve these goals, self-monitoring of blood glucose may need to be obtained 5–7 times daily, particularly in women who are on multishot regimens with a sliding scale for insulin dosing or who are utilizing an insulin pump. Additional testing is indicated when symptoms of hypoglycemia develop. Blood glucose testing at 2 or 3 A.M. will evaluate for evidence of nocturnal hypoglycemia allowing for dietary or insulin adjustments to aid in prevention.

DISPLAY 14-3

Diabetes in Pregnancy Education Checklist

Name:_____ DOB:_____ Age:_____

Diabetes Type:_____ Age at Diagnosis:_____

Diabetes Educator:_____

The patient with diabetes and pregnancy will demonstrate the following:

Expected Outcome	Date
Understanding of diabetes, role of glucose and insulin transport	
Understanding related to the significance to pregnancy of 3-hour GTT results (GDM)	
Understanding effect pregnancy has on diabetes control including role of placental hormones	
Understanding of potential outcomes of uncontrolled blood glucose—macrosomia, polyhydramnios, preterm delivery, IUFD, neonatal hypoglycemia, ketoacidosis, birth trauma, cesarean delivery	
Understanding of significance of Hgb A1c for spontaneous abortion and congenital defects	
Ability to appropriately utilize reflectance meter including quality controls	
Use of autolancet to obtain blood sample	
Understanding of diabetic diet (diet diary first week) and role of exercise with safety guidelines	
Appropriate recording technique of blood glucose values and abnormal reactions	
Understanding of glycemic goals for treatment	
Knowledge of onset and peak times of prescribed insulin	

The glucose level that precipitates hypoglycemic reactions should be determined because this varies in individuals with diabetes. Some diabetics may have difficulty tolerating normal blood glucose levels because they are accustomed to extreme hyperglycemia. The level at which symptomalogy develops with hypoglycemia will determine the intensity of initial therapy. As the patient adjusts to a new lower mean blood glucose level, the level at which symptoms develop should decrease, allowing the individual to better tolerate normoglycemia.

Type 1 diabetics may not develop hypoglycemic reactions until blood glucose levels are very low, indicating a lack of awareness compared to Type 2 diabetics, who may exhibit symptoms at 70 mg/dL. Hypoglycemia unawareness develops in Type 1 diabetes as a result of defective glucose counterregulation due to insufficient glucagon and epinephrine release in response to hypoglycemia (Amiel, Sherwin, Simonson, & Tamborlane, 1988; Cryer & Gerich, 1990). Glucagon, which is released from the alpha cells of the pancreas in response to hypoglycemia,

DISPLAY 14-3 (continued)

Expected Outcome	Date
Appropriate inspection and storage of insulin	
Ability to draw up insulin appropriately (single or mixed dose)	
Appropriate identification of timing of injection, injection sites, rotation, and injection technique	
Identification of signs and symptoms of hypoglycemia	
Appropriate treatment for hypoglycemia with documented low blood glucose (patient and support person)	
Support person demonstrates knowledge of glucagon use and appropriate administration—provided prescription for two with refills	
Understands need to check ketones daily with first void (pregestational) and with BG values of ≥180 mg/dL	
Identification of the signs and symptoms of ketoacidosis and need to report persistent N/V, illness, infection, persistent hyperglycemia or recurrent insulin reactions	
Understanding of appropriate sick day management (provided written guidelines)	
Schedule of antepartum testing	
Significance of GDM for future pregnancies and development of overt diabetes later in life and risk minimizing interventions	
Significance of diabetes and development of long-term complications related to poor control	

Level of Comprehension:_____ Learning Impediments:_____

Family Support: _____

Previous Education: _____

enhances hepatic release of glucose. Impaired glucagon secretion frequently develops after 2–5 years of IDDM (Levandoski, Santiago, & White, 1993). Epinephrine assumes a primary role in recovery from hypoglycemia when glucagon secretion is impaired by increasing hepatic production of glucose and decreasing glucose utilization (Levandoski, Santiago, & White, 1993). Diminished epinephrine secretion usually does not occur until later in the course of diabetes (Levandoski, Santiago, & White, 1993). Hypoglycemia unawareness may also be a manifestation of autonomic neuropathy (American Diabetes Association [ADA], 1996). Women with hypoglycemia unawareness should be treated carefully, because the absence of symptoms at dangerously low blood glucose values can result in injury or death. Frequent blood glucose monitoring is critical for these women and should be mandatory prior to participating in high-risk activities such as driving, exercising, or bathing.

An assessment of how the woman treats hypoglycemia and whether there is a pattern of occurrence, particularly nocturnal hypoglycemia, should be made. Women with diabetes may overtreat and may not understand appropriate management of hypoglycemia, resulting in rebound hyperglycemia. Ingestion of 10–15 grams of carbohydrate (1/2 cup of fruit juice, 1 cup of milk, 1/2–3/4 cup of regular soda) for mild reactions and 15–30 grams for moderate reactions will usually raise blood glucose within 15–20 minutes (Levandoski, Santiago, & White, 1993). Retesting the blood glucose approximately 15 minutes after treatment will determine if more carbohydrates are needed. If so, an additional 15 grams should be consumed. If hypoglycemia develops near a snack or meal time, then treatment should consist of consumption of the usual carbohydrates from the snack or meal. Severe reactions may require administration of glucagon and family members and significant others should be instructed on the technique. Two glucagon kits should be immediately available with prescriptive refills. Frequent contact with the diabetes nurse or diabetes healthcare provider during insulin adjustments may reduce the incidence of hypoglycemia reactions.

Nocturnal hypoglycemia may be due to an excessive dose of intermediate acting insulin prior to dinner or the need for more carbohydrates and protein in a bedtime snack. The individual with diabetes may need to awaken at 2 or 3 A.M. to obtain a glucose measurement to determine the exact response to insulin manipulation so adjustments can be made accordingly. Nocturnal hypoglycemia should be treated aggressively to prevent the development of more serious sequelae. Nocturnal hypoglycemia accounts for over 50% of all episodes of severe hypoglycemia and may be due in part to patients not awakening to early warning signs (Levandoski, Santiago, & White, 1993).

Pregnant women with pregestational diabetes are asked to perform ketone checks daily from the first voided urine and when blood glucose levels exceed 180 mg/dL. Evidence of ketones in the urine should be reported to their healthcare provider. Women with nausea and vomiting are instructed on "sick day" management, which replaces carbohydrates normally ingested in solid form with liquids and soft foods containing an equal amount of carbohydrates. Written instructions for sick day management should be provided. During these periods, women may need to check their blood glucose levels more frequently. Hospitalization will be required for women who become dehydrated or are unable to eat for prolonged periods of time due to the risk of development of hypoglycemia or ketoacidosis. Infection is the primary cause of diabetic ketoacidosis, so women are instructed to observe and report promptly any signs and symptoms of infection. Stress in pregnant women with diabetes may also result in elevations in blood glucose. Intensive management may be a source of stress for the woman, so that frequent evaluation of the woman's adaptation to the diabetic program should be explored to identify these feelings, allowing ventilation. Family support and support from healthcare providers gives an important source of motivation and satisfaction for women involved in intensive diabetic management. Pregnant women with Types 1 and 2 diabetes will probably require more frequent contact with the diabetes nurse, sometimes as often as every other day for guidance with insulin adjustments and to evaluate the response to adjustments. Well-controlled diabetic gravidas may only need weekly contact to review blood glucose values.

Insulin Therapy

If diet therapy and exercise fail to control maternal glycemia in gestational diabetes, then insulin therapy is begun after education for self-administration. Refer to Display 14-3 for educational guidelines for insulin therapy. This instruction can usually be done in an outpatient setting and does not require hospitalization. Human insulin should be used exclusively in pregnancy and during the reproductive years due to possible stimulation of anti-insulin antibodies that may cross the placenta and contribute to fetal macrosomia (Menon et al., 1990). Most women with gestational diabetes can be controlled with 1–2 injections daily of a mixed dose of an intermediate acting insulin (NPH or lente) and a short acting insulin (regular). Education should include a discussion of the types of insulin with duration and peak of action of the types to be used. The importance of eating meals and snacks to avoid hypoglycemia should be stressed. If regular insulin is given, women are instructed to eat 30 minutes later. Women with GDM should be educated about how to check their insulin bottles for the expiration date and to discard any bottles that have any clumping, frosting, precipitation, or change in clarity or color. They should be taught to store unused bottles in the refrigerator and to use open bottles within 30 days. Site selection and rotation should be discussed. Most gestational diabetics can use the abdomen exclusively in pregnancy, avoiding a 2-inch area surrounding the umbilicus. Absorption from the abdomen is the most rapid and most consistent, followed by the arms, thighs, and buttocks. Arms and thighs should not be used on a day that these limbs will be exercised. One region should be used before going to the next region even in the abdomen, such as upper or lower. For women who are visually impaired or who are very afraid of needles, a pen device with insulin-containing cartridges can be used. Jet injectors may be used also but are considerably more expensive and cause some discomfort at the site. Hands should be washed prior to each injection. Good hygiene precludes the need for alcohol cleansing of the skin. Alcohol that has been used to cleanse the skin should be allowed to air dry to avoid stinging with injection. Alcohol should, however, be used to cleanse the tops of the insulin bottles. Insulin should be rolled gently in the hand to mix and not shaken to prevent bubbles from forming inside the bottle. Women need to learn the technique for correctly drawing up mixed-dose insulins. Syringes that the patient can read easily should be used. The markings on the 50-unit and 30-unit insulin syringes may be too small for some women to see, requiring the use of devices that magnify the markings. The markings on the 100-unit syringe are larger and may be adequate for interpretation. Aspiration at the site is not necessary. The site should not be massaged after injection. If the site bleeds, mild pressure should be applied and the blood glucose should be checked more frequently due to increased or decreased

absorption of the insulin. Women on insulin therapy should be taught the signs and symptoms of hypoglycemia and appropriate treatment although hypoglycemic reactions are rare in gestational diabetes who are compliant. Disposal of syringes and lancets should be in a puncture-resistant disposable container. The appropriate disposal of needles should be determined by contacting the local trash disposal authorities. The educational session ends when the woman with gestational diabetes demonstrates correct technique for drawing up and administering insulin. Contact with the diabetes nurse should occur within 2 days of insulin therapy initiation and then weekly for insulin adjustments unless untoward reactions are occurring or dosing adjustments are needed more frequently. Written materials that review the information covered in the education session alleviate anxiety and provide a resource for review.

Women with Type 2 diabetes usually require two insulin injections daily to normalize blood glucose levels. Three to four injections daily may be required to control blood glucose in pregnant women with Type 1 diabetes. Institution of intensive insulin therapy may require hospitalization for women who have been in poor control. During hospitalization, intensive assessment and correction of knowledge deficits should be incorporated into care in preparation for home self-monitoring. Most women are willing to incorporate intensive management of diabetes into their care due to the desire for a healthy baby. Those women who are well controlled or who have been in a preconception program may be managed on an outpatient basis. Hypoglycemia can be a serious complication of intensive insulin management. Untoward effects in the fetus from maternal hypoglycemia have not been demonstrated (Steel, Johnston, & Hepburn, 1990). Pattern management is encouraged rather than treating elevations after the fact. Insulin requirements will increase as gestation progresses as the levels of placental contra-insulin hormones rise. Insulin requirements in the first trimester (0.7 U/kg of ideal body weight) may be lower due to fetal siphoning of glucose and nausea and vomiting. The second trimester usually requires 0.8 U/kg dosing, increasing to 0.9 U/kg in the third trimester (Homko & Khandelwal, 1996). If insulin requirements decrease dramatically in the third trimester, fetal/placental compromise should be suspected and monitored very closely (Miller, 1994). When a very high dosage of insulin is required (>100 U/daily), glycemic control will best be achieved by using multiple injections initially. Intensive insulin therapy usually consists of more than two injections of insulin daily. Possible combinations of regimens include:

- short- and intermediate-acting insulin prebreakfast and predinner
- short-acting insulin before each meal plus intermediate insulin at bedtime
- short- and intermediate-acting insulin before breakfast plus short-acting insulin before dinner plus intermediate-acting insulin at bedtime
- long-acting insulin at bedtime and short-acting insulin before each meal and at bedtime (Miller, 1994)

Continuous Subcutaneous Insulin Infusion (CSII)

When multi-injection regimens fail to achieve glycemic control in very motivated and compliant women, the subcutaneous insulin infusion pump can be an option. The pump is programmed to deliver basal rates of buffered regular insulin to control the blood glucose during a given time over 24 hours. Multiple basal rates can be programmed. Boluses are given for meals and snacks based on preprandial blood glucose values and the number of carbohydrates to be consumed. The use of the pump in pregnancy is controversial because pregnancy is ketosis-prone. Pump malfunction could lead to the rapid development of diabetic ketoacidosis. The use of the pump also requires more frequent blood glucose checks (6–8 times daily) and nocturnal checks to assure pump function. Women who are using the pump prior to pregnancy may continue do so with pregnancy if they are willing to accept the increased demands for glucose testing to assure their safety.

FETAL SURVEILLANCE AND TIMING OF DELIVERY

Specific guidelines are lacking for the most appropriate methods or gestational age to begin fetal assessment of diabetic pregnancies. Most caregivers begin antenatal testing in the third trimester when the risk of perinatal mortality is greatest. Fetal death in the final weeks of pregnancy has been associated with poor glycemic control, hydramnios, and fetal macrosomia (Landon & Gabbe, 1996). Fetal demise may occur at an earlier gestational age in diabetic women with vascular disease, preeclampsia, or intrauterine growth retardation (Landon & Gabbe, 1996).

The easiest and most convenient method of fetal assessment is daily fetal movement counting where the mother counts fetal movements after a meal. The test is considered reactive if the fetus moves 10 times in a 2-hour period. Fetal movement counting can be started at 28 weeks in women with pregestational diabetes or in women with GDM who have complications such as hypertension but is almost always used adjunctively with other testing.

The nonstress test (NST) is the most frequently used screening test for evaluating fetal well-being in diabetic gravidas. Women with poorly controlled diabetes or with vascular complications may have testing started weekly at 28 weeks and twice weekly at 32 weeks. Women with diet-controlled gestational diabetes (A1) may not require testing until 40 weeks if there are no complications and they have been well controlled. Insulin-dependent gestational diabetics (A2) should undergo twice weekly testing at 32 weeks gestation without complications and at 28 weeks with complications. The American College of Obstetricians and Gynecologist (ACOG) recommends initiating a program of fetal surveillance during the third trimester with the timing and frequency based on the degree of risk present (ACOG, 1994). A nonreactive NST requires further testing, usually a contraction stress test or a biophysical profile.

Diabetic women (Types 1 and 2) who have been well controlled without complications and with reassuring antenatal testing may safely await delivery until 39 weeks gestation in well-dated pregnancies. Women with gestational diabetes mellitus who have maintained euglycemia and have not developed complications may await spontaneous labor, although most will be electively delivered by 41 weeks gestation. Those women with vascular disease who have worsening hypertension, intrauterine growth retardation, or nonreassuring fetal testing warrant early delivery. Delivery prior to 39 weeks carries a risk of delivering an infant with immature lungs, therefore most physicians opt for amniocentesis and lung maturity studies before induction of labor or cesarean section. Poor metabolic control or history of stillbirth are also indications for amniocentesis and scheduled delivery. Suspected macrosomia as an indication for delivery is controversial and contributes to the high cesarean section rate (50%) in women with diabetes (Landon & Gabbe, 1996).

INTRAPARTUM MANAGEMENT

When the pregnant diabetic is admitted in spontaneous labor or for elective delivery, attention should be directed at the maternal and fetal condition. A thorough history should be obtained that includes information regarding overall glucose control, episodes of hypoglycemia or ketoacidosis, and vascular complications of diabetes such as retinopathy, nephropathy, hypertension, or neuropathy. The current diabetic regimen should be reviewed and timing of last meal and last insulin injection recorded, noting the expected insulin peak. The glucose level that induces hypoglycemic reactions should also be recorded. Women with diabetes should not receive anything by mouth during labor or induction due to the higher risk of operative delivery. Intravenous access should be established early to allow for prompt treatment of hypoglycemia and to administer insulin when necessary. Maintenance of euglycemia extends into the intrapartum period to prevent neonatal hypoglycemia. The pregnant woman with diabetes needs to know how her diabetes will be managed during labor and any concerns she may have should be addressed soon after

admission. Blood glucose should be checked on admission and then every 1–2 hours with the initial value correlated to a laboratory determined glucose. Intravenous regular insulin is begun when blood glucose levels reach 120 mg/dL via a controlled infusion device piggybacked into a primary line. The primary intravenous solution should be 0.9% sodium chloride with a glucose-containing solution as the secondary line with an infusion rate based on blood glucose values. For prehydration for conduction anesthesia or for boluses for treatment of hypotension or fetal heart rate abnormalities, the nonglucose containing solution should be infused to avoid the development of maternal hyperglycemia.

The prenatal record should be reviewed, noting abnormal laboratory values that might be evidence of pregnancy-induced hypertension. The Hgb A1c value or glycosylated hemoglobin will provide an indicator of overall glucose control for the 4–6 weeks preceding the determination. The initial prenatal vital signs should be compared to current vital signs noting any significant increase in the blood pressure. Examination of previous ultrasound findings may reveal evidence of hydramnios or fetal macrosomia. Women with hydramnios are at increased risk for fetal cord prolapse with rupture of the membranes. Evidence of fetal macrosomia should alert the nurse to be prepared for shoulder dystocia at delivery. Labor aberrations such as arrest of descent or secondary uterine inertia may be early indications of cephalopelvic disproportion associated with macrosomia.

Continuous fetal monitoring should be initiated on admission and observed for patterns associated with uteroplacental insufficiency. The left lateral recumbent position should be maintained as much as possible to improve uterine perfusion. Neonatal resuscitative supplies should be immediately available and a neonatal team called when indicated.

Many women with diabetes will be electively induced. Cervical ripening may be indicated for those with unfavorable Bishop scores. Oxytocin administration should follow appropriate protocols (see Display 14-4, "Protocol for the Nursing Management of the Intrapartum Woman with

Insulin-Dependent Diabetes). Oxytocin administration requires a separate solution and infusion device when concomitantly administered with insulin.

Maintenance of euglycemia (60–120 mg/dL) continues into the intrapartum period with the goal of providing maternal nutrition during labor and preventing neonatal hypoglycemia. Women who are well controlled antenatally usually do not need insulin during labor. Blood glucose levels should be checked every 1–2 hours with a calibrated and quality-control-verified meter. Insulin should be started and titrated according to the institution's algorithm when blood glucose exceeds 110 mg/dL. Some women with Type 1 diabetes will need intravenous insulin on admission for spontaneous labor. (See Display 14-5.) They should have nothing by mouth in labor due to the higher risk for operative delivery. The American College of Obstetricians and Gynecologists recommends beginning insulin at 1 U/hr for blood glucose values of 100–140 mg/dL, 1.5 U/hr for glucose levels of 141–180 mg/dL, 2.0 U/hr for glucose values of 181–220 mg/dl, and 2.5 U/hr for values >220 (ACOG, 1994). Some institutions use dosages that are much higher. Regardless of the insulin algorithm, the key is close monitoring of glucose levels in labor. The concentration of the insulin mixture is also based on institution protocol. When a woman with diabetes is admitted in spontaneous labor, her last insulin dose should be ascertained to determine when the peak will occur. During the expected peak time, blood glucose levels should be checked more closely monitoring for evidence of hypoglycemia. Glucose, when administered to women with diabetes during labor, should be considered a medication and be administered via a controlled infusion device piggybacked into a primary line of nonglucose solution (0.9% sodium chloride). When boluses of fluid are indicated such as prehydration for an epidural, a nonglucose solution should be used. Insulin solutions, utilizing regular insulin only, are also titrated via a controlled infusion device.

The woman with Type 1 diabetes who is scheduled for a cesarean section or induction should be scheduled early in the day, omitting the morning dose of insulin. Glucose and insulin should be instituted according to the intrapartum protocol. Women with gestational diabetes, Type 2, or well-controlled Type 1, diabetes may not need insulin for a scheduled cesarean section. Blood glucose levels should be monitored closely and insulin or glucose begun as indicated. Induction of labor is managed in much the same way as scheduled cesarean sections by withholding the morning insulin dose, using glucose and insulin during the induction as indicated.

POSTPARTUM MANAGEMENT

Insulin requirements drop dramatically with delivery of the placenta when placental contra-insulin hormones are no longer being produced. Insulin infusions should be discontinued immediately after delivery to avoid profound hypoglycemia. Oral intake should be initiated as soon as possible. Insulin should be resumed when fasting blood glucose levels are >110 mg/dL and 2 hours postprandial levels exceed 150–180 mg/dL. When blood glucose values are abnormal, oral hypoglycemics should be reinstituted for women who were controlled by these drugs pregestationally. Women with gestational diabetes require blood glucose testing after delivery. If the woman has required insulin during pregnancy for achievement of euglycemia, the blood glucose should be checked on the day of delivery and the following day. If insulin is required, the woman should be considered a diabetic and managed with diet, oral hypoglycemics and insulin as required. If the woman had diet-controlled gestational diabetes, she should be evaluated at 6 weeks postpartum for Type 2 diabetes if she is not breastfeeding.

For women with Type 1 diabetes, the insulin infusion should be discontinued immediately after delivery. Blood glucose should be checked every 4 hours if NPO or preprandial if on a regular diet. Subcutaneous insulin should be initiated as indicated by blood glucose values. Tight glycemic control is no longer necessary although some women with pregestational diabetes may have difficulty reverting to prepregnancy

DISPLAY 14-4

Protocol for the Nursing Management of the Intrapartum Woman with Insulin-Dependent Diabetes

PURPOSE
To outline the nursing priorities and care specific to the intrapartum woman with insulin-dependent diabetes.

LEVEL
Interdependent

SUPPORTIVE DATA
Maternal morbidity and mortality are increased in the presence of Type 1 or Type 2 diabetes mellitus. The fetus is at risk for congenital anomalies, intrauterine fetal demise, macrosomia, intrauterine growth retardation, and hypoglycemia, and the mother with diabetes is at risk for infections, diabetic ketoacidosis, accelerated hypoglycemia, operative delivery, and postpartum hemorrhage. Achievement of euglycemia during the intrapartum period may decrease fetal and maternal complications.

CONTENT

Insulin Adminstration

1. Induction of labor and scheduled cesarean section.
    a. Withold usual insulin dosage and diet on the morning of the scheduled procedure.
    b. Intravenous solution of 5% dextrose to be infused at 125 ml/ hour if blood glucose <100 mg/dL. Use 0.9% normal saline if blood glucose >140 mg/dL (ACOG, 1994).
    c. Begin insulin infusion if blood glucose level >120 mg/dL or if patient using a subcutanous insulin infusion pump, titrate based on blood glucose algorithm.

2. Spontaneous labor
    a. Withhold insulin dosage.
    b. Patient must not have anything orally.
    c. Note time and type of last insulin injection being alert to peak action.
    d. Intravenous solution of 5% dextrose to be infused at 125 ml/hour with active labor or for blood glucose levels of <100 mg/dL. Use normal saline for blood glucose levels of >140 mg/dL.
    e. Begin insulin infusion if blood glucose level is >120 mg/dL.
    f. Continue subcutaneous insulin infusion pump titrated to blood glucose.

3. Prepare insulin infusion as specified in "Procedure for Intravenous Insulin Administration," Display 14-5.

4. Intravenous insulin dosage is titrated to patient's blood glucose values.

5. Intravenous insulin infusion is discontinued prior to delivery to decrease the incidence of postpartum hypoglycemia.

6. Dextrose 50% is maintained at the bedside in the event of profound hypoglycemia.

DISPLAY 14-4 (continued)

Nursing Assessments

1. Assess maternal vital signs hourly unless condition or stage of labor indicate otherwise.
2. Assess temperature every 4 hours.
3. Maintain hourly intake and output.
4. Assess urine for ketones
   a. Hourly if indwelling catheter is inserted.
   b. At every void without an indwelling catheter.
5. Examine skin over insulin injection sites noting the following:
   a. Bruising
   b. Areas of hypertrophy.
   c. Signs of inflammation or cellulitis
6. Examine feet noting the following:
   a. Lesions
   b. Ulcers
   c. Lower extremity pulses
   d. Level of sensation
7. Assess for signs and symptoms of urinary tract infection or upper respiratory infection.

Blood Glucose Monitoring

1. Assess blood glucose level on admission.
2. Review patient's home blood glucose monitoring record to assess baseline values and evaluate trends and individual responses.
3. When the patient has nothing orally, check blood glucose level every 2 hours.
4. When the patient is receiving intravenous insulin, check blood glucose level hourly.
5. Assess blood glucose level if signs and symptoms of hypoglycemia occur.

Fetal Monitoring

1. Initiate fetal heart rate monitoring.
2. Encourage lateral recumbent position to increase uterine perfusion.
3. Refer to "Guidelines for Fetal Heart Rate Monitoring," pages 414–416.

Complications

1. Monitor for signs and symptoms of hypoglycemia.
   a. Cold, clammy skin
   b. Shaking
   c. Sweating
   d. Mental confusion or anxiety
   e. Light-headedness
   f. Pallor
   g. Numbness of tongue or lips
2. Monitor for signs and symptoms of diabetic ketoacidosis.
   a. Blood glucose of >300 mg/dL
   b. Presence of ketonuria
   c. Altered level of consciousness
   d. Kussmaul's respirations
   e. Acetone breath

DISPLAY 14-4 (continued)

NURSING INTERVENTIONS

Hypoglycemia

1. If the patient is symptomatic, obtain blood glucose, discontinue insulin infusion, and notify physician.

2. If blood glucose value is 60 mg/dL, initiate treatment.

3. Treatment of hypoglycemia
   a. For the conscious patient taking food by mouth:
      *Give 10–15 grams of carbohydrate such as 8 oz. of skim milk, or 1/2 cup of fruit juice or other snack such as 4 peanut butter or cheese crackers.
      *If hypoglycemia occurs preceding a meal, serve meal immediately.
      *Recheck blood glucose in 15 minutes.
      *If blood glucose level is still <60 mg/dL. give another 15 grams of carbohydrate.
   b. For the conscious patient who must have nothing orally, but who is receiving 5% dextrose intravenously, do the following:
      *Administer 300 ml of 5% dextrose over 10–15 minutes.
      *Recheck blood glucose level after administering bolus.
   c. For the unconscious patient, do the following:
      *Notify physician.
      *Administer 10 ml 50% dextrose over 5 minutes. Subsequent doses may be necessary.
      *Blood pressure, pulse, and respirations must be taken every 5 minutes until stable.
      *Recheck blood glucose level every 5–15 minutes until >80 mg/dL.

Diabetic Ketoacidosis

1. Obtain values of blood glucose and urine ketones and notify physician.

2. Establish clear airway.
   a. Administer oxygen at 8–10 liters/minute via a nonrebreathing face mask.
   b. Obtain arterial blood gases.
   c. Anticipate need for intubation and mechanical ventilation.
   d. Apply pulse oximeter to monitor oxygen saturations and titrate oxygen to maintain saturations of 95%.

3. Insert indwelling catheter and obtain urine for culture and sensitivity.

4. Discontinue beta agonists if being administered and withold corticosteroids if ordered.

5. Begin fluid resuscitation. The usual recommended schedule includes the following:
   a. Administer 1000–2000 ml of normal saline over the first hour as ordered by the physician.
   b. Decrease fluids to 200–250 ml/hour.
      *If sodium level is <155 mEq/liter, use 0.9% sodium chloride and if >155 mEq/liter, use 0.45% sodium chloride.
      *If blood glucose level is 200 mg/dL or less, use 5% dextrose.
   c. Anticipate need for invasive hemodynamic monitoring.
   d. Assess for signs or symptoms of pulmonary edema.
      *dyspnea
      *tachypnea
      *wheezing
      *cough (with or without frothy sputum) or "tickle in throat"

DISPLAY 14-4 (continued)

   e. Assess for hypovolemia
      *decrease in blood pressure
      *increase in pulse rate
      *urine output <30 ml/hour
      *slow capillary refill
      *decrease in central venous and pulmonary capillary wedge pressure if monitoring is initiated

6. Begin intravenous insulin infusion concomitantly with fluid resuscitation per physician order. The usual recommended dose is the following:
   a. 10–20 U regular insulin bolus intravenously.
   b. Follow with 5–10 U per hour.
   c. If blood glucose has not fallen by 10% in first hour, double the dosage of insulin.
   d. If blood glucose level is <200 mg/dL, decrease insulin dose to 1–2 U per hour.
   e. Intravenous insulin dosage is titrated to blood glucose level.
   f. Monitor blood glucose every 15–20 minutes.
   g. Monitor for signs and symptoms of hypoglycemia.
   h. Monitor for signs and symptoms of cerebral edema (especially if blood glucose level has decreased at a rate >75–100 mg/dL hour).
      *headache
      *vomiting
      *deteriorating mental status
      *widening of pulse pressure due to rise in intracranial pressure
      *bradycardia
      *sluggish pupillary light reflex
   i. Notify physician of signs and symptoms of cerebral edema or hypoglycemia immediately.

7. Apply cardiac monitor and assess for the following:
   a. ST segment depression
   b. Inverted T waves
   c. Appearance of U waves after T waves

8. Monitor serum potassium levels.
   a. Anticipate need for potassium replacement for <3.0 mEq/L.
   b. Potassium replacement is discontinued if urinary output is <40 ml/hour.

9. Monitor serum bicarbonate levels.
   a. Anticipate need for intravenous bicarbonate if pH is <7.10.
   b. The usual recommended dose is 44 mEq sodium bicarbonate over 2 hours.

methods of care and loosening of control. Intravenous glucose should be continued until oral intake is resumed. The sooner the mother is fed, the sooner the return to a prepregnancy state with a decrease in insulin requirements. The insulin dose after delivery is usually 50–60% of the end of pregnancy dose or 0.4–0.6 U/kg daily based on postpartum weight. The caloric requirements for women with pregestational diabetes should be recalculated in the postpartum period and adjustments for breastfeeding made. Women with Type 1 diabetes are encour-

DISPLAY 14-4 (continued)

10. Obtain blood, urine, and sputum cultures as ordered.

11. Administer antibiotics as ordered.

12. Ensure that resuscitative equipment is immediately available.

DOCUMENTATION

1. Pertinent maternal and fetal assessments.

2. Initiation of protocols used in patient care.

3. All nursing and medical interventions and patient's response.

4. Insulin dosage in units per hour.

5. Initial and subsequent insulin dosages, as well as times of dosage changes.

6. Time, indication, and results of glucose monitoring.

7. Physician notification including indication and response.

REFERENCES

ACOG. (1994). Diabetes and pregnancy. ACOG Technical Bulletin, No. 200.

AWHONN. (1993). Didactic content and clinical skills verification for professional nurse providers of basic, high-risk, and critical care intrapartum nursing. Washington, DC: AWHONN.

Chauhan, S. P., & Perry, G. P. (1995). Management of diabetic ketoacidosis in the obstetric patient. Obstetrics and Gynecology Clinics of North America, 22(1), 143–155.

Harvey, M. G. (1992). Diabetic ketoacidosis during pregnancy. Journal of Perinatal and Neonatal Nursing, 6(1), 1-13.

Homko, C. J., & Khandelwal, M. (1996). Glucose monitoring and insulin therapy during pregnancy. Obstetrics and Gynecology Clinics of North America, 23(1), 47–75.

Luzi, L, Barrett, E. J., Groop, L. C., Ferrannini, E., & DeFonzo, R. A. (1988). Metabolic effect of low-dose insulin therapy on glucose metabolism in DKA. Diabetes, 36, 1470–1477.

Miller, E. H. (1994). Management of diabetes in pregnancy. Seminars in Perinatology, 18 (5), 414–431.

Rodgers, B. D., & Rodgers, D. E. (1991). Clinical variables associated with diabetic ketoacidosis during pregnancy. Journal of Reproductive Medicine, 36, 797–799.

Whiteman, V. E., Homko, C. J., & Reece, E. A. (1996). Mangement of hypoglycemia and diabetic ketoacidosis in pregnancy. Obstetric and Gynecology Clinics of North America, 23, 87–107.

aged to breastfeed but must be alert to signs and symptoms of hypoglycemia and may need to eat a snack prior to breastfeeding to prevent occurrence of hypoglycemia.

Postpartum care of the newly delivered diabetic woman should include close observation of vaginal bleeding due to the increased risk of postpartum hemorrhage particularly in women who have had large infants, prolonged labors, or polyhydramnios. The incidence of puerperal infection is higher in diabetic women so nurses should be alert to signs and symptoms of infection in the postpartum period (Jacobson & Cousins, 1989).

Early infant contact may allay fears and anxieties the mother may have regarding her infant's well-being. Breastfeeding is encouraged in Types 1 and 2 diabetes, and GDM with appropriate dietary adjustments made for lactation. Nurses should be alert to signs and symptoms of hypoglycemia during or after breastfeeding in women with pregestational diabetes who are insulin dependent. A snack prior to feeding time may help avoid the development of hypoglycemia.

Glucose intolerance in women with GDM persists for a variable period of time after delivery. High body mass index and higher fasting blood glucose values in women with previous GDM are factors associated with diabetes that persist after delivery (Coustan, Carpenter, O'Sullivan, & Carr, 1993). Women with previous GDM should have a 75-gram, 2-hour oral glucose tolerance test (OGTT) at their 6-week postpartum check-up (ADA, 1996; Metzger, 1991). Lactation may affect the results of the OGTT, so the test should be delayed until after weaning in women who are breastfeeding. The diagnosis of diabetes is based on a FBS >126 mg/dL on two occasions or a 1–2 hour value >200 mg/dL (ADA, 1997). During the postpartum examination, women with previous GDM should be advised of the 50% risk for development of GDM in subsequent pregnancies and encouraged to obtain early prenatal care. Ideally, women with previous GDM should be tested for diabetes prior to conception to allow for preconception care in those with overt disease. Women with a history of GDM have a 50–75% risk of developing overt diabetes in 10–15 years after the index pregnancy (O'Sullivan, 1991). This risk may be reduced by attaining and maintaining ideal body weight.

The importance of preconception care and glycemic control to reduce the incidence of spontaneous abortion and congenital defects should be stressed at the postpartum visit. Contraceptive options should be explored and a joint decision made about an appropriate and acceptable method of birth control. When pregnancy is being considered, contraception should be continued until the woman with pre-existing diabetes can have her diabetes evaluated and receive appropriate preconception care.

DIABETIC KETOACIDOSIS

Diabetic ketoacidosis (DKA) is a potentially life-threatening complication of uncontrolled diabetes. The development of DKA is more common in pregnant women with overt diabetes (1.73%) than in women with gestational diabetes (0.7%) (Kilvert, Nicholson, & Wright, 1993). Improved glycemic control has decreased the incidence of DKA in diabetic gravidas regardless of type. Significant morbidity and mortality for both mother and fetus occur as a result of DKA. Fetal loss, which includes spontaneous abortion and intrauterine fetal death with maternal DKA, has been reported as high as 22% (Kilvert, Nicholson, & Wright, 1993). Prevention of DKA with intensive management is the treatment goal for care of women with diabetes during pregnancy.

Ketoacidosis occurs as a result of insulin deficiency, which causes excess plasma glucose, inadequate glucose uptake by the periphery, and enhanced gluconeogenesis (glycogen conversion to glucose). Osmotic diuresis accompanies hyperglycemia (>300 mg/dL) resulting in significant urinary losses of potassium, sodium, and water. As alternate substrates are utilized for energy production such as lipolysis, hepatic oxidation of fatty acids increases the formation of ketone bodies. Due to the decreased buffering capacity of pregnancy, ketoacids will quickly overwhelm the maternal system.

Predisposing factors for the development of diabetic ketoacidosis in pregnancy are placental production of insulin antagonists, lowered buffering capacity, and accelerated starvation. Development of DKA in pregnancy usually occurs secondarily as a result of infection, stress, emesis, dehydration, steroid administration, and the use of adrenergic agonists in the treatment of preterm labor. Infections, particularly of the urinary tract, are the most common cause of DKA in pregnancy (Harvey, 1992). Poor compliance with the diabetic regimen has also been noted as a contributory factor in DKA as well as subcutaneous insulin infusion pump failure (Rodgers & Rodgers, 1991).

The clinical presentation of DKA in pregnancy includes vomiting, anorexia, abdominal pain,

DISPLAY 14-5

Procedure for Intravenous Insulin Administration

PURPOSE
To outline nursing responsibility in the safe adminstration of insulin by continuous infusion.

SUPPORTIVE DATA
Infants of women with diabetes are at risk for development of neonatal hypoglycemia. Euglycemia during the intrapartum period may decrease the incidence and severity of neonatal hypoglycemia. Continuous insulin is titrated to the patient's blood glucose level during the intrapartum period. The usual dosage for intravenous insulin is 0.25–2.5 U/hour to maintain a blood glucose level of 60–110 mg/dL. Continuous insulin infusion is also administered for diabetic ketoacidosis. The usual insulin infusion rate is 5–10 U/hour of regular insulin with an initial bolus of 10–20 U.

EQUIPMENT
Intravenous fluids as prescribed   Infusion pump
Regular insulin   Appropricte intravenous tubing

PROCEDURE	KEY POINTS
1. Prepare equipment.	
a. Check physician's order for correct drug, dosage, route, and intravenous fluid.	A physician's order is necessary to initiate infusion.
b. A primary line for infusion of an appropriate intravenous maintenance solution should be established.	A primary line is necessary to maintain intravenous access should intravenous insulin be discontinued.
c. Obtain regular insulin from the the pharmacy, add medication, and label bag with date, dosage, time, and signature of registered nurse.	Regular insulin is added to normal saline to produce a concentration of 1 cc normal saline = 1 U regular insulin. (100 U regular insulin added to 100 ml normal saline)
d. Place insulin solution on an infusion pump and flush 50 ml of solution through cassette or tubing and discard.	An infusion pump is required to ensure accurate flow rate and precise titration of intravenous insulin. Flushing the tubing allows the insulin binding sites on polyvinylchloride tubing to become saturated, preventing the admixture from being robbed of insulin during infusion.

DISPLAY 14-5 (continued)

PROCEDURE	KEY POINTS
e. Piggyback insulin into primary intravenous line at the port closest to patient.	Insulin is easily titrated according to blood glucose levels if administered via a secondary line, rather than added to the mainline intravenous solution. Other medications may be given through the distal port without altering the insulin infusion flow rate.
f. Ensure that 50% dextrose is available at the bedside.	In the event severe hypoglycemia occurs, 50% dextrose is administered.
2. Prepare patient. a. Identify patient by name and identification band and check for allergies.	
b. Assess patient's level of understanding and acceptance of procedure. c. Explain procedure, equipment, and nursing care involved to patient and significant others.	Individualized patient teaching is necessary to meet the needs of the patient and family for information and emotional support.
d. Review signs and symptoms of hypo- and hyperglycemia and instruct patient to notify nursing staff of any of the following: shaking, numbness of the tongue or lips; severe hunger; lightheadedness, cold, clammy skin; and nausea or vomiting.	The pregnant woman with diabetes is at risk for both diabetic ketoacidosis and accelerated hypoglycemia.

3. Perform baseline nursing assessments.
  a. Record patient's baseline temperature, pulse, respirations, and blood pressure.
  b. Baseline laboratory evaluations: blood glucose, urine ketones.
	Maternal and fetal baseline information is necessary to establish presence or absence of preexisting complications.

4. Begin insulin infusion. 5. Document primary and secondary line infusions. 6. Document initial dosage and time. 7. Continue care by initiating "Protocol for the Nursing Management of the Intrapartum Woman with Insulin-Dependent Diabetes," page 243.	Insulin must be documented in units per hour.

DISPLAY 14-5 (continued)

REFERENCES

ACOG. (1994). Diabetes and pregnancy. ACOG Technical Bulletin, No. 200.

AWHONN. (1993). Didactic content and clinical skills verification for professional nurse providers of basic, high-risk, and critical care intrapartum nursing. Washington, DC: AWHONN.

Chauhan, S. P., & Perry, G. P. (1995). Management of diabetic ketoacidosis in the obstetric patient. Obstetrics and Gynecology Clinics of North America, 22(1), 143–155.

Harvey, M. G. (1992). Diabetic ketoacidosis during pregnancy. Journal of Perinatal and Neonatal Nursing, 6(1), 1–13.

Homko, C. J., & Khandelwal, M. (1996). Glucose monitoring and insulin therapy during pregnancy. Obstetrics and Gynecology Clinics of North America, 23(1), 47–75.

Luzi, L, Barrett, E. J., Groop, L. C., Ferrannini, E., & DeFonzo, R.A. (1988). Metabolic effect of low-dose insulin therapy on glucose metabolism in DKA. Diabetes, 36, 1470–1477.

Miller, E. H. (1994). Management of diabetes in pregnancy. Seminars in Perinatology, 18 (5), 414–431.

Rodgers, B. D., & Rodgers, D. E. (1991). Clinical variables associated with diabetic ketoacidosis during pregnancy. Journal of Reproductive Medicine, 36, 797-799.

Whiteman, V. E., Homko, C. J., & Reece, E. A. (1996). Mangement of hypoglycemia and diabetic ketoacidosis in pregnancy. Obstetric and Gynecology Clinics of North America, 23, 87–107.

polyuria, and polydipsia. Clinical symptoms of acidosis include weakness, malaise, headache, and hyperventilation. Kussmaul respirations develop as a result of the body attempting to correct the metabolic acidosis by reducing the level of carbon dioxide. A fruity odor to the breath indicates large amounts of acetone in the blood. The diagnosis of DKA is confirmed based on laboratory findings of plasma glucose >300 mg/dL (although DKA can develop in pregnancy at levels much lower), an arterial pH of <7.3, and plasma bicarbonate level below 15 mEq/L (Kitabchi, Young, Sacks, & Morris, 1979). The hematocrit and urea nitrogen levels are usually elevated due to dehydration. The leukocyte count may also be elevated even in the absence of infection as a result of dehydration, hemoconcentration, and the increase in cortisol and catecholamine levels (Whiteman, Homko, & Reece, 1996). Due to this, band neutrophil elevation should be used as an indicator of infection.

Prompt diagnosis and aggressive management of DKA is indicated to reduce the adverse perinatal outcomes. Immediate goals for therapy are correction of dehydration, hyperglycemia, and electrolyte imbalance. The fluid deficit in DKA may be as high as 10 liters. Peripheral access should be obtained with a large bore catheter. If this is too difficult, then placement of a central venous line or Swan-Ganz catheter becomes necessary to allow rapid administration of a high volume of fluid and hemodynamic monitoring. In the first hour, 1000–2000 milliliters (ml) of isotonic saline should be infused. The rate after that should be based on hemodynamic status but usually is 250–500 ml per hour. Hydration restores intravascular volume, allowing improved tissue perfusion and insulin delivery as well as lowering blood glucose due to the effects of hemodilution. When plasma glucose levels fall to 200–250 mg/dL, the saline infusion should be changed to a solution containing 5%

dextrose to prevent hypoglycemia which could result in cerebral edema.

A low-dose continuous infusion of 5–10 units (U) of regular insulin per hour is the recommended treatment regimen for DKA after a bolus of 10–20 U has been administered (Luzi, Barrett, Groop, Ferrannini, & DeFronzo, 1988). An infusion pump should be utilized to administer the insulin via a piggybacked line, which can be regulated without affecting the rate of fluid administration. If the serum glucose does not fall by 10% after the first hour, the insulin dosage should be doubled. Once the blood glucose reaches 200–250 mg/dL, the insulin infusion should be reduced and maintained at 1–2 U per hour and continued for 12–24 hours after the DKA resolves. A subcutaneous injection of regular insulin should be administered at least one hour prior to discontinuance of the insulin infusion (Whiteman, Homko, & Reece, 1996).

In women with anuria or oliguria, a foley catheter should be inserted to allow accurate determination of urine output. A urine specimen for urinalysis and culture should be obtained to rule out a urinary tract infection as the cause of DKA. Placement of a nasogastric tube to prevent aspiration with vomiting is necessary in the lethargic or comatose patient. A peripheral arterial catheter should be placed in severely acidotic women to allow frequent blood gas determinations and laboratory assessments. Oxygenation should be monitored continuously by a pulse oximeter and oxygen should be delivered via a nonrebreathing face mask to mantain oxygen saturations of 95% after the initial blood gas has been drawn. Continuous electrocardiographic (ECG) monitoring is necessary to detect changes associated with hypokalemia such as peak T waves (Chauhan & Perry, 1995). A falsely elevated serum potassium may be present on admission but as the acidosis resolves and glucose uptake of the cells improves, potassium rapidly shifts back into the cells leading to a serum deficit. Potassium replacement should be started after the potassium status is known and the patient has adequate urinary output. Potassium levels will need to be obtained serially during the course of treatment to avoid wide fluctuations of normal. Bicarbonate is

administered at a pH of 7.10 and discontinued when the pH reaches 7.20 (Whiteman, Homko, & Reece, 1996). Too aggressive alkalinization can interfere with oxygen delivery to the tissues and lead to alkalosis with more serious sequelae.

Continuous fetal monitoring during maternal DKA may reveal signs of a seriously compromised fetus. Nonreactive fetal heart rates, repetitive late decelerations, and tachycardia may denote fetal jeopardy but are not necessarily indications for immediate delivery, which could result in maternal deterioration. In utero resuscitation by stabilizing maternal hyperglycemia and metabolic acidosis, and improving hydration status usually resolve evidence of fetal compromise (Chauhan & Perry, 1995).

Preterm contractions may also accompany DKA in pregnancy. Beta adrenergics for treatment of preterm labor are contraindicated in DKA due to their anti-insulin activity (Rodgers & Rodgers, 1991). Hydration may resolve uterine activity but if required, magnesium sulfate is the tocolytic of choice for treatment of preterm labor in DKA. Corticosteroids to accelerate fetal lung maturity are also contraindicated in DKA because of the associated risk of hyperglycemia.

REFERENCES

Adams, M. M., Bruce, F. C., Shulman, H. B., Kendrick, J. S., & Brogan, D. J. (1993). The PRAMS Working Group: Pregnancy planning and preconception counseling. Obstetrics and Gynecology, 82, 955–959.

American Diabetes Association. (1995). Gestational diabetes mellitus [Position statement]. Diabetes Care, 18(Suppl. 1), 24–25.

American Diabetes Association. (1996). Preconception care of women with diabetes. Diabetes Care, 19(Suppl. 1), 525–528.

American Diabetes Association. (1997). Report of the expert committee on the diagnosis and classification of diabetes mellitus. Diabetes Care, 20, 1183–1197.

American Dietetic Association. (1993). Position of the American Dietetic Association: Use of nutritive and nonnutritive sweeteners. Journal of the American Dietetic Association, 93, 816–821.

Amiel, S. A., Sherwin, R. S., Simonson, D. C., & Tamborlane, W. V. (1988). Effect of intensive insulin therapy on glycemic thresholds for counterregulatory hormone release. Diabetes, 37, 901–907.

Artal, R., Wiswell, R., & Romen, Y. (1985). Hormonal response to exercise in diabetic and non-diabetic patients. Diabetes, 39 (Suppl. 2), 78–80.

Boden, G. (1996). Fuel metabolism in pregnancy and in gestational diabetes mellitus. Obstetrics and Gynecology Clinics of North America, 23, 1–10.

Bourbon, J. R., & Farrell, P. M. (1985). Fetal lung development in the diabetic pregnancy. Pediatric Research, 19, 253–267.

Buchanan, T. A., & Kitzmiller, J. L. (1994). Metabolic interactions of diabetes and pregnancy. Annual Review of Medicine, 45, 245–260.

Buchanan, T. A., Metzger, B. E., & Freinkel, N. (1990). Accelerated starvation in late pregnancy: A comparison between obese women with and without gestational diabetes mellitus. American Journal of Obstetrics and Gynecology, 162, 1015–1020.

Carr, S., Coustan, D. R., Martelly, P., Broscoe, F., & Rotondo, L. (1989). Precision of reflectance meters in screening for gestational diabetes. Obstetrics and Gynecology, 73, 727–731.

Carpenter, M. W. (1993). Metabolic changes in gestational diabetes. Clinics in Perinatology, 20, 583–591.

Carpenter, M. W., & Coustan, D. R. (1982). Criteria for screening tests for gestational diabetes. American Journal of Obstetrics and Gynecology, 144, 768–773.

Catalano, P. M., Tyzbir, E. D., Wolfe, R. R., Calles, J., Roman, N. M., Amini, S. B., & Sims, E. A. (1993). Carbohydrate metabolism during pregnancy in control subjects and women with gestational diabetes. American Journal of Physiology, 264, 60–67.

Chauhan, S. P., & Perry, K. G., Jr. (1995). Management of diabetic ketoacidosis in the obstetric patient. Obstetrics and Gynecology Clinics of North America, 22, 143–155.

Cordero, L., & Landon, M. B. (1993). Infant of the diabetic mother. Clinics in Perinatology, 20, 635–648.

Cousins, L., Rigg, L., Hollingsworth, D., Brink, G., Aurand, J., & Yen, S. S. (1980). The 24-hour excursion and diurnal rhythm of glucose, insulin, and C-peptide in normal pregnancy. American Journal of Obstetrics and Gynecology, 136, 483–488.

Coustan, D. R., Carpenter, M. W., O'Sullivan, P. S., & Carr, S. R. (1993). Gestational diabetes: Predictors of subsequent disordered glucose metabolism. American Journal of Obstetrics and Gynecology, 168, 1139–1145.

Cryer, P. E., & Gerich, J. E. (1990). Hypoglycemia in insulin dependent diabetes mellitus: Insulin excess and defective glucose counterregulation. In H. Rifkin & D. Porte, Jr. (Eds.), Ellenberg and Rifkin's diabetes mellitus: Theory and practice (pp. 526–546). New York: Elsevier.

Czeizel, A. E., & Dudas, I. (1992). Prevention of the first occurrence of neural tube defects by periconceptional vitamin supplementation. New England Journal of Medicine, 327, 1832–1835.

Diabetes and pregnancy. (1994). ACOG Technical Bulletin, No. 200.

Engelgau, M. M., Herman, W. H., Smith, P. J., German, R. R., & Aubert, R. E. (1995). The epidemiology of diabetes and pregnancy in the U.S., 1988. Diabetes Care, 18, 1029–1033.

Greene, M. F. (1993). Prevention and diagnosis of congenital anomalies in diabetic pregnancies. Clinics in Perinatology, 20, 533–547.

Hagay, Z. J. (1994). Diabetic ketoacidosis in pregnancy: Etiology, pathophysiology and management. Clinical Obstetrics and Gynecology, 37, 39–49.

Hagay, Z. J., & Reece, E. A. (1992). Diabetes mellitus in pregnancy. In E. A. Reece, J. C. Hobbins, M. J. Mahoney, & R. H. Petrie (Eds.), Medicine of the fetus and mother (pp. 982–1020). Philadelphia: Lippincott.

Hare, J. W. (1994). Diabetic complications of diabetic pregnancies. Seminars in Perinatology, 18, 451–458.

Harvey, M. G. (1992). Diabetic ketoacidosis during pregnancy. Journal of Perinatal and Neonatal Nursing, 6, 1–13.

Homko, C. J., & Khandelwal, M. (1996). Glucose monitoring and insulin therapy during pregnancy. Obstetrics and Gynecology Clinics of North America, 23, 47–74.

Jacobson, J. D., & Cousins, L. (1989). A population-based study of maternal and perinatal outcome in patients with gestational diabetes. American Journal of Obstetrics and Gynecology, 161, 981–986.

Jovanovic-Peterson, L. (1993). Medical management of pregnancy complicated by diabetes. Alexandria, VA: American Diabetes Association.

Kilvert, J. A., Nicholson, H. O., & Wright, A. D. (1993). Ketoacidosis in diabetic pregnancy. Diabetic Medicine, 10, 278–281.

Kitabchi, A. E., Young, R., Sacks, H., & Morris, L. (1979). Diabetic ketoacidosis: Reappraisal of therapeutic approach. Annual Review of Medicine, 30, 339–357.

Kitzmiller, J. L., & Combs, C. A. (1996). Diabetic nephropathy and pregnancy. Obstetrics and Gynecology Clinics of North America, 23, 173–203.

Kitzmiller, J. L., Gavin, L. A., Gin, G. D., Jovanovic-Peterson, L., Main, E. K., & Zigrang, W. D. (1991). Preconception care of diabetics: Glycemic control prevents congenital anomalies. Journal of the American Medical Association, 265, 731–736.

Klein, B. E., Moss, S. E., & Klein, R. (1990). Effect of pregnancy on progression of diabetic retinopathy. Diabetes Care, 13, 34–40.

Knopp, R. H., Magee, M. S., Raisys, V., Benedetti, T. J., & Bonet, B. (1991). Hypocaloric diets and ketogenesis in the management of obese gestational diabetic women. Journal of the American College of Nutrition, 10, 649–667.

Landon, M. B., & Gabbe, S. G. (1996). Fetal surveillance and timing of delivery in pregnancy complicated by diabetes mellitus. Obstetric and Gynecology Clinics of North America, 23, 109–123.

Landon, M. B., Gabbe, S. G., & Sachs, L. (1990). Management of diabetes mellitus and pregnancy: A survey of obstetricians and maternal-fetal specialists. Obstetrics and Gynecology, 75, 635-640.

Langer, O., Brustman, L., Anyaegbunam, A., & Mazze, R. (1987). The significance of one abnormal glucose tolerance test value on adverse outcome in pregnancy. American Journal of Obstetrics and Gynecology, 157, 758–763.

Lavin, J. P., Barden, T. P., & Miodovnik, M. (1981). Clinical experience with a screening program for gestational diabetes. American Journal of Obstetrics and Gynecology, 141, 491–494.

Lesser, K. B., & Carpenter, M. W. (1994). Metabolic changes associated with normal pregnancy and pregnancy complicated by diabetes mellitus. Seminars in Perinatology, 18, 399–406.

Levandoski, L. A., Santiago, J. V., & White, N. H. (1993). Hypoglycemia. In V. Peragallo-Dittko, K. Godley, & J. Meyer (Eds.), A core curriculum for diabetes education (pp. 349–372). Chicago: American Association of Diabetes Educators.

Lindsay, M. K., Graves, W., & Klein, L. (1989). The relationship of one abnormal glucose tolerance test value and pregnancy complications. Obstetrics and Gynecology, 73, 103–106.

Luzi, L., Barrett, E. J., Groop, L. C., Ferrannini, E., & DeFronzo, R. A. (1988). Metabolic effect of low-dose insulin therapy on glucose metabolism in diabetic ketoacidosis. Diabetes, 37, 1470–1477.

Magee, M. S., Knopp, R. H., & Benedetti, T. J. (1990). Metabolic effects of 1200 kcal. diet in obese pregnant women with gestational diabetes. Diabetes, 39, 234–240.

Management of diabetes in pregnancy. (1986, May). ACOG Technical Bulletin, No. 86.

Matheson, D., & Efantis, J. (1989). Diabetes and pregnancy: Need and use of intensive therapy. Diabetes Educator, 15, 242–248.

Marquette, G. P., Klein, V. R., & Niebyl, J. R. (1985). Efficacy of screening for gestational diabetes. American Journal of Perinatology, 2, 7–9.

Menon, R. K., Cohen, R. M., Sperling, M. A., Cutfield, W. S., Mimouni, F., & Khoury, J. C. (1990). Transplacental passage of insulin in pregnant women with insulin-dependent diabetes mellitus. Its role in fetal macrosomia. New England Journal of Medicine, 323, 309–315.

Mestman, J. H., & Schmidt-Sarosi, C. (1993). Diabetes mellitus and fertility control: Contraception management issues. American Journal of Obstetrics and Gynecology, 168, 2012–2020.

Metzger, B. E. (1991). Summary and recommendations of the Third International Workshop-

Conference on Gestational Diabetes Mellitus. Diabetes, 40(Suppl. 2), 197–201.

Miller, E. H. (1994). Metabolic management of diabetes in pregnancy. Seminars in Perinatology, 18, 414–431.

Miller, E., Hare, J. W., Cloherty, J. P., Dunn, P. J., Gleason, R. E., Soeldner, J. S., & Kitzmiller, J. L. (1981). Elevated maternal hemoglobin A1c in early pregnancy and major congenital anomalies in infants of diabetic mothers. New England Journal of Medicine, 304, 1331–1334.

National Diabetes Data Group (1979). Classification and diagnosis of diabetes mellitus and other categories of glucose intolerance. Diabetes, 28, 1039–1057.

Neiger, R., & Coustan, D. R. (1991). The role of repeat glucose tolerance tests in the diagnosis of gestational diabetes. American Journal of Obstetrics and Gynecology, 165, 787–790.

Neiger, R., & Kendrick, J. (1994). Obstetric management of diabetes in pregnancy. Seminars in Perinatology, 18, 432–450.

O'Sullivan, J. B. (1991). Diabetes mellitus after gestational diabetes mellitus. Diabetes, 40(Suppl. 2), 131–139.

O'Sullivan, J. B., & Mahan, C. M. (1964). Criteria for the oral glucose tolerance test in pregnancy. Diabetes, 13, 278–285.

Plovie, B. (1991). Diabetes in pregnancy (Series 2, Module 10). New York: March of Dimes.

Reece, E. A., Gabrielli, S., & Abdalla, M. (1988). The prevention of diabetes associated birth defects. Seminars in Perinatology, 12, 292–301.

Reece, E. A., & Homko, C. J. (1994) Infant of the diabetic mother. Seminars in Perinatology, 18, 459–469.

Reece, E. A., Homko, C. J., & Hagay, Z. (1995, July). When the pregnancy is complicated by diabetes. Contemporary Obstetrics and Gynecology, 43–61.

Reece, E. A., Homko, C. J., & Hagay, Z. (1996). Diabetic retinopathy in pregnancy. Obstetric and Gynecology Clinics of North America, 23, 161–171.

Rizzo, T., Metzger, B. E., Burns, W. J., & Burns, K. (1991). Correlation between antepartum maternal metabolism and child intelligence. New England Journal of Medicine, 325, 911–916.

Rodgers, B. D., & Rodgers, D. E. (1991). Clinical variables associated with diabetic ketoacidosis during pregnancy. Journal of Reproductive Medicine, 36, 797–800.

Rosenn, B., Miodovnik, M., Combs, C. A., Khoury, J., & Siddiqi, T. A. (1991). Pre-conception management of insulin-dependent diabetes: Improvement in pregnancy outcome. Obstetrics and Gynecology, 77, 845–849.

Speelman-Rhiley, D. (1993). Psychosocial assessment and support. In V. Peragallo-Dittko, K. Godley, & J. Meyer (Eds.), A core curriculum for diabetes education (pp. 27–51). Chicago: American Association of Diabetes Educators.

Steel, J. M., Johnstone, F. D., Hepburn, D. A., & Smith, A. F. (1990). Can prepregnancy care of diabetic women reduce the risk of abnormal babies? British Medical Journal, 301, 1070–1074.

White, P. (1949). Pregnancy complicating diabetes. American Journal of Medicine, 7, 609.

Whiteman, V. E., Homko, C. J., & Reece, E. A. (1996). Management of hypoglycemia and diabetic ketoacidosis in pregnancy. Obstetrics and Gynecology Clinics of North America, 23, 87–107.

Willhote, M. B., Bennert, H. W., Palomake, G. E., Zaremba, M. M., Herman, W. H., Williams, J. R., & Spear, N. H. (1993). The impact of preconception counseling on pregnancy outcomes. The experience of the Maine Diabetes in Pregnancy Program. Diabetes Care, 16, 450–455.

Wason, C. J. (1993). Pregnancy: Preconception to postpartum. In V. Peragallo-Dittko, K. Godley, & J. Meyer (Eds.), A core curriculum for diabetes education (pp. 393–444). Chicago: American Association of Diabetes Educators.

CHAPTER 15

Acute Renal Failure in Pregnancy

Shirley M. Griffith

"Bones can break, muscles can atrophy, glands can loaf, even the brain can go to sleep without immediate danger to survival. But, should kidneys fail, neither bone, muscle, nor brain could carry on."
Homer Smith, PhD (Toto)

Acute renal failure (ARF) is a rare but life-threatening complication of pregnancy. It is defined as a sudden impairment or decline in renal function, associated with an increase in serum blood urea nitrogen (BUN) and creatinine. It is frequently, but not always associated with oliguria, hyperkalemia, and sodium and water retention (Crandall, 1989). It is often reversible, but if prolonged, may lead to a need for chronic dialysis or renal transplantation.

Significant physiologic changes associated with the renal system occur during normal pregnancy. The alterations are described in Chapter 1. In addition to anatomic adaptations, renal function undergoes change, evidenced by adjustments in laboratory parameter reference ranges. A comparison of normal values in selected renal laboratory parameters for pregnant and nonpregnant patients is presented in Table 15-1. This chapter addresses the etiology of ARF during pregnancy, classifications, and strategies for management.

ETIOLOGY

The incidence of acute renal failure during pregnancy requiring dialysis is reported to be 1:10,000–15,000 pregnancies. Milder forms of renal insufficiency are noted more frequently (Shemin & Chazan, 1989). The causes of renal failure during pregnancy are presented in Display 15-1.

Severe PIH/HELLP Syndrome

Pregnancy-induced hypertension (PIH) and HELLP syndrome (hemolysis, elevated liver enzymes, and low platelets) are disease processes that affect approximately 8% of all pregnancies (ACOG, 1996). The symptoms associated with PIH and HELLP that relate to kidney function include hypertension, edema, proteinuria, renal vasospasm, and intravascular volume depletion. Renal insufficiency secondary to PIH or HELLP syndrome can also result in increased serum BUN and creatinine. ARF from these two disease processes is rare, but accounts for a substantial percentage of the cases of pregnancy-related ARF. When it does occur, it is usually manifested as acute tubular necrosis (ATN); however, almost all cases are reversible.

Obstruction

Acute renal failure resulting from obstruction is a relatively rare occurrence in pregnancy. The most common reasons for obstruction are compression from the gravid uterus, renal calculi, or compression from a retroperitoneal bleed. (See Display 15-2.)

Acute renal failure attributed to uterine compression is generally seen in the third trimester, most often with multiple gestations or polyhydramnios. The patient usually experiences an acute onset of flank pain, nausea, vomiting, and anuria. The diagnosis is established by ultrasound or radiologic studies, possibly an x-ray of the kidneys, ureters, and bladder (KUB), or an intravenous pyelogram (IVP). The treatment of choice usually is delivery, depending on fetal gestational age and pulmonary maturity. In cases of prematurity, treatment options include position changes, decompressive amniocentesis, or the placement of ureteral stents or nephrostomy tubes.

Renal calculi are a relatively common cause of severe abdominal pain in pregnant women. They can lead to renal failure if they are bilateral, or unilateral in the patient who has only one functioning kidney. The patient usually presents with pain characteristic of renal colic. Though diagnosis may be confirmed by ultrasound, usually a KUB or IVP is required. The treatment generally is directed toward relief of the obstruction, and may require surgery or the placement of ureteral stents.

Volume Contraction/Decreased GFR

The most common causes of hypovolemia or volume contraction in pregnancy are hemorrhage, hyperemesis, and volume shifts. The treatment for conditions leading to hypovolemia includes prompt intravascular fluid and blood replacement. This is essential for recovery and prevention of progression from prerenal to intrarenal failure.

Acute Infection/Sepsis

Renal failure secondary to sepsis results from associated volume contraction, hypotension from vasodilation, or nephrotoxins released by the causative organism. Each of these can lead to renal ischemia, the precursor to actual ARF.

Pyelonephritis occurs in 1–2.5% of all pregnancies and is caused by an ascending infection from untreated bactevria. In pyelonephritis there is evidence of abnormal renal function, which can result in abnormally-low creatinine

TABLE 15-1.   Normal Renal Laboratory Values in the Pregnant and Nonpregnant Woman

Parameter	Pregnant	Nonpregnant
Serum BUN	5–12 mc/dl	10–20 mg/dl
Serum Creatinine	<1.0 mg/dl	<1.5 mg/dl
Serum Uric Acid	1.2–4.5 mg/dl	1.5–6.0 mg/dl
Serum Osmolality	275–280 mOsm	285–295 mOsm
Serum Sodium	130–140 meq/L	136–145 meq/L
Serum Potassium	3.3–4.1 meq/L	3.5–5.0 meq/L
Urine Protein	<300 mg/day	<150 mg/day
Urine Creatinine Clearance	120–160 cc/min	91–130 cc/min
Urine Sodium	Not documented	80–180 meq/L
Urine Creatinine	Not documented	1–2 g/L

Note. BUN >13 or creatinine >.08 in pregnancy warrants further evaluation.

DISPLAY 15-1

Etiologies of Acute Renal Failure in Pregnancy

1. PIH/HELLP Syndrome
2. Obstruction
3. Volume Contraction/Decreased Glomerular Filtration Rate
   Hemorrhage/DIC
   - Placenta Previa
   - Abruptio Placentae
   - Amniotic Fluid Embolism
   - Acute Fatty Liver of Pregnancy
   - Uterine Atony
   - Retained Intrauterine Fetal Demise
   - Retained Placenta
   Dehydration
   - Hyperemesis
   Extravascular Volume Shifts
4. Acute Infection/Sepsis
5. Acute Fatty Liver of Pregnancy
6. Lupus Nephritis
7. Postpartum Renal Failure/Hemolytic Uremic Syndrome (HUS)

DISPLAY 15-2

Etiologies of Obstructive Renal Failure in Pregnancy

Mechanical	Functional
Edema	Diabetic Neuropathy
Renal Calculi	Neurogenic Bladder from Spinal Cord Injury
Tumors (i.e., cervical)	
Urethral Strictures	Compression from Gravid Uterus
Blood Clots	
Obstruction of Catheter	

clearance values and thus increased serum levels of creatinine. In addition, pyelonephritis, like any other bacterial infection, can lead to sepsis, thus further increasing the risk of ARF.

Prior to the legalization of abortion, septic abortions accounted for numerous cases of ARF; however, both are rarely seen today. The other pregnancy-related infection that can lead to sepsis and all of its related complications is chorioamnionitis.

The goal of treatment in these cases is eradication of the underlying infection and supportive therapy until the infection resolves. In most cases, renal function will return when the infection is resolved.

Acute Fatty Liver of Pregnancy

Acute fatty liver (AFL) of pregnancy was first described in 1934 as a case report and then in 1940 as a unique clinical entity (Shemin & Chazan, 1989). It is seen most often after the 35th week of pregnancy and is characterized by microvesicular fatty infiltration of the centrilobular hepatocytes of the liver.

According to Shemin and Chazan (1989), the estimated incidence of AFL of pregnancy is 1:13,000 pregnancies. Clinical symptoms include fatigue, jaundice, vomiting, and abdominal pain. Patients frequently exhibit signs of disseminated intravascular coagulation (DIC) secondary to liver failure. Sixty percent also experience ARF, though the reasons for renal compromise are unclear.

Prior to 1970 this disease process was associated with an 80% mortality rate. Since 1970 these statistics have reversed and today the survival rate is documented as 80% (Hou, 1991). Though most patients with AFL and ARF recover, residual renal deficiency is frequently noted (Hou, 1991). In the presence of documented AFL of pregnancy, delivery is the treatment of choice, followed by symptomatic supportive therapy until full recovery takes place.

Lupus Nephritis

According to Hou (1991), with the exception of diabetic nephropathy, lupus nephritis is the most common glomerular disease seen in pregnancy. Hou also notes that few diseases are as capable of producing renal failure so fulminant, and yet potentially treatable.

Various studies have revealed that patients with active lupus at the time of conception are at increased risk of renal insufficiency and ARF. Patients in remission for 6–12 months prior to conception exhibit fewer lupus flares and thus are at decreased risk for renal dysfunction. Aggressive treatment is generally initiated once lupus nephritis is diagnosed. Treatment includes administration of prednisone 60 mg po QD, and hospitalization is often warranted because of the risk of other concomitant complications. If renal function does not improve, cytotoxic drugs are considered. If the pregnancy has reached 34 weeks of gestation, delivery is generally recommended, as the fetal mortality rate approaches 50% in the face of renal insufficiency. The significant risk for fetal demise is attributed to acute renal failure, hypertension, and placental vasculopathy (Hou, 1991).

According to Ferris (1990), many cases of lupus nephropathy during pregnancy can be attributed to the adverse effects of hypertension or superimposed PIH. It is difficult to distinguish the etiology of the nephropathy without thorough evaluation of laboratory results. Such tests include antinuclear antibodies (ANA), Complement (C3 and C4, CH50), and anti-DNA antibody levels. In most cases the patient is treated based on the assumption that the etiology is PIH.

According to Jaffe (1985), patients with diabetic nephropathy usually have accentuated proteinuria as a result of vascular disease. They do not, however, usually suffer renal consequences as a result of pregnancy or delivery. Therefore ARF is usually not associated with this disease process.

Idiopathic Postpartum Renal Failure/Hemolytic Uremic Syndrome

Idiopathic postpartum renal failure, also commonly referred to as hemolytic uremic syndrome (HUS), is a rare but highly lethal form of ARF that was first described in the 1950s (Gasser, Gautier, Stack, Siebenmann, & Oechlin, 1955). It can occur during the intrapartum period or anytime within the first 10 weeks postpartum, and is most often seen in women with otherwise uncomplicated pregnancies. According to Hou, the mortality rate, prior to 1979 was 61%. Of those who survive, 90% require long-term dialysis or renal transplantation. Many patients have some prodromal flu-like symptoms, nausea, vomiting, hematuria, and proteinuria. This course rapidly progresses to ARF, which is most often oliguric in nature. Additionally, most patients exhibit significant hypertension, microangiopathic (hemolytic) anemia, and 75% experience thrombocytopenia.

The primary event in HUS appears to be endothelial damage, which leads to disruption of endothelial cell processes that prevent thrombogenesis. This leads to the formation of microthrombi in the vessels of many organs. Jaffe (1985) has documented an association with certain drugs including oxytocin, ergots, and oral contraceptives, as well as with patients with retained placentas. However, there are no data to support any of these as causing the disorder.

Presumptive diagnosis of HUS may be made based on the presence of active urinary sediment, along with quantitative evaluation for the presence of hemoglobin but absence of red blood cells. A definitive diagnosis can only be made based on renal biopsy results.

Plasmapheresis has recently been added to the list of potential treatments for this type of ARF, based on the theory that a plasma factor may be responsible for promoting platelet aggregation. Thus, if the factor can be removed and be replaced by fresh plasma, restoration of renal function is possible (Krane, 1988). There are currently no prospective randomized trials to support this therapy, but because of the otherwise poor prognosis associated with this condition, it may represent a reasonable therapy (Hou, 1991).

CLASSIFICATION

Renal failure is classified as one of three types: prerenal, intrarenal, or postrenal, depending upon the physiologic location of the insult. ARF is also categorized as either anuric, oliguric, nonoliguric, or polyuric, defined by the amount of urine that is produced in a 24-hour period. Anuria refers to production of less than 100 cc of urine per 24 hours. Oliguria refers to less than 400 cc urine production in 24 hours, and non-oliguric renal failure indicates greater than 400 cc per 24 hours. The final term, polyuria, designates those patients in ARF who excrete more than 6 liters of urine in a 24-hour period.

In order to better appreciate the different aspects of each etiology of ARF, see Figure 15-1 for a review of the anatomy of the kidney. Each kidney is made up of approximately 1 million nephrons. The nephrons are the individual functional units of the kidney, each having the capa-bility to produce urine. Each nephron is made up of a glomerulus and a long tubule (see Figure 15-2). The glomerulus is the structure through which fluid is filtered from the blood. The tubule filters the waste products out of the blood and produces urine on its way to the pelvis of the kidney.

Prerenal Failure

Prerenal failure is an insult that occurs before the blood reaches the kidneys. It is most often a cardiovascular problem that results in hypoperfusion of the kidneys. The most common cause is hemorrhage and resultant impaired oxygen transport. Though the structure of the kidneys themselves is normal, they are unable to properly filter blood. (See Display 15-3.)

This type of renal failure is the most common form associated with pregnancy and can often be reversed if adequate perfusion is re-established in a timely fashion. If the decreased perfusion and oxygen transport persists, irre-

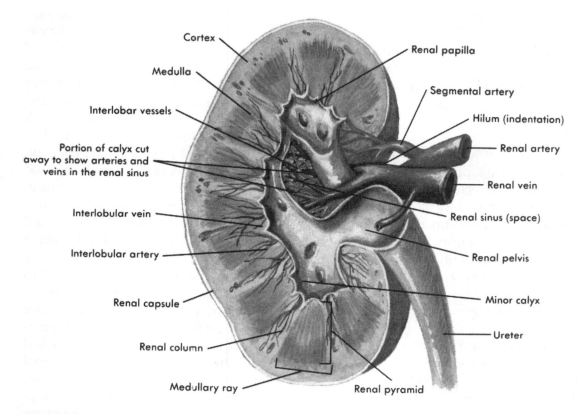

Figure 15-1. Longitudinal section of the kidney and ureter. The cortex forms the outer part of the kidney, and the medulla forms the inner part. A central cavity called the renal sinus contains the renal pelvis. The renal columns of the kidney project from the cortex into the medulla and are separated by the pyramids.

versible ischemic damage may occur. This results in progression to intrarenal failure or acute tubular necrosis (ATN).

Prerenal failure may be distinguished from intrarenal failure based on evaluation and comparison of various laboratory values. In prerenal failure the body retains sodium and water in an attempt to maintain an adequate circulating volume. This results in a low urinary excretion of sodium and very concentrated urine that has a high osmolality and specific gravity. The elevation in serum levels of blood urea nitrogen (BUN) and creatinine are seen because an inadequate volume of blood reaches the kidneys in order for these substances to be filtered out. (See Table 15-2.)

Intrarenal Failure

Intrarenal failure assumes intrinsic damage to the nephrons that results in deterioration of actual renal function. Intrarenal failure can be the end result of either glomerular nephritis or ATN. ATN in turn can be caused by either ischemia or nephrotoxicity. The diagnosis of intrarenal failure is one of exclusion, and is only made when both pre- and postrenal failure have been ruled out.

Glomerular nephritis accounts for 25% of the cases of intrarenal failure (Crandall, 1989). Rare cases have resulted from papillary necrosis, interstitial nephritis, or polyarteritis. In glomerular nephritis, antigen/antibody complexes get

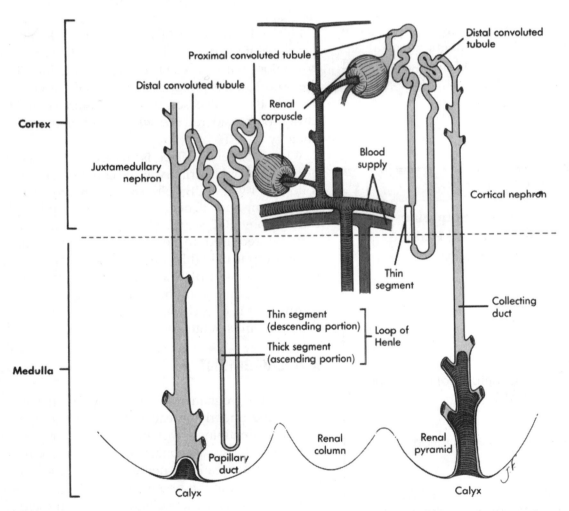

Figure 15-2. Functional unit of the kidney—the nephron. The juxtamedullary nephrons (those near the medulla of the kidney) have loops of Henle that extend deep into the medulla of the kidney, whereas other nephrons do not.

trapped in the basement membrane of the glomerulus, causing inflammation and injury.

ATN secondary to ischemia can be anticipated if the patient's mean arterial pressure (MAP) is below 60–70 mmHg in the afferent arterioles, or if circulation is interrupted for more than 30 minutes (Crandall, 1989). Ischemic injuries damage tubular epithelium as well as the cells of the basement membrane. Basement membrane cells do not have the ability to regenerate, thus ischemia in this portion of the nephron can lead to irreparable damage.

Nephrotoxicity results from the intake of substances that directly damage the renal tubules. These substances range from heavy metals to ions, and also include various medications. (See Display 15-4.) Injuries from medications usually affect the renal tubules but avoid the basement membrane, therefore making this a more reversible type of ATN. Treatment targets flushing the necrotic cells out of the tubules and allowing time for healing and tissue regeneration. Frequently osmotic diuretics are utilized in addition to the administration of large quantities of intravenous fluid.

In intrarenal failure, serum BUN and creatinine rise because the damage to the renal tubules prevents them from adequaate filtration of substances, even if adequate perfusion exists.

Postrenal Failure

Postrenal failure is caused by the obstruction or disruption of the flow of urine from the urinary tract. The obstruction can occur anywhere from the calyces to the urethral meatus. For renal failure to occur, the obstruction must be bilateral, unless the patient has only one functioning kidney. The causes of postrenal failure are either mechanical or functional and were reviewed in Table 15-3. This type of renal failure is highly reversible if the obstruction is relieved in a timely fashion, but can result in intrarenal failure if the obstruction is prolonged. Though it accounts for only 10% of all cases, postrenal failure should always be considered first when determining the etiology of ARF.

When postrenal failure is suspected, evaluation begins with urinary tract catheterization, followed by a KUB, ultrasound, intravenous pyelogram, and, if necessary, a computerized tomography (CT scan). On occasion, surgery may be required to relieve the obstruction. Urine output is highly variable in this type of renal failure, and BUN and creatinine are both elevated. Urine sodium can be high if the obstruction is of a chronic nature, but is low if the problem is acute.

MANAGEMENT

ARF during pregnancy is treated by first determining the underlying cause. Goals of therapy include maintaining euvolemia, avoiding hyperkalemia, acidosis, hyponatremia, and hypocalcemia. Serum creatinine needs to be maintained below 2 mg/dl in the pregnant patient, because of the concomitant association of intrauterine fetal death with higher levels (Knuppel, Montenegro, & O'Brien, 1985). Adequate nutri-

DISPLAY 15-3

Hemodynamic Sequelae Leading to Prerenal Failure in Pregnancy

Impaired Cardiac Function
- Cardiogenic Shock
- Pulmonary Embolism
- Hypotension

Vasodilation
- Sepsis (pyelonephritis, chorioamnionitis, septic abortion)
- Anaphylaxis

Intravascular Volume Contraction
- Hemorrhage
- GI Losses (hyperemesis)
- Volume Shifts (third spacing fluid, which depletes intravascular volume)

TABLE 15-2. Differential Diagnosis of Prerenal and Intrarenal Failure

Lab Values	Prerenal	Intrarenal
BUN:Creatinine Ratio	20–40:1	10–15:1
Urine Sodium	<20 meq/L	>40 meq/L
Urine Concentration	Concentrated	Dilute
Urine Osmolality	>500 (High)	<300 (Low)
Urine Specific Gravity	>1.020 (High)	<1.010 (Low)
Urine Sediment	Normal/Hyaline Casts	Abnormal (Cellular Casts & Debris)
Fractional Excretion of Sodium (FENa)*	≤ 1%	>1%

*FENa not accurate when done within 8 hours of administration of Lasix.

tion must also be maintained as well as avoiding hyper- and hypotension. If the patient is undelivered, fetal well-being is assessed dependent upon gestational age. Dialysis may also be indicated.

In order to more accurately assess central hemodynamic status, particularly preload, a pulmonary artery catheter is recommended during initial evaluation and stabilization. This also assists with management of the patient with hypertension, as elevated blood pressure may be caused by fluid overload, or as a compensatory response in cases of intravascular volume depletion (Hou, 1991). A pulmonary artery catheter capable of measuring continuous mixed venous oxygen saturation (SvO$_2$) permits assessment of oxygen transport status. This may be especially helpful in determining renal perfusion.

Euvolemia is maintained by careful administration of a predetermined total fluid volume. To calculate the total volume of fluid necessary for each patient, the patient's total volume of urine for a 24-hour period should be added to a calculated figure of 6–8 cc/kg/day. If the patient is febrile, adjustments may be necessary to compensate for insensible water loss.

The use of diuretics in ARF remains somewhat controversial as data generally indicate neither benefit nor harm. Because patients with non-oliguric renal failure generally have a better prog-

nosis than those with oliguric failure, an attempt to increase urine output with diuretics may be considered. The one exception to this is the patient with PIH or HELLP syndrome. Unless intravascular volume overload has been documented by central hemodynamic monitoring, repetitive use of diuretics should be avoided in this population of women. It should also be noted that any patient who receives repeated high doses of lasix can experience hearing loss.

DISPLAY 15-4

Nephrotoxic Drugs that May Lead to ATN

1. Aminoglycosides
   - Gentamycin
   - Tobramycin
   - Kanamycin
   - Amikaci
2. Radiological Contrast Dyes
3. Acetaminophen
4. Nonsteroidal Anti-inflammatory Drugs

DISPLAY 15-5

General Guidelines for Initiation of Dialysis

1. Hyperkalemia (K+ > 5.6 meq/L)
2. Fluid Overload
3. Hyponatremia
4. Severe Metabolic Acidosis
5. Uremic Complications
   - BUN >100 mg/dL
   - Bleeding
   - CNS Symptoms
   - Severe Nausea or Vomiting

The acute loss of renal function may lead to many secondary metabolic complications, the most common of which is hyperkalemia. It is a significant potential risk because of the association with cardiac dysrythmias. Depending on the degree of severity, hyperkalemia can be treated in a multitude of ways. Any potassium >6.8 meq/L needs to be treated acutely, and should not be delayed until dialysis can be initiated. Acidosis can also occur and bicarbonate should be administered to keep the bicarbonate level between 18–22 meq/L and the pH >7.2. Chronic and severe acidosis is treated with dialysis (see Display 15-5). A serum sodium below 125 meq/L also requires dialysis, and if it is below 120 meq/L, the administration of hypertonic saline during dialysis is also necessary. In the event of hypocalcemia, oral supplements can be given. Intravenous calcium supplements are reserved for those patients who exhibit carpal pedal spasm or a positive Chvostek's sign. Chvostek's sign is illicited by tapping the facial nerve. Ipsilateral contraction of the facial muscles is a positive test result.

Some care providers support the use of prophylactic dialysis even when these symptoms are not present. Supporters believe that this decreases the mortality rate, however, there is a lack of substantial supportive data.

Optimal nutrition in the course of ARF is critical. The oral route is preferable, but parenteral nutrition can be used when the patient is unable to eat. Protein intake should be of high biologic value, and limited to 0.6 gms/kg/day if the patient is being managed without dialysis. This requirement increases to 1.5 gms/kg/day if dialysis has been instituted, because of amino acid loss associated with dialysis. Total caloric requirements are calculated using the patient's ideal body weight.

If the patient is receiving any drug therapy, the doses need to be adjusted to renal failure doses. Finally, because infection is the leading cause of death in renal failure, prevention and treatment of infection is of utmost importance.

CASE STUDY

To illustrate concepts related to ARF during pregnancy, including identification, etiology, assessment data, and management, excerpts from a case study are presented next.

The patient is a 32-year-old woman transported to a tertiary care obstetric facility 16 hours after a spontaneous vaginal delivery. Her diagnoses included severe PIH, HELLP syndrome, DIC, eclampsia, and ARF.

Blood and urine samples were obtained for laboratory evaluation. An ammonia level was also evaluated secondary to the patient's jaundice to rule out AFLP and was within normal limits.

An intraarterial catheter and pulmonary artery catheter were also placed. Initial hemodynamic and laboratory data are presented in Display 15-6. These data indicated that the patient was centrally hypovolemic, with a low cardiac output, and therefore poor renal perfusion.

Treatment included administration of 3 liters of crystalloid solution intravenously. This resulted in improved cardiac output, a lowered systemic vascular resistance (SVR), and increasd preload. However, the patient demonstrated persistent oliguria despite normalization of intravascular volume. There was also no change in urine output following administration of furosemide. A dopamine infusion of 3 mcg/kg/min, considered a dosage within the range to facilitate renal perfusion, also failed to improve renal function.

DISPLAY 15-6

Case Study: Patient Assessment Data

Hemodynamic	Laboratory
CVP-2 mm Hg	BUN 11 mg/dl
PAP-12/4 mm Hg	Creatinine 1.0 mg/dl
PCWP-4 mm Hg	Bilirubin 13 mg/dl
Cardiac Output—5.4 l/min	LDH 3200 U/l
SVR-1748 dyne/sec/cm-5	Magnesium 7.1 mg/dl
PVR-39 dyne/sec/cm-5	SGOT 1603 U/l
	Platelets 48,000
	PT 15 sec.
	PTT 30 sec.
	Fibrinogen 155 mg/dl

DISPLAY 15-7

Case Study Update: Assessment Data

Laboratory	Hemodynamic	Urinalysis
BUN 30 mg/dl	CVP-5 mm Hg	Urine Sodium 101 meq/l
Creatinine 2.9 mg/dl	PAP-23/15 mm Hg	Urine Creatinine 250 mg/l
Uric Acid 9.0 mg/dl	PCWP-15 mm Hg	Muddy Brown Casts
	C.O.-8.43 l/min	
	SVR-1043 dyne/sec/-5	RBCs too numerous to count (TNTC)
	PVR-25 dyne/sec/-5	FENa 0.8%

Laboratory results were repeated following these treatment measures and are presented in Display 15-7. They indicated worsening renal function. The diagnosis of intrarenal failure/ATN was made and a renal consult was obtained.

The recommendations of the renal consultation team were implemented and included discontinuation of dopamine, maintenance of euvolemia with a total intravenous fluid intake of 56 cc/hr, and initiation of hemodialysis. Hemodialysis was initiated on Hospital Day 3 and repeated on Hospital Day 4. The patient remained persistently oliguric and hemodialysis was repeated on Hospital Day 6.

On Day 7 the patient exhibited a significant increase in spontaneous urine output for the first time, totaling 444 cc in 24 hours. A diagnosis of nonoliguric failure was made at that time. Her laboratory results indicated that her BUN and creatinine remained significantly elevated so a left subclavian dialysis catheter was placed that day in anticipation of the need for prolonged therapy.

On Hospital Day 11 the patient's BUN was 55 mg/dl and creatinine 7.2 mg/dl. Her urine output had increased to more than 2 liters the previous day and she was discharged home with plans for follow-up dialysis.

SUMMARY

Though acute renal failure associated with pregnancy is relatively rare, it is a serious, potentially life-threatening medical condition that requires a multidisciplinary approach to care. Because prerenal failure is the most common type of ARF in pregnancy, it is also essential that patients at risk be identified early and treated aggressively, in order to prevent progression of the disease process to intrarenal failure. With good assessment skills and appropriate management, the prognosis for full recovery is greatly enhanced.

REFERENCES

Asrat, T., & Nageotte, M. (1990). Renal failure in pregnancy. Seminars in Perinatology, 14(1), 59–67.

Burrow, G. N., & Ferris, T. F. (1988). Medical complications during pregnancy (3rd ed.). Philadelphia: W. B. Saunders.

Crandall, Betty Irwin (1989). Nephrology Nursing: Concepts and Strategies. In Beth Tamplet Ulrich (Ed.), Acute renal failure (pp. 45–60). Norwalk, CT: Appleton & Lange.

Dafnis, E., & Sabatini, S. (1992). The effects of pregnancy on renal function: Physiology and pathophysiology. The American Journal of the Medical Sciences, 303(3), 184–205.

Davison, J., & Dunlop, W. (1980). Renal hemodynamics and tubular function in normal human pregnancy. Kidney International, 18, 152–161.

Ferris, T. F. (1990). Advanced internal medicine. St. Louis, MO: Year Book Medical.

Garret, M. G. (1995). The nutritional management of acute renal failure. Journal of Clinical Nursing, 4, 377–382.

Gasser, C., Gautier, E., Steck, A., Siebenmann, R., & Oechlin, R. (1955). Hamolytish-uramische syndrome. Medizinechen Wochenschrift, 85, 905–909.

Grunfeld, J. P., & Pertuiset, N. (1987). Acute renal failure in pregnancy: 1987. American Journal of Kidney Diseases, 9(4), 359–62.

Hou, S. (1991). Critical care obstetrics (2nd ed.). Boston: Blackwell Scientific.

Jaffe, D. J. (1985). Postpartum evaluation of renal function. Clinical Obstetrics and Gynecology, 28(2), 298–309.

Knuppel, R., Montenegro, R., & O'Brien, W. (1985). Acute renal failure in pregnancy. Clinical Obstetrics and Gynecology, 28(2), 288–296.

Krane, N. K. (1988). Acute renal failure in pregnancy. Archives of Internal Medicine, 148, 2347–2357.

Lindheimer, M., & Katz, A. (1991, February). OB renal problems. Contemporary Obstetrics and Gynecology, 76–94.

Neumann, M., & Urizar, R. (1994). Hemolyic uremic syndrome: Current pathophysiology and management. ANNA Journal, 21(4), 137–143.

Paller, M. S. (1995). Medical complications during pregnancy (4th ed.). Philadelphia: W. B. Saunders.

Shemin, D., & Chazan, J. (1989). Acute renal failure in pregnancy. Rhode Island Medical Journal, 72. 125–127.

Sibai, B. M., & Ramadan, M. K. (1993). Acute renal failure in pregnancies complicated by hemolysis, elevated liver enzymes, and low platelets. American Journal of Obstetrics and Gynecology, 168, 1682–1690.

CHAPTER 16

Thyroid Disorders in Pregnancy

Jamie Caldwell

Thyroid disease complicates up to .3% of pregnancies (Davis, Lucas, Hankins, Roach, & Cunningham, 1989). Although the incidence is low, prompt recognition and treatment are necessary to ensure optimal maternal–fetal outcomes. Pregnancy has a significant impact on maternal thyroid function. An understanding of changes in function of the thyroid gland during pregnancy is required to correctly interpret thyroid function tests and to recognize and manage thyroid disorders. Alteration in thyroid hormone levels affects the maternal metabolic state and results in widespread systemic effects, with perinatal outcome dependent upon the severity of illness at delivery. Early treatment with resulting euthyroid status at delivery is associated with good pregnancy outcomes, whereas failure to correct thyroid dysfunction increases the risk of preeclampsia, heart failure, and adverse perinatal outcomes (Davis et al., 1989; Davis, Leveno, & Cunningham, 1988; Millar et al., 1994).

THYROID HORMONES

Thyroid function includes regulation of metabolic rate by secretion of thyroid hormones triiodothyronine (T_3) and thyroxine (T_4). These hormones increase basal metabolic rate and oxygen consumption, and promote normal growth and central nervous system development of the fetus. Thyroxine is the predominate circulating thyroid homone and is produced exclusively in the thyroid gland. The majority of T_3 is converted from T_4 in peripheral tissues, with only a small amount secreted from the thyroid gland. T_3 is responsible for most of the activity mediated by the thyroid gland. Iodine, derived from dietary sources, is necessary for the synthesis of thyroid hormone.

Thyroid hormones are transported in the blood bound to plasma proteins, primarily to thyroxine binding globulin (TBG) and in small amounts to prealbumin and albumin. Less than 1% of thyroid hormone is free (unbound) in plasma, with only the free hormone physiologically active. Stable blood levels are maintained by protein-bound hormones, which serve as a reservoir to replace free T_3 and T_4 as needed.

The regulation of thyroid hormones involves a negative feedback mechanism. The thyroid gland is directly regulated by the anterior pituitary gland and indirectly by the hypothalamus, which releases thyroid-releasing hormone (TRH). Thyroid-stimulating hormone (TSH) then is secreted from the anterior pituitary, controlling the synthesis and release of thyroid hormones. Increased levels of free thyroid hormones suppress TSH release.

THYROID FUNCTION IN PREGNANCY

Changes in thyroid function occur related to varying metabolic demands and hormonal changes that occur with pregnancy. The thyroid gland becomes moderately enlarged because of hyperplasia of the glandular tissue and increased vascularity. However, normal pregnancy does not cause significant thyromegaly, and any goiter recognized during pregnancy should be considered pathologic (Lowe & Cunningham, 1991). A marked increase in circulating levels of TBG occurs in response to high estrogen levels. This increase peaks at 20 weeks gestation, and remains at double baseline values throughout the remainder of the pregnancy (Glinoer et al., 1990). In addition, increased levels of human chorionic gonadotropin are associated with thyroid stimulation (Lazarus, 1993). As a result, total serum T_3 and T_4 are elevated, although the values remain within normal nonpregnant range. The biologically active thyroid hormones, free T_4 and T_3, remain within normal range throughout pregnancy. Serum levels of TSH also remain within normal range, with considerable variation seen during gestation (Glinoer et al., 1990). A decreased availability of iodide for the maternal thyroid is related to increased renal clearance and loss to the fetoplacental unit. Consequently, low iodine intake during pregnancy increases the incidence of goiter.

ETIOLOGY

Thyroid disorders are most commonly seen in women of childbearing age. Hyperthyroidism, also known as thyrotoxicosis, is a condition resulting from the effects of excessive secretion of thyroid hormones. An increase of basal metabolic rate and oxygen consumption occurs in response to an excess thyroid hormone concentration. The most common cause of hyperthyroidism in pregnancy is Graves disease, an organ-specific autoimmune process associated with thyroid-stimulating antibody (TSAb) activity. These antibodies mimic TSH in their ability to stimulate thyroid function, and are responsible for thyroid hyperfunction and growth in Graves disease (Lowe & Cunningham, 1991). TSAb activity frequently declines during pregnancy as suppression of the maternal immune response occurs in response to fetal cytokines (ACOG, 1993; Burrow, 1993). Consequently, patients with Graves disease may have a relapse of their hyperthyroidism in the

postpartum period. Transient elevation of thyroid hormones is seen in women with hyperemesis gravidarum, with a spontaneous return to normal values following resolution of hyperemesis (Mestman, 1991; Millar et al., 1994). Other less common causes of hyperthyroidism include hydatidiform mole and trophoblastic disease.

Hypothyroidism occurs when circulating levels of thyroid hormones are inadequate, resulting in a slowing of metabolic processes. Primary hypothyroidism results when the thyroid gland fails to synthesize and secrete sufficient amounts of thyroid hormone. Thyroid failure may occur following thyroidectomy or thyroid ablation with radioactive iodine in the treatment of Graves disease, or may result from an autoimmune process (Hashimoto's thyroiditis). Other rare causes include pituitary and hypothalamic failure. Because overt hypothyroidism is often associated with infertility, its occurance during pregnancy is infrequent. The incidence of gestational hypertension and low-birth-weight infants is increased in cases of untreated maternal hypothyroidism (Davis et al., 1988; Leung, Millar, Koonings, Montoro, & Mestman, 1993).

Transient postpartum thyroid dysfunction affects 5–10% of women during the first year following delivery (Mestman, Goodwin, & Montoro, 1995). The most common cause is autoimmune chronic thyroiditis. Risk factors include a personal or family history of thyroid or autoimmune disease and a positive test early in pregnancy or shortly after delivery for microsomal autoantibodies. The clinical course varies, but most commonly transient hyperthyroidism is followed by transient hypothyroidism and then recovery. Fatigue is the most common manifestation. Because the symptoms are vague and nonspecific, it is infrequently diagnosed. It is usually self-limiting, although thyroxine therapy may occassionally be necessary for 4–6 weeks (Wood, 1994).

DIAGNOSIS

Recognition of hyperthyroidism in pregnancy may be difficult because commonly associated signs and symptoms are also found with normal pregnancy. Changes in thyroid function affect many different body systems, with signs and symptoms reflecting changes in metabolic state (Display 16-1). The clinical picture of the pregnant patient with excess or deficiency of thyroid hormones varies with the severity of the disease. Diagnosis is verified by laboratory findings. Familiarity with values is necessary when interpreting the results of laboratory data in order to differentiate expected changes of normal pregnancy from pathological changes. No single test is relied on exclusively because of endogenous and exogenous factors that may affect findings. Values of commonly used tests and changes associated with normal pregnancy, hyperthyroidism, and hypothyroidism are listed in Table 16-1. The measurement of total serum levels includes free and protein-bound hormones. Serum levels of free thyroid hormone are the most accurate indications of changes in thyroid activity. Hyperthyroidism is confirmed by the presence of decreased TSH and elevated concentrations of free thyroid hormones in the blood. However, suppression of serum TSH has been reported during the first trimester of normal pregnancies and in patients with hyperemesis gravidarum (Mestman, 1991). Calculation to index free T_4 (FT_4I) and T_3 (FT_3I) adjusts values for pregnancy-related changes in TBG and serum albumin and correlates well with the actual free T_4 concentration (Mestman, 1991). Hypothyroidism is confirmed by laboratory findings of decreased concentrations of total and free T_4 and an elevated serum TSH value. The measurement of radioiodine uptake by the thyroid is contraindicated during pregnancy because of the potential for damage to the fetal thyroid gland.

MATERNAL COMPLICATIONS

The presence of excess thyroid hormones dramatically affects the cardiovascular system. The positive chronotropic and inotropic effects of thyroid hormones on cardiac function create a dramatic increase of cardiac workload. These changes are a direct result of the effect of thyroid hormones on the heart (Mestman, 1991). In addition, an increased sensitivity to and number of catecholamine receptors in cardiac muscle cells occurs in the presence of excessive thyroid hormones. Hemodynamic function of the thyrotoxic pregnant patient reflects a hyperdynamic state. A 65% elevation of cardiac output, a 21% increase in heart rate, and a 35% reduction in systemic vascular resistance (SVR) have been found in pregnant thyrotoxic women (Easterling, Schmucker, Carlson, Millard, & Benedetti, 1991). Despite clinical improvement

DISPLAY 16-1

Clinical Signs and Symptoms

Hyperthyroidism	Hypothyroidism
Resting tachycardia, palpitations, dyspnea, atrial fibrillation, increase in cardiac output and contractility, cardiac enlargement	Bradycardia, decreased cardiac output
Fine tremors of hands, weight loss, muscle weakness	Weight gain, muscle cramps and weakness
Exopthalmos, staring gaze	Dull, apathetic appearance
Nervousness, anxiety, chronic fatigue	Easily fatigued, lethargy
Thyromegaly, auscultation of thyroid bruit	
Skin warm and moist, heat intolerant, diaphoresis	Cool, dry skin, cold intolerant

TABLE 16-1. Diagnostic Tests of Thyroid Function

Test	Normal Value	Normal Pregnancy	Hyperthyroid	Hypothyroid
Total serum T_4	5–12 ug/dl	Increased	Increased	Decreased
Free T_4	0.8–2 ng/dL	No change	Increased	Decreased
Total serum T_3	75–235 ng/dl	Increased	Increased	Decreased
Thyroid-stimulating hormone	0.3–6 mU/L	No change	Decreased	Increased

as evidenced by normalization of thyroid hormone levels and heart rate following treatment, hemodynamic function remains hyperactive in these patients. Therefore, they continue to be at risk for the development of complications (Easterling et al., 1991 Mestman, 1991). The hemodynamic changes that occur with uncontrolled hyperthyroidism are consistent with the cardiovascular changes associated with pregnancy-induced hypertension (Davis et al., 1989; Easterling et al., 1991). Data suggest that lack of control of hyperthyroidism significantly increases the maternal risk of severe preeclampsia (Easterling et al., 1991; Millar et al., 1994).

Exposure of the heart to excessive thyroid hormones may cause cardiomegaly and ventricular dysfunction (Davis, 1989; Lowe & Cunningham, 1991; Mestman, 1991). Electrocardiogram (EKG) changes including atrial fibrillation and left ventricular hypertrophy have been found in patients with hyperthyroidism (Mestman, 1991). Congestive heart failure is the primary cause of maternal morbidity in acute cases of thyrotoxicosis, and occurs when the ventricles are no longer able to maintain a sufficient cardiac output to meet the metabolic needs of the body.

Thyroid crisis or "storm" is a rare but potentially life-threatening occurence during pregnancy. Progression to stupor and then coma may occur if treatment is not begun. Most cases occur in patients with untreated or uncontrolled hyperthyroidism at time of delivery or when other physiologic stress may occur. The outpouring of catecholamines that occurs with complications such as pregnancy-induced hypertension, anemia, or infection may precipitate cardiac failure and/or thyroid crisis. Clinical manifestations occur in response to a marked hypermetabolism and excessive adrenergic response. In addition to exaggerated signs and symptoms of hyperthyroidism, thyroid crisis is characterized by central nervous system manifestations and hyperthermia (Display 16-2). Elevations of thyroid hormone values are seen, although no correlation exists between the severity of the disease state and the increased level of thyroid hormone (Mestman, 1991).

A collaborative approach to care that includes the perinatal nurse, obstetrician, perinatologist, and anesthesiologist is most beneficial in caring for the patient with complications. Management of maternal complications requires rapid and aggressive interventions. Care is focused on reduction of thyroid hormone output and beta-adrenergic blockade. If heart failure or thyroid storm develops, a loading dose of 600–1000 mg of PTU is given orally or by nasogastric tube, followed by 150–300 mg every 6 hours (ACOG, 1993; Mestman, 1991). In addition to antithyroid drugs, treatment with pharmacologic agents, which are administered only during the acute phase of thyrotoxicosis for short-term therapy, is begun (Table 16-2). Iodides administered in large amounts transiently inhibit thyroid hormone formation and release with a rapid response. They are administered 1 hour after the initial dose of PTU to avoid excess hormone stores within the thyroid gland. Iodide may be given orally as potassium iodide or Lugol's solution, or intravenously as sodium

DISPLAY 16-2

Signs and Symptoms of Thyroid Crisis or "Storm"

Fever >100°F	Agitation
Congestive heart failure	Delirium
Vomiting	Stupor
Diarrhea	Coma

iodide. Propranolol is a beta-adrenergic blocker that inhibits catecholamine effects and decreases heart rate and anxiety. Propranolol also blocks the conversion of T_4 to T_3. Its use requires careful assessment prior to administration to patients with congestive heart failure. The negative inotropic effects of beta-adrenergic blockade may directly depress myocardial contractility and block compensatory adrenergic stimulation of the heart, resulting in cardiac decompensation. Its use is also contraindicated in patients with asthma and for long-term therapy because of potential fetal effects. These effects may include intrauterine growth retardation, impaired response to anoxic stress, and fetal bradycardia. Adrenal glucocorticoid agents inhibit the conversion of T_4 to T_3 and provide glucocorticoid in case of adrenal insufficiency. Hydrocortisone, prednisone, or dexamethasone is administered in divided doses. Propranolol, iodides, and glucocorticoid agents are discontinued after resolution of acute symptoms, whereas antithyroid drugs are continued to achieve and maintain a euthyroid state.

Treatment is directed toward identification and aggressive treatment of possible precipitating factors. In the presence of heart failure, cardiac workload and oxygen consumption are reduced as complications such as hypertension, infection, and anemia are treated and resolved. The patient is assessed for concomitant preeclampsia. Blood products are administered to correct anemia, and broad-spectrum antibiotic therapy is begun for treatment of infection following collection of blood and urine cultures.

FETAL EFFECTS

The fetal thyroid gland is able to synthesize thyroid hormone beginning at 10–12 weeks gestation. The extent of transfer of maternal thyroid hormone to the fetus is controversial. Lower levels of thyroid hormone have been found in cord serum than in maternal serum, indicating that although placental transfer occurs it is not enough to maintain concentrations in the newborn within normal limits (Mestman et al., 1995). Antithyroid medications, iodides, and thyroid-stimulating immunoglobins cross the placenta without difficulty. TSH does not cross the placenta in significant amounts (Burrow, 1993).

An increased occurance of SGA neonates born to women with poorly controlled hyperthyroidism has been attributed to both prematurity (Davis et al., 1989; Millar et al., 1994) and to growth retardation caused by a prolonged maternal history of Graves disease (Mitsuda et al., 1992). The thyroid-stimulating antibodies present in Graves disease cross the placenta and place the fetus and neonate at risk for thyrotoxicosis. This condition is suggested by a maternal history of thyrotoxicosis, the presence of thyroid-stimulating antibodies, and persistent fetal tachycardia (Lazarus, 1993). Thyrotoxicosis occurs in about 1% of these neonates, but usually resolves within 2–3 months of life with the disappearance of maternal immunoglobulin (Millar et al., 1994). Follow-up studies have found no adverse effects on children exposed in utero to antithyroid medications during pregnancy. These include effects on neonatal thyroid function, neonatal outcome, long-term growth, and intellectual development (Wing, Millar, Koonings, Montoro, & Mestman, 1994; Burrow, Klatskin, & Genel, 1978).

Thyroid hormones are necessary for normal neurologic development of the fetus, and inadequate amounts of thyroid hormone may result in mental retardation (cretinism). Although an increased incidence of small for gestational age and stillborn infants is seen in patients with untreated hypothyroidism, infants of treated mothers are generally without evidence of thyroid dysfunction or other related complications (ACOG, 1993; Leung et al., 1993).

TABLE 16-2. Pharmacological Treatment of Thyroid Crisis or "Storm" in Pregnancy

Medication	Dosage
1. Propylthiouracil	Loading: 600–1000 mg orally then 300 mg every 6 hrs
2. Sodium iodide	.5–1 g intravenously every 8 hrs
3. Propranolol	40–80 mg every 4–6 hrs orally or 1 mg/min, intravenously, up to 10 mg/4hrs
4. Dexamethasone or Hydrocortisone	2 mg every 6 hrs, intravenously or orally 100 mg intravenously every 8 hrs
5. Acetaminophen	325 mg rectally every 3 hrs

Screening of newborns for congenital hypothyroidism is now routine. Early adequate treatment is essential to ensure normal mental and physical development of the neonate.

Fetal well-being is assessed throughout pregnancy for signs of fetal compromise, such as intrauterine growth retardation and fetal tachycardia. Fetal complications are rarely seen in the patient who maintain metabolic control.

MANAGEMENT

Risks to the pregnant woman and her fetus with untreated thyroid disease are significant. Early diagnosis and treatment to obtain prompt maternal metabolic control positively affect maternal–fetal outcomes. The goal of treatment for hyperthyroidism is to decrease the overproduction of thyroid hormone by blocking its synthesis and by inhibiting the peripheral conversion of T_4 to T_3. Antithyroid drugs are the treatment of choice for hyperthyroidism during pregnancy. Because these drugs cross the placenta and may cause fetal hypothyroidism and goiter, the goal of treatment is to use the lowest dose possible to maintain a maternal euthyroid state. A mildly thyrotoxic range of the mother is maintained with serum thyroxine levels in the upper normal range (Lazarus, 1993). Hyperthyroidism is generally treated with either propylthiouracil (PTU) or methimazole. Both block the synthesis, but not the release, of thyroid hormones. In addition, PTU inhibits the conversion of T_4 to T_3

in the periphery. Once the thyroid gland becomes depleted of stored hormone, a euthyroid state is attained. This typically occurs within 4–6 weeks, although some clinical improvement may be seen within the first week of treatment (Burrow, 1993). Reports of an increased incidence of congenital fetal scalp defects associated with methimazole have limited its use during pregnancy in the past, although more recent studies have found no evidence of related teratogenic effects in this group (Wing et al., 1994). Because PTU is protein-bound, there is little transplacental transfer and it is found in lesser concentrations in breastmilk than methimazole (Wing et al., 1994). Mothers requiring antithyroid medication may breastfeed, although monitoring of neonatal thyroid function is indicated related to the potential risk of neonatal hypothyroidism (Committee on Drugs, 1983; Cooper, 1987). Maternal side effects of antithyroid drugs are uncommon, but may include skin rash, pruritis, nausea, and agranulocytosis as a rare but serious complication.

Thyroidectomy may be indicated for the patient who has a hypersensitivity to or a history of poor compliance with antithyroid medications. Medical control of thyroid hormone is required prior to surgery. Subtotal thyroidectomy is most commonly performed during the second trimester, in order to avoid the risk of spontaneous abortion or preterm labor.

Hypothyroidism is most commonly treated with levothyroxine, a synthetic thyroid preparation.

Recent data have shown the need for an increase in the dosage during pregnancy in women with hypothyroidism, although there is considerable individual variation in the requirement during pregnancy (McDougall & Maclin, 1995; Mandel, Larsen, Seeley, & Brent, 1990; Wood, 1994). The increase in required dosage during pregnancy is thought to be related to the increase in serum concentrations of TBG, which results in decreased serum concentrations of free T_3 and T_4 (Wood, 1994). Periodic monitoring of TSH and thyroxine values is recommended throughout the pregnancy to determine the need for adjustment of dosage (McDougall & Maclin, 1995).

NURSING CARE ISSUES

The obstetric nurse formulates appropriate diagnoses as they relate to the patient in order to guide nursing interventions and assist evaluation of patient outcomes. A list of potential nursing diagnoses related to care of the intrapartum obstetric patient affected by thyroid disease is provided in Display 16-3. Priorities of care are determined by the severity of the disease.

Uncontrolled thyrotoxicosis during pregnancy creates profound physiologic changes that require frequent multisystem assessment. Care during thyroid crisis includes close monitoring of the cardiovascular system, which is critical as the system responds to a hypermetabolic state and heightened sensitivity to adrenergic receptors. Ongoing evaluation of cardiac function includes the use of electrocardiograph monitoring for observation of changes in heart rate and rhythm. Blood pressure may be monitored continuously through the use of an intraarterial line, which also is useful for frequent blood and arterial blood gas sampling. The use of a pulmonary artery catheter (PAC) provides a more complete hemodynamic assessment by measuring preload, afterload, cardiac output, and contractility. These measures guide treatment and are used to evaluate the patient's response to treatment. Fiberoptic capacities of the PAC allow the additional assessment of oxygen transport and consumption on a continual basis. Because the patient is at risk for cardiac failure, close monitoring for signs and symptoms of pulmonary edema is indicated. These include dyspnea,

DISPLAY 16-3

Nursing Diagnoses for the Obstetric Patient with Thyroid Disease

Hyperthyroidism
1. Alteration in metabolism, related to excessive thyroid hormone production and adrenergic hyperactivity.
2. Potential for increased oxygen demands and cardiac workload, related to an increase in metabolic demands and anxiety.
3. Potential for congestive heart failure, related to increased preload due to decreased diastolic filling time or ventricular dysfunction.
4. Potential for maternal and family anxiety, related to hospitalization during pregnancy.
5. Knowledge deficit regarding hyperthyroidism and its management.

Hypothyroidism
1. Ineffective thermoregulation, related to slowed metabolism.
2. Activity intolerance, related to decreased metabolic rate.
3. Knowledge deficit regarding hypothyroidism and its management.

crackles at the lung bases, persistant cough productive of pink sputum, and an increase in left preload (pulmonary capillary wedge pressure). Cardiogenic pulmonary edema may occur as a result of left ventricular dysfunction, shortened diastolic filling time resulting from tachycardia, or increased venous return to the heart (preload). The goal of treatment for cardiogenic pulmonary edema is reduction of preload, including diuresis and minimization of fluid intake. Ventilatory support involving tracheal intubation and mechanical ventilation may be required until the pulmonary edema is resolved.

Respiratory assessment includes monitoring of arterial blood gases and arterial oxygen percent saturation. Maintenance of adequate oxygenation for the patient and her fetus is reflected by an arterial oxygenation saturation of greater than 95%. Respiratory rate and the use of accessory muscles provide an indication of respiratory effort. Measures to meet an increased oxygen demand include the use of supplemental oxygen, and positioning to improve cardiac output and facilitate oxygen delivery. For example, an upright position for the patient in congestive heart failure decreases preload and increases cardiac output.

Hyperthermia results from the accelerated metabolic state of thyrotoxicosis. In the febrile patient, the reduction of body temperature lowers oxygen consumption. A cooling blanket, tepid baths, and administration of acetaminophen are indicated for patients with a body temperature higher than 102°F (39°C.). Aspirin is contraindicated because it may increase the concentration of free thyroxine. Additional nursing care also includes assessment for fetal heart rate responses appropriate for gestational age and assessment for signs of preterm labor.

Patient education is critical and is provided in a multidisciplinary approach that includes all caregivers. Specific educational needs are identified by the patient and her care providers. These include recognition of signs and symptoms of her disease and the need to report changes promptly, the purpose and potential side effects of medications, identification of nutritional needs, and an understanding of the importance of continued medical follow-up care. Information about the effects of the disease on her pregnancy and fetus is included. This knowledge enables her to actively participate in the management of her care and disease. Psychosocial needs are identified and incorporated into the care plan, with the focus of care including the woman, her fetus, and her significant others. Anxiety and fear for the health of the mother and fetus are experienced commonly with the presence of complications. During hospitalization, explanation and reassurance decrease anxiety that is experienced for the health of the mother and fetus and the fear of potential loss. Supportive measures include provision of frequent updates of maternal and fetal conditions to the patient and her family, avoidance of unnecessary separation of the woman and her significant other, and provision of a quiet, calm environment.

Close patient follow-up is important. As a euthyroid state is reached, correction of maternal heart rate, weight, and improvement of symptoms should be noted. Clinical symptoms indicating poor control, poor adherence to treatment, or cardiac compromise are indications for hospitization for further maternal and fetal evaluation.

REFERENCES

American College of Obstetricians and Gynecologists. (1993). Thyroid disease in pregnancy. Technical Bulletin No. 181. Washington, DC: Author.

Burrow, G. (1993). Thyroid function and hyperfunction during gestation. Endocrine Review, 14, 194–202.

Burrow, G., Klatskin, E., & Genel, M. (1978). Intellectual development in children whose mothers received propylthiouracil during pregnancy. Yale Journal of Biological Medicine, 51, 151.

Committee on Drugs, American Academy of Pediatrics. (1983). The transfer of drugs and other chemicals into human breast milk. Pediatrics, 72, 375.

Cooper, D. (1987). Antithyroid drugs: To breast-feed or not to breast-feed. American Journal of Obstetrics and Gynecology, 157, 234–235.

Davis, L., Leveno, K., & Cunningham, G. (1988). Hypothyroidism complicating pregnancy. Obstetrics and Gynecology, 72, 108–112.

Davis, L., Lucas, M., Hankins, G., Roark, M., & Cunningham, G. (1989). Thyrotoxicosis complicating pregnancy. <u>American Journal of Obstetrics and Gynecology</u>, <u>160</u>, 63–70.

Easterling, T., Schmucker, B., Carlson, K., Millard, S., & Benedetti, T. (1991). Maternal hemodynamics in pregnancies complicated by hyperthyroidism. <u>Obstetrics and Gynecology</u>, <u>78</u>, 348–391.

Glinoer, D., De Nayer, P., Bourdoux, P., Lemone, M., Robyn, C., Van Steirteghem, A., Kinthaert, J., & Lejuene, B. (1990). Regulation of maternal thyroid during pregnancy. <u>Journal of Clinical Endocrinology and Metabolism</u>, <u>71</u>, 276–287.

Lazarus, J. H. (1993). Treatment of hyper- and hypothyroidism during pregnancy. <u>Journal of Endocrinological Investigation</u>, <u>16</u>, 391–396.

Leung, A., Millar, L., Koonings, P., Montoro, M., & Mestman, J. (1993). Perinatal outcome in hypothyroid pregnancies. <u>Obstetrics and Gynecology</u>, <u>81</u>, 349–353.

Lowe, T., & Cunningham, F. (1991). Pregnancy and thyroid disease. <u>Clinical Obstetrics and Gynecology</u>, <u>34</u>, 72–81.

Mandel, G., Larsen, P., Seeley, E., & Brent, G. (1990). Increased need for thyroxine during pregnancy in women with primary hypothyroidism. <u>The New England Journal of Medicine</u>, <u>323</u>, 91–96.

McDougall, R., & Maclin, N. (1995). Hypothyroid women need more thyroxine when pregnant. <u>The Journal of Family Practice</u>, <u>41</u>, 238–240.

Mestman, J. (1991). Severe hyperthyroidism in pregnancy. In S. Clark, D. Cotton, G. Hankins, & J. Phelan (Eds.), <u>Critical care obstetrics</u> (pp. 307–328). Boston: Blackwell Scientific.

Mestman, J., Goodwin, T., & Montoro, M. (1995). Thyroid disorders of pregnancy. <u>Endocrinology and Metabolism Clinics of North America</u>, <u>24</u>, 41–71.

Millar, L., Wing, D., Leung, A., Koonings, P., Montoro, M., & Mestman, J. (1994). Low birth weight and preeclampsia in pregnancies complicated by hyperthyroidism. <u>Obstetrics and Gynecology</u>, <u>84</u>, 946–949.

Mitsuda, N., Tamaki, H., Amino, N., Hosono, T., Miyai, K., & Tanizawa, O. (1992). Risk factors for developmental disorders in infants born to women with Graves disease. <u>Obstetrics and Gynecology</u>, <u>80</u>, 359–363.

Wing, D., Millar, L., Koonings, P., Montoro, M., & Mestman, J. (1994). A comparison of propylthiouracil versus methimazole in the treatment of hyperthyroidism in pregnancy. <u>American Journal of Obstetrics and Gynecology</u>, <u>170</u>, 90–95.

Wood, A. (1994). Thyroxine therapy. <u>The New England Journal of Medicine</u>, <u>331</u>, 174–180.

CHAPTER 17

Acute Fatty Liver of Pregnancy

Donna Jean Ruth and Renee Jones

Acute fatty liver of pregnancy (AFLP) is a rare disorder of unknown etiology, first identified as a specific clinical entity by Sheehan in 1940 (Sheehan, 1940). A disease unique to the third trimester of pregnancy, it is characterized by accumulation of microvascular fat deposits in the hepatic parenchyma, resulting in acute liver failure, coagulopathy, and encephalopathy. The incidence of AFLP is about 1:14,000 (Poctros, Pettus, & Reynolds, 1983). As recently as 1980, fetal and maternal mortality rates as high as 85% were reported. However, with increased awareness, earlier recognition, and aggressive management, the mortality from AFLP has been reduced to 18–25% (Kaplan, 1985).

ETIOLOGY

The cause of AFLP remains unknown. A variety of theories have been suggested to explain AFLP. These include nutritional deficiencies, hepatitis, environmental factors, Reye's syndrome, a variant of preeclampsia, and genetic factors. Nutritional deficiencies have been suggested by a variety of sources as a possible cause of AFLP, although supportive data have not been reported. It has also been suggested that AFLP may represent a stage in the development of acute viral hepatitis. However, evaluation of liver biopsy in patients with AFLP has failed to demonstrate any progression from the

histologic changes associated with AFLP to the inflammation and necrosis associated with acute viral hepatitis, nor have patients been found to have serologic changes associated with viral infections, or viral particles isolated in biopsy material (Duff, 1991). Environmental factors have also been put forth as a possible cause of AFLP—specifically, exposure to a variety of drugs. Tetracycline is known to inhibit protein synthesis, which results in fat deposits in the liver. Clinical symptoms of tetracycline-induced AFL and AFLP are identical. Thus, a careful history related to drug use is essential in identification of patients with drug-induced fatty liver disease versus patients with AFLP. Reye's syndrome has AFLP also been theorized as a potential trigger for AFLP. Electron microscopy reveals enlargement of the mitochondria in both disorders, but a more detailed exam of patients with AFLP shows very dense bodies in the mitochondria that are absent in those with Reye's syndrome (Barton et al., 1990).

A more common theory is that AFLP is actually an atypical presentation of preeclampsia (Minakami & Okan, 1988). Although preeclampsia is present in approximately half the patients with AFLP, there are several characteristics that establish them as separate clinical entities that may occur concurrently. Evidence of fatty infiltration of the liver on ultrasound, CT scan, or MRI suggests AFLP (Rofsky & Fleischer, 1995). The PT, PTT, fibrinogen and platelet count, and

276

serum glucose levels are abnormal in AFLP. In preeclampsia/HELLP syndrome, PT, PTT, fibrinogen, and serum glucose levels are normal, with only the platelet count being low. The intravascular hemolysis present in patients with HELLP syndrome does not appear until late in the course of AFLP. Finally, histologic changes in the liver reveal the differences in the two disease processes. The patient with AFLP typically demonstrates fat deposits and the patient with preeclampsia/HELLP syndrome demonstrates inflammation, necrosis, and fibrin deposits (Rolfs & Ishak, 1985).

In addition, current research indicates there may be a genetic component to AFLP. Several studies suggest a link between AFLP and fetuses who have Long Chain 3-Hydroxyacyl Coenzyme A Dehydrogenase Deficiency (LCHAD). LCHAD is caused by an enzyme defect in the beta-oxidation cycle. This results in an inability of the body to break down fatty acids into a usable energy source. Women who are carriers for LCHAD may develop AFLP if the fetus has LCHAD (Sims et al., 1995; Treems et al., 1996). This intriguing link requires further investigation but shows promise in identifying a potential trigger for AFLP.

ANATOMY AND PHYSIOLOGY

Central to any discussion of AFLP is a review of the anatomy and physiology of the liver. The largest solid internal organ in the body is the liver, weighing about three pounds (Guyton & Hall, 1996). It lies in the right upper quadrant of the abdomen underneath the diaphragm. The liver is divided into right and left lobes with the right being the larger lobe. Within the lobes are numerous lobules and hepatocytes, the functional unit of the liver. Surrounding the liver is a tough membrane, known as the Glisson's capsule.

The liver is unique in that it has a dual blood supply. The hepatic artery provides 350 ml of oxygenated blood to the liver, making it the chief source of oxygen. The portal vein delivers 1100 ml of nutrient rich blood from the gastrointestinal system, making proteins, fats, and carbohydrates available for the many metabolic functions of the liver. The blood exits the liver through the central vein into the hepatic vein

and finally to the inferior vena cava (Guyton & Hall, 1996).

Within the liver there are 50,000–100,000 lobules (Fig. 17-1). The lobules, which are the functional unit in the liver, contain two types of cells, the hepatocytes and Kupffer cells. These lobules lie adjacent to the central vein. Branching off from the central vein are the sinusoids. The sinusoids serve as a reservoir of blood and are where exchange of oxygen, nutrients, and waste takes place. Between the sinusoids are the lobules, which contain the hepatocytes. Substances produced by the hepatocytes are secreted into the sinusoids and drained to the central vein. Adjacent to the hepatocytes are the bile canaliculi, which drain bile from the hepatocytes into the bile duct. Also along the lobules are the Kupffer cells. These cells are tissue macrophages that phagocytize bacteria and foreign substances that enter the liver via the portal vein.

The liver is an organ that is essential for the maintenance of life, as it is involved in almost every metabolic function of the body. Functions of the liver may be divided into three major categories: vascular functions for the storage and filtration of blood, metabolic functions, and secretory functions.

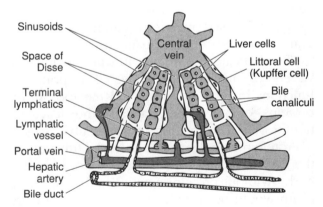

Figure 17-1. Basic structure of a liver lobule, showing the hepatic cellular plates, the blood vessels, the bile-collecting system, and the lymph flow system composed of the spaces of Disse and the interlobular lymphatics.

Reprinted from Guyton, Taylor, & Granger (1975). As modified from Elias: Circulatory Physiology, Vol. 2: Dynamics and Control of the Body Fluids. Philadelphia: W. B. Saunders.

The liver serves as both a reservoir and a filter for blood. About 1100 ml of blood from the portal vein drains into the liver sinusoids each minute. An additional 350 ml flow into the sinusoids from the hepatic artery. Total blood flow averages 1500 ml per minute (Guyton & Hall, 1996). The pressure in the hepatic vein and portal vein are low to allow blood to flow through the liver with little resistance. Should pressure in the hepatic vein increase, the liver becomes a reservoir for blood and becomes engorged and edematous. During times of stress the liver will shunt blood back into the systemic circulation. Also, one must remember that with liver injury the result is rapid, massive blood loss into the abdomen.

The liver also serves as a blood filtration system. The inner surfaces of the sinusoids contain Kupffer cells. These cells, which are highly phagocytic, engulf foreign material and bacteria in the blood as it flows through the liver. As a result, the blood circulates back into the systemic circulation cleansed of bacteria and foreign material. Also, the porous endothelial lining of the sinusoids allows large quantities of lymph to drain to the space of Disse, which connects to the lymphatic system. This system allows for drainage of lymph, plasma proteins, and excess fluid. Any increase in pressure in the hepatic vessels results in an increase in fluid moving into the lymphatic system, overwhelming its ability to drain it, and eventually causing ascites.

The next category of liver function includes a variety of metabolic activities. The principal functions include synthesis and metabolism of proteins, carbohydrates, fat, and the deactivation or biotransformation of many substances.

Protein metabolism is an essential function of the liver because proteins are not stored in the body. Without protein metabolism by the liver, death would occur in a matter of days. Protein metabolism results in the deamination of amino acids, the formation of urea, and the formation of plasma proteins.

Every protein is made up of amino acids arranged in a specific sequence. If one is absent the synthesis of a protein may not be possible. The liver takes up the amino acids from the portal vein and converts them into various proteins. Once the cells have reached the capacity for accepting proteins, the excess amino acids can be degraded and used for energy or changed to glycogen and stored. This process is known as deamination.

Ammonia is produced as a result of the deamination process. Ammonia is also produced by the action of bacteria in the gut. The liver converts ammonia into urea, which can then be excreted by the kidneys. Without this conversion the ammonia level will rapidly rise, resulting in hepatic coma and death.

The liver also synthesizes plasma proteins. Virtually all the plasma proteins, with the exception of gammaglobulin, are formed in the hepatic cells. Plasma proteins such as prothrombin, fibrinogen, and factor VII are essential in the clotting cascade. Albumin is responsible for maintaining the colloid oncotic pressure. Significant coagulopathy and changes in colloid oncotic pressure will result from disruptions in liver functions.

Carbohydrate metabolism is also conducted by the liver. Through carbohydrate metabolism the liver regulates the circulating level of glucose. As the blood enters the liver via the portal vein, glucose is converted to glycogen and stored in the hepatocytes via the process of glycogenesis. Glycogen can be converted back to glucose as needed. This process is known as glycogenolysis. Once glycogen stores have been depleted the liver can convert proteins and fats to glucose through the process of gluconeogenesis. This is known as the liver's glucose buffer function. Disruptions in liver function will interfere with this function and result in profound hypoglycemia.

The principal site for fat synthesis is the liver. Specifically, the liver is responsible for betaoxidation of fatty acids, the formation of acetoacetic acid, the formation of the lipoproteins, synthesis of cholesterol and phospholipids, and the conversion of excess carbohydrates and proteins to fat. Phospholipids are essential to maintain cell wall integrity. Lipoproteins are required for lipid transport. Cholesterol is formed into bile salts. The excess carbohydrates and proteins stored as adipose tissue can be broken down to glycerol and fatty acids to be used as energy.

Another metabolic function of the liver is the biotransformation or the deactivation of numerous substances by the liver. The result of the deactivation process is an inactive substance, which is then bound to a variety of substances and excreted via the urine or feces. Many drugs such as antibiotics, analgesics, anti-inflammatory drugs, diuretics, sedatives, and cardiovascular drugs are deactivated by the liver. The hormones testosterone, estrogen, aldosterone, and cortisol are all metabolized by the liver. Liver failure may result in toxic levels of substances generally deactivated by the liver.

The final category of liver function is the secretory function. Bile is produced by the hepatocytes in the liver and stored in the gall bladder. It is released into the intestines when needed to aid in digestion. Bile salts are also manufactured by the liver. Bile salts are required for the emulsification of fat in the intestines. Bile salts are also essential for the absorption of vitamins A, D, E, and K. Vitamins may be stored in the liver, specifically vitamins A, D, and B_{12}, for up to one year.

The liver is also responsible for the excretion of bilirubin. Bilirubin is formed during the destruction of red blood cells. The hepatocytes remove bilirubin from the blood and chemically modify it to make it soluble in aqueous solutions. The conjugated bilirubin is then secreted by the hepatocytes into the bile. The bile is secreted into the intestines where it is converted to urobilinogen and excreted in the feces. Urobilinogen that enters the systemic circulation is excreted by the kidneys.

When faced with the enormity of the liver's contribution to the functions of the body, it is clear that liver failure will result in severe multisystem organ dysfunction.

CLINICAL PRESENTATION

Early recognition and prompt delivery have improved the outcome for both mother and fetus; therefore, it is imperative that the patient with AFLP be diagnosed and treated aggressively. Patients with AFLP most often present with clinical manifestations of the disease in the third trimester of pregnancy. The average gestational age at time of onset is 35–36 weeks (Baker & Cefalo, 1985; Riely et al., 1987). It is most com-

mon in first pregnancies, and more frequent in twin gestations and in those with male fetuses. The onset is insidious and nonspecific. Initial signs and symptoms include anorexia, lethargy, malaise, headache, tachycardia, nausea, and vomiting. Central nervous system symptoms include restlessness, mental confusion, asterixis, seizure, and coma. The patient may develop right upper quadrant pain and ascites as the fluid accumulates in the liver and abdomen. Fever is generally not present until the later stages of the disease. Jaundice is generally only present in the later stages of the disease. As the liver failure worsens, the patient may develop generalized edema, gastrointestinal hemorrhage, disseminated intravascular coagulation (DIC), renal failure, pancreatitis, pleural effusions, profound hypoglycemia, and hepatic coma. The patient with AFLP will require laboratory assessment to help establish the diagnosis and severity of the disease process. Laboratory analysis should include tests that assess function of the hematologic, hepatic, and renal systems (Display 17-1).

Hematologic abnormalities common to patients with AFLP include anemia, leukocytosis, coagulopathy, and thrombocytopenia. The patient may be anemic as a result of gastrointestinal bleeding, intravascular hemolysis, or the pregnancy itself. The WBC is generally elevated and may be as high as 30,000 mm (Kaplan, 1985). If the patient has acute hepatic failure, synthesis of plasma proteins may be impaired, resulting in significant coagulopathy. Prothrombin time (PT) and partial thromboplastin time (PTT), which measure the speed of the extrinsic and intrinsic clotting pathways, respectively, are prolonged. If the patient has developed DIC, the platelet count and fibrinogen will be decreased and fibrin degradation products will be increased.

Liver function tests will provide the clinician with information regarding hepatic function. Tests include serum glutamic oxaloacetic transaminase (SGOT) or aspartate aminotransferase (AST), serum glutamic pyruvic transaminase (SGPT), or alanine aminotransferase (ALT), lactic dehydrogenase (LDH), alkaline phosphates, bilirubin, and ammonia. These values are not affected by pregnancy except for the serum alkaline phosphate. This value is increased because of

DISPLAY 17-1

AFLP Laboratory Analysis

Hematologic
Anemia
Leukocytosis
Thrombocytopenia
WBC >15,000

Coagulation
PT, PTT prolonged
Fibrinogen decreased

Hepatic Function
SGOT (or AST) increased (100–1000 u/L)
SGPT (or ALT) increased higher than SGOT
LDH markedly increased
Alkaline phosphatase 3x to 4x normal
Bilirubin increased
Ammonia increased

Biochemical
Hypoglycemia

Renal Function
BUN increased
Uric acid increased
Creatinine increased

Urinalysis
Creatinine clearance decreased
Urine sodium decreased
Proteinuria
Urine output decreased

the process of a heat-stable alkaline phosphate produced in the placenta.

The SGOT and SGPT are moderately elevated in AFLP, indicating liver damage. The SGPT is more specific and generally exceeds the increased value of the SGOT, which ranges between 100 and 1000 U/L. The LDH will be significantly elevated related to its presence in large quantities in liver tissue.

Alkaline phosphatase is three to four times normal in pregnancy. The enzyme is produced in the liver and excreted in the bile. The level rises with bile duct injury or cholestasis. This value may be nonspecific in patients with AFLP.

The serum bilirubin is usually < 10 mg/dl unless hemolysis or renal failure are present. Total bilirubin is a measure of the liver's ability to conjugate and excrete bile. When the level of unconjugated bilirubin is elevated, there may be

significant intrahepatic cellular damage. If the conjugated bilirubin is increased, this is an indication of biliary obstruction.

Serum ammonia level is mildly increased early in the course of AFLP. As the liver failure worsens, the ammonia levels may reach levels ten times normal. If ammonia is not converted to urea and levels continue to rise, hepatic coma results.

Hypoglycemia is also common in patients with AFLP. As the liver fails, its ability to convert glycogen to glucose fails and results in profound hypoglycemia, coma, and death if not reversed.

The patient with AFLP may also present with renal dysfunction. Laboratory analysis of blood urea nitrogen (BUN), creatinine, and uric acid should be assessed. During pregnancy BUN, creatinine, and uric acid are all excreted more effectively than in the nonpregnant adult because of the 50% increase in glomerular filtration rate. In patients with AFLP the BUN may be increased to 18 mg/dl over a normal pregnancy value of 8.2 mg/dl. The creatinine and uric acid levels are increased. The creatinine clearance and urine volume are decreased.

Other diagnostic studies that may be helpful to the clinician include ultrasound, computerized tomography scans, and liver biopsy. Ultrasound and CT scans have been suggested as alternatives to liver biopsy because they are safe, noninvasive, and readily available. However, the sensitivity and specificity in diagnosis of AFLP has not been established (Campillo et al., 1986; Maben et al. 1988; McKee et al., 1986; Purdie & Waters, 1988; Van & Podrasky, 1990).

Liver biopsy may be the key to diagnosis. The biopsy with a special stain for fat will reveal the fat deposits characteristic of AFLP. The fat deposits are free fatty acids rather than triglycerides. The nuclei of the cells remain in a central location and are normal in size and appearance (Varner & Rinderknecht, 1980). Liver biopsy may not be done at the bedside unless the PT is within 3 seconds of control and the platelet count is greater than 60,000 ml³ (Mabie, 1992).

DIFFERENTIAL DIAGNOSIS

A common clinical dilemma is diagnosing AFLP. The clinician must also consider hepatitis, cholestasis, and PIH/HELLP syndrome as working diagnoses.

Hepatitis may resemble AFLP initially; however, serologic tests can establish the diagnosis of hepatitis A, B, or D. Also, as discussed previously, the anatomic changes that occur in the liver with AFLP and hepatitis are very different. Delivery does not alter the course of hepatitis.

Patients with cholestasis of pregnancy usually present with pruritus and jaundice. In AFLP jaundice does not develop until late in the disease. In cholestasis, alkaline phosphatase levels are elevated and in AFLP they are not (Duff, 1991). Also, the hallmark anatomic change associated with cholestasis of pregnancy is biliary stasis, which is absent in AFLP.

The differential diagnosis between AFLP and PIH/HELLP syndrome is the most challenging

and in many cases may not be possible, based on clinical signs and symptoms. PIH/HELLP syndrome may occur concurrently with AFLP, making the laboratory assessments less useful. If AFLP occurs without PIH/HELLP syndrome, the laboratory analysis is useful. In AFLP the PT, PTT, fibrinogen, platelet count, and serum glucose levels are all abnormal. In patients with PIH/HELLP syndrome, only the platelet count will be abnormal.

The treatment for both AFLP and PIH/HELLP syndrome is supportive care and delivery. While the diagnosis is being determined, the patient should be prepared for delivery. Remission of AFLP does not occur without delivery of the fetus.

CLINICAL MANAGEMENT AND TREATMENT

The management of AFLP remains maternal stabilization followed by delivery and supportive care (Usta, Barton, & Amon, 1994). Early recognition, early delivery, and better supportive care have all helped to improve fetal and maternal outcome with AFLP.

Assessment should begin with a complete history. The patient's chief complaint should be ascertained and evaluation conducted for the presence or absence of other signs and symptoms. Review of past medical history, family history, and social history should be assessed as well. Other assessments should include vital signs, level of consciousness, electrocardiographic monitoring, skin color, breath sounds, urine output, oxygen saturation, and fetal assessments. Fetal heart rate monitoring or biophysical monitoring should be done concurrently with maternal evaluation. This is essential because of the increased risk of fetal compromise including stillbirth in pregnancies complicated by AFLP (Varner & Rinderknecht, 1980; Moise & Shah, 1987).

The patient with AFLP should be hospitalized. Once the diagnosis of AFLP has been made, preparation for delivery should begin. Remission of the disease generally does not begin until delivery has been achieved (Hon et al., 1984). Although cesarean section has been recommended as the most expeditious route of delivery, there are no studies to support that immediate cesarean section offers significant benefit over vaginal delivery. Vaginal delivery may be preferable because it offers less stress to the maternal system. Decisions regarding the mode of delivery should be based on a thorough assessment of both maternal and fetal status and the favorability of the cervix for an induction of labor. Careful monitoring of the fetus during labor is required because of high incidence of fetal distress in AFLP patients (Moise & Shah, 1987).

If cesarean section is performed, many anesthesiologists prefer general anesthesia because of the risk of coagulopathy. However, the choice of the anesthetic agents must be done carefully because many of the agents used in general anesthesia are hepatotoxic. If the coagulopathy can be corrected, spinal anesthesia has been proposed as an alternative, to avoid the adverse effects of general anesthesia on a diseased liver (Ebert et al., 1984).

The use of a pulmonary artery catheter may be necessary to assess hemodynamic function. In addition to providing important information regarding the hemodynamic status of the patient, the use of a pulmonary artery catheter can also provide essential data regarding oxygen transport in these critically ill patients.

Careful attention to nursing care of these patients is essential. The general goal of management is supportive until resolution of the disease process can occur. Specific assessment and interventions are performed with knowledge of complications common in patients with liver failure. See Display 17-2 for a list of potential nursing diagnoses.

Frequent laboratory assessment of liver function is necessary. Following trends in liver function allows the clinician to track progression and resolution of the disease. With liver failure and the disruption in the production of plasma proteins, the patient is at risk for development of significant coagulopathy and DIC. Signs and symptoms of DIC include oozing from venipuncture sites, bleeding gums, epistaxis, hematuria, bruising, and increased vaginal bleeding. DIC is treated with aggressive volume replacement and restoration of adequate oxygen transport to tissues. Crystalloid solution, fresh frozen plasma, platelets, vitamin K, and packed red blood cells may all be necessary in volume replacement.

The patient with AFLP may also develop significant pulmonary complications. Assessment of pulmonary status includes respiratory rate, quality of respirations, breath sounds, and oxy-

DISPLAY 17-2

Nursing Diagnoses

Potential for infection related to

- indwelling urinary catheter
- IV sites
- decreased action of liver to filter bacteria

Alteration in fluid volume (deficit) related to disseminated intravascular coagulation

Impaired gas exchange related to pulmonary edema

Ineffective breathing patterns related to decreased central nervous system function

Alteration in nutrition; less than body requirements related to inability of liver to process protein, fat, or carbohydrates

Alterations in family process related to intensive care setting

gen saturation via pulse oximetry should be performed frequently depending on specific patient condition. Tachypnea, tachycardia, decreased breath sounds, coughing, anxiety, and decreased oxygen saturation are all signs of pulmonary compromise. AFLP patients are at risk for both cardiogenic and noncardiogenic pulmonary edema. Cardiogenic pulmonary edema may be iatrogenic related to fluid volume replacement. Noncardiogenic pulmonary edema may be related to changes in colloid oncotic pressure and increased pulmonary capillary permeability. Chest x-ray and arterial blood gases may confirm the diagnosis of pulmonary edema. A pulmonary artery catheter allows measurements that differentiate between cardiogenic and noncardiogenic pulmonary edema. Supplemental oxygen via face mask or nasal cannula may be necessary. Often to maintain adequate ventilation and oxygenation the patient may require intubation and mechanical ventilation (Baker & Cefalo, 1985).

Disturbances in carbohydrate metabolism result in difficulty maintaining blood glucose levels greater than 60 mg/dl. Blood glucose levels should be checked every 1–2 hours. Signs and symptoms of hypoglycemia include exhaustion, headaches, irritability, confusion, and coma. The patient requires administration of an intravenous solution that contains 5–20% dextrose. An ampule of 50% dextrose should be kept at the bedside for immediate administration as necessary.

Disturbances in protein metabolism may lead to neurologic abnormalities as ammonia builds up in the body. The goal is to provide the patient with adequate nutrition but limit the amount of ammonia produced. Signs and symptoms of ammonia toxicity include altered level of consciousness, asterixis, headache, seizures, and hepatic coma. Protein intake may be restricted or eliminated. Enemas may be given to promote colonic emptying and reduce the amount of ammonia produced in the bowel. Total parenteral nutrition may be necessary with low protein formulas.

Renal failure is common in patients with AFLP. Frequent assessment of renal function should be done. Hourly urine output measure-

ments are essential. Urine output greater than 30 ml/hr generally indicates adequate renal perfusion. Renal damage may occur, which results in the inability of the kidneys to concentrate urine, thus urine specific gravity should be monitored. Creatinine, BUN, and uric acid levels should also be assessed. Patients with AFLP may require dialysis in the face of acute renal failure.

The ability of the liver to deactivate drugs and other substances may be impaired. Any medication or substance that requires hepatic metabolism must be withheld from the patient with AFLP. The action of the Kupffer cells in the filtration of foreign substances and bacteria may also be disrupted. Meticulous attention to sterile and aseptic techniques may help minimize the risk of nosocomial infection.

Patients with AFLP may develop ascites, which can be treated with administration of diuretics, sodium restriction, or paracentesis. Electrolyte disturbances should be corrected as necessary. The gastric pH should be maintained at levels greater than 5.0 to prevent stress ulcers. The administration of H_2 receptor blockers and antacids may help to prevent stress ulcers as well (Duff, 1991).

Emotional support for the patient and family is crucial. The family and patient need simple explanations regarding prognosis, equipment, procedures, and plan of care. The patient and family may be very anxious and should be encouraged to participate in the overall care and support of the patient. Following delivery the clinician should encourage bonding as the maternal and neonatal condition allow.

Remission of the disease is generally observed within 2–3 days following delivery (Riely, 1987). Recovery of hepatic, renal, and neurologic function is usually complete. Infants do not show signs of hepatic dysfunction. AFLP is unlikely to occur in subsequent pregnancies.

AFLP is a potentially reversible disease, therefore liver transplantation is generally utilized as a last resort, and thus has a limited role in the treatment of patients with AFLP. There has been one case reported of liver transplantation for AFLP (Ockner et al., 1990). A multidisciplinary team should be involved in any decision to transplant an AFLP patient (Mabie, 1992).

SUMMARY

AFLP is a rare but potentially fatal complication of the third trimester of pregnancy. Morbidity and mortality have decreased in recent years because of earlier recognition and aggressive management. It is important to have a good understanding of AFLP because prompt diagnosis and immediate treatment may improve maternal and fetal outcome.

REFERENCES

Baker, V. V., & Cefalo, R. L. (1985). Fulminant hepatic failure in the third trimester of pregnancy. Journal of Reproductive Medicine, 30, 229–252.

Barton, J. R., Sibai, B. M., Mabie, W. C., et al. (1990). Recurrent acute fatty liver of pregnancy. American Journal of Obstetrics and Gynecology, 163, 534–536.

Campillo, B., Bernuan, J., Wite, M. O., et al. (1986). Ultrasonography in acute fatty liver of pregnancy. Annals of Internal Medicine, 105, 383–384.

Duff, P. (1991). Acute fatty liver of pregnancy. In S. L. Clark, D. B. Cotton, G. D. V. Hankins, & J. P. Phelan (Eds.), Critical care obstetrics (2nd ed., pp. 484–497). Boston: Blackwell.

Ebert, E. C., Sun, E. A., Wright, S. H., et al. (1984). Does early diagnosis and delivery in acute fatty liver of pregnancy lead to improvement in maternal and infant survival? Dig Dis Science, 29, 453–459.

Guyton, A. C., & Hall, J. E. (1996). The liver as an organ. In A. C. Guyton & J. E. Hall, Textbook of medical physiology (9th ed., pp. 883–888). Philadelphia: W. B. Saunders.

Hon, S. H., Levin, S., Ahola, S., et al. (1984). Acute fatty liver of pregnancy: Survival with early cesarean section. Dig Dis Science, 29, 449–452.

Kaplan, M. M. (1985). Acute fatty liver of pregnancy. New England Journal of Medicine, 13, 49–61.

Mabie, W. C. (1992). Acute fatty liver of pregnancy. Gastroenterology Clinics of North America, 21 (4), 951–959.

Maben, W. C., Dacus, J. V., Sibai, B. M., et al. (1988). Computed tomography in acute fatty liver of pregnancy. American Journal of Obstetrics and Gynecology, 158, 142–145.

McKee, C. W., Weir, P. E., Foster, J. H., et al. (1986). Acute fatty liver of pregnancy and diagnosis by computed tomography. British Medical Journal, 292, 291–292.

Minakami, H., & Okan, S. T. (1988). Preeclampsia: A microvascular fat disease of the liver? American Journal of Obstetrics and Gynecology, 159, 1043–1048.

Moise, K. J., & Shah, D. M. (1987). Acute fatty liver of pregnancy: Etiology of fetal distress and fetal wastage. Obstetrics and Gynecology, 67, 482–485.

Ockner, S. A., Brunt, E. M., Cohn, S. M., et al. (1990). Fulminant hepatic failure caused by acute fatty liver of pregnancy treated by orthotopic liver transplantation. Hepatology, 11, 59–64.

Poctros, P. J., Pettus, R. L., & Reynolds, T. B. (1983). Idiopathic fatty liver of pregnancy: Findings in ten cases. Medicine, 63, 449–452.

Purdie, J. M., & Waters, B. N. J. (1988). Acute fatty liver of pregnancy: Clinical features and diagnosis. Australian and New Zealand Journal of Obstetrics and Gynecology, 28, 62–67.

Riely, C. A. (1987). Acute fatty liver of pregnancy. Seminars in Liver Disease, 7(1), 47–54.

Riely, C. A., Latham, R. S., Romero, R., et al. (1987). Acute fatty liver of pregnancy. Annals of Internal Medicine, 106, 703–708.

Rofsky, N. M., & Fleischer, H. (1995). CT and MRI of diffuse liver disease. Seminars in Ultrasound, CT and MRI, 16(1), 16–33.

Rolfs, D. B., & Ishak, T. G. (1985). Acute fatty liver of pregnancy: A clinicopathologic study of 35 cases. Hepatology, 5, 1149–1158.

Sheehan, H. L. (1940). The pathology of acute yellow atrophy and delayed chloroform poisoning. Journal of Obstetrics and Gynaecology British Empire, 47, 49–61.

Sims, H. F., Brackett, J., Powell, C., et al. (1995). The molecular basis of pediatric long chain 3-hydroxyacyl CO-A dehydrogenase deficiency associated with maternal acute fatty liver of pregnancy. Proceedings of the National Academy of Science, 92, 841–847.

Treems, W. R., Sharp, M. E., Hale, D. E., et al. (1996). Acute fatty liver of pregnancy, hemolysis, elevated liver enzymes and low platelet syndrome and long chain 3-hydroxyacyl CO enzyme A dehydrogenase deficiency. American Journal of Gastroenterology, 49, 393–397.

Usta, I. M., Barton, J. R., & Amon, E. A. (1994). Acute fatty liver of pregnancy: An experience in the diagnosis and management of fourteen cas-es. American Journal of Obstetrics and Gynecology, 171(5), 1342–1347.

Van, L. L. & Podrasky, A. (1990). Computed tomography and ultrasonographic findings in women with acute fatty liver of pregnancy. Journal of Reproductive Medicine, 35, 815–817.

Varner, M., & Rinderknecht, N. K. (1980). Acute fatty metamorphosis of pregnancy: A maternal mortality and literature review. Journal of Reproductive Medicine, 24, 177–180.

CHAPTER 18

Autoimmune Disorders in Pregnancy

Patricia M. Sauer

Under normal situations, the immune response is initiated when a foreign organism or antigen invades the body. Macrophages, which are stored in the lymphoid tissue, phagocytize most invading organisms and pass antigens by cell-to-cell contact to chemical mediators, called lymphokines. The lymphokines present the antigen to B-lymphocytes and T-lymphocytes. The lymphocytes are cloned and activated. Helper T-lymphocytes secrete lymphokines, which further activate the B-lymphocytes resulting in an increased quantity of antibodies. The antibodies enter the bloodstream, target their specific antigen, and form antigen–antibody complexes. Antibodies eliminate foreign organisms by either directly attacking them or by triggering the complement system. The complement system consists of proteins (C1–C9, B, and D) that are normally inactive, but become activated by an antigen–antibody reaction. A portion of the antibody that becomes activated combines with one of these proteins in the complement system and mobilizes a cascade of events, which produces multiple products that help eliminate the foreign organism. The complement system protects the body from the invading organism through actions that include phagocytosis; rupture of the invading organism's surface; migration of neutrophils and macrophages to the region of the antigen; activation of mast cells, which release substances that inactivate the antigen; and the

inflammatory process. Cytotoxic or killer T-lymphocytes, in addition to antibodies, are also capable of directly destroying the invading organism. The suppressor T-lymphocytes regulate the activity of helper and cytotoxic T-lymphocytes and therefore prevent an excessive immune reaction that may potentially destroy the body's tissues (Feinberg & Gonik, 1991; Guyton & Hall, 1996). Refer to Figure 18-1 for an overview of the normal immune response.

The immune system normally does not develop an immune reaction against the body's tissues because of its ability to recognize the body's cells. However, in autoimmune disorders the body may fail to recognize its own proteins and promote destruction of the body's own tissues. Regulation of the immune response is impaired, most likely because of decreased suppressor T-lymphocytic activity. Additionally, cytotoxic T-lymphocytes destroy the body's cells. Autoantibodies, or antibodies that are directed against the body's proteins and tissues, promote cellular and tissue damage by immune complex reactions (Boumpas et al., 1995; Sala, 1993).

The incidence of autoimmune disorders in the general population is 5–7%. Autoimmune disorders peak around the time of puberty and generally occur with higher frequency in females (Floyd & Roberts, 1992). Understanding the pathophysiology, management, and the effects of autoimmune disorders and therapies on pregnancy facilitates the obstetric nurse in providing

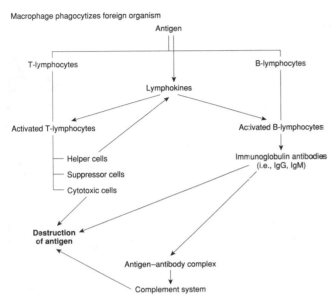

Figure 18-1. Normal immune response.

comprehensive care to the woman with an autoimmune disorder. This chapter focuses on systemic lupus erythematosus, antiphospholipid syndrome, and autoimmune thrombocytopenia. Chapter 19 will focus on AIDS.

SYSTEMIC LUPUS ERYTHEMATOSUS

Incidence

Systemic lupus erythematosus (SLE) is a multi-system collagen vascular disease that primarily affects women of childbearing age. It is more prevalent in African Americans, Asian Americans, and Hispanics than in Anglo-Americans (Hahn, 1994; Sala, 1993). SLE is estimated to occur in 1:1660–2952 deliveries (Gimovsky & Montoro, 1991; Sala, 1993).

Etiology and Pathophysiology

The cause of SLE is basically unknown, but genetic predisposition and sexual gender most likely influence the development of the disease. Additionally, certain environmental factors, such as ultraviolet light or possibly a virus, may trigger the development of autoantibodies that promote cellular and tissue damage (Hahn, 1994). SLE involves an exaggerated immune response (increased B-lymphocyte activity with subse-

quent antibody formation) that goes unregulated most likely because of either decreased suppressor T-lymphocyte activity or abnormal increase in helper T-lymphocyte activity. Autoantibodies form immune complexes with specific antigens. Immune complexes are inadequately cleared from the circulation and promote tissue damage by activating the complement system and promoting the inflammatory response (Boumpas et al., 1995a).

Definition and Diagnosis

SLE is typically diagnosed when at least four criteria for clinical manifestations are exhibited. These criteria are widely published (Floyd & Roberts, 1992; Gimovsky & Montoro, 1991; Hahn, 1994; Sala, 1993) and are summarized in Display 18-1. SLE may involve one organ system initially, but typically involves multiple body systems. Most individuals experience periods of exacerbation and remission (Hahn, 1994).

Clinical Manifestations

Permanent organ system sequelae occurs in 10% of all pregnancies (Gimovsky & Montoro, 1991). Exacerbation of SLE (lupus flare) is manifested by a variety of organ system involvement. The renal system is the most commonly affected body system in SLE. Impaired renal function results from reaction of autoantibodies against antigens on renal basement membranes and precipitation of immune complexes in the renal vasculature and glomeruli. Renal deterioration ensues because of inflammatory-mediated cellular necrosis, and eventually, fibrosis. Hypertension has also been associated with renal deterioration (Boumpas et al., 1995a). Appearance of proteinuria or casts in the urine may reflect renal tissue damage. Additionally, elevations in serum creatinine and blood urea nitrogen as well as oliguria support the suspicion of renal impairment.

Skin and joint involvement manifest frequently in individuals with SLE. Malar or "butterfly" rash may be seen over the cheeks and bridge of the nose, and may also involve the chin and ears. Discoid lesions (raised, scaly, erythematous patches) may be disfiguring and appear on sun-exposed areas (Hahn, 1994). Photosensitivity is associated with anti-Ro and SS-A antibodies and

DISPLAY 18-1

ARA Criteria for Diagnosis of SLE*

- Malar rash ("butterfly")—erythema that is flat or raised and is typically present over the cheeks and bridge of the nose
- Discoid rash—erythematous raised, scaly patches
- Photosensitivity
- Oral or nasopharyngeal ulcers
- Arthritis involving two or more peripheral joints characterized by tenderness, swelling, or effusion
- Serositis—described as pleuritis or pericarditis
- Renal disorder
- Neurologic disorder—seizures or psychosis without other identifiable cause
- Hematologic disorder—hemolytic anemia, thrombocytopenia, or lymphopenia
- Immunologic disorder (i.e., positive antibodies for anti-Sm, false positive VDRL)
- Abnormal titer of antinuclear antibodies (ANA)

*American Rheumatism Association Criteria for Diagnosis of SLE
Presence of at least four clinical manifestations supports the diagnosis of SLE

is seen in one third to two thirds of individuals with SLE. Ultraviolet light may initiate the development of autoantibodies that promote cellular damage of the skin. Joint involvement may be manifested as arthralgia, arthritis, or occasionally with the development of nodules and joint deformities (Boumpas et al., 1995b).

Central nervous system involvement includes a spectrum of behavioral disturbances that include depression, anxiety, mood swings, psychosis, and cognitive impairment (Hahn, 1994). Cerebral vascular accidents and convulsions may also manifest (Sala, 1993). Neuropsychiatric disease may result from primary events, such as deposition of immune complexes in brain tissue and blood vessels, or occur from secondary events such as the multisystem effects of SLE or complications from therapy. Hypertension is also common in SLE and has been associated with progression of renal deterioration. Hyperlipidemia, induced either by steroid therapy or by intracellular cholesterol accumulation from immune com-

plexes, combined with hypertension, increases the individual's risk for atherosclerotic disease and myocardial ischemia. Valvular lesions (stenosis or regurgitation) have been seen with increased frequency and may result in hemodynamic disturbances that necessitate valve replacement (Boumpas et al., 1995a).

Pulmonary manifestations include pleurisy and pleural effusions. Signs and symptoms consistent with lupus pneumonitis include fever, dyspnea, and cough (Hahn, 1994). Pulmonary manifestations may arise from acute alveolar–capillary injury as increased complement split products activate neutrophils that aggregate in the pulmonary vasculature, impairing oxygenation. Pulmonary hypertension is uncommon but may develop from vascular occlusion secondary to vasoconstriction and platelet aggregation from inflammatory processes (Boumpas et al., 1995a). Hematologic system involvement may also be manifested. Autoantibodies may react directly with antigens on cellular surfaces, such as erythrocytes or platelets, resulting in destruction. Hemolytic anemia and lymphopenia are common. Thrombocytopenia may also be evident, but is usually mild (Hahn, 1994).

Laboratory Manifestations

Antinuclear antibodies (ANA) are directed against nuclear cellular components. ANA is positive in 90–95% of individuals with SLE. ANA may occur in normal states (in low titers), such as in the elderly. A positive ANA may also manifest in other autoimmune diseases, chronic inflammatory processes, or viral infections. Certain drugs can induce positive ANA results ("lupus-like syndrome") (Hahn, 1994). Therefore, a positive ANA does not confirm SLE. However, a negative ANA makes the diagnosis of ANA unlikely (Treseler, 1988). Because the presence of ANA is not specific for SLE, once a positive SLE is identified, several additional antibody screens are performed. Antibodies to double-stranded DNA (anti-dsDNA) and to smooth-muscle antigen (anti-Sm) are more specific for SLE (Hahn, 1994).

Serum complement levels (C3 and C4) indicate consumption of immune complexes. Elevated or normal serum compliment levels indicate that immune complexes are being cleared. During exacerbation, immune complexes are not cleared from the body. Therefore, decreasing serum complement levels are consistent with exacerbation of the disease (lupus flare) (Floyd & Roberts, 1992; Gimovsky & Montoro, 1991; Rubbert, Pirner, Wildt, Kalden, & Manger, 1992). Additional laboratory findings that are consistent with lupus flare include increasing anti-DNA and rising ANA titer (Boumpas et al., 1995b; Gimovsky & Montoro, 1991). Lupus anticoagulant (LAC) and anticardiolipin antibodies (ACLA) are antiphospholipid antibodies that are found in some individuals with SLE (Kaaja, Julkunen, Viinikka, & Ylikorkala, 1993) and play a role in thrombosis. They are associated with significant perinatal morbidity and mortality (Adams, Druzin, Edershiem, Bond, & Kogut, 1992; Hayslett, 1992). Antiphospholipid antibodies and the antiphospholipid syndrome are discussed later in this chapter.

Laboratory findings, in addition to clinical manifestations, may be helpful in the determination of particular organ system involvement with lupus exacerbation. For example, renal involvement may be manifested by cellular casts in the urine, increased proteinuria, elevated serum creatinine, and decreased creatinine clearance. Hemolytic anemia, leukopenia, or thrombocytopenia may reflect hematologic involvement.

Maternal–Fetal Implications

Although it is disputed as to whether or not pregnancy is associated with an increased incidence of lupus flare (Petri, Howard, & Repke, 1991; Rubbert et al., 1992; Urowitz, Gladman, Farewell, Sterwart, & McDonald, 1993; Wong, Chan, & Lee, 1991), it is generally accepted that the frequency of lupus exacerbation during pregnancy is decreased as long as the disease was inactive at the time of conception (Gimovsky & Montoro, 1991; Hayslett, 1992; Urowitz et al., 1993). Active disease at the onset of pregnancy carries an increased risk of either lupus flare or continuation of active SLE (Hayslett, 1992). There is no laboratory or clinical prediction of impending lupus flare. However, hypertension prior to pregnancy is associated with a three- to fourfold increase in the incidence of lupus flare during pregnancy (Gimovsky & Montoro, 1991).

Impaired uteroplacental oxygen delivery occurs in SLE because of immune complex deposition along the trophoblastic membranes (Sala, 1993) and decidual and placental vascular thrombosis (Weiner, Lorber, & Blumenfeld, 1992). The fetus is at significant risk for hypoxemia and intrauterine fetal demise, especially if the disease flares or remains active during pregnancy (Floyd & Roberts, 1992; Rubbert et al., 1992; Weiner et al., 1992). Fetal survival is reduced significantly in the presence of hypertension and renal deterioration (Gimovsky & Montoro, 1991; Hayslett, 1991; Rubbert et al., 1992). Perinatal loss is lessened as long as the disease remains in remission or treatment is employed to control organ system manifestations (Weiner et al., 1992).

The onset of SLE during pregnancy or the postpartum period is often severe in presentation (Hayslett, 1992) and associated with a higher incidence of nephrotic syndrome and/or thrombocytopenia (Varner, Meehan, Syrop, Strottmann, & Goplerud, 1983). Hypertension and proteinuria, in addition to any number of multisystem manifestations that are consistent with both superimposed preeclampsia and SLE, may promote difficulty in differentiating superimposed preeclampsia from lupus flare. Determination of serum complement levels, ANA titer, and anti-DNA titer may be helpful. However, the increased incidence of fetal mortality in both lupus flare and superimposed preeclampsia may necessitate delivery of the fetus regardless of the definitive diagnosis.

Preterm delivery occurs with higher frequency in women with SLE in comparison to the normal population (Floyd & Roberts, 1992; Rubbert et al., 1992; Johnson, Petri, Witter, & Repke, 1995). Preterm delivery may be attributed to medically indicated delivery of the preterm fetus secondary to maternal or fetal complications. Preterm delivery may also occur as a result of the disease process. There is a noted increase in the incidence of premature rupture of membranes in women with SLE, possibly from weakening of connective tissue structures within the amniotic membranes (Johnson et al., 1995).

Neonatal lupus may manifest as cutaneous changes with or without systemic or cardiac involvement such as congenital heart block and is associated with antibodies to SS-A/Ro and SS-B/La (Floyd & Roberts, 1992; Waltuck & Buyon, 1994). Transplacental passage of maternal autoantibodies into the fetal circulation may react with fetal autoantigens, form immune complexes, and promote fetal tissue destruction (Boumpas et al., 1995; Waltuck & Buyon, 1994). Complete heart block is rare and occurs as a result of binding of the autoantibodies to the fetal cardiac conduction system (Waltuck & Buyon, 1994). Congenital heart block may be permanent and many infants require insertion of a pacemaker in the first months of life (Fox, Lumb, & Hawkins, 1990; Waltuck & Buyon, 1994). Mortality for these infants is approximately 30% (Boumpas et al., 1995b; Waltuck & Buyon, 1994). Noncardiac manifestations of neonatal lupus typically involve cutaneous changes; the skin of the newborn may be red and scaly with atrophic lesions of the face and upper thorax (Boumpas et al., 1995b). Symptoms usually resolve within 6 months to 1 year of age. The occurrence of neonatal lupus does not have any correlation with severity of maternal disease (Boumpas et al., 1995b; Floyd & Roberts, 1992; Waltuck & Buyon, 1994).

Treatment

A stimulus or stressful event may trigger the immune response, resulting in inflammation and tissue damage. Glucocorticoids, such as prednisone or hydrocortisone, inhibit the immune response by suppressing the activity of antibodies and T-lymphocytes. They alleviate inflammation by stabilizing cell membranes. As a result of stabilization of cell membranes, the release of damaging proteolytic enzymes that promote cellular damage is reduced (Guyton & Hall, 1996). Prednisone in daily doses of 40–60 mg for 2–3 weeks is generally given to women with lupus flare (Scott & Branch, 1994). Doses are increased in increments of 5–10 mg/day until symptoms are controlled. Doses may need to be as high as 2 mg/kg/day. Once symptoms are controlled, the dose is tapered to the lowest possible dose (Floyd & Roberts, 1992; Gimovsky & Montoro, 1991). Prednisone does not cross the placenta as readily as dexamethasone or betamethasone. Therefore, it is preferred for maternal treatment (Gimovsky & Montoro, 1991). In some clinical situtations, such as fetal heart block, dexamethasone may be administered to reduce inflammatory changes of the fetal heart that may be responsible for producing the conduction abnormality (Waltuck & Buyon, 1994). Chronic administration of corticosteroids may suppress the hypothalamic–pituitary–adrenal axis and render the individual incapable of adapting to physiologic stress because of decreased secretion of endogenous glucocorticoids (cortisol). Therefore, corticosteroid coverage is necessary during times of stress. Labor is certainly a stressful event and may necessitate administration of corticosteroids throughout the intrapartum period, particularly if previous exacerbations have occurred or if complications arise during labor. In this situation, hydrocortisone in three doses of 100 mg is administered intravenously. Immunosuppressive agents such as azathioprine may be necessary for the control of symptoms associated with lupus flare. When given, azathioprine is generally given in doses of 1–2 mg/kg/day. Immunosuppressive agents are generally limited to severe, life-threatening SLE exacerbation (Gimovsky & Montoro, 1991) because of potential teratogenicity and a potential for neonatal immunosuppression (Goldman, Mientus, Kutzer, Mulvihill, & Medsger).

ANTIPHOSPHOLIPID SYNDROME

Incidence

Primary antiphospholipid syndrome (APS) is an autoimmune disorder characterized by systemic abnormalities that occur as a result of vascular occlusion. Anticardiolipin antibody (aCL) and the lupus anticoagulant (LAC) are antiphospholipid antibodies (aPL) that have been associated with APS. Anticardiolipin antibody has been identified in 2–21% of the general population and the lupus anticoagulant has been identified in 0.27–5% of the general population (Pathson et al., 1993; Out et al., 1992).

Etiology and Pathophysiology

Anticardiolipin antibody and lupus anticoagulant are closely related antibodies (Love & Santoro, 1990) that are directed against phospholipids. Antiphospholipid antibodies bind to membranes of phospholipids or promote platelet activation and therefore predispose to the formation of platelet thrombi on vessel walls. Activated platelets help the initiation of the clotting cascade and formation of fibrin (Hayslett, 1992). Thrombosis from platelet aggregration is also promoted by an imbalance between the prostaglandins prostacyclin (inhibits platelet aggregation) and thromboxane (promotes platelet aggregation) in favor of thromboxane (Kaaja et al., 1993; Silviera et al., 1992). Fibrinolysis, a system that regulates the clotting cascade to prevent excessive thrombosis, is inhibited (Kaplan, Cartash, Pizzarello, & Furie, 1992), promoting further thrombus formation.

Definition and Diagnosis

Primary antiphospholipid syndrome is defined as the occurrence of the lupus anticoagulant and anticardiolipin antibodies combined with evidence of arterial or venous thrombosis, thrombocytopenia, or recurrent fetal loss (Perez & McClendon, 1992). Secondary antiphospholipid syndrome is described as the presence of aPL in a subset of individuals who have SLE. Women with secondary antiphospholipid syndrome have a higher incidence of fetal loss compared to women who have SLE without aPL (Adams et al., 1992; Boumpas et al., 1995a; Hayslett, 1992). In addition to the exclusion of SLE for the diagnosis of primary antiphospholipid syndrome, other exclusionary diagnoses include infections, certain drug reactions, and other connective tissue diseases (Perez & McClendon, 1992). Positive aPL without symptoms do not indicate APS (Boumpas et al., 1995b).

Clinical Manifestations

Multiple body systems are adversely affected by vascular occlusion that occurs secondary to arterial or venous thrombosis. Venous thrombosis has a propensity to occur in the left leg, possibly due to compression of the left iliac vein by the right iliac artery as they cross. Venous thrombosis in the lower extremities occurs with equal frequency in all three trimesters and may be manifested by leg swelling and complaints of pain. Leg swelling and pain are common complaints in the third trimester of pregnancy and are most likely caused by compression of the common iliac veins by the enlarged uterus, which may mimic venous thrombosis. Therefore, objective testing to confirm the presence of thrombosis is indicated (Ginsberg & Hirsch, 1992).

Hemolytic anemia may reflect hematologic involvement in APS. Thrombocytopenia is common and results from increased platelet consumption that occurs secondary to binding of aPL to platelet phospholipids. Renal failure with hypertension may also occur in APS as a result of occlusion of the renal microvasculature with thrombi. Renal impairment can range from mild presentation to end-stage renal failure

(Amigo, Torres, Robles, Bochicchio, & Reyes, 1992). Cerebral infarction is a more common manifestation of APS (Perez & McClendon, 1992) and may occur from thrombus formation in the cerebral microvasculature.

Thrombosis may predispose the individual to the development of coronary artery occlusion or valvular disease. Nonbacterial vegetative growth on the heart valves (verrucous endocarditis) can lead to ischemic events, mitral insufficiency, myocardial dysfunction, and pericardial effusion. Thrombi within the cardiac chambers has been documented, although it is rare, and may occur secondary to myocardial dysfunction (Kaplan et al., 1992). Uteroplacental involvement occurs from placental thrombosis and infarction (Out et al., 1992; Silver et al., 1993) and may be manifested by severe intrauterine fetal growth restriction, placental abruption, and fetal death. Clinical manifestations consistent with uteroplacental involvement are further discussed later in this chapter under the heading of "Maternal–Fetal Implications."

Laboratory Manifestations

Determination of aPL includes measurement of LAC and aCL of either IgG or IgM class. Venous thromboses and thrombocytopenia are strongly associated with IgG aCL (Segovia, 1992). A very high titer of IgG aCL is also strongly associated with an increased incidence of perinatal loss (Pattison, Chamley, McKay, Liggins, & Butler, 1993). Lupus anticoagulant is determined by laboratory measurement based on prolongation of phospholipid-dependent clotting tests. Based on this description of laboratory measurement and the term "lupus anticoagulant," one would expect a propensity for bleeding. However, for unexplained reasons, LAC prolongs the partial thromboplastin time (PTT) in vitro, but promotes systemic and placental thrombosis in vivo (MacLean, Cumming, McCall, Walker, & Walker, 1994). Unexplained prolongation in the PTT warrants evaluation for aPL (Perez & McClendon, 1992).

Interlaboratory variation in the measurement of aPL has been documented and may occur as a result of performance of different coagulation tests or a lack of standardization for cutoff values that determine whether the results are positive or negative. Although there is general agreement on high levels of aCL, there is more variation as to when to consider lower values positive. There is less variation in results for LAC, which is appropriately classified as positive or negative. Because of variation in laboratory measurement, it is recommended that positive aPL be confirmed by another laboratory, unless titers are very high (Peaceman, Silver, MacGregor, & Socol, 1992).

Maternal–Fetal Implications

Pregnancy can exacerbate the disease process of APS because of the propensity for thrombosis due to the hypercoagulable state of pregnancy (Hochfeld et al., 1994). Thrombosis in the uteroplacental vessels impairs oxygen delivery to the fetus. Severe fetal compromise (spontaneous abortion and fetal death) is of considerable consequence; pregnancy loss occurs in >60% of women with APS (Branch, Silver, Blackwell, Reading, & Scott, 1992; Silviera et al., 1992) who do not receive treatment. Treatment improves fetal survival somewhat (Branch et al., 1992; Caruso et al., 1993; Silviera et al., 1992) yet the pregnancy remains at considerable risk. Severe fetal intrauterine growth restriction, oligohydramnios, and elevated resistance in the umbilical arteries are findings consistent with impaired uteroplacental perfusion that may precede intrauterine fetal death (Caruso et al., 1993; Mari & Wasserstrum, 1991).

The disease process may create a hostile intrauterine environment for the fetus, necessitating early delivery. A high incidence of preterm delivery has been noted in these women (Caruso et al., 1993; Cowchock, Reece, Balaban, Branch, & Plouffe, 1992) and occurs either from initiation of labor to preserve maternal and fetal well-being or from premature rupture of membranes. Premature rupture of membranes is quite common (Caruso et al., 1993; Cowchock et al., 1992) and is thought to occur with higher frequency in women treated with steroids. Subclinical chorioamnionitis or glucocorticoid effects on collagen in women treated with corticosteroids may be responsible for premature rupture of membranes (Cowchock et al., 1992). Women with APS are at significant risk for the development of severe preeclampsia (Hochfeld et al., 1994; Landy, Kessler, Kelly, & Weingold, 1992), which may also necessitate early delivery.

Treatment

Low-dose aspirin may be given alone or in combination with corticosteroids or heparin (Scott & Branch, 1994) for the prevention of thrombosis. Aspirin (Lockshin, Druzin, & Qamar, 1989) and heparin (Cowchock et al., 1992; Silver et al., 1993) are preferred over corticosteroids and combined therapy with heparin and corticosteroids (Scott & Branch, 1994). Low-dose aspirin (<150 mg) may be given daily. Heparin may be given subcutaneously to promote anticoagulation in patients with APS. Higher doses (5000 units subcutaneously every 12 hours or intravenous heparin infusion) may be necessary throughout pregnancy for previous venous thrombosis or history of pulmonary embolus in a previous pregnancy (Peaceman, Silver, MacGregor, & Socol, 1992). Other approaches to the management of APS, such as intravenous immunoglobulin, have been investigated (Spinnato, Clark, Peirangeli, & Harris, 1995), but are not considered standard treatment.

AUTOIMMUNE THROMBOCYTOPENIA

Incidence

Autoimmune thrombocytopenia (ATP), which has also been referred to as idiopathic thrombocytopenia purpura (Druzin & Stier, 1994; Mofada et al., 1994) occurs frequently in women of childbearing age. It is the most common autoimmune disorder of pregnancy (Pillai, 1993) and is estimated to occur once or twice in 1000 deliveries (Cook, Miller, Katz, & Cefalo, 1991).

Etiology and Pathophysiology

Underproduction of platelets, increased destruction of platelets, or sequestration of platelets within the enlarged spleen may result in thrombocytopenia. Autoimmune thrombocytopenia typically is caused by maternal factors, or antiplatelet antibodies (Burrows & Kelton, 1995; Yong, Donahue, Hegde, & Linch, 1992) that accelerate platelet destruction. Platelet destruction occurs primarily as a result of binding of maternal platelet associated IgG (PAIgG) antibodies to platelet surface antigens. Platelet destruction also results from binding of IgM antibodies to platelet surface antigens. The IgM antibodies destroy the platelets directly or by activating the complement system. Activation of phagocytes and positive feedback of lymphokines provide feedback that promotes platelet destruction as a result of complement activation (Yong et al., 1992). Fetal platelet destruction can potentially occur as IgG antibodies, unlike IgM, can cross the placenta and attach to fetal platelets. The affected fetus can be born with dangerously low platelet levels and is at risk for serious complications (Cook et al., 1990).

Definition and Diagnosis

Autoimmune thrombocytopenia is a diagnosis that is derived when other medical conditions that may be responsible for a decreased platelet count are excluded. Twenty-one percent of women with thrombocytopenia will most likely have hypertension (Burrows & Kelton, 1993). In addition to hypertensive disorders, SLE, APS, disseminated intravascular coagulation (DIC), human immunodeficiency virus (HIV), drug-induced thrombocytopenia, and laboratory artifact may be responsible for thrombocytopenia (Silver, Branch, & Scott, 1995).

Incidental thrombocytopenia, or pregnancy-associated thrombocytopenia, is a mild thrombocytopenia (platelets <150 × 10⁹/l but usually >100 × 10⁹/l) (Pillai, 1993), accounts for greater than 70% of thrombocytopenia in pregnant women (Silver et al., 1995). Platelet survival is decreased in normal pregnancy because of an accelerated state of fibrinolysis, an adaptive response that maintains the placental–uterine interface (Pillai, 1993). Platelet count is rarely less than 80 × 10⁹/l, and women do not demonstrate propensity for bleeding (Silver et al.,

1995). Platelet destruction may increase near term. Therefore, decreased platelet count in the first half of pregnancy is more consistent with ATP as opposed to incidental thrombocytopenia (Pillai, 1993).

Clinical and Laboratory Manifestations

Routine evaluation of complete blood cell counts in the antepartum period has facilitated recognition of thrombocytopenia in pregnancy (Pillai, 1993; Silver et al., 1995). Mild thrombocytopenia (platelet count 100–150 × 10^9/l) in the absence of other hematologic abnormalities, lymphadenopathy, splenomegaly, preeclampsia, and drugs known to induce thrombocytopenia are more consistent with incidental thrombocytopenia (Pillai, 1993). In the presence of thrombocytopenia, circulating platelets are younger and therefore more effective. Bleeding times generally remain normal with lower platelet counts (Druzin & Stier, 1994). Severe drops in platelet counts (<50 × 10^9/l during the antepartum period or <20 × 10^9/l near the time of delivery) (Pillai, 1993) may be associated with propensity for bleeding; however, steroids are usually administered, reducing the risk to the mother. The primary concern with ATP is that of transplacental passage of maternal PAIgG to the fetus and resultant fetal thrombocytopenia.

Maternal–Fetal Implications

Significant thrombocytopenia (platelet count <50 × 10^9/l) predisposes the fetus or infant to hemorrhagic complications, such as intracranial hemorrhage (ICH). Although neonatal ICH is rare, the potential for its occurrence continues to be the fundamental issue that guides antepartum and intrapartum management decisions. Approximately 10–16% of women with ATP deliver infants with a platelet count <50 × 10^9/l (Burrows & Kelton, 1993; Garmel, Craigo, Morin, Crowley, & D'Alton, 1995; Yamada & Fujimoto, 1994). Neonatal platelet counts of less than 20 × 10^9/l is uncommon with an incidence of <0.2% (Burrows & Kelton, 1993). Neither maternal platelet count nor maternal antiplatelet antibody (PAIgG) levels are predictors of fetal or neonatal thrombocytopenia (Pillai, 1993; Cook et al., 1991;

Silver et al., 1995; Burrows & Kelton, 1993; Yamada & Fujimoto, 1994; Kaplan, 1990; Daffos, Forestier, Kaplan, & Cox, 1988). Because fetal descent during vaginal delivery may predispose the severely thrombocytopenic fetus to ICH, determination of fetal platelet count prior to delivery is ideal. Scalp sampling, at one time performed during labor to determine fetal platelet count, does not yield accurate estimates of fetal platelet count. Samples are often inaccurate because the specimen is often clotted or contaminated by maternal blood or amniotic fluid (Cook et al., 1991; Silver et al., 1995; Yamada & Fujimoto, 1994). If the fetal sample is contaminated in any manner, the sample may induce activation of the clotting cascade and platelet aggregation, leading to incorrect diagnosis of thrombocytopenia (Daffos et al., 1988). Cordocentesis is an acceptable method for obtaining fetal platelet count prior to delivery, but controversy exists as to whether evaluation of fetal platelet count by cordocentesis can be justified based on the low incidence of ICH (Cook et al., 1991; Silver et al., 1995). However, because the literature is blurred as to the relationship of severe thrombocytopenia with consistent cut-off values (e.g., <50 × 10^9/l versus <20 × 10^9/l) and its impact on the incidence of ICH, cordocentesis may be considered an acceptable approach to guide decision regarding the mode of delivery (Garmel et al., 1995; Kaplan et al., 1990; Daffos et al., 1988; Moise et al., 1988).

Cesarean delivery was at one time recommended for women with ATP, because passage of the fetus through the birth canal was thought to be the inciting mechanism for fetal intracranial hemorrhage (Silver et al., 1995). More recent studies have failed to demonstrate a correlation between mode of delivery and incidence of neonatal ICH (Mofada et al., 1994; Cook et al., 1991; Burrows & Kelton, 1993; Silver et al., 1995; Moise et al., 1988). Silver and colleagues (1995) note that it is difficult to attribute neonatal ICH to labor and delivery events based on earlier studies, because the timing of determination of neonatal ICH is not specified or evaluation of ICH was performed at an inappropriate interval (several days after delivery instead of immediately after delivery). Additionally, neonatal platelet count typically declines within the first few days of life, increasing the risk of morbid or hemorrhagic events secondary to thrombocytopenia (Garmel et al., 1995). Neonatal ICH, therefore, may occur several days after delivery when the neonatal platelet count reaches a nadir and may not necessarily be impacted by the mode of delivery. Burrows and Kelton (1993) note a potential bias in the studies that were included in their meta-analysis to be that of a failure to identify the timing of platelet sampling and timing of the determination of neonatal ICH.

Neonatal ICH is an extremely rare complication of ATP. In a prospective study of more than 15,000 deliveries over a 7-year period (Burrows & Kelton, 1993), ICH did not occur in any infant delivered from a woman with ATP. Neonatal ICH and fetal morbidity and mortality in this study occurred in infants with alloimmune thrombocytopenia, which is a serious fetal disorder without maternal consequence that complicates 1:5000 deliveries (Burrows & Kelton, 1993) and is caused by platelet-specific antibody (PLAl) that targets fetal platelets. It is similar to Rh-isoimmunization except that in alloimmune thrombocytopenia, first children are often affected (Scott & Branch, 1994). Platelet and HLA typing are not routinely tested during pregnancy. Therefore, women are usually referred to maternal–fetal specialists for evaluation because of a history of a previous affected newborn or sisters with affected children. Cordocentesis is the only method for evaluation of this disease (Daffos et al., 1988).

Treatment

Prednisone is administered to women with ATP if maternal platelet count falls below $20 \times 10^9/l$ during the antepartum period or below $50 \times 10^9/l$ when the woman approaches delivery (Pillai, 1993). Prednisone is typically administered in divided daily doses of 1–2 mg/kg for 2–3 weeks. The dose is usually tapered over 2-week intervals to maintain the platelet count about $50 \times 10^9/l$. The spleen provides a major source for the production of antiplatelet antibodies and is a major site for the destruction of damaged platelets. Thrombocytopenia that is unresponsive to corticosteroid therapy may necessitate splenectomy. Splenectomy is avoided during pregnancy, if at all possible, because of the risks to the pregnancy and fetus (Scott & Branch, 1994). Splenectomy does not necessarily prevent thrombocytopenia in the fetus because antibodies to platelets are produced in other sites. Additionally, splenectomy may be associated with a higher incidence for ATP because it is possible that the spleen removes the immune complexes that are responsible for the destruction of platelets. Free antiplatelet antibodies in the circulation may actually increase as a result of removal of the spleen (Yamada & Fujimoto, 1994).

ASSESSMENT

A comprehensive review of the woman's history and thorough assessment of all body systems facilitate the obstetric nurse in anticipating potential complications that may occur during the antepartum, intrapartum, or postpartum periods. The woman is questioned about periods of exacerbations and remissions, particularly if she is diagnosed with either SLE or APS. Specific information regarding the woman's symptoms and organ system involvement, medication usage, and occurrence of exacerbations of the disease prior to pregnancy and during the current pregnancy is sought in the review of her history. The obstetric nurse should also ascertain the woman's level of understanding about her disease and the impact of pregnancy on the disease process in order to identify any educational needs.

Assessment of body systems is accomplished in an attempt to identify organ system involvement. On admission, vital signs should be evaluated. Elevation of temperature is noted because women with SLE are at risk for infection, either from the disease process or from the effects of glucocorticoid therapy. Assessment of respiratory rate and pattern facilitates gathering of information regarding pulmonary status. Hypertension is common in individuals with

SLE, and APS and blood pressure should therefore be measured frequently during labor. Because thrombocytopenia is often associated with hypertension (Burrows & Kelton, 1993), women with ATP should also be screened for elevations in blood pressure. Additionally, detection of clinical findings consistent with preeclampsia (refer to the chapter on hypertensive disorders in this text) should be recognized promptly and brought to the attention of the physician. Serum complements may be ordered by the physician if it is difficult to distinguish clinical findings consistent with lupus exacerbation versus preeclampsia. Serum complement values are often reviewed for evidence of a trend toward lower levels (Sala, 1993), necessitating more than one determination.

The cardiopulmonary system should be assessed by questioning the patient about any symptoms of exertional dyspnea as well as any diagnostic work-up findings, such as findings from an echocardiogram that may have been ordered to further investigate cardiopulmonary complaints. The diagnostic reports are reviewed for documentation of impaired myocardial function. Heart sounds should be auscultated for gallops or murmurs. Lung sounds are ausculated for wheezes, crackles, or friction rub. Intake and output are measured and fluid balance is documented. Hemoglobin oxygen saturation (SaO_2) as well as electrocardiogram (ECG) should be monitored continuously if there are any complaints of shortness of breath, chest pain, or dyspnea. The obstetric nurse should note any history of prosthetic heart valves, pericarditis, or endocarditis.

Renal involvement is common in women with SLE (Boumpas et al., 1995a). Therefore, review of any evaluation of renal function during the antepartum period is important. Results obtained from 24-hour urinalysis during the antepartum period should be scrutinized for any evidence of increasing proteinuria or decreased creatinine clearance. Urine output is measured at a frequency determined to be appropriate based on baseline renal function. On admission, a urinalysis and blood chemistry should be obtained and scrutinized for proteinuria, elevated serum creatinine, and elevated blood urea nitrogen as well as other abnormalities. Results are compared to baseline values during pregnancy.

The woman should be questioned about any history of mood swings, depression, psychosis, or seizures. Complaints of dizziness or headache require further investigation. Additionally, subtle mental status changes noted by the nurse or significant other may indicate central nervous system involvement and should receive serious attention. Hematologic involvement should be assessed by reviewing complete blood count for any evidence of anemia or thrombocytopenia. The nurse should evaluate the patient for bruising and ask her if she has noted increased bleeding tendencies. Because of the significant risk for thrombosis, particularly with SLE and APS, the nurse should evaluate for calf tenderness and lower-extremity edema. The woman should be assessed throughout pregnancy for preterm uterine contractions and premature rupture of membranes because of an increased risk for preterm delivery. Infection may occur secondary to glucocorticoid therapy (Scott & Branch, 1994). Therefore, the nurse should explore for signs of infection (e.g. elevated temperature, complaints of uterine tenderness, foul-smelling vaginal discharge).

Impaired oxygen delivery to the fetus can be anticipated with SLE (Sala, 1993; Weiner et al., 1992) and APS (Branch et al., 1992; Caruso et al., 1993; Mari & Wasserstrum, 1991; Silviera et al., 1992). Ultrasound reports should be reviewed for documentation of fetal intrauterine growth restriction, oligohydramnios, or abnormal Doppler flow studies. Antepartum testing, including nonstress testing, biophysical profile, and Doppler velocimetry, generally begins around 26 weeks (Sala, 1993). The frequency of fetal evaluation is determined by activity of the disease process. Because labor is a vulnerable time for a fetus already stressed, continuous fetal heart rate monitoring during labor is recommended. Fetal heart rate should be monitored for the evidence of well-being. The presence of nonreassuring FHR findings should be communicated immediately to the patient's physician and appropriate nursing interventions should be initiated.

DISPLAY 18-2

Laboratory Findings Consistent with SLE and APS

Laboratory Value	Comments
ANA	• Positive ANA does not confirm SLE, however a negative result makes the diagnosis of SLE unlikely.
Anti-SM antibodies	• More specific for SLE
anti-dsDNA	• More specific for SLE
Serum Complements (C3, C4)	• Indicate consumption of immune complexes • Levels decrease with SLE exacerbation.
Lupus Anticoagulant (LAC)	• May be present in some individuals with SLE who have secondary antiphospholipid syndrome • Positive LAC combined with presence of symptoms is associated with primary APS. • Promotes systemic and placental thrombosis • Associated with high perinatal morbidity and mortality
Anticardiolipin antibody (ACLA)	• May be present in some individuals with SLE who have secondary antiphospholipid syndrome • Positive ACLA combined with presence of symptoms is associated with primary APS • Venous thrombosis and thrombocytopenia associated with ACLA of IgG class • Associated with fetal loss
SS-A/Ro	Associated with neonatal lupus
SS-B/La	Associated with neonatal lupus

Source: Author

PLAN FOR NURSING CARE AND INTERVENTIONS

Nursing care of the woman with autoimmune disease is centered upon astute assessment of body systems and supportive interventions. Abnormal assessment findings should be communicated to appropriate healthcare members. Supportive interventions strive to alleviate tissue damage that is mediated by the hyperactive immune response and preserve maternal end-organ perfusion and fetal oxygenation. Impaired end-organ perfusion may occur in autoimmune disorders as a result of immune complex deposition along the blood vessels (in SLE) or from obstruction of the microvasculature secondary to thrombosis (in APS). Oxygen delivery to the maternal organs, including the uteroplacental system, may be reduced. Oxygenation may be promoted with pharmacologic therapy, such as corticosteroids, which attempts to reduce inflammatory changes and suppress the immune response that promotes immune complex deposition. Additional interventions, such as lateral positioning, oxygen administration, and bedrest may also be necessary. Delivery of the fetus occurs when uterine perfusion is inadequate (intrauterine growth retardation, oligohydramnios, or fetal heart rate abnormalities). The need for frequent fetal evaluation and potential for early delivery to promote maternal and fetal well-being may result in a great deal of anxiety in the woman and her family. Information regarding evaluation methods and interventions is provided and the woman is supported emotionally. The nurse should provide information that is supported by a professional understanding of the disease process.

REFERENCES

Adams, D., Druzin, J. L., Edersheim, T., Bond, A., & Kogut, E. (1992). Condition specific antepartum testing: Systemic lupus erythematosus and associated serologic abnormalities. American Journal of Reproductive Immunology, 29.

Amigo, M. C., Torres, R. G., Robles, M., Bochicchio, T., & Reyes, P. A. (1992). Renal involvement in primary antiphospholipid syndrome. Journal of Rheumatology, 18, 8.

Boumpas, D. T., Austin, H. A., Fessier, B. J., Balow, J. E., Klipper, J. H., & Lockshin, M. D. (1995a). Systemic lupus erythematosus: Emerging concepts part 1: Renal, neruopsychiatric, cardiovascular, pulmonary, and hematologic disease. Annals of Internal Medicine, 122, 12.

Boumpas, D. T., Fessler, B. J., Austin, H. A., Balow, J. E., Klippel, J. H., & Lockshin, M. D. (1995b). Systemic lupus erythematosus: Emerging concepts part 2: Dermatologic and joint disease, the antiphospholipid antibody syndrome, pregnancy and hormonal therapy, morbidity and mortality, and pathogenesis. Annals of Internal Medicine, 123, 1.

Branch, D. W., Silver, R. M., Blackwell, J. L., Reading, J. C., & Scott, J. R. (1992). Outcome of treated pregnancies in women with antiphospholipid syndrome: An update of the Utah experience. Obstetrics and Gynecology, 80, 4.

Burrows, R. F., & Kelton, J. G. (1993). Fetal thrombocytopenia and its relation to maternal thrombocytopenia. New England Journal of Medicine, 329, 20.

Burrows, R. F., & Kelton, J. G. (1993). Pregnancy in patients with idiopathic thrombocytopenic purpura: Assessing the risks of the infant at delivery. Obstetrics and Gynecology Survey, 48, 12.

Caruso, A., DeCarolis, S., Ferrazzani, S., Valesini, G., Caforio, L, & Mancuso, S. (1993). Pregnancy outcome in relation to uterine artery flow velocity waveforms and clinical characteristics in women with antiphospholipid syndrome. Obstetrics and Gynecology, 82, 6.

Cook, R. L., Miller, R. C., Katz, V. L., & Cefalo, R. C. (1991). Immune thrombocytopenic purpura in pregnancy: A reappraisal of management. Obstetrics and Gynecology, 78, 4.

Cowchock, F. S., Reece, E. A., Balaban, D., Branch, D. W., & Plouffe, L. (1992). Repeated fetal losses associated with antiphospholipid antibodies: A collaborative randomized trial comparing prednisone with low-dose heparin treatment. American Journal of Obstetrics and Gynecology, 158, 4.

Daffos, F., Forestier, F., Kaplan, C., & Cox, W. (1988). Prenatal diagnosis and management of bleeding disorders with fetal blood sampling.

American Journal of Obstetrics and Gynecology, 158, 4.

Druzin, M. L., & Stier, E. (1994). Maternal platelet count at delivery in patients with idiopathic thrombocytopenic purpura, not related to perioperative complications. Journal of the American College of Surgeons, 179.

Feinberg, B. B., & Gonik, B. (1991). General precepts of the immunology of pregnancy. Clinical Obstetrics and Gynecology, 34, 1.

Floyd, R. C., & Roberts, W. E. (1992). Autoimmune disease in pregnancy. Obstetric and Gynecology Clinics of North America, 19, 2.

Fox, R., Lumb, M. R., & Hawkins, D. F., (1990). Persistent fetal sinus bradycardia associated with maternal anti-Ro antibodies. Case report. British Journal of Obstetrics and Gynecology. 97.

Frank, M. M., & Lawley, T. J. (1994). Immune-complex diseases. In K. J. Isselbacher, E. Braunwald, J. D. Wilson, J. B. Martin, A. S. Fauci, & D. L. Kasper (Eds.), Harrison's principles of internal medicine (pp. 1638–1643). New York: McGraw-Hill.

Garmel, S. H., Craigo, S. D., Morin, J. M., Crowley, J. M., & D'Alton, M. E. (1995). The role of percutaneous umbilical blood sampling in the management of immune thrombocytopenic purpura. Perinatal Diagnosis, 15.

Gimovsky, M. L., & Montoro M. (1991). Systemic lupus erythematosus and other connective tissue diseases in pregnancy. Clinical Obstetrics and Gynecology, 34, 1.

Ginsberg, J. S., & Hirsch, J. (1992). Use of antithrombotic agents during pregnancy. Chest, 102, 4.

Goldman, R. R., Mientus, J. M., Kutzer, J. E., Mulvihill, J. J., & Medsger, T. A. (1993). Pregnancy outcome in women with systemic lupus erythematosus treated with immunosuppressive drugs. Journal of Rheumatology, 20, 7.

Guyton, A. C., & Hall, J. E. (1996). The adrenocorticoal hormones. In Textbook of medical physiology (9th ed., pp. 957–970). Philadelphia: W. B. Saunders.

Guyton, A. C., & Hall, J. E. (1996). Resistance of the body to infection: 1. Leukocytes, granulocytes, the monocyte-macrophage system, and inflammation. In Textbook of medical physiology (9th ed., pp. 435–443). Philadelphia: W. B. Saunders.

Hahn, B. H. (1994). Systemic lupus erythematosus. In K. J. Isselbacher, E. Braunwald, J. D. Wilson, J. B. Martin, A. S. Fauci, & D. L. Kasper (Eds.), Harrison's principles of internal medicine (pp. 1643–1648). New York: McGraw-Hill.

Hayslett, J. P. (1992). The effect of systemic lupus erythematosus on pregnancy and pregnancy outcome. American Journal of Reproductive Immunology, 28.

Hayslett, J. P. (1991). Maternal and fetal complications in pregnant women with systemic lupus erythematosus. American Journal of Kidney Diseases, 22, 2.

Hochfeld, M., Druzin, M. L., Maia, D., Wright, J., Lambert, R. E., & McGuire, J. (1994). Pregnancy complicated by primary antiphospholipid syndrome. Obstetrics and Gynecology, 83, 5.

Johnson, M. J., Petri, M. Witter, F. R., Repke, J. T. (1995). Evaluation of preterm delivery in a systemic lupus erythematosus pregnancy clinic. Obstetrics and Gynecology, 86, 3.

Kaaja, R., Julkunen, L., Viinikka, O., & Ylikorkala, (1993). Production of prostacyclin and thromboxane in lupus pregnancies: Effect of small dose of aspirin. Obstetrics and Gynecology, 81, 3.

Kaplan, S. T., Cartash, E. K., Pizzarello, R. A., & Furie, R. A. (1992). Cardiac manifestations of the antiphospholipid syndrome. American Heart Journal, 124, 5.

Kaplan, C., & Cox, W. (1988). Prenatal diagnosis and management of bleeding disorders with fetal blood sampling. American Journal of Obstetrics and Gynecology, 158, 4.

Kaplan, C., Daffos, F., Forestier, F., Tertian, G., Catherine, N., Pons, J. C., & Tchernia, G. (1990). Fetal platelet counts in thrombocytopenic pregnancy. Lancet, 336.

Landy, J. J., Kessler, C., Kelly, W. K., & Weingold, A. B. (1992). Obstetric performance in patients with the lupus anticoagulant and/or anticardiolipin antibodies. American Journal of Perinatology, 9, 3.

Lockshin, M. D., Druzin, M. L., & Qamar, T. (1989). Prednisone does not prevent recurrent fetal death in women with antiphospholipid antibody. American Journal of Obstetrics and Gynecology, 160, 2.

Love, P. E., & Santoro, S. A. (1990). Antiphospholipid antibodies: Anticardiolipin and the lupus anticoagulant in systemic lupus erythematosus (SLE) and in non-SLE disorders. American College of Physicians, 112, 9.

MacLean, M. A., Cumming, G. P., McCall, F., Walker, I. D., & Walker, J. J. (1994). The prevalence of lupus anticoagulant and anticardiolipin antibodies in women with a history of first trimester miscarriages. British Journal of Obstetrics and Gynecology, 101.

Mari, G., & Wasserstrum, J. (1991). Flow velocity waveforms of the fetal circulation preceding fetal death in a case of lupus anticoagulant. American Journal of Obstetrics and Gynecology, 164, 3.

Mofada, A. S. M., Osman, M. E. E., Kides, E., Kareem, A., Momen, A., Abdullah, S. A. H., & Mobaireek, K. A. (1994). Risk of thrombocytopenia in the infants of mothers with idiopathic thrombocytopenia. American Journal of Perinatology, 11, 6.

Out, H. J., Bruinse, H. W., Christiaens, G. C. M. L., Vliet, M. V., deGroot, P. G., Nieuwenhuis, K., & Derkson, R. H. W. M. (1992). A prospective, controlled multicenter study on the obstetric risks of pregnant women with antiphospholipid antibodies. American Journal of Obstetrics and Gynecology, 167, 1.

Pattison, J. S., Chamley, L. W., McKay, E. J., Liggins, G. C., Butler, W. S. (1993). Antiphospholipid antibodies in pregnancy: Prevalence and clinical associations. British Journal of Obstetrics and Gynecology, 100.

Peaceman, A. M., Silver, R. K., MacGregor, S. N., & Socol, M. L. (1992). Interlaboratory variation in antiphospholipid antibody testing. American Journal of Obstetrics and Gynecology, 166, 6.

Perez, R. E., & McClendon, J. R. (1992). Primary antiphospholipid syndrome and multiorgan arterial and venous thromboses. Journal of Rheumatology, 19, 8.

Petri, M., Howard, D., & Repke, J. (1991). Frequency of lupus flare in pregnancy. The Hopkins Lupus Pregnancy Center experience. Arthritis Rheumatology, 34, 12.

Pillai, M. (1993). Platelets and pregnancy. British Journal of Obstetrics and Gynecology, 100.

Rubbert, A., Pirner, K., Wildt, L., Kalden, J. R., & Manger, (1992). Pregnancy course and complications in patients with systemic lupus erythematosus. American Journal of Reproductive Immunology, 28.

Sala, D. J. (1993). Effects of systemic lupus erythematosus on pregnancy and the neonate. Journal of Perinatal and Neonatal Nursing, 7, 3.

Scott, J. R., & Branch, D. W. (1994). Immunologic disorders. In R. K. Creasy & R. Resnik (Eds.), Maternal-fetal medicine. Principles and practice (3rd ed., pp. 467–481). Philadelphia: W. B. Saunders.

Segovia, D. A. (1992). Clinical manifestations of the antiphospholipid syndrome. Journal of Rheumatology, 19, 11.

Silver, R. K., MacGregor, S. N., Scholl, J. S., Hobart, J. M., Neerhof, M. G., & Ragin, A. (1993). Comparative trial of prednisone plus aspirin versus aspirin alone in the treatment of anticardiolipin antibody-positive obstetric patients. American Journal of Obstetrics and Gynecology, 173, 2.

Silver, R. M, Branch, D. W., & Scott, J. R. (1995). Maternal thrombocytopenia in pregnancy: Time for a reassessment. American Journal of Obstetrics and Gynecology, 173, 2.

Silviera, L. H., Hubble, C. L., Jara. L. J., Saway, S., Osuna, P. M., Seleznick, M. J., Angel, J., O'Brien, W., & Espinoza, L. R. (1992). Prevention of anticardiolipin antibody-related pregnancy losses with prednisone and aspirin. American Journal of Medicine, 93.

Spinnato, J. A., Clark, A. L., Peirangeli, S. S., & Harris, E. N. (1995). Intravenous immunoglobulin therapy for the antiphosholipid syndrome in pregnancy. American Journal of Obstetrics and Gynecology, 172, 2.

Treseler, K. (1988). Collagen-vascular diseases or syndromes. In Clinical laboratory and diagnostic tests. Significance and nursing implications (2nd ed., pp. 433–440). Norwalk, CT: Appleton & Lange.

Urowitz, M. B., Gladman, D. D., Farewell, V. T., Sterwart, J., & McDonald, J. (1993). Lupus and pregnancy studies. Arthritis Rheumatology, 36, 10.

Varner, M. W., Meehan, R. T., Syrop, C. H., Strottmann, M. P., & Goplerud, C. P. (1983).

Pregnancy in patients with systemic lupus erythematosus. <u>American Journal of Obstetrics and Gynecology</u>, <u>145</u>, 8.

Waltuck, J., & Buyon, J. P. (1994). Autoantibody-associated congenital heart block: Outcome in mothers and children. <u>American College of Physicians</u>, <u>120</u>, 7.

Weiner, Z., Lorber, M., & Blumenfeld, Z. (1992). Umbilical and uterine artery flow velocity waveforms in pregnant women with systemic lupus erythematosus treated with aspirin and glucocorticoids. <u>American Journal of Reproductive Immunology</u>, <u>28</u>.

Wong, K. L., Chan, K. Y., & Lee, C. P. (1991). Outcome of pregnancy in patients with systemic lupus erythematosus. A prospective study. <u>Archives of Internal Medicine</u>, <u>151</u>.

Yamada, H., & Fujimoto, S. (1994). Perinatal management of idiopathic thrombocytopenic purpura in pregnancy: Risk factors for passive immune thrombocytopenia. <u>Annals in Hematology</u>, <u>68</u>.

Yong, B. K., Donahue, R. E., Hegde, U., & Linch, D. C. (1992). Human macrophage colony-stimulating factor levels are elevated in pregnancy and in immune thrombocytopenia. <u>Blood</u>, <u>80</u>, 11.

CHAPTER 19

Human Immune Deficiency Virus and Acquired Immune Deficiency Syndrome

Mimi Jones and Tonda Verdejo

Over the last decade, acquired immune deficiency syndrome (AIDS) has emerged as a disease process that presents a significant threat to women of childbearing age. Infection with human immune deficiency virus (HIV), once thought to be limited to specific groups of high-risk individuals and their sexual partners, is now identified with greater frequency in the general population, including pregnant women. According to the Centers for Disease Control (CDC, 1997), adult/adolescent women with AIDS comprised 20% of the total cases reported in 1996, an increase of 7.5% above cases reported in females in 1992 (CDC, 1995). In addition, there are many HIV-positive women of childbearing age, known and unknown, without clinical evidence of AIDS.

Chu, Hanson, and Jones (1996) followed a cohort of HIV-positive patients from January 1990 through August 1994 that consisted of women, ages 15–44, diagnosed as either HIV positive or with clinical evidence of AIDS. At the onset of the study 14% of the women were pregnant. In each subsequent year of the study, the group displayed a pregnancy rate of 5.8%. Although these pregnancy rates are lower than those found in the HIV-negative population, the evidence is compelling that there are significant medical, social, and economic complications associated with this disease process and pregnancy each year.

Pregnant women with HIV and AIDS, both diagnosed and undiagnosed, present unique challenges for the perinatal healthcare team. When known, the presence of HIV/AIDS infection confers high-risk status to the pregnancy. This diagnosis creates a crisis for the patient and her support system, while presenting the opportunity for therapeutic intervention that may improve the ultimate outcome. When HIV/AIDS infection is undiagnosed, the pregnant patient is vulnerable to potentially fatal AIDS-related illnesses and is at increased risk for neonatal transmission.

This chapter provides current information regarding HIV/AIDS in an effort to enhance the ability of perinatal nurses to effect optimal maternal and neonatal outcomes. Pathophysiology and epidemiologic content are reviewed. Specific strategies that facilitate the identification of infected patients are suggested. Current management recommendations are presented, including techniques that the nurse can use to limit the risk of neonatal exposure. The chapter closes with several case studies to illustrate critical points.

HUMAN IMMUNODEFICIENCY VIRUS AND AIDS

Immune Physiology

Normal immune function is the result of the complex interplay among a variety of cell types and biologic substances. Immune response may be divided into two broad categories: innate immunity and acquired immunity.

Innate immunity refers to the body's overall ability to resist all types of invaders. Examples include the natural barrier provided by the skin, the toxic properties of gastric acid secretions, the phagocytotic action of white blood cells and macrophages, as well as the action of chemical compounds found in the blood that are capable of destroying invading organisms (Guyton, 1991).

Acquired immunity involves the body's ability to mount a targeted response to a specific invading organism and is achieved through the function of several systems or components. The first component is a complex complement system that consists of a variety of proteins, many of which possess enzymatic activity. The complement system eliminates the antigen by various methods including phagocytosis, lysis, agglutination, neutralization, chemotaxis, activation of mast cells, and induction of the inflammatory response. The complement system is most often activated by an antigen/antibody reaction (Guyton, 1991).

The second type of acquired immunity, cell-mediated immunity, involves the activity of two types of lymphocytes: B lymphocytes and T lymphocytes (see Figure 19-1). Both of these cell types develop during the embryonic period in fetal hemopoietic tissue and undergo a process of differentiation before migrating to various sites in the lymphatic system. Lymphocytes are found with great abundance in lymphatic tissue such as lymph nodes, spleen, tonsils, adenoids, and bone marrow. An antigen, successful in invading a host, is first phagocytized and digested by circulating macrophages.

Then the macrophages deliver pieces of the antigen directly to B and T lymphocytes located in these lymphatic tissues (Guyton, 1991).

When confronted with the antigen, B lymphocytes enlarge and become lymphoblasts. Some of the lymphoblasts become "memory cells" that protect the individual from subsequent disease caused by the same organism. Most of the lymphoblasts, however, become plasma cells, which in turn produce antigen-specific antibodies, also known as immunoglobulins. These immunoglobulins are distributed throughout the lymphatic and circulatory systems and represent approximately 20% of total plasma proteins. The five types of immunoglobulins, IgM, IgG, IgA, IgD, and IgE, function in two distinct ways to eliminate the invading organism. Antibodies can directly eliminate antigens through agglutination, precipitation, neutralization, or lysis. In addition, antibodies indirectly eliminate invaders by activating the complement system described previously (Guyton, 1991).

In the same way that B lymphocytes are stimulated by the presence of the antigen, T lymphocytes are also activated. Similar to B lymphocytes, T lymphocytes have an abundance of antigen-specific receptor sites. When binding occurs, "memory" T cells are produced and activated T cells are released into the lymph. There are three types of activated T cells. Helper T cells represent the greatest percentage of activated T cells and function as the regulator of overall immune response. Helper T cells secrete interleukins and interferon, substances that are required for normal immunity. Cytotoxic T cells, also known as killer cells, are capable of mounting a direct attack on the invading organism. Suppressor T cells function in a regulatory capacity by managing the actions of both helper T cells and cytotoxic T cells (Guyton, 1991).

Pregnancy induces an immunosuppressed state to protect the developing fetus from maternal antibody response. This phenomenon occurs without rendering the pregnant woman unduly susceptible to infections. However, there is evidence to suggest that certain viral infections are more severe in pregnancy (Isada & Grossman, 1991). Pregnancy results in an elevation in leukocytes, with third trimester values increasing

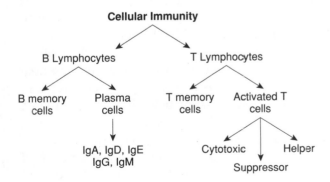

Figure 19-1. Cellular immune function.

to a mean of 10,000 mm³. There is conflicting information in the literature regarding the effect of pregnancy on lymphocyte levels. Some authors report no change in CD4+ lymphocyte counts, some report a decrease, and still others report an increase (Johnstone, Thong, Bird, & Whitelaw, 1994). A normal CD4 cell count in a nonpregnant woman ranges from 800–1200 mm³ (Lewis, Collier, & Heitkemper, 1996). Johnstone and colleagues (1994) report a decrease during pregnancy in CD4+ cells of approximately 100 mm³, attributing the change to the migration of CD4+ cells to lymphatic tissues early in gestation.

As this simplified review indicates, normal immunologic capacity results from a network of intricate pathways and complex processes designed to eliminate pathogenic organisms and prevent reinfection. The system works to prevent illnesses extrinsic to the individual, such as those caused by invading bacteria and viruses, as well as preventing organisms consistent with the normal flora of the host from becoming pathologic. When one or more of the steps is altered or eliminated, an individual lacks the ability to mount an immunologic response and is vulnerable to a host of infections.

PATHOPHYSIOLOGY

Virology

The organism responsible for HIV infection and AIDS is classified as a retrovirus. Retroviruses are unique in that they alter the genetic code of susceptible host cells. The name retrovirus refers to

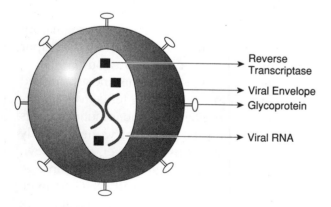

Figure 19-2. HIV virion.

Reverse Transcriptase

Viral Envelope

Glycoprotein

Viral RNA

the unusual, "backwards" step found in the life cycle of this family of viruses, in which the viral RNA is returned to a viral DNA state, a reversal of the usual genetic process. There are several retroviruses responsible for human pathology including *Oncovirinae,* which is responsible for several types of leukemia and *Spumavirinae,* also known as human foamy virus (Sweet & Gibbs, 1995).

The HIV virion is a simple organism, consisting of three basic components (Smith & Rogers, 1996). As Figure 19-2 illustrates, the central core contains two RNA strands and an essential enzyme called reverse transcriptase. The genes found on the strands of RNA provide the genetic material necessary to produce infection as well as regulatory genes that control the degree of viral production. This inner area is surrounded by layers of protein, which in turn are covered by a viral envelope consisting of two lipid layers embedded with protruding glycoproteins. These glycoproteins function as the primary binding site between HIV and the host cells.

When introduced into a host, the HIV virion is distributed throughout the body via the circulatory system, seeking cells that have CD4 receptor sites on their cell membrane. CD4 receptor sites are found on cells central to immunologic function, most commonly T-lymphocytes, monocytes, and macrophages, as well as lymphoidal tissue. When the target cell is located, a series of complex biological processes occur that allow attachment of the virus to the host cell and facilitate ultimate infection as shown in Figure 19-3 (Smith & Rogers, 1996).

Initially, the viral glycoprotein binds to the CD4 receptor site. The two cell membranes fuse and the viral RNA enters the host cell. Once inside the host cell cytoplasm, the viral RNA is disassembled. Through the action of reverse transcriptase, the viral RNA becomes viral DNA, which is then transported into the nucleus of the host cell. The viral DNA contains the essential genetic content necessary to produce infection. With additional enzymatic action, the viral DNA is integrated with the host cell DNA and is referred to as the provirus. The provirus may remain inactive for an indeterminate amount of time, contributing to the varying degrees of latency associated with early HIV infection.

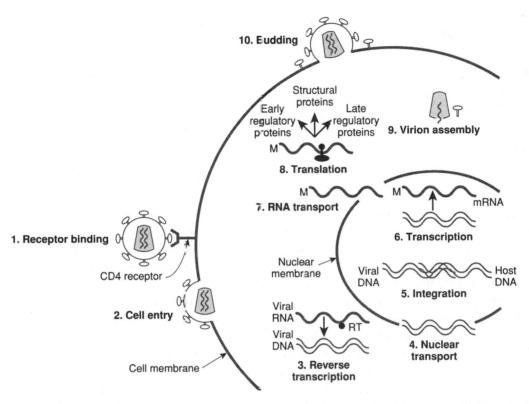

Figure 19-3. Viral replication cycle. From "Immunopathogenesis and detection of HIV infection in women and newborns," by D. K. Smith and M. F. Rogers, 1996, Clinical Obstetrics and Gynecology, p. 80. Reprinted with permission.

The trigger for active viral replication is unknown. Once activated, however, the provirus generates viral messenger RNA (mRNA), which is released into the cytoplasm of the host cell. Here, the inner core of the replicated virus is assembled and then covered by layers of protein. This bundle migrates to the host cell membrane where it is released through a process called budding. During budding, surface glycoproteins are embedded into the viral envelope, completing the production of the virion and ending the cycle of viral replication. HIV replication results in the death of the host cell. Over time, this continued reduction in the number of CD4+ cells results in diminished function of the immune system, rendering the infected host susceptible to a variety of opportunistic illnesses.

Two distinct viral types associated with immunodeficiency have been identified. HIV-1 is the virus associated with the majority of HIV and AIDS cases diagnosed worldwide. HIV-2 is found primarily in patients originating from Africa or with African contacts. However, antibodies to HIV-2 have been detected in individuals from other parts of the world, including Europe and the United States. HIV-2 produces immunodeficiency similar to that associated with HIV-1. It is possible for an individual to be infected with both of the HIV types (Sweet & Gibbs, 1995). Unless otherwise stated in this chapter, the term HIV refers to infection with HIV-1.

Disease Progression

It is well known that HIV is transmitted by direct contact with infected blood and body fluids. There are a variety of mechanisms by which this can occur, including exposure to contaminated needles, sexual contact with an infected partner, transmission during pregnancy, and receipt of infected blood products and tissues. Figure 19-4 summarizes the source of HIV infection in adult and adolescent females for 1996 as reported to the CDC (CDC, 1996a and b). Heterosexual contact and injection drug use are the modes of transmission most often implicated in female infection. Perinatal transmission is responsible for 91% of pediatric AIDS cases (CDC, 1996a and b).

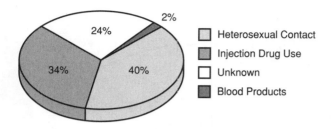

Figure 19-4. Exposure by category in adult and adolescent females 1996.

As noted previously, HIV has a distinct affinity for CD4 receptors. CD4 receptors are abundant on cells involved in immune response, particularly T lymphocytes, as well as B lymphocytes and macrophages. Quantification of CD+T cells, along with the monitoring of trends indicative of increasing or decreasing levels, represents the primary parameter used to determine the degree of an individual's immunocompromise. CD4 cell counts provide guidance for the initiation of antiretroviral and prophylactic therapy and serve as a prognostic indicator for individuals with HIV (CDC, 1997). In addition to monitoring CD4 cell counts, healthcare providers are using measure-

ment of viral load with increased frequency to evaluate patients and provide information regarding the effectiveness of treatment (HIV/AIDS Treatment Information Service, 1997). Viral load, or viremia, refers to the amount of HIV RNA in the blood. The Consensus Statement on Antiretroviral Therapy for HIV infection in 1996 (Carpenter et al., 1996) reported that high viral loads (>50,000 HIV RNA copies/mL) are associated with a greatly increased risk of clinical disease progression. They suggest that viral levels have greater predictive value than CD4 cell counts related to disease progression and are acceptable measures for both initiation and modification of antiretroviral therapy.

It is useful, considering the nature of HIV and the progressive degree of immunocompromise, to view the disease process as existing along a continuum. Pantaleo, Graziosi, and Fauci (1993) describe the disease progression commonly found in individuals with HIV infection as outlined in Figure 19-5. Primary HIV infection is generally followed by an initial decline in the CD4+T lymphocytes, a rapid rise in the presence

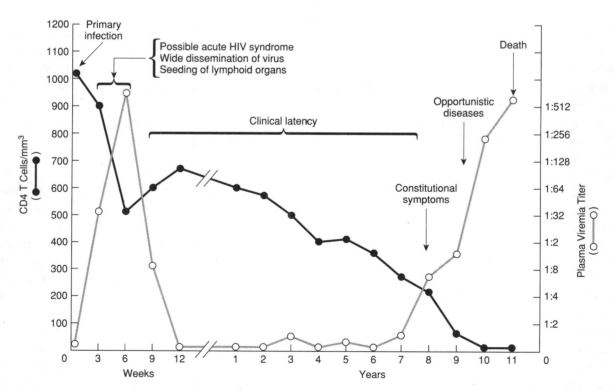

Figure 19-5. Disease progression. From "The immunopathogenesis of human immunodefiency virus infection," by G. Pantaleo, C. Graziosi and A Fauci, 1993, <u>New England Journal of Medicine</u>, p. 331. Reprinted with permission.

of the virus in the blood and, for some individuals, the emergence of an acute illness similar to mononucleosis. It is important to note, however, that up to 30% of those with acute infection may remain asymptomatic. During this period of acute illness, which can last up to 3 months, there is wide dissemination of the virus to lymphatic tissue throughout the body. Once in the lymphatic tissue, the virus is trapped within the matrix of lymphoidal cells and cannot escape. As the body mounts an antigen specific immune response to HIV, the viral load in the blood begins to decrease.

As the acute illness resolves and the degree of viremia diminishes, individuals enter the second phase of the disease process, which is described as a period of clinical latency. Although clinically quiet, the virus is microbiologically very active in the lymphatic tissue where rapid viral replication occurs. During this period, which can last up to 10 years, the most common physical finding is generalized lymphadenopathy. There is a progressive, prolonged decline in the CD4 T lymphocyte level that occurs even though the level of the virus in the blood is extremely low. Toward the end of the period of clinical latency, the matrix of the lymphatic tissue is destroyed, losing its ability to contain the virus. At this point, the virus reemerges in the blood, resulting in an increased viral load.

The emergence of an AIDS-defining illness signals the end of the period of clinical latency. This occurs when the level of circulating CD4 T lymphocytes is so low, approximately 400 mm^3, that constitutional disease becomes evident. This is accompanied by the presence of opportunistic infections and specific AIDS-related illnesses that are the hallmarks of profound immunosuppression. Display 19-1 summarizes these infections as outlined by the American College of Obstetricians and Gynecologists (ACOG, 1997).

The effects of pregnancy on the progression of HIV are unclear. Sweet and Gibbs (1995) summarize the existing literature, citing studies that support no acceleration of the disease progression of HIV during pregnancy, as well as studies that indicate exactly the opposite. A review article published by the Royal College of Obstetrics and Gynecology (RCOG, 1996) reports that the current consensus is that pregnancy does not significantly alter the progression of HIV. Likewise, studies evaluating the effect of HIV on pregnancy indicate that in the United States, positive serostatus is not related to any adverse outcome other than the risk of perinatal transmission (Sweet & Gibbs, 1995).

Diagnosis

The diagnosis of HIV infection, in individuals without clinical evidence of AIDS (such as decreased levels of CD4+ cells and the presence of an AIDS-defining illness), requires laboratory confirmation that the virus is present. This can be determined either indirectly through the identification of viral specific antibodies, or directly via viral cultures or antigen detection tests (Sweet & Gibbs, 1995). The indirect method is used most frequently and can be divided into two basic types of tests: screening and diagnostic.

The enzyme-linked immunosorbent assay (ELISA) is the standard screening test used to detect HIV antibodies. Serum from the individual is placed in test wells containing viral antigens. If HIV antibodies are present in the blood they will attach to the antigen. A reagent is then added that will bind to the antigen/antibody complex producing a change in color that can be detected and quantified. If there is no change in color, the test is considered to be negative or nonreactive. However, a negative ELISA requires subsequent testing to confirm that the individual is, in fact, not infected. A period of up to several months exists, following infection with HIV, before the immune response occurs (Fauci & Lane, 1994). During this period, antibodies are undetectable. For this reason, the CDC recommends that an individual with a negative result return for follow-up screening with a repeat ELISA in 3–6 months. A repeated negative ELISA indicates absence of infection, assuming that no new exposure to the virus has occurred (CDC, 1987).

The ELISA is considered to be positive or reactive if a dramatic change occurs with the addition of the reagent to the sample. Small amounts of antibodies result in weak color changes, in which case the results are reported as inconclusive or indeterminate. Positive and

DISPLAY 19-1

AIDS-Related Illnesses

AIDS-Indicator Conditions

Bacterial infections, multiple or recurrent

Candidiasis of bronchi, trachea, or lungs

Candidiasis of esophagus

Carcinoma, invasive cervical

Coccidioidomycosis, disseminated or extrapulmonary

Cryptococcosis, extrapulmonary

Cryptosporidiosis, chronic intestinal

Cytomegalovirus disease other than retinitis

Cytomegalovirus retinitis

Herpes Simplex, with esophagitis, pneumonitis, or chronic mucocutaneous ulcers

Histoplasmosis, disseminated or extrapulmonary

HIV encephalopathy (dementia)

HIV wasting syndrome

Immunosuppression, severe HIV related

Isosporiasis, chronic intestinal

Kaposi sarcoma

Lymphoid interstitial pneumonia and/or pulmonary lymphoid hyperplasia

Lymphoma, Burkitt (or equivalent term)

Lymphoma, immunoblastic (or equivalent term)

Lymphoma, primary in brain

Mycobacterium avium-intracellulare or *Mycobacterium kansasii,* disseminated or extrapulmonary

Mycobacterium tuberculosis, disseminated or extrapulmonary

Mycobacterium tuberculosis, pulmonary

Mycobacterial disease, other, disseminated or extrapulmonary

Pneumocystis carinii pneumonia

Pneumonia, recurrent

Progressive multifecal leukoencephalopathy

Salmonella septicemia, recurrent

Toxoplasmosis of brain

Source: CDC, 1994.

inconclusive ELISA results should be followed with an additional test to confirm the presence of infection and eliminate the possibility that a false positive ELISA has occurred. The test most commonly used for this purpose is the Western Blot, which identifies the antibody reaction with several of the antigenic components of the virus. There are three primary antigens present on the HIV virion, each with a distinct molecular weight. When present, the antibody in the sample reacts with the antigen in the reagent, forming weighted bands or darkened areas on the Western Blot. In order to be considered positive, the Western Blot must demonstrate bands to two of the three HIV antigens.

Direct confirmation of HIV infection is accomplished through identification of viral particles or viral culture. The simplest direct test involves the ELISA technique. In this case the ELISA is selective for specific components of the HIV antigen, not the HIV antibody as is the case with the screening ELISA. Viral cultures are also used to directly identify the presence of HIV using peripheral blood cells. Additionally, polymerase chain reaction (PCR) identifies the presence of HIV proviral DNA and RNA and has been particularly useful in determining the presence of infection in neonates. Figure 19-6 illustrates an algorithm published by Fauci and Lane (1994) that summarizes an appropriate testing scheme for the diagnosis for HIV-1 and HIV-2 applicable in the general population. Care providers may need to proceed to confirmatory Western Blot

testing more rapidly in the pregnant population, in order to identify those patients who are truly HIV positive and might benefit from treatment.

Epidemiology

To interpret the epidemiologic literature regarding HIV infection and AIDS, the reader must have a clear understanding of the terms used for reporting. The Centers for Disease Control report infection and demographic information for both HIV and AIDS. Even though these terms represent the clinical progression of the same disease entity, they are not used interchangeably. In 1993, the CDC issued the Revised Classification System for HIV Infection and Expanded Surveillance Case Definition for AIDS Among Adolescents and Adults (CDC, 1992). The new system integrates CD4+ cell counts with the presence of clinical illness and is presented in Table 19-1. CD4+ cell counts are divided into three categories. Counts <200/µL indicate the progression of HIV infection to AIDS. The clinical conditions associated with immunodeficiency have likewise been divided into three categories reflecting the nature of symptomatology and the presence of AIDS-indicator conditions. (The reader is directed to the CDC document for details regarding both symptomatic and AIDS-indicator conditions.) This matrix results in nine mutually exclusive categories that provide the framework currently used by the CDC in monitoring the disease (see Table 19-1).

Several other factors impact the interpretation of epidemiologic information. Although the number of HIV cases is important, only 28 states currently report information regarding newly diagnosed HIV infections. In addition, HIV-positive individuals are only reported by these states if the test was performed by a healthcare provider. Individuals who receive anonymous testing, including those who select home testing, are not included in the statistics reported by the CDC. All states, however, report newly diagnosed cases of AIDS. Consequently, the literature that summarizes actual epidemiologic trends tends to reference AIDS cases. Information that presents national epidemiology concerning HIV infection is based on estimates and, according to the CDC, does not reflect the entire scope of the problems associated with infection (CDC, 1995a).

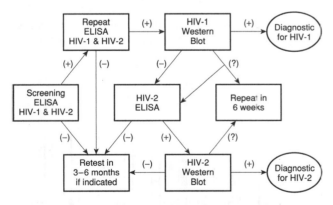

Figure 19-6. Testing algorithm. From Harrison's Principles of Internal Medicine by A. Fauci and C. Lane 1994. New York. McGraw-Hill. Reprinted with permission.

TABLE 19-1. CDC HIV/AIDS Classification System

| | Clinical Categories | | |
CD4+ T cell Categories	A Asymptomatic, acute (primary) HIV or primary generalized lymphadenopathy	B Symptomatic, not A or C conditions	C AIDS-indicator conditions
1. ≥500 µl	A1	B1	C1
2. 200–499 µl	A2	B2	C2
3. <200 µl (AIDS-indicator cell count)	A3	B3	C3

Source: CDC (1993).

In reviewing the epidemiologic information regarding AIDS in the United States, it is clear that both the scope and demographic nature of the illness are changing. As of June 1996, just over 548,000 cumulative cases of AIDS had been reported to the CDC. As Figure 19-7 illustrates, the number of total reported AIDS cases increased steadily throughout the 1980s and into the early 1990s. In 1993, the number of reported cases increased dramatically. This abrupt change does not reflect an actual increase in the number of cases, but rather the change in the diagnostic criteria used to distinguish AIDS from HIV infection as referenced in the previous paragraph. Since 1994, the total number of new AIDS cases reported to the CDC has stabilized in the United States, as illustrated in Figure 19-7, at between 60,000 and 70,000 per year.

Although the rate of increase in new cases of AIDS seems to have stabilized, the demograph-

ic characteristics of the illness have changed dramatically over time. As illustrated in Figure 19-8, the CDC reports that the rate of newly reported AIDS cases increased among women until 1994, at which point the number plateaued. In 1985, women represented 7% of cases reported annually, increasing to 20% in 1996 (CDC, 1996a and b). As Figure 19-9 indicates, the disease is more commonly diagnosed in African American women and those of Hispanic origin. In 1995, AIDS was the third leading cause of death in all women, ages 25–44, but the leading cause of death in African American women (Gwinn & Wortley, 1996).

Additionally, pediatric infection continues to be of great concern to healthcare providers; however, as Figure 19-10 demonstrates, the rate of infection in this age group seems to be decreasing. Eight hundred children were reported to the CDC with AIDS in 1995, a

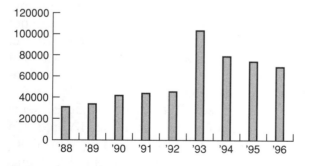

Figure 19-7. Reported AIDS cases by year.

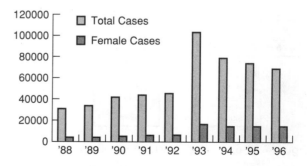

Figure 19-8. AIDS cases in females by year.

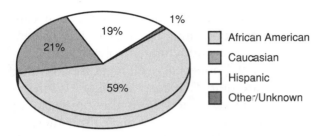

Figure 19-9. Ethnic/racial distribution of AIDS, 1996.

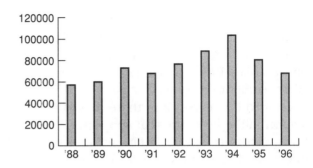

Figure 19-10. Pediatric AIDS cases by year.

decrease from 1,049 in 1996. This reduction is attributed by the CDC to several factors (CDC, 1996a and b) and probably reflects lower rates of neonatal transmission due to improved perinatal management.

MANAGEMENT OF HIV AND AIDS IN PREGNANCY

As the population of pregnant women with HIV infection increases, so does the opportunity to identify, through research, optimal methods of treatment. Findings allow obstetric care providers to offer an array of interventions designed to improve maternal health and protect the infant from viral transmission. In recent years, recommendations for management of the pregnant patient with HIV have been published by several organizations. Research continues in a variety of academic centers, focusing on appropriate assessment of the HIV pregnant patient and treatment modalities designed to limit perinatal transmission. Current research is focusing on treatment protocols that limit perinatal transmission while maximizing maternal health. Lindsay (1996) identified three major advancements that have had a positive impact on limiting perinatal transmission over the last several years. The first relates to the importance of offering HIV screening to all pregnant women. The second involves the use of anti-retroviral therapy in the HIV-positive pregnant woman. The final advancement relates to the increased effort to identify, through research, the major determinants of perinatal transmission.

Screening

Prior to 1994, screening for HIV infection was based on recommendations issued by the CDC (CDC, 1987), which advocated targeted screening of women of childbearing age based on the presence of identifiable risk factors. These risk factors included the use of IV drugs, prostitution, sexual contact with partners at risk, residence in a community or country with a high prevalence of HIV infection, and transfusion with a blood product between 1978 and 1985. The recommendations stated that the primary purpose of HIV screening was to identify *uninfected* individuals so that they might engage in behavioral changes that would limit their risk of infection. The CDC extended the recommendation for counseling and testing to pregnant women suggesting that, in addition to risk reduction behavior in noninfected individuals, recognition of HIV infection would allow the pregnant woman to receive appropriate medical care, plan for the medical care of her infant, and make family planning decisions (CDC, 1987). Additionally, knowledge of HIV status provided the woman of early gestation the opportunity to make the decision to continue or terminate her pregnancy. In practice, there was minor emphasis placed on widespread perinatal screening by healthcare providers outside of geographic areas with a high prevalence of cases, primarily because there was little therapeutic advantage to be gained from knowing a pregnant woman's HIV status.

This position regarding screening changed dramatically in April 1994 with the release of a report (CDC, 1994a) that presented the results of a multicentered, placebo-controlled clinical trial conducted by agencies of the National Institutes of Health. The study, known as the AIDS Clinical Trial Group (ACTG) Protocol 076, found that the rate of transmission from mother to infant was reduced from 22.5% to 8.3% by the administration of ZDV to pregnant and laboring women and their exposed neonates after delivery. Display 19-2 summarizes the study design and treatment protocol.

Prior to this revelation, there was little information in the literature that supported interventions directed toward diminishing perinatal infection. The remarkable results of ACTG 076 finally provided those caring for HIV-positive pregnant women with tangible recommendations for care that could improve newborn outcomes. The basic premise upon which antiretroviral therapy is based rests on the assumption that the healthcare provider knows the HIV status of the pregnant patient and that the HIV-positive patient consents to antiretroviral therapy. Consequently, HIV screening is being performed with increased frequency prior to and during pregnancy.

Screening for HIV has a direct impact on all perinatal nurses, regardless of practice setting. Screening is best accomplished preconceptually or early in gestation that centrally involves perinatal nurses in offices, clinics, or other outpatient settings. On the other hand, a number of pregnant women do not obtain prenatal care and may first encounter the issue of HIV screening in the acute care setting, involving both inpatient perinatal nurses as well as nurses in other patient care units. The responsibility for screening may be delegated from the physician or nurse practioner to the staff nurse. This must be done in accordance with state law and organizational policy, and must include the components identified by the CDC (1993) for testing in the general population: performance of a personalized risk assessment, creation of a risk reduction plan, pretest counseling, and informed consent. Based on the findings of ACTG 076, CDC issued additional recommendations for counseling and voluntary testing for all pregnant women (CDC, 1995a) as has the ACOG (1997). Display 19-3 summarizes these guidelines for perinatal HIV testing.

Assessment

Once diagnosed, the HIV-positive pregnant patient requires standard prenatal, intrapartal, and postpartal assessments, as well as evaluation of additional parameters associated with her disease process. Care providers must monitor indi-

DISPLAY 19-2

ACTG Protocol 076 Summary

Patient Eligibility
- Had not received antiretroviral treatment during the current pregnancy
- Had no clinical indications for maternal antepartum antiretroviral therapy
- Had a CD4+ T-lymphocyte count >200 μl at the initial assessment

Zidovudine Regimen
- Oral administration of 100 mg ZDV five times a day, initiated at 14–34 weeks gestation and continued for the remainder of the pregnancy
- During labor, intravenous administration of ZDV in a loading dose of 2 mg per kg body weight given over 1 hour, followed by a continuous infusion of 1 mg per kg body weight per hour until delivery
- Oral administration of ZDV to the newborn (ZDV syrup at 2 mg per kg body weight per dose given every 6 hours) for the first 6 weeks of life, beginning 8–12 hours after birth

Source: CDC (1994a).

cators of maternal status, such as CD4+ cell counts and viral load, as well as the patient's response to antiretroviral therapy via serial complete blood counts. In addition, the patient must receive ongoing evaluation for the presence of opportunistic infections and AIDS-defining illnesses. Finally, enhanced fetal assessment is warranted to monitor fetal growth and status in utero. Display 19-4 outlines appropriate assessment parameters for the HIV-positive pregnant patient.

Antiretroviral Treatment

In addition to highlighting the importance of widespread HIV screening of pregnant patients, ACTG Protocol 076 resulted in specific recommendations from the United States Public Health Service concerning the use of antiretroviral therapy in pregnancy to reduce the likelihood of perinatal transmission (CDC, 1994a). ZDV is currently the only antiretroviral agent approved for use by the Food and Drug Administration, although studies are ongoing regarding the use of additional drugs in pregnancy. ZDV interrupts replication of HIV through inhibition of the action of reverse transcriptase (Minkoff & Augenbraun, 1997). Display 19-5 outlines the

current CDC recommendations for the use of ZDV in pregnancy. The most common adverse effect associated with ZDV is suppression of the bone marrow function resulting in anemia. Hemoglobin and hematocrit levels should be monitored at frequent intervals in pregnant patients and neonates receiving ZDV. There are additional reverse transcriptase inhibitors, such as zalcitabine, stavudine, and lamivudine, used in the general HIV-positive population. These drugs, however, have not been evaluated for use in pregnancy

The obvious goal of antiretroviral treatment is to reduce maternal viral load. As previously defined, viral load (viral burden, viremia) is the quantity of the HIV RNA or virus that is found in the blood. Research has demonstrated, and healthcare providers are aware, that patients with high levels of HIV in the blood progress to AIDS more rapidly (Donovan, Bush, Markowitz, Baxa, & Saravolatz, 1996). There is increasing evidence that associates the degree of maternal viral load with the risk of perinatal transmission. Weiser and colleagues (1994) followed 19 pregnant women and their infants and identified HIV titers as the major determinant of perinatal trans-

DISPLAY 19-3

CDC Guidelines for Perinatal HIV Testing

1. Care providers should ensure that all pregnant women are counseled and encouraged to be tested for HIV infection.
2. HIV testing should be voluntary.
3. Counseling and testing should be offered cs early in pregnancy as possible.
4. Uninfected pregnant women who continue to engage in risk-taking behavior should be encouraged to avoid further exposure and receive follow-up testing during the third trimester.
5. Pregnant women who do not seek prenatal care should be promptly assessed for HIV infection at the initial encounter.
6. Women who do not receive testing should be encouraged to have their children tested.
7. Pregnant women should be provided access to other HIV prevention and treatment services as needed.

DISPLAY 19-4

Assessment Parameters for the HIV-Positive Pregnant Woman

Routine Prenatal Assessment

- Health history and physical exam
- Complete cell blood count with differential
- Hepatitis B surface antigen
- Triple screen (as desired by patient)
- Rubella (if non-immune)
- STD screening (serology, gonorrhea, chlamydia)
- Urinalysis
- PAP smear
- PPD for tuberculosis

HIV Specific Assessment

- Cytomegalovirus titers
- Toxoplasmosis titers
- Hepatic/Renal profile
- Lymphocyte profile (total and % CD4 cell count)
- HIV viral load

mission. Rouzioux and colleagues (1993) found an association between both the occurrence and timing of transmission and the severity of maternal infection. Dickover and colleagues (1996) noted increased perinatal transmission with plasma HIV-1 RNA levels above 50,000 copies/mL. They recommended that interventions be directed toward reducing the viral load to 20,000 copies/ml or below to achieve the greatest level of protection.

Although the results from ACTG 076 were encouraging and offered pregnant HIV-positive patients an intervention to reduce the likelihood of infection, the study raised as many, if not more, questions than it answered. ZDV is not 100% successful at preventing perinatal trans-

mission, and the long-term risks associated with its use, for both the mother and the infant, are not precisely known. A theoretical risk exists that ZDV treatment in women during pregnancy might contribute to the emergence of a resistant HIV strain suggesting that the drug may be less effective if used at a later date. Additionally, long-term studies on the effects of intrauterine and neonatal exposure of infants to ZDV have not been completed. These considerations should be presented to the woman during the informed consent process, along with the anticipated benefits, to assure that she has the opportunity to make the best decision about treatment options.

In their article on antiretroviral therapy in pregnancy, Minkoff and Augenbraun (1997) note that pregnancy creates a set of unique, ethical concerns for patients and care providers that have the potential to create negative maternal outcomes. They note that women with HIV who are pregnant receive the option for ZDV treatment with or without the clinical conditions that would indicate the need for antiretroviral therapy in the absence of pregnancy. In other words, pregnancy enhances the woman's access to this treatment. However, this treatment is specifically directed toward reducing the risk of perinatal transmission, without regard to long-term maternal well-being. On the other hand, pregnancy will likely exclude the same woman from newly developed treatment regimes, including the use of protease inhibitors and combination drug therapy, which might improve her long-term prognosis. Minkoff and Augenbraun (1997) suggest that care providers consider the option of combination therapy when the maternal CD4+ cell count falls below 500. Research is currently underway at major medical centers evaluating the use of protease inhibitors and combination therapy during pregnancy. It is likely that additional recommendations will be forthcoming that will provide reassurance concerning new drug treatment in pregnancy. In the meantime, pregnant HIV-positive women should be presented, whenever possible, with the option to participate in available research protocols designed to specifically evaluate new management regimes during pregnancy.

DISPLAY 19-5

CDC Recommendations for Perinatal ZDV

Antepartum Period

Beginning at 14 weeks:

ZDV, 100 mg po, 5 times per day
(Alternative schedule: 200 mg po, TID)

Intrapartum Period

Loading dose:

2 mg/kg of body weight, IV over 1 hour, followed by

Maintenance Dose:

1 mg/kg of body weight, IV until delivery

Neonatal Treatment

2 mg/kg of body weight, po every 6 hours, beginning at 8–12 hours of life, for the first 6 weeks of life.

Additional Determinants of Perinatal Transmission

It is well documented that HIV can be passed from mother to fetus or mother to newborn during the perinatal period. What is less clear is at what point during pregnancy infection actually occurs and which specific clinical conditions, in addition to viral load, either enhance or retard infectivity.

Orloff, Simonds, Steketee, and St. Louis (1996) propose a method to determine the timing of infection. They divided perinatal transmission into three categories—in utero, intrapartum, and postpartum—and determined the point at which infection most likely occurred by using direct isolation of HIV. If, through the use of polymerase chain reaction and isolation of actual virus, the infant blood was found to be infected within the first 48 hours after birth, the infection was classified as occurring in utero. If blood tests taken within 48 hours of birth were negative for the presence of the virus and sub-

sequent tests taken within the next several days of life were positive, the infant was thought to have acquired the infection during the intrapartum period. If initial infant testing was negative but follow-up tests became positive at a later date, the infection was classified as occurring during the postpartum period.

Rouzioux and colleagues and the French Collaborative Study Group (1993) estimated that 65% of infants with perinatally acquired HIV were infected during the intrapartum period. Orloff and colleagues (1996) estimated that 25–50% of HIV-positive infants were infected prior to the intrapartum period. Mandelbrot and colleagues (1996) evaluated the fetuses of 28 HIV-positive pregnant women electing to terminate their pregnancies. Using direct viral isolation techniques, they found none of the 28 to be infected with HIV, concluding that perinatal transmission, in general, occurs late in gestation. A relatively small percentage of infants become infected during the postpartum period.

The timing of perinatally acquired HIV is important when considering the mode of transmission and possible strategies to limit transmission. A variety of interventions have been evaluated and studied. Because the majority of perinatally acquired HIV infections seem to occur late in gestation or during the intrapartum period, most of the recommendations are directed toward this particular point along the continuum. Landesman and colleagues (1996) and Minkoff and colleagues (1995) identified an increased risk of transmission in the presence of low CD4 counts and rupture of membranes for greater than 4 hours. ACOG (1997) recommends that artificial rupture of membranes and the use of fetal scalp electrodes be avoided. In addition, they caution against the use of maneuvers that could cause fetal skin abrasions or injury during delivery. Bardeguez (1996) recommends that care providers avoid scalp pH determination as well.

There has been considerable speculation and research evaluating the effectiveness of performing a cesarean birth to reduce the chance of transmission. Theoretically, operative delivery might decrease the risk of intrapartum infection. Lin and colleagues (1996) demonstrated that the least amount of microinfusion from mother to infant occurs during elective cesarean delivery. The authors stated that this finding may have implications for reducing perinatal transmission of blood-borne viruses. Data are unclear, however, regarding the effectiveness of performing a cesarean section to prevent transmission. In a prospective, observational study, Landesman and colleagues (1996) identified no significant benefit in cesarean versus vaginal delivery. This is in conflict with results from the European Collaborative Study (1994), which demonstrated a reduction in perinatal transmission associated with cesarean delivery. In a review of prospective studies evaluating the mode of delivery and the risk of transmission, Dunn and colleagues (1994) concluded that available data do not support the routine use of cesarean birth for HIV-infected women. Currently, there is no official recommendation calling for cesarean births in pregnancies complicated by HIV. ACOG (1996) suggests that care providers use methods other than cesarean birth to protect the infant from vaginal secretions, such as avoiding rupture of the membranes.

The greatest risk for transmission during the postpartum period is associated with the practice of breastfeeding. Most of the data surrounding breastfeeding and HIV transmission comes from studies of African and European women conducted in the late 1980s and early 1990s (Cutting, 1994; European Collaborative Study, 1992). In 1992, the World Health Organization (WHO) published recommendations regarding the practice of breastfeeding by HIV-positive women (WHO, 1992). When applied to the economic, social, and epidemiologic climate in the United States, this consensus statement advises women with HIV to choose an alternate method to breastfeeding for feeding their infants. This recommendation is supported by ACOG (1997) as well as the American Academy of Pediatrics (AAP, 1997).

CASE PRESENTATIONS

The HIV pregnant patient may present for health care in a variety of settings under a wide range of circumstances. A patient may seek care knowing that she is HIV positive or she may be unaware of her HIV status. If HIV positive she may share the information with her provider, or choose to withhold the information and decline testing. The HIV-positive patient may present without signs of immunocompromise or may exhibit symptoms indicating infection, such as lymphadenopathy. If the disease has progressed to the point that opportunistic illnesses are present, the patient may require services ranging from outpatient management to critical care. The following case presentations are included to illustrate these points.

Case #1

B. W., a 28-year-old, Caucasian gravida 4, para 2-0-1-2, presented to the emergency department on January 22, 1996. She was approximately 27 weeks and 2 days gestation, which was confirmed by an ultrasound performed at her initial clinic visit, one week prior to this encounter. Her primary complaint was a productive cough, accompanied by increasing shortness of breath and intermittent, worsening mid-scapular back pain. She had previously experienced two, full-term, unremarkable vaginal deliveries. She denied all substance use and reported having a supportive family network, including an involved partner. Her outpatient clinic record indicated late entry into prenatal care. Display 19-6 summarizes the findings from her admission physical exam and initial testing. Additionally, B. W. was found to have extensive oral candida. A quick speculum exam was negative for ferning and nitrazine. The wet mount was positive for trichomoniasis, clue cells indicating bacterial vaginosis, numerous WBCs, and copious yeast. A sputum sample was obtained, as well as blood and genital cultures. She was begun on antibiotic and antifungal agents. B. W. responded to 40% O_2 via face mask with her SaO_2 increasing to 95%. She denied the presence of uterine contractions, and the biophysical profile provided reassurance of fetal well-being. She was transferred from the ED to the Medical Intensive Care Unit (MICU).

A careful review of her prenatal record indicated that B. W. had been counseled at her first prenatal visit, in accordance with organizational policy, about both the availability and desirabil-

DISPLAY 19-6

Significant Initial Findings for B. W.

Physical Exam

HR 140; RR 38; BP 143/68; T 103

Oxygen Saturation: 88% on room air

Fetal Heart Rate: 160 bpm

Auscultation indicated diminished breath sounds in both bases

Chest x-ray revealed bilateral basilar alveolar infiltrates

Laboratory Findings

Complete Blood Count

    Hemoglobin: 9.7

    Hematocrit: 29.5

    WBCs: 0.8

Arterial Blood Gases:

    ph: 7.5 pCO_2: 25 PO_2: 62

Blood Chemistry

    potassium   2.9

ity of HIV screening for pregnant women. She declined testing at that time, but indicated that she would reconsider testing at a later date. In light of her significant candida infection, her physician again approached her about HIV testing while in the MICU. At this time she consented to be tested. Her CD4 count was 20/mm³. The viral load was not determined. After lengthy discussion, she confirmed that she had been HIV positive for 3 years. She indicated that the source of her infection was a former partner with a history of IV drug use. He had been diagnosed as being HIV positive prior to the beginning of their relationship and died from AIDS-related complications 2 years ago. B. W. refused permission to inform her family or her current partner concerning her HIV status. The State Public Health Department was notified in accordance with existing statutes. Infectious Disease Service was consulted and, with her consent, she was begun on ZDV, 200 mg IV Q 8 hours.

While in the intensive care unit, B. W. was managed by a care team that included physicians from Maternal–Fetal Medicine, Pulmonary Medicine and Infectious Disease, MICU nursing and respiratory care staff, the OB/GYN, and Pulmonary Clinical Nurse Specialists. Pastoral Care, Social Services, Pharmacy, Nutritional Support, and Physical Therapy were also involved. This collaborative approach was critical in the management of B. W.'s care. There were numerous issues surrounding her refusal to disclose her HIV status to her family members and her partner. The Ethical Support Team was consulted and assisted team members, not only in clinical decision making, but also with the various personal conflicts that emerged over the course of her 3-week hospital stay.

Over the next several days, B. W's pulmonary status continued to deteriorate and on Hospital Day 3, she was intubated and placed on the ventilator. Her blood cultures were positive for Group B streptococcus and *Staphylococcus epidermidis,* however, her sputum cultures remained negative. Based on these findings and her radiographic studies, the physicians made the diagnosis of adult respiratory distress syndrome (ARDS) and communicated the dire nature of her prognosis to her family without revealing her HIV status. Throughout this period of time, she continued to have reassuring fetal testing despite the precarious nature of her status. Over the next week, B. W. had periods of O_2 desaturation, and on Hospital Day 10, B. W. developed a pneumothorax requiring chest tube placement.

At this point, the members of her care team felt that two critical decisions needed to be made. The first concerned the fetus and the point at which intervention via cesarean section would best be accomplished. The second involved disclosure of B. W.'s HIV status to her mother, who was now making all healthcare decisions for her daughter. A patient care conference was held and, after lengthy discussion, made the decision to inform B. W.'s mother of her HIV status. Her mother was shocked at the diagnosis and consented to a cesarean delivery. A female infant weighing 2 pounds, with Apgar scores of 5 and 8, was delivered via cesarean section on Hospital Day 11 and was transferred to the Neonatal Intensive Care Unit. B. W. had an unremarkable postoperative recovery and was returned to MICU.

It quickly became evident that B. W.'s partner, S. R., would need to be informed about the risk of HIV infection to his infant. The NICU staff felt that consent for ZDV treatment in the infant was necessary, as long-term effects of the treatment were unknown. B. W.'s mother was reluctant to provide the consent and elected to inform S. R. of the problem. After a discussion with the physicians, S. R. consented to the administration of ZDV to his daughter and requested an HIV test for himself. Following discharge from the NICU, ongoing management for the infant was arranged with a university-affiliated pediatric HIV/AIDS program in an adjacent state. The family reports that B. W.'s daughter is HIV positive, but that she is currently doing well. She lives with her maternal grandmother and her two older sisters.

B. W. continued to be managed by the team following delivery; however, her condition progressively deteriorated. On Hospital Day 20, the family elected to discontinue all therapeutic measures and she died shortly after the ventilator was removed on Hospital Day 21. B. W. never saw her newborn child.

Case #2

On September 1, 1996, S. S., a 24-year-old, gravida 6, para 3-0-2-3, African American female presented to the OB clinic at approximately 12 weeks gestation for her initial prenatal visit. Her history was significant for three previous uncomplicated vaginal deliveries with two subsequent elective abortions. Her three children were 7, 6, and 4 years of age, and she was currently in a 6-month-long relationship with the father of this current pregnancy. She admitted to occasional use of marijuana and cocaine, but denied the use of crack and reported no injection drug use. In fact, she reported that her drug use had diminished significantly over the last several months since meeting her current partner. She stated that he did not use drugs. She had no physical complaints but reported a history of abnormal PAP smears. Routine prenatal tests were obtained and she consented to HIV screening as well as a urine drug screen.

At her return clinic visit, S. S. was informed that both the ELISA and Western Blot indicated that she was HIV positive. Her urine drug screen was negative and other routine lab tests were normal. This diagnosis was given to S. S. at a time when other members of the healthcare team were present to provide emotional support and assist her in coping with this devastating news. She was unable to grasp the complex information required for posttest counseling. Consequently, a follow-up appointment was made for the next day and the HIV case manager drove S. S. home.

At her visit the next day she was accompanied by A. C., her partner. S. S. had informed him of her test results the night before the visit. He was visibly upset, but supportive, and expressed concern about the health of S. S., the infant, and himself. Her partner said he had heard that there were new treatments available and wanted to be tested as soon as possible. The physician, nurse practitioner, and HIV case manager reviewed the disease process and specifically addressed the issue of perinatal transmission. The couple had questions about the likelihood of transmission to the baby and asked about the option of terminating the pregnancy. A. C. was particularly concerned that new treatment might not be available for S. S. because she was pregnant. After significant discussion, they reached the mutual decision to continue with the pregnancy. A. C. was referred for HIV screening.

Display 19-7 summarizes the additional lab work that was ordered for S. S. Based on her CD4 cell count, S. S. was classified as having AIDS. At her next visit, she was referred for colposcopy to further evaluate her abnormal PAP smears and for a chest x-ray to establish a baseline radiographic profile. A PPD was administered to test for tuberculosis. Vaccinations against *Hemophilius* B influenza and the Pneumovax were administered. The hepatitis B vaccine series was begun. S. S. was provided the opportunity to transfer care to a center offering experimental protocols using combination antiretroviral therapy in pregnancy, but elected to continue care in the clinic. In accordance with the ACTG 076 protocol, S. S. was begun on ZDV, 100 mg 5 times per day. Due to an allergy to Septra, she was placed on

CD4 cell count has risen to 482 and her viral load has decreased to <10,000. A. C.'s initial HIV test was negative, as were two consecutive ELISA. Their daughter likewise remains free of infection.

SUMMARY

HIV is a dynamic illness that produces a wide variety of outcomes. Continued attention to prevention of infection may result in a reduction in the number of new HIV infections. Advances in medical management may impede the progression of the disease from HIV to AIDS, changing the nature of the infection from one that is uniformly fatal to chronic in nature. Advances in the management of HIV in pregnancy will most surely result in a continued decrease in perinatal transmission and an improvement in overall maternal status.

Perinatal nurses possess the ability to improve maternal and neonatal outcomes through research-based practice. We make this contribution through efforts to gain current knowledge regarding new treatment protocols and management recommendations. Even more importantly, however, we have the opportunity to enhance patient care by providing the emotional support and nurturing that is often missing from the lives of these women.

REFERENCES

American Academy of Pediatrics. (1997). Report of the Committee on Infectious Diseases (24th ed., pp. 279–304).

American College of Obstetricians and Gynecologists. (1997). Human immunodeficiency virus infections in pregnancy. Education Bulletin, 232, 2–8.

American Psychological Association. (1994). Publication Manual (4th ed.). Washington, DC: American Psychological Association.

Bardeguez, A. D. (1996). Management of HIV infection for the childbearing age woman. Clinical Obstetrics and Gynecology, 39(2), 344–360.

Carpenter, C. L., Fischl, M. A., Hammer, S. M., Hirsch, M. S., Jacobsen, D. M., Katzenstein, D. A., Montaner, J. S., Richman, D. D., Saag, M. S., Schooley, R. T., Thompson, M. A., Vella, S., Yeni,

DISPLAY 19-7

Additional Laboratory Evaluation for S. S.

CD4+ cell count	179 µL
HIV viral load	41,347
Hepatitis panel	negative
Cytomegalovirus	IgG positive IgM negative
Toxoplasmosis	IgG negative IgM negative

Pentamidine, 300 mg via nebulizer every 28 days for *Pneumocystis carinii* prophylaxis.

S. S.'s antepartum course was relatively uneventful. She had one upper respiratory infection that was treated with erythromycin. She also underwent several ultrasounds to monitor fetal growth. Her physician ordered serial CBCs with differential as well as periodic CD4 cell counts and measurements of viral load. All of these remained stable throughout the pregnancy, giving no indication of worsening illness. Her glucose tolerance test at 28 weeks was normal. She made the decision to undergo postpartum tubal ligation and signed the required consent form.

At 39 weeks the patient presented to Labor and Delivery for evaluation of labor. When examined, her cervix was 3 cm, 100%, with the vertex at -2 station. She was having irregular contractions with intact membranes. Due to the need to control the delivery circumstances and because she was multiparous, she was admitted to the hospital. Intravenous ZDV treatment was initiated following the ACTG 076 protocol. The Neonatal Intensive Care Unit was notified of her admission. S. S. labored with intact membranes and external fetal monitoring for 4 hours and 45 minutes and delivered a female over an intact perineum.

S. S. elected to bottle-feed her infant daughter. During her postpartum course, S. S. was begun on combination antiretroviral therapy. Currently, her

P. G., & Volberging, P. A. (1996). Antiretroviral therapy for HIV infection in 1996. Journal of the American Medical Association, 276(2), 146–153.

Centers for Disease Control and Prevention. (1987). Public health service guidelines for counseling and antibody testing to prevent HIV infection and AIDS. Morbidity and Mortality Weekly Review, 36(31), 509–515.

Centers for Disease Control and Prevention. (1992). 1993 revised classification system for HIV infection and expanded surveillance case definition for AIDS among adolescents and adults. Morbidity and Mortality Weekly Review, 41(RR-17), 1–19.

Centers for Disease Control and Prevention. (1993). Recommendations for HIV testing services for inpatients and outpatients in acute-care hospital settings. Morbidity and Mortality Weekly Review, 42(RR-2), 1–17.

Centers for Disease Control and Prevention. (1994a). Zidovudine for the prevention of HIV transmission from mother to infant. Morbidity and Mortality Weekly Review, 43(16), 285–289.

Centers for Disease Control and Prevention. (1994b). Recommendations of the U.S. Public Health Service Task Force to reduce perinatal transmission of human immunodeficiency virus. Morbidity and Mortality Weekly Review, 43(RR-11), 1–20.

Centers for Disease Control and Prevention. (1995a). HIV/AIDS Surveillance Report, 7(2), 2–39.

Centers for Disease Control and Prevention. (1995b). First 500,000 AIDS cases—United States. Morbidity and Mortality Weekly Review, 44(46), 849–853.

Centers for Disease Control and Prevention. (1995c). U.S. Public Health Service recommendations for human immunodeficiency virus counseling and voluntary testing for pregnant women. Morbidity and Mortality Weekly Review, 44(RR-7), 1–14.

Centers for Disease Control and Prevention. (1996a). HIV/AIDS Surveillance Report, 8(1), 1–28.

Centers for Disease Control and Prevention. (1996b). HIV/AIDS Surveillance Report, 8(2), 2–39.

Centers for Disease Control and Prevention. (1997a). 1997 revised guidelines for performing CD4 + T cell determinations in persons infected with human immunodeficiency virus (HIV). Morbidity and Mortality Weekly Review, 46(RR-2), 1–24.

Centers for Disease Control and Prevention. (1997b). Update: Trends in AIDS incidence, deaths and prevalence—United States, 1996. Morbidity and Mortality Weekly Review, 46(8), 165–173.

Chu, S. Y., Hanson, D. L., Jones, J. L., and the Adult/Adolescent HIV Spectrum of Disease Project Group. (1996). Pregnancy rates among women infected with human immunodeficiency virus. Obstetrics and Gynecology, 87(2), 195–198.

Cutting, W. A. M. (1994). Breastfeeding and HIV—A balance of risks. Journal of Tropical Pediatrics, 40, 6–11.

Dickover, R. E., Garratty, E. M., Herman, S. A., Sim, M., Plaeger, S., Boyer, P. J., Keller, M., Deveikis, A., Stiehm, E. R., & Bryson, Y. J. (1996). Identification of levels of maternal HIV-1 RNA associated with risk of perinatal transmission. Journal of the American Medical Association, 275(8), 599–605.

Donovan, R. M., Bush, C. E., Markowitz, N. P., Baxa, D. M., & Saravolatz, L. D. (1996). Changes in virus load markers during AIDS-associated opportunistic diseases in human immunodeficiency virus-infected person. Journal of Infectious Disease, 174, 401–403.

Dunn, D. T., Newell, M. L., Mayaux, M. J., Kind, C., Hutto, C., Goedert, J. J., Andiman, W., & Perinatal AIDS Collaborative Transmission Studies. (1994). Mode of delivery and vertical transmission of HIV-1: A review of prospective studies. Journal of Acquired Immune Deficiency Syndromes, 7(10), 1064–1066.

European Collaborative Study (1992). Risk factors for the mother-to-child transmission of HIV-1. Lancet, 339, 1007–1012.

Fauci, A. S., & Lane, C. (1994). Human immunodeficiency virus (HIV) disease: AIDS and related disorders. In K. J. Isselbacher, E. Braunwald, J. D. Wilson, J. B. Martin, A. S. Fauci, & D. L. Kasper (Eds.), Harrison's principles of internal medicine, Vol.2 (13th ed.). New York: McGraw-Hill.

Guyton, A. C. (1991). Textbook of medical physiology (8th ed.). Philadelphia: W. B. Saunders.

Gwinn, M., & Wortley, P. M. (1996). Epidemiology of HIV infection in women and newborns. Clinical Obstetrics and Gynecology, 39(2), 292–304.

HIV/AIDS Treatment Information Service. (1997). Understanding viral load. Fact Sheet.

Isada, N. B., & Grossman, J. H. (1991). Perinatal infections. In S. G. Gabbe, J. R. Niebyl, & J. L. Simpson (Eds.), Obstetrics: Normal and problem pregnancies. New York: Churchill Livingstone.

Johnstone, F. D., Thong, K. J., Bird, A. G., & Whitelaw, J. (1994). Lymphocyte subpopulations in early human pregnancy. Obstetrics and Gynecology, 83(6), 941–946.

Landesman, S. H., Kalish, L. A., Burns, D. N., Minkoff, H., Fox, H. E., Zorrilla, C., Garcia, P., Fowler, M. G., Mofenson, L., & Tuomala, R. (1996). Obstetric factors and the transmission of human immunodeficiency virus type 1 from mother to child. The New England Journal of Medicine, 334(25), 1617–1623.

Lewis, S. M., Collier, I. C., & Heitkemper, M. M. (1996). Medical-surgical nursing: Assessment and management of clinical problems (4th ed.). St. Louis, MO: Mosby.

Lin, H., Kao, J., Hsu, H., Mizokami, M., Hirano, J., Chen, D. (1996). Least microtransfusion from mother to fetus in elective cesarean delivery. Obstetrics & Gynecology, 87(2), 244–248.

Lindsay, M. K. (1996). HIV infection in women. Clinical Obstetrics and Gynecology, 39, 2.

Mandelbrot, L., Brossard, Y., Aubin, J., Bignozzi, C., Krivine, A., Simon, F., & Dommergues, M. (1996). Testing for in utero human immunodeficiency virus infection with fetal blood sampling. American Journal of Obstetrics and Gynecology, 175(2), 489–493.

Minkoff, H., & Augenbraun, M. (1997). Antiretroviral therapy for pregnant women. American Journal of Obstetrics and Gynecology, 176(2), 478–489.

Minkoff, H., Burns, D. N., Landesman, S., Youchah, J., Goedert, J. J., Nugent, R. P., Muenz, L. R., & Willoughby, A. D. (1995). The relationship of the duration of ruptured membranes to vertical transmission of human immunodeficiency virus. American Journal of Obstetrics and Gynecology, 173(2), 585–589.

Orloff, S. L., Simonds, R. J., Skeketee, R. W., & St. Louis, M. W. (1996). Determinants of perinatal HIV-1 transmission. Clinical Obstetrics and Gynecology, 39(2), 386–395.

Pantaleo, G., Graziosi, C., & Fauci, A. S. (1993). The immunopathogenesis of human immunodeficiency virus infection. New England Journal of Medicine, 328(5), 327–335.

Rouzioux, C., Costagliola, D., Burgard, M., Blanche, S., Mayaux, M., Griscelli, C., Valleron, A., & the HIV Infection in Newborns French Collaborative Study Group. (1993). Timing of mother to child HIV-1 transmission depends on maternal status. AIDS, 7(Suppl. 2), 49–51.

Royal College of Obstetrics and Gynecology. (1996). HIV and pregnancy. British Journal of Obstetrics and Gynaecology, 103, 1184–1190.

Smith, D. K., & Rogers, M. F. (1996). Immunopathogenesis and detection of HIV infection in women and newborns. Clinical Obstetrics and Gynecology, 39(2), 277–291.

Sweet, R. L., & Gibbs, R. S. (1995). Infectious diseases of the female genital tract (3rd ed.). Baltimore: Williams & Wilkins.

Weiser, B., Nachman, S., Tropper, P., Viscosi, K. H., Grimson, R., Baxter, G., Fang, G., Reyelt, C., Hutcheon, N., & Burger, H. (1994). Quantitation of human immunodeficiency virus type 1 during pregnancy: Relationship of viral titer to mother-to-child transmission and stability of viral load. Procedure of the National Academy of Science, 91, 8037–8041.

World Health Organization. (1992). Constitution on HIV transmission and breastfeeding, Geneva. Weekly Epidemiologic Record, 67, 177–184.

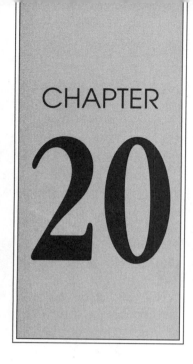

CHAPTER 20

Trauma in Pregnancy

Jane Daddario

INCIDENCE AND SIGNIFICANCE

Trauma is the most frequent cause of death in women aged 35 years or less. The increased frequency has had a significant impact on our society, not only in terms of human loss but in economic cost as well. Following heart disease, cancer, and stroke, trauma is the fourth leading cause of death among all age groups in the United States.

The magnitude of this problem has also been felt within the obstetric community. Trauma is the leading cause of death among women of childbearing age. One in every 12 pregnant women sustains a significant traumatic injury (Laverly & Staten-McCormick, 1995). Most injuries that bring pregnant women to the hospital are minor and have no impact on the outcome of the pregnancy. Trauma, however, is responsible for 20% of nonobstetric-related deaths of pregnant women (Clark, Cotton, Hankins, & Phelan, 1994). It has been estimated that accidental injury occurs in 7% of all pregnancies, with the distribution of reported cases increasing as pregnancy progresses (Huzel & Remsburg-Bell, 1996; Patterson, 1984; Rozycki, 1990). Approximately 8.8% of injuries occur during the first trimester, 40% in the second, and the remaining 52% in the third trimester of pregnancy (Clark et al., 1994). The true incidence of accidental injury probably is underestimated because early pregnancy is often unrecognized in the emergency room, especially if the woman is unconscious (Vaizey, Jacobson, & Cross, 1994).

Several causes of traumatic injury may be readily identified. Motor vehicle accidents, responsible for 48,700 deaths in 1987 alone, have greatly increased mortality in the general population (Trunkey, 1990). The majority of obstetric trauma is the result of motor vehicle accidents. McAnena, Moore, and Marx (1990) reported that motor vehicle accidents accounted for 75% of all blunt trauma in pregnancy. Though often associated with minor injuries, motor vehicle accidents cause death nearly 10 times more frequently than other sources of trauma. Falls, burns, firearm injuries, and domestic violence are other sources of trauma in pregnancy. Although most traumatic injuries during pregnancy are minor in nature, significant morbidity and mortality may be encountered. An understanding of the impact of trauma on the mother and fetus and the social problems surrounding the injury facilitates nursing assessment and the development of an appropriate plan of care. Foreknowledge of not only typical traumatic injuries but also associated complications allows few surprises for the nurse who encounters a pregnant trauma victim.

Maternal Morbidity and Mortality

Maternal mortality is most often due to injuries sustained from motor vehicle accidents, specifically head injuries followed by multiple internal injuries, which lead to hypovolemic shock and exsanguination (Schwab & Shaikh, 1985). These injuries tend to worsen if the victim is ejected from the vehicle. Acute spinal cord injury may be sustained by the pregnant woman resulting in serious maternal morbidity, especially due to cardiopulmonary dysfunction (Gilson, Miller, Clevenger, & Curet, 1995). Head and spinal cord injuries will continue to occur because pregnant women do not always see the need to use the shoulder harness with the lap belt when driving. Despite reports that the fetal skull can be fractured by being crushed between the seat belt and the sacral promontory, research data supports the benefits of seat belt use during pregnancy (Clark et al., 1994). There is no evidence that seat belts increase the risk of fetal loss (Hendey & Votey, 1994). Airbags may cause maternal injuries, such as abrasions to the face, neck, and chest, but they have been shown to reduce injuries overall, especially when used in conjunction with a lap and shoulder belt (Hendey & Votey, 1994).

Other life-threatening injuries that may be encountered in the multiple trauma victim include dissection of major thoracic and abdominal vessels, pleural space intrusion, liver and splenic lacerations, bowel perforation, multiple extremity fractures, and pelvic hematomas or fractures. Certain injuries and associated complications are unique to the pregnant trauma victim. They include uterine damage, placental abruption, and amniotic fluid embolism. Disseminated intravascular coagulation may also develop in the presence of a large placental abruption, significant hemorrhage, or intrauterine fetal demise.

Blood supply to the pelvic organs is greatly increased during pregnancy. It is not uncommon following blunt or penetrating abdominal trauma for a transplacental fetal–maternal hemorrhage to occur. In a study of 32 pregnant trauma patients, the incidence of fetal–maternal hemorrhage was 28%, with a mean blood loss of 16 cc and a range from 5–40 cc (Boehm, 1990; Sokal, Katz, Lell, & Fox, 1980). Uterine rupture, which occurs less than 1% of the time, has been reported in association with accidents involving deceleration forces that tear the uterus away

from its fixation point and cases where pregnant women were run over by moving vehicles causing extreme compression of the abdomen (Clark et al., 1994; Crosby, 1983; Landers, Newland, & Penney, 1989). However, placental abruption is much more likely to occur than is uterine rupture and has been reported as late as 5 days following the initial injury (Dees & Fuller, 1989; Smith, 1987). Studies demonstrate that abruptio placentae occurs in 40–50% of patients with major traumatic injuries and up to 5% of patients with minor injuries (Goodwin & Breen, 1990; Pearlman, Tintinalli, & Lorenz, 1990). Neufeld (1993) reported a maternal death rate less than 1%, but fetal loss was seen in 20–30% of the cases reviewed (Neufeld, 1993). The placenta is less elastic than the uterus, and force directed to the uterus can result in shearing of the placenta, producing abruptio placentae or uterine rupture (Hill & Lense, 1996). Hypoxia and blood loss may compromise the fetus, with resulting neurologic sequelae or death. The extent of uterine damage may make repair impossible, necessitating an emergency hysterectomy (Hill & Lense, 1996). Though no statistics are available regarding the incidence of preterm labor and premature rupture of membranes secondary to trauma, any injury resulting in hypoxic insults may increase such risk.

A review of significant trauma statistics in the general population also helps anticipate the concomitant impact on maternal outcome. Direct cerebral and high spinal cord injuries account for approximately 50% of all trauma deaths (Lewis, 1984). Traumatic brain injury has an annual death rate that approximates 30 per 100,000 population and accounts for 44% of the injury death rate worldwide (Kraus, 1991). The incidence of traumatic brain injury ranges from 152 to 430 cases per 100,000 per year depending on the population studied and catchment area (Kraus, 1991). Traumatic brain injury in pregnancy is poorly delineated. Blunt abdominal trauma sustained during motor vehicle accidents has been the focus of attention of researchers regarding the pregnant trauma patient.

Thoracic trauma is the primary cause of death in 25% of all fatal accidents and is a concurrent injury in 50% (Trunkey, 1984). Blunt trauma accounts for the majority of these injuries and is most often due to the impact of a steering wheel or dashboard during a motor vehicle accident. Pregnant drivers who wear improperly placed seat belts or none at all are susceptible to such complications as pneumothorax, flail chest, pericardial tamponade, hemothorax, ruptured diaphragm, tension pneumothorax, great vessel dissection, and pulmonary or myocardial contusions.

The penetrating injuries most frequently encountered are gunshot wounds and stabbing injuries. If the current trends of violence continue in this country, by the year 2003 the number of people killed by firearms will exceed the number of people killed in motor vehicle accidents (MMWR, 1994). Penetrating trauma, however, is becoming more and more common, especially in urban areas. In 1991, six states (California, Louisiana, Maryland, Nevada, Texas, and Virginia) and the District of Columbia, had more deaths as the result of firearms than of motor vehicle accidents (MMWR, 1994). The extent of tissue damage from a firearm depends largely on the kinetic energy involved. For example, low-velocity missiles or knives generally produce less significant bleeding and tissue destruction than high-velocity weapons (Hinkle & Betz, 1995).

Associated injuries resulting from firearms include open pneumothorax, pericardial tamponade, hemothorax, and great vessel dissection. There is a high frequency of internal organ injury with gunshot wounds. Intraabdominal organs may also be affected if the path taken by the penetrating object transects the diaphragm. The full bladder is vulnerable to penetrating injury as pregnancy advances. Penetrating abdominal wounds may be produced by a variety of objects yet are most often caused by bullets (Hinkle & Betz, 1995). The uterus often serves as a protective shield to other organs though the fetus may be placed in a position of greater susceptibility. Maternal mortality from bullet wounds was low in 77 cases reported, whereas fetal mortality ranged from 41–71% and was dependent on gestational age (Sandy & Koerner, 1989).

Stab wounds are the second most frequent type of penetrating abdominal injury and are generally less severe than bullet wounds because the bowel is likely to slide away from the penetrating object. Injuries to the bowel are less common in pregnant women because the enlarged uterus displaces and protects the intestines. The extent of injury is greater with multiple stab wounds, especially those to the bowel. Patterns of injury may be predicted by following the path of the instrument involved. Perinatal mortality for all intrauterine wounds approximates 40% (Sandy & Koerner, 1989).

As mentioned earlier in this chapter, abdominal trauma may result from either blunt or penetrating sources. The uterus and urinary bladder are at reduced risk of injury in the first trimester because they are confined to the bony pelvis. As gestation advances, the potential risk of injury increases. The uterus remains a pelvic organ until 12 weeks and is well protected from abdominal injury. It is not until about the thirteenth to fourteenth week gestation that the uterus is considered an abdominal organ (Vaizey et al., 1994). There is an overall increase in blood flow to the uterus during pregnancy from 60 ml/min to 600 ml/min. At term, a volume equivalent to the mother's entire circulating blood volume passes through the uterus every 10 minutes, thus increasing the potential for massive blood loss in late pregnancy when abdominal trauma occurs (Vaizey et al., 1994).

Blunt injuries, in addition to uteroplacental damage discussed previously, may include genitourinary trauma such as bladder rupture, urethral lacerations, and renal contusion or avulsions. Genitourinary trauma to a woman is rarely reported by the urologist (Levin & Edson, 1994).

Pelvic fractures continue to cause significant morbidity and mortality and remain the third most common injury in motor vehicle accidents (Esposito, 1994). There is an increased incidence of extensive retroperitoneal hemorrhage due to engorged pelvic veins. The pelvis usually fractures in two places due to the bony ring structure. Such injury does not necessarily preclude vaginal delivery.

There are 2.2 million patients each year in the United States who suffer burn injuries and seek medical attention. Of these patients, less than 4% are pregnant (Laverly & Staten-McCormick, 1995). Pregnant women may sustain burn trauma, but less than 0.1% suffer a thermal injury severe enough to warrant hospital admission (Esposito, 1994; Fox & Fabian, 1990; Lavin & Polsky, 1983; Rozycki, 1990). The majority of burn injuries occur in the home versus industry. Injury may be due to contact with hot objects, electric currents, or exposure to chemicals. Fetal death may be as high as 36% with serious thermal burns in the first trimester. Preterm labor may be experienced by second and third trimester patients (Clark et al., 1994). Common household electrical injuries are probably underreported. Intrauterine fetal death, decreased fetal movement, and oligohydramnios at delivery has been reported in six patients who sustained a household electrical injury (Clark et al., 1994). Inhalation injury and carbon monoxide intoxication may complicate the clinical picture if there was prolonged exposure to flames, heated gases, or smoke. Fetal acidosis and hypoxia result from the collection of carbon monoxide in the fetal compartment (Mighty, 1994).

In the absence of inhalation injury, maternal survival depends on the extent and depth of the burn (Deitch, Rightmire, Clothier, & Blass, 1985). Thermal injuries sustained as a result of an explosion may also be accompanied by significant blunt or penetrating trauma. Although thermal injury may result in superficial destruction of the skin and underlying tissue, alteration of virtually every organ system may occur. The pregnant burn victim is especially vulnerable to intravascular volume deficit and hypoxia (Crosby, 1983; Deitch et al., 1985; Rozycki, 1990; Taylor, Plunkett, McManus, & Pruitt, 1976). Maternal mortality is expected to range 50–90% when burns exceed 70–80% of the total body surface area in women of childbearing age. Prognosis of the mother and fetus is good when pregnant patients sustain less than 30% total body surface area (Laverly & Staten-McCormick, 1995). When prognostic factors are assessed, maternal outcome is not influenced by the pregnancy itself (Rode et al., 1990)

Fetal Morbidity and Mortality

The most common cause of fetal death in cases of trauma is maternal death. The second leading cause is placental abruption, which

has been reported in 59% of patients involved in severe motor vehicle accidents. The incidence of placental abruption occurs more frequently when the pregnant woman is ejected from a motor vehicle or strikes the steering column (Civil, Talucci, & Schwab, 1988; Clark et al., 1994). It has been documented that placental laceration, although rare, has always been associated with fetal loss (Stuart, Harding, & Davies, 1980). Kissinger and colleagues (1991) demonstrated in a review of 93 injured pregnant patients that the incidence of fetal death increased following maternal shock, pelvic fracture, and hypoxia. Rapid compression and expansion of the uterus produce shearing forces that tear an essentially rigid placenta from the flexible uterine wall. Maternal and fetal bleeding ensue and fetal death results from exsanguination of the fetal blood volume into the uterine cavity (Civil et al., 1988). Hoff and colleagues (1991) confirmed in a review of 73 pregnant patients that changes in maternal heart rate, systolic blood pressure, or hematocrit were not associated with fetal death. Predictors of fetal demise were worsening injury severity score, maternal fluid requirements, hypoxia, and acidosis. Fetal injury is most common in the third trimester, when the fetal head is engaged in the pelvis. Fetal skull fracture and intracranial damage may be the result of severe maternal pelvic trauma (Hill & Lense, 1996). The fetus is more susceptible to injury from gunshot and stab wounds than the mother.

Perinatal mortality secondary to noncatastrophic trauma does not greatly increase if the fetus is healthy prior to the insult (Fries & Hankins, 1989). The frequency of direct fetal injury following trauma is unknown. Though it is uncommon to have a serious fetal injury in the absence of maternal injury, studies demonstrate that fetal injuries may be diagnosed with the uterus intact (Agran, Dunkle, Winn, & Kent, 1987).

Amniotic fluid provides a cushioning effect, and in cases of minor blunt trauma the fetus usually survives intact. As the uterus rises out of the pelvis, the fetus becomes more vulnerable. The most common direct fetal injuries are skull fractures and intracranial hemorrhage

(Agran et al., 1987; Stuart et al., 1980). Fetal skull fractures are most often associated with motor vehicle accidents and result from fetal impact against the sacral prominence of the symphysis pubis, as well as from forward flexion of the torso over the gravid uterus. Other reported fetal fractures include the mandible, clavicle, vertebrae, and long bones (Bowdler, Faix, & Elkins, 1987).

As previously noted, trauma may result in rupture of the amniotic membranes. If a rupture occurs and the fetus is preterm or not engaged in the maternal pelvis, a cord prolapse may occur resulting in compression and fetal compromise. Maternal hypovolemia or hypotension may result in significant reduction in uteroplacental perfusion, thus contributing to fetal hypoxia or acidemia. Abdominal trauma secondary to battering has been reported to cause significant fetal heart rate abnormalities. Regardless of the severity of maternal injury, fetal heart rate abnormalities may serve as predictors of fetal head trauma (Sokal et al., 1980).

The fetus, if injured but alive and beyond 24 weeks, is potentially salvageable. Gestational age has a significant impact on decision making with regard to timing of delivery. In the best of circumstances, cesarean delivery is not likely to result in a surviving infant prior to 24 weeks gestation. However, when the pregnancy has achieved 26 weeks gestation, the survival rate is expected to be greater than 50% (Laverly & Staten-McCormick, 1995).

Etiology

Many social issues contribute to the overall high incidence of trauma. Drunk driving, nonuse of vehicle restraints or helmets, prevalence of handguns, and domestic violence crime associated with drugs are just a few. Factors that have led to the high incidence of maternal injuries include increased societal mobility, presence of women in the workplace throughout pregnancy, entrance of women into jobs previously held by men, and exposure to violent behavior (Daddario, 1989).

Traumatic injuries result from mechanical, electrical, or thermal injuries to organs or tissues (Halpern, 1989). Mechanical or kinetic energy is responsible for the vast majority of injuries. Certain patterns of injury may be expected to occur depending on the mechanism of the event. Knowledge of these injury patterns will guide the nursing assessment and encourage a high index of suspicion for possible injuries that may not be immediately visible. An accident in which the body is subjected to a significant amount of kinetic energy is likely to produce serious or critical injuries. The Committee on Trauma of the American College of Surgeons (1968) lists the following as some mechanisms that involve significant energy absorption:

1. Falls of 20 feet or more.
2. Motor vehicle accidents in which a change in speed of 20 mph has occurred, major vehicular damage is present, rollover is involved, passenger is ejected, or death of occupant within either car occurs.
3. Pedestrian hit at speed of 20 mph or more.

DOMESTIC VIOLENCE

Incidence and Significance

Domestic violence is a significant problem in our society. A detailed discussion of all the issues surrounding domestic violence and its impact on pregnancy is beyond the scope of this chapter. This chapter reviews the incidence of abuse, identification of victims, screening tools used with pregnant women, and problems with time constraints in the clinical setting. Intervention strategies used by healthcare providers that impact outcomes are briefly discussed.

Statistics vary depending on the populations studied. The facts about domestic violence are startling and clearly demonstrate that this is a serious health problem faced by healthcare providers.

"In the United States, every nine seconds a woman somewhere is physically abused by her partner. Approximately 4 million (7%) American women who are married or living with someone as a couple are physically abused, and 20 million (37%) are verbally or emotionally abused by their partner. The U.S. Department of Justice estimates that 95% of assaults on spouses or ex-spouses are committed by men against women. About 1 in 5 women victimized by their spouse or ex-spouse reported they had been a victim of a series of at least three assaults in the previous six months. 25% to 45% of battered women have been battered during pregnancy, increasing the incidence of miscarriage, preterm labor, and low birthweight. Over half of women murdered in the U.S. are killed by their intimate male partners. 92% of women who have been physically abused by their partners did not discuss the incident with their physicians; 57% did not discuss the abuse with anyone." (Furniss, 1997)

Rape, sexual assault, and sexual abuse are all part of the problem. Therefore, until ruled out, battery should be considered a possible cause of trauma in female patients who do not have clear histories (Helton, 1986; McLeer, Anwar, Herman, & Maquiling, 1989). Many emergency department visits are the result of domestic violence. Approximately 30% of women treated for injuries in emergency departments in this country are the result of abuse (MMWR, 1993). Previous studies have demonstrated that emergency department staff often fail to recognize battering as the cause of symptoms and injuries presented. Often the need for protection and psychological support is not addressed. Roberts, Lawrence, Otoole, and Raphael (1997) reviewed the medical records of 324 patients who disclosed domestic violence in a screening questionnaire and compared the results with those of a random sample of emergency department controls. They found that victims of domestic violence had made more emergency department and outpatient visits, were more likely to have had psychiatric treatment, had higher rates of alcohol abuse, and attempted suicide during the previous five years.

Suicide attempts in pregnant women are rarely successful. The incidence during pregnancy is similar to data reported on nonpregnant women of comparable age. Frequency of suicide attempts in pregnant women increases with the diagnosis of pregnancy, or early in the third trimester. These attempts are made most commonly by teenagers, primigravidas, the emotionally immature, and unmarried women with poor socioeconomic support (Sherer & Schenker, 1989). Early involvement of psychiatric support and intervention is paramount to a successful maternal/fetal outcome.

Violence often begins in pregnancy and escalates as gestation advances. Recent studies of battering during pregnancy report that the prevalence ranges anywhere from 1–25% before pregnancy (Campbell, 1995; Christian, 1995; Laverly & Staten-McCormick, 1995; Parker, McFarlane, & Soleken, 1994). Newberger and colleagues (1992) cite data that during the first four months of pregnancy there are 154 acts of violence per 1,000 pregnant women and that during the fifth through ninth months of pregnancy violence increases to 170 of 1,000 pregnant women. Variability of statistics is partially dependent on inquiry methods and sampled demographics (Campbell, 1995). The partner's jealousy of the unborn child, anger about the pregnancy, or anger toward the woman have been attributed to increased abuse during pregnancy. The higher likelihood of unplanned pregnancies and short intervals between births are believed to be the result of sexual abuse. Data support that the prevalence of physical or sexual abuse during pregnancy is similar for African American and Caucasian women and lower for Latina women (Campbell, 1995). Campbell (1995) found that the most common mental health correlates are depression and anxiety.

Sexual assault is reported to have little immediate physical effect on the outcome of pregnancy. Satin, Hemsell, Stone, Theriot, and Wendel (1991) studied 114 cases of sexual assault in pregnant women over a 5-year period, and concluded that these cases were accompanied by less physical trauma than in nonpregnant women. It is important that victims of sexual assault be examined by a specialist so that forensic evidence is not missed. Careful screening for sexually transmitted diseases is part of the physical examination (Satin et al., 1991; Vaizey et al., 1994).

Screening

Careful screening and identification are critical in addressing the problems of domestic violence. It is common for women who are being abused to be reluctant to admit to violence in the relationship because of shame, fear, and a belief that health providers will not understand or be able to help. Women are often hesitant to fill out forms stating that they have been abused, yet they will often admit to abuse when verbally questioned by a sensitive healthcare provider. Universal screening of all prenatal patients for domestic violence should be a standard of care. Nurses should be trained to perform universal screening for abuse in order to meet the needs of the pregnant woman.

A number of screening tools have been developed and studied with different populations of pregnant women. The Nursing Research Consortium on Violence and Abuse developed the Abuse Assessment Screen, which uses five questions to assess remote and recent history of sexual and physical abuse as well as fear of the abuser (Norton, Peipert, Zierler, Lima, & Hume, 1995). The Abuse Assessment Screen is used with pregnant as well as nonpregnant women (Display 20-1). In a study of 334 women, the Abuse Assessment Screen was compared with the routine social service interview. The Abuse

DISPLAY 20-1

Questions Included in the Abuse Assessment Screen

1. Have you ever been emotionally or physically abused by your partner or someone important to you?   Yes No

2. Within the last year, have you been hit, slapped, kicked, or otherwise physically hurt by someone?   Yes No

    If yes, by whom? (circle all that apply)

    Husband Ex-husband Boyfriend Stranger Other Multiple

    Number of times:

3. Since you've been pregnant, have you been hit, slapped, kicked, or otherwise physically hurt by someone?   Yes No

    If yes, by whom? (circle all that apply)

    Husband Ex-husband Boyfriend Stranger Other Multiple

    Number of times:

    Mark area of injury on the body map. (body map included)

    Score the most severe incident to the following scale:

    1 = Threats of abuse, including use of a weapon
    2 = Slapping, pushing; no injuries and/or lasting pain
    3 = Punching, kicking, bruises, cuts, and/or continuing pain
    4 = Beaten up, severe contusions, burns, broken bones
    5 = Head, internal, and/or permanent injury
    6 = Use of weapon, wound from weapon

4. Within the past year, has anyone forced you to have sexual activities?   Yes No

    If yes, by whom? (circle all that apply)

    Husband Ex-husband Boyfriend Stranger Other Multiple

    Number of times:

5. Are you afraid of your partner or anyone you listed above?   Yes No

Assessment Screen detected a higher rate of violence in each category, and violence in the last year and during the current pregnancy (Norton et al., 1995).

Data support that repeated questioning on multiple visits increases detection of violence. Asking direct questions about abuse during the assessment screen seems to be a significant factor in detection. How and when to ask questions is an acquired art (Chez, King, & Brown, 1997). The experienced clinician must learn techniques and clues to look for during the assessment (Display 20-2).

There are many myths regarding domestic violence. One common myth is that violence occurs more often in certain social, cultural, and ethnic groups (Chez et al., 1997). Another myth is that violence occurs only in dysfunctional families. Often, healthcare providers will not screen a family that appears problem-free. Clues may be found in the behavior of the patient and family. Emotional abuse is part of the abuse cycle. Controlling, coercive, and intimidating behaviors are common among abusers. Many women victims do not recognize these behaviors as abuse; however, characteristic signs of abuse may be

DISPLAY 20-2

Assessing Emotional Violence

These signs are characteristic of emotional abuse:

- Partner ridicules or ignores the woman's feelings.
- Partner ridicules or insults the woman's religion, race, heritage, class, or most valued beliefs.
- Partner withholds approval, appreciation, or affection as punishment.
- Partner uses name-calling or constant shouting.
- Partner insults or drives away the woman's family or friends.
- Partner humiliates the woman in public or private.
- Partner keeps the woman from working.
- Partner refuses to do his share of the chores or pay his share of the bills.
- Partner takes money from, steals property from, or otherwise controls the financial affairs of the woman.
- Partner threatens to withdraw financial support from the dependent woman.
- Partner tells others about the woman's sexual affairs in order to embarrass or humiliate her.
- Partner harasses the woman about affairs he imagines she is having.
- Partner raises his voice to dominate a conversation or to assert control.
- Partner uses size or body to threaten or intimidate.
- Partner punishes or deprives children when angry at the woman.
- Partner threatens to kidnap their children if the woman has left him.
- Partner abuses pets to hurt or intimidate the woman.
- Partner threatens to kill himself if the woman doesn't do what he wants.
- Partner threatens to physically hurt the woman or her family.

Chez, R. A., King, M. C., & Brown, J. (1997, Spring). Homing in on abuse: What to ask and how to listen. Contemporary Nurse Practitioner (pp. 20–28).

identified when making an assessment (Hinkle & Betz, 1995).

Complications and Associated Problems

Studies on violence in pregnancy reveal that there is an increased incidence among abused women of cigarette smoking, alcohol use, history of drug use, poor weight gain, poor nutrition, emotional problems, posttraumatic stress disorder, and lack of a support system (Campbell, 1995). Exacerbations of chronic illnesses such as diabetes, hypertension, and asthma resulting from abuse-related stress can place the fetus at risk for impaired growth and development (Greenberg, McFarlane, & Watson, 1997). Many of the pregnancies are unplanned, and there is a lack of involvement with the father of the infant. Outcomes of these pregnancies indicate inadequate prenatal care, increased rates of low birth weight, miscarriage, complications of pregnancy, postpartum depression, child abuse once the baby is born, and homicide (Campbell, 1995; Christian, 1995). Recent research suggests that low birth weight is the result of smoking, substance use, and physical abuse during pregnancy (Institute of Medicine, 1985; McFarlane, Parker, & Soeken, 1996; Slutsker, Smith, Higginson, & Fleming, 1993; U.S. Dept. of Health and Human Services, 1991). High-risk pregnancy status should be assigned to the battered pregnant woman (Rozycki, 1990).

Using a five-question screen to detect physical abuse in pregnancy, researchers found ethnic-specific interrelationships regarding the increased use of tobacco, alcohol, and illicit drugs. The study sampled 1203 African American, Hispanic, and Caucasian pregnant women from public prenatal clinics in two urban settings. Tobacco use had the highest prevalence among Caucasian women, alcohol/illicit drug use was highest among African American women, and Hispanic women had the lowest prevalence rates of physical and substance abuse. Low infant birth weights were associated significantly with Caucasian and African American women who had been abused. There were no effects on birth weight among the Hispanic women studied. Using

more than one substance has a compounding effect on birth weight. Refusing to use substances with the abuser caused physical abuse to begin or escalate for many of the women in the study. Self-medication with tobacco, alcohol, and illicit drugs may be used as a mechanism to cope with the abuse. The abusive partner may supply the drugs or finances for its purchase, making it more difficult for the woman to leave because of her increasing drug addiction. Data suggest that abuse, smoking, alcohol, and illicit drug use are intertwined for many women. Offering the woman options for safety and abuse prevention may empower her to reduce or stop substance use. Nurses have the opportunity to develop clinical protocols integrating assessment and intervention for physical abuse, smoking, and substance use that impact healthy outcomes for pregnant women and their infants (McFarlane et al., 1996).

Intervention

Interventions planned for the abused woman should be considered within the woman's cultural orientation (Campbell, 1995). Healthcare providers must offer supportive care, not inappropriate interventions. Advising, forcing choices, criticizing the victim or her husband, using scare tactics to elicit a response, or inciting anger in the woman are not acceptable behaviors on the part of the provider and may actually place the woman at risk for additional or escalating violence. Appropriate nursing behaviors include providing emotional support, exploring options, listening empathetically, allowing verbalization of feelings, and positively supporting all decisions the woman makes (Christian, 1995).

In many of our primary care facilities, healthcare providers find it difficult to spend adequate time with women who disclose abuse. Reimbursement issues and time constraints are a reality within our current healthcare delivery system. Other patients may be waiting. Asking the woman to talk to someone else in the office or to come back during the week for a longer appointment may be an alternative. Safety is a major focus of intervention. It is important to always ask the woman if it is safe for her to have referral information in her possession. Often the abuser will search the victim's personal belongings and question her about her conversation with the healthcare provider. Suggesting that she call the domestic violence hotline or going to a nearby shelter may be a priority. Unless the woman is at a point of awareness, acknowledgment, or change, she may not be willing to use the resources (Chez et al., 1997). Several actions available to the healthcare provider include assisting the woman to examine her options, talking with her about the components of a healthy relationship, and teaching the skills for explaining what is wanted in a relationship (Hinkle & Betz, 1995). Ending an abusive situation may be complicated by denial, inertia, and even grief (Chez et al., 1997). It is important that the woman realize that she is not responsible for the abuse nor does she provoke it. She must make choices about her own behavior and how she wants to live her life because she cannot change the abuser. Often the woman feels she cannot change and she has no options (Chez et al., 1997). Therefore, change may be difficult, slow, and occur in stages. It is important for the nurse to remember the woman will not make changes until she is ready.

Physical abuse is assault and is illegal in the United States. It is critical that all healthcare providers are aware of state laws concerning domestic violence, sexual assault, and protective orders. Many abused women are not aware that marital status does not protect the abuser. Assault by a spouse is a crime and the abuser can be prosecuted (McFarlane et al., 1996).

The nurse must document the abuse. It is essential that the information is captured on a written document. A standard abuse assessment form can be used, noting the frequency and severity of present and past abuse. The location and extent of injury, pain reported, days absent from work, treatments, interventions, any discussion of an escape plan, and shelter assistance offered/declined must be documented. The nurse should record a statement of no history or threat of abuse if none exists and record any educational materials given to the woman (McFarlane et al., 1996).

Nurses must be aware of the resources in their area and be prepared to provide telephone numbers and referrals for women who screen positive for domestic violence. Women need educational material on abuse just as would be provided them for nutrition or stress management (Chez et al., 1996). The problem of domestic violence in pregnancy requires energy, time, and continuous attention. Nurses have a responsibility to become better informed. It is only by detection of battering during pregnancy that nurses will have the opportunity to intervene and protect the lives of the mother and her unborn child.

FRAMEWORK FOR ACCEPTED THERAPY

The mechanism of injury, gestational age of the fetus, and associated complications determine the maternal–fetal response to trauma. Certain physiologic and anatomic changes of pregnancy may significantly mask and influence patterns of injury and patient responses. For these reasons, such changes should be considered in planning care for the pregnant trauma patient. (See Table 20-1.)

Obstructions and reductions in blood flow from trauma are poorly tolerated by the mother and fetus as pregnancy is considered a high-flow, low-resistance cardiovascular state. Hemorrhage may go unnoticed because the increased blood volume may mask hypotension. The pregnant woman may lose up to 35% of her circulating blood volume before signs of shock are evident, and for this reason does not have the same ability to compensate for blood loss (Mighty, 1994; Bremer & Cassata, 1986). Therefore, correcting hypovolemia is a priority.

The difference in the ratio of plasma to red blood cells results in a decrease in hematocrit and albumin concentration. Due to decreased colloid osmotic pressure, the pregnant woman is vulnerable to leakage of plasma into the extravascular compartment. Thus, vigorous fluid resuscitation may increase the likelihood of pulmonary edema. However, the risk of volume overload should not prevent intravascular volume replacement but rather promote careful calculation in order to decrease capillary leakage. If the pregnant trauma patient requires immediate surgery under conduction anesthesia, additional

TABLE 20-1. Changes to Consider in Planning Care for Pregnant Trauma Patients

Physioanatomic Changes During Pregnancy	Clinical Impact
Cardiovascular	
Blood volume increased by 50%	May lose 30–35% of blood volume before shock is evident
Plasma volume increased more than red blood cells; heart rate increases 15–20 beats per minute	Physiologic anemia
Decreased systemic vascular resistance; cardiac output increased by 50%	May not develop cool, clammy skin
Respiratory	
Respiratory rate increased; tidal volume increased 30–40%; functional residual capacity decreased 25%	Compensated respiratory alkalosis
Metabolic rate and oxygen consumption increased	Reduced oxygen reserve; less tolerant of hypoxia
Chest wall broadened and diaphragm elevated	Thoracostomy performed above the normal site
Peripheral edema, dyspnea, and third heart sound present	May clinically mimic congestive ventricular failure
Abdominal viscera displaced and compressed; stretched abdominal musculature; decreased bowel sounds	Increased risk of liver or splenic rupture; abdominal injury may be masked or mimicked by pregnancy; altered patterns of referred pain; rebound tenderness may be present or absent
Decreased gastric motility; prolonged gastric emptying time; incompetent esophageal sphincter	Increased risk of aspiration
Pelvic venous congestion	Increased risk of hemorrhage
Protruding uterus and/or bladder	Increased risk of injury
Hematologic	
Increased clotting factors VII, VIII, IX, and X; increased fibrinogen level	Hypercoagulability

fluid administration may be required in order to stabilize the blood pressure because of blood sequestered in the dilated vascular beds.

Oxygen reserve is decreased as a result of increased metabolic rate, thus enhancing the risk of maternal and fetal hypoxia. The chronic compensated respiratory alkalosis of pregnancy also decreases blood-buffering capacity. Associated alterations in arterial blood gas values should be considered when caring for these women. For example, the pregnant trauma patient with a pCO_2 of 40 mm Hg may indeed have respiratory acidemia. Therefore, hypoventilation should

be considered even though such a value in the nonpregnant woman would be normal.

The uterine vasculature has both alpha and beta receptors but, due to the vasodilatory state of pregnancy, there is no uteroplacental vasoconstriction to impede blood flow. Perfusion pressure determines blood flow to the uterus because the uteroplacental vascular bed functions as a dilated, passive, low-resistance system (Lee & Mezzadri, 1990). Every 8–11 minutes the total circulating blood volume flows through the uterus, thus making the potential for bleeding a major consideration. Because of stretching of the abdominal wall and displacement of intraabdominal organs, diminished response to peritoneal irritation may be observed, complicating patient assessment.

Administration of oxygen and vasopressors alone will not improve blood flow to the uterus and placenta during hemorrhage or hypotensive episodes. Blood flow will be enhanced only through restoration and maintenance of circulating blood volume (Clark et al., 1994; Pimentel, 1991). Once the pregnant woman experiences hypovolemic shock, compensatory mechanisms become activated. The uterus is then treated as a nonvital organ with blood shunted away to the brain, heart, kidney, and lungs. Fetal hypoxemia, metabolic acidemia, and death may ensue (Clark et al., 1994; Dees & Fuller, 1989).

ASSESSMENT

There is high risk for the pregnant patient with trauma because the normal anatomic and physiologic changes that have occurred as a result of her pregnancy will frequently mask serious derangements in maternal physical integrity and homeostasis. The trauma victim's initial contact with medical and nursing personnel often occurs in the emergency department setting, where lack of familiarity with obstetric principles and normal changes associated with pregnancy is common. Conversely, medical and nursing obstetric specialists may be unfamiliar with the principles of trauma stabilization and management. Therefore, the most effective strategy in providing the highest quality of care for the pregnant trauma victim requires collaboration between the emergency trauma and obstetric specialists. The nurse, well-grounded in both obstetric and trauma care, is invaluable in assuring coordination of care for this patient population.

Maternal Assessment

The trauma assessment may be conceived as a "two-tier" system, more generally known as primary and secondary surveys. Initial emphasis is placed on the primary survey, in which life-threatening conditions are identified and resuscitation of vital signs is undertaken. Upon stabilization of vital signs, a secondary survey is per-

formed. This includes a detailed head-to-toe examination, management of non-life-threatening injuries, and continual reassessment of the patient's condition.

Primary Survey

The ABC's of initial trauma management are encompassed in the primary survey, which may be accomplished within minutes when performed efficiently and with a directed approach. Correctly applied, the primary survey includes simultaneous assessment and intervention when significant, immediate life-threatening injuries are present. Assessment and treatment priorities for the trauma patient should follow these steps:

1. Airway maintenance (and concurrent control of the cervical spine).
2. Assessment of breathing and circulation.
3. Control of hemorrhage and treatment of shock.

Assessment of the airway includes the basics: look, listen, and feel for movement of air. For the conscious patient, airway assessment can be accomplished at a glance; that is, the talking or shouting patient obviously has an open airway. An unconscious patient requires a closer assessment and may need assistance in gaining an airway.

Breathing and circulation may be assessed simultaneously because attention is directed to the neck and chest during this step of the primary survey. After establishing an adequate airway, assessing respiratory function by evaluating its rate and quality follows. Indications of distress include tachypnea, bradypnea, use of accessory muscles, shallow or painful respirations, asymmetric chest excursion, dyspnea, and inability to move air despite an open airway. Any of these symptoms should trigger suspicion of such chest injuries as pneumo- or hemothorax, tension pneumothorax, rib fracture or flail chest, and open sucking chest wounds.

Following assessment of respiratory rate and quality, attention should be directed to the neck. The trachea must be inspected and its position—whether or not it is midline—noted. Deviation of the trachea to either side may indicate the presence of tension pneumothorax or massive hemothorax. The neck veins must be assessed for flatness or distention. The former will accompany hypotension, pneumothorax, or cardiac tamponade. The presence of edema, subcutaneous air, or discoloration must also be noted.

Assessment of circulation is performed concurrently with assessment of breathing in the primary survey. It is important to note that time-consuming blood pressure measurement need not be performed during the primary survey in order to diagnose shock. Palpation of the pulse of the carotid artery indicates a systolic pressure of at least 60 mm Hg. The pulse of the femoral artery may be palpated if systolic pressure is at least 70 mm Hg. Palpation of the pulse of the radial artery, indicating a systolic pressure of at least 80 mm Hg, can be performed while visually inspecting the thorax (Schwab & Shaikh, 1985). Blood volume in the pregnant patient is increased by 50% (2000 mL). She may compensate well for hypovolemic shock until 25–35% of her volume is lost. Blood loss up to 1500 mL may occur before cardiovascular instability becomes apparent (Laverly & Staten-McCormick, 1995; Pimentel, 1991). Significant compromise in uterine blood flow may exist in the presence of a normal-appearing blood pressure (Mighty, 1994).

The chest is assessed for contusions, asymmetric excursion, paradoxical breathing, deformities, or open sucking wounds. The thorax is then palpated, and the presence of pain, rib instability, or subcutaneous emphysema is noted. Breath sounds must be auscultated; if decreased or absent on one side, percussion may indicate pneumothorax (hyperresonance) or hemothorax (dullness). Heart sounds should be briefly assessed to ascertain if they are distant or muffled. Pericardial tamponade will muffle heart sounds. Several life-threatening thoracic injuries should be detected during the primary survey. All demand immediate intervention to avoid catastrophe. Table 20-2 briefly describes each injury and its suggested initial management.

Circulatory assessment is completed by observing the patient's skin color and temperature, determining her mental status, and measuring capillary refill through a nail blanch test. Poor circulatory status is reflected in the patient who is cool, pale, agitated, and has prolonged capillary refill.

The third step of the primary survey should already have been initiated by other members of the trauma team by the time the first two steps have been assessed. External bleeding must be controlled. Direct pressure and pressure bandages control most sources of peripheral bleeding; vessel ligature or tourniquets are rarely necessary.

Secondary Survey

After resuscitation measures have been initiated, the secondary survey is performed. For the gravid patient, this includes a thorough head-to-toe examination with special attention given to the abdominal and pelvic assessment.

A brief neurologic assessment will reveal level of consciousness and sensorimotor function. Use of the mnemonic *AVPU* aids in rapid determination of level of consciousness:

A = *A*lert and oriented
V = Responds to *V*erbal stimulus
P = Responds only to *P*ain
U = *U*nresponsive

Although this is a very basic method for evaluating a patient's level of consciousness, its simplicity will promote clear communication about the patient's neurologic status among all caregivers. Descriptive labels such as lethargic, obtunded, or vegetative are subjective and are often interpreted differently by personnel involved in patient care. This method relies solely on objective assessment and enhances continuity. Early assessment is important, because establishing a baseline will assist in recognizing signs of deterioration.

After determining level of consciousness, examine the head for contusions, lacerations, and bony deformities. Basilar skull fractures are often accompanied by bleeding from the ear or nose, postauricular swelling and discoloration (Battle's sign), and periorbital edema and ecchymosis ("raccoon eyes"). The pupils must be evaluated for equality, reactivity to light, and accommodation. A portable cross-table lateral x-ray of the cervical spine, the radiograph of choice for initial evaluation of the cervical vertebrae, should be taken at this time.

TABLE 20-2. Life-Threatening Thoracic Injuries

Type of Injury	Clinical Manifestations	Interventions
Airway obstruction	1. Profound shock 2. Cyanosis 3. No air movement	If attempts to clear airway with finger sweep, modified jaw thrust, suction, or laryngoscopy fail, perform immediate surgical cricothyrotomy
Tension pneumothorax	1. Cyanosis and acute respiratory distress 2. Profound shock 3. Trachea devicted away from affected side 4. Jugular vein distention 5. Breath sounds absent and decreased on affected side 6. Hyperresonance on affected side	Immediately relieve tension by inserting 14-gauge needle into fifth intercostal space, midaxillary line, on affected side; use chest tube for long-term management
Flail chest	1. Respiratory distress 2. Multiple unstable rib fractures 3. Paradoxical respirations 4. Poor air movement despite open airway	Internally stabilize rib fractures by immediate intubation with positive pressure ventilation
Open pneumothorax	1. Respiratory distress 2. Open sucking chest wound 3. Subcutaneous emphysema	Cover immediately with petrolatum gauze or any airtight dressing; use chest tube for long-term management, and observe closely for development of tension pneumothorax
Pericardial tamponade	1. Profound shock 2. Tightly distended jugular 3. Muffled heart sounds	Perform immediate pericardiocentesis or prompt thoracotomy with pericardial decompression and repair of myocardial injury
Massive hemothorax	1. Profound shock 2. Respiratory distress 3. Breath sounds decreased or absent on affected side 4. Dullness to percussion on affected side	Immediately use chest tube with aggressive blood volume replacement, autotransfusion

Sensorimotor function may be easily evaluated in the conscious patient. If the patient is unconscious, how she responds to painful stimuli will indicate function. Withdrawal from or localization of pain indicates an intact sensorimotor system. Decorticate or decerebrate posturing accompanies deep cerebral hemispheric or upper brainstem injury. Spinal cord injury will produce flaccid paralysis below the level of the lesion. Spinal cord injury and any accompanying neurologic deficit or neurogenic shock may be difficult to diagnose in the woman with an altered or absent level of consciousness. A high index of suspicion of neurogenic shock should be maintained in the presence of refractory hypotension unresponsive to aggressive fluid replacement when there is no apparent source of blood loss. A relative bradycardia may accompany the hypotension (Fox & Fabian, 1990).

The Glascow Coma Scale is a common method for evaluating and monitoring neurologic status (Display 20-3). It has been shown to be a valid tool in predicting final outcome for head-injured victims (American College of Surgeons Committee on Trauma, 1993). Scores are derived by selecting the numerical value for the *best* response in three components of the evaluation and by calculating a total. An initial score of 8 or higher predicts a 94% favorable outcome, and scores of 3 and 4 predict only a 10% favorable outcome (American College of Surgeons Committee on Trauma, 1993; Campbell, 1985).

The secondary survey should be continued by moving down the body. A thorough reassessment of the chest and circulation is performed, including a portable anteroposterior radiograph of the thorax. This is followed by an abdominal and pelvic exam. Abdominal pain, tenderness, or distention may not be observed in the pregnant patient, and peritoneal signs may be confusing or unreliable, even in the presence of significant organ injury. The most common cause of intraperitoneal hemorrhage is splenic rupture (Laverly & Staten-McCormick, 1995). If intraabdominal hemorrhage is suspected, the most reliable assessment tool in the trauma room is the diagnostic peritoneal lavage (Auerbach, 1979; Baker, 1982; Higgins, 1988; Mighty, 1994). It is 94–98% accurate in detecting intraperitoneal bleeding

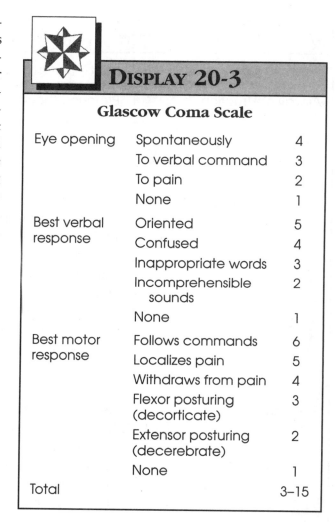

DISPLAY 20-3

Glascow Coma Scale

Eye opening	Spontaneously	4
	To verbal command	3
	To pain	2
	None	1
Best verbal response	Oriented	5
	Confused	4
	Inappropriate words	3
	Incomprehensible sounds	2
	None	1
Best motor response	Follows commands	6
	Localizes pain	5
	Withdraws from pain	4
	Flexor posturing (decorticate)	3
	Extensor posturing (decerebrate)	2
	None	1
Total		3–15

(Mighty, 1994). Results are positive for intraperitoneal bleeding if the returned fluid is bloody. The fluid may also be examined microscopically. The following are criteria for a positive result:

1. More than 100,000 red blood cells per millimeter.
2. More than 500 white blood cells per millimeter.
3. Presence of bile, intestinal contents, or bacteria.
4. Amylase level greater than 1.5 times the patient's serum amylase level (Cummings & Cummings, 1984; Higgins, 1988; Mighty, 1994).

Culdocentesis may be the individual physician's method of choice in evaluating intraperitoneal fluid, but should only be performed by someone thoroughly experienced with this procedure.

Abdominal and pelvic assessment assumes greater significance for the pregnant trauma victim. By this point in the secondary survey, maternal stabilization should be under way, if not already accomplished. Assessment of the uterus, fetus, and pelvis will provide some indication of fetal viability and well-being, and it is at this junction that collaboration between trauma and obstetric specialists provides a critical enhancement of patient outcome. Fetal assessment will be discussed later in this chapter.

A uterine assessment pertinent to the trauma victim includes measurement of fundal height to provide an estimate of gestational age; palpation of the uterus for tenderness and contraction frequency, intensity, duration, and resting tone; assessment of fetal heart rate; and performance of a vaginal exam to assess for lacerations, cervical status, and pelvic fracture. Evidence of bony fragments in the vaginal vault may be indicative of a pelvic fracture (Mighty, 1994). Any vaginal bleeding or amniotic fluid leakage must be noted.

Pelvic bony structures should be evaluated clinically and radiographically. Significant, comminuted pelvic fractures may be obviously unstable when anteroposterior or medial pressure is manually applied at the iliac crests and pubic symphysis. An anteroposterior radiograph of the pelvis will reveal less obvious fractures and should be performed as part of the secondary survey. Blunt trauma forceful enough to produce fractures will usually result in at least two disruptions of the pelvic ring, with a potential loss of 6 to 8 U of blood (McQuillan & Wiles, 1988). Assessment of the urethral meatus for obvious tissue damage or bleeding must be made. If these are absent, a urinary catheter should be inserted to monitor urine output and to rule out hematuria. Trauma to the liver and spleen, often associated with rib fractures, occurs in up to 25% of severe motor vehicle accidents (Laverly & Staten-McCormick, 1995). Preterm labor may occur as a result of the trauma or secondary to therapeutic interventions, especially surgery.

An assessment of the extremities for soft tissue or skeletal injury completes the secondary survey. Crush injury may be life-threatening and is the result of prolonged pressure to the limbs, which leads to severe impairment of myocyte integrity and rhabdomyolysis. Injury occurs as the result of individuals trapped under fallen debris during earthquakes, bombings, fires, and other disasters. Skeletal muscles of victims are subjected to prolonged strain leading to a dissolution of the integrity of the muscle cell membrane and derangement of cellular transport (Schoenfeld et al., 1995). After pressure has been removed from a trapped limb, within hours or days after injury, extracellular fluid volume enters damaged muscle cells (Odeh, 1991). Potassium, phosphate, myoglobin, and other cell products leak from damaged muscle cells resulting in severe hyperkalemia, which may lead to cardiac arrest. Lactic acidosis, disseminated intravascular coagulopathy, may also occur as a result of leakage, thromboplastin release, and renal tubule damage caused by myoglobin release from muscle cells. An integrated trauma team approach is necessary for the management of the pregnant victim of a crush injury. A surgeon, obstetrician, orthopedist, and nephrologist will play an important role in the management of this patient (Schoenfeld et al., 1995).

Injuries of the musculoskeletal system may appear dramatic, but rarely pose an immediate threat to life. Hip fractures or dislocations may be clinically evident if the lower extremity on the affected side appears shorter or longer and is rotated medially or laterally. Significant hemorrhage from femur fractures or any open fracture may occur. Assessment of the neurovascular function of an affected extremity includes evaluation of sensation, movement, color, capillary refill, swelling, and distal pulses.

Finally, optimal care of the pregnant trauma victim is promoted by a psychosocial assessment and the provision of emotional support for her and her family. Although an acute trauma resuscitation phase demands strict attention to the patient's physical condition, as much time as possible should be spent in determining the victim's emotional status and extended support system and in reassuring the pregnant woman that aggressive care offers the fetus the best chance for survival. Extreme physical stress and fear have been shown to influence physiologic function during pregnancy and have been correlated with increased uterine activity and termination of pregnancy (Buchsbaum, 1986). The pregnant patient and her family should be kept informed of her progress and the status of her baby and should be allowed to express their fear and anxiety within a supportive milieu. Family members should also be allowed to stay with the patient whenever appropriate.

Fetal Assessment

During initial maternal stabilization efforts, fetal assessment should address estimation of gestational age and evidence of well-being. More thorough assessment modalities may be implemented as maternal response permits. Medical and nursing personnel with expertise in obstetrics should be actively involved in this process as soon as possible.

The last menstrual period, fundal height, and biometric evaluation by ultrasonography may be used to assess the gestational age of the fetus. Due to the degree of injury, many trauma victims may be unable to provide precise dates for their last menstrual period, thus making this method unreliable. Fundal height measurement and ultrasound assessments are more practical, and accuracy of ultrasound is enhanced by early and serial sonograms.

Evidence of well-being and identification of stressors may be elicited by assessment of fetal heart rate responses. Examination by real time ultrasonography confirms the presence or absence of fetal heart activity and serves as an immediate indicator of fetal status. Ultrasound determinations of the biparietal diameter (BPD), femur length, and fetal abdominal circumference will allow for assessment of gestational age within 2–3 weeks in the second and third trimesters. Estimation of probable fetal weight within 10% can also be obtained in the last two trimesters (Laverly & Staten-McCormick, 1995).

Further assessment of fetal heart rate responses may be via auscultation or electronic fetal monitoring. Auscultation permits calculation of a baseline rate in beats per minute and may allow detection of marked changes in rate. By approximately 8–12 weeks gestation, fetal heart tones should be audible by Doppler and by a fetoscope by 16–19 weeks gestation. However, auscultation with a fetoscope following blunt abdominal trauma may be difficult. Electronic fetal monitoring permits evaluation of baseline rate, variability, and periodic patterns.

A marked sinusoidal pattern has been identified frequently in fetuses who are severely anemic (Higgins & Garite, 1984). It has been observed that sinusoidal oscillations of more than 25 beats per minute are closely associated with poor fetal/neonatal outcome (Higgins & Garite, 1984). Other characteristics that indicate compromise include repetitive late, variable, or prolonged decelerations; absent variability; and tachycardia or bradycardia. In a hypovolemic patient, classic late decelerations may be alleviated by prompt volume replacement and repositioning. It should be remembered that placental abruption—a common cause of uteroplacental insufficiency in the obstetric trauma patient—though usually occurring within 48 hours of the injury, has been reported as late as 5 days (Bondurant, Boehm, Fleischer, & Machin, 1984; Bremer & Cassata, 1986; Higgins & Garite, 1984; Stuart et al., 1980). Other tests that may be used to assess fetal status include ultrasonography, computerized tomography, magnetic resonance imaging, and percutaneous umbilical blood sampling.

Early diagnosis of traumatic fetal head injury may necessitate sequential ultrasound examinations to confirm intracranial bleeding. Massive acute intracerebral hematomas have been readily diagnosed by ultrasound in the antepartum period (Bondurant et al., 1984). It is important to realize, however, that slowly developing intracranial hemorrhages may require serial ultrasound over 3–5 days for detection (Donn, Barr, & McLeary, 1984).

It is crucial that diagnostic studies be initiated as soon as possible. The risk of radiation exposure during x-rays may be decreased by shielding the woman's abdomen with a lead apron and limiting the actual number of films for each individual view. Computed tomography scanning may be helpful in assessing direct fetal injury, as well as maternal intraabdominal bleeding, following blunt trauma. In some institutions, it has been used in place of peritoneal lavage, for the diagnosis of internal hemorrhage. A concern expressed about computed tomography is radiation dosage. The estimated absorbed dose of 2 mGy (0.2 rad) is about half that of standard pelvimetry (Civil et al., 1988). To date, in animal and human data, exposure between 5 and 10 rads has not indicated an increase in gross congenital anomalies or intrauterine growth retardation (Esposito, Gens, Smith, & Scorpio, 1989). There is limited radiologic exposure for the fetus with computed tomographic scanning (CT). This technology can be employed as an important diagnostic tool in trauma (Grumbach, Mechlin, & Mintz, 1985).

Magnetic resonance imaging (MRI) is a non-invasive technology used for imaging of structural fetal defects as well as fetal function, as it has the ability to detect some enzyme defects. Its major advantage over ultrasound is its ability to define soft tissue structures in the maternal pelvis. Magnetic resonance imaging (MRI) has an important role in assessing the pregnant trauma victim, because maternal abdominal and pelvic structures can be more easily visualized than they are with ultrasound, which can be complicated by obesity and gas. Magnetic resonance imaging (MRI) is probably safer than computed tomography because it does not require ionizing radiation (Hill & Lense, 1996).

Percutaneous umbilical blood sampling (PUBS) or cordocentesis may be used to assess fetal acid-base status and hematocrit. This procedure is frequently used to diagnose coagulopathies, hemoglobinopathies, hemophilias, congenital infections, and to obtain a rapid fetal karyotyping. Cordocentesis allows direct access to fetal circulation, thus assisting the physician in determining the severity of fetal injury as well as in plan management for transfusion (Dunn, Weiner, & Ludomirski, 1988).

The interval between maternal death and delivery directly influences the survival rate of the infant. Many studies indicate that surviving infants may not suffer sequelae if they are delivered within 5 minutes of maternal death (Lee & Mezzadri, 1990). Uncertainty about the time of the mother's death is not a contraindication to perimortem cesarean section. Neonatal outcome is critically affected by the elapsed time after the mother's death and gestational age of the fetus.

Katz supports data that an interval of less than 10 minutes between maternal death and delivery correlates with good neonatal survival (Katz, Dotters, & Droegemueller, 1986). Beyond 2–4 minutes, the chances of successful resuscitation of the mother diminishes. The obstetric nurse has approximately 4 minutes from time of insult to restore hemodynamic stability (Lee & Mezzadri, 1990). The cardiopulmonary resuscitation team must ensure that there are pauses to determine the presence and status of the fetal heartbeat. It is recommended that the fetus be delivered, regardless of gestational age, if the mother does not respond to open- or closed-chest massage within 15 minutes and is declared dead.

POTENTIAL PROBLEMS RELATED TO THE PREGNANT TRAUMA PATIENT

Maternal Hemodynamic Stability

- Maternal hemorrhagic shock secondary to traumatic injury
- Maternal hemorrhage and shock secondary to uterine damage
- Maternal hemorrhage and shock secondary to placental abruption
- Maternal hemorrhage and shock secondary to bladder rupture
- Maternal hemorrhage and shock secondary to penetrating trauma
- Decreased cardiac output related to vena cava compression by the enlarged uterus

Adequate Maternal Pulmonary Function

- Venous stasis and pulmonary emboli related to coagulation alterations and immobility
- Inadequate airway related to obstruction
- Impaired gas exchange related to pulmonary contusion
- Alteration in ventilation related to pleural space injuries
- Alteration in ventilation related to bony thorax fractures

Fetal Well-Being

- Fetal hypoxia secondary to maternal shock
- Fetal hypoxia secondary to uterine damage

- Fetal hypoxia secondary to placental abruption
- Premature rupture of membranes
- Onset of preterm labor
- Direct fetal injury secondary to maternal trauma
- Fetal injury secondary to penetrating trauma
- Emergency delivery secondary to fetal compromise and/or uterine or placental injuries
- Alteration in uteroplacental perfusion related to cardiovascular compromise secondary to maternal positioning

Psychosocial Well-Being

- Maternal and family anxiety related to sudden hospitalization during pregnancy
- Maternal and family anxiety related to pending surgical procedures and possible fetal injury or death
- Alteration in maternal–infant bonding related to patient's condition and fetal outcome
- Alteration in maternal–infant bonding related to maternal injuries and clinical condition

TREATMENT OF THE PREGNANT TRAUMA PATIENT

In addition to the management principles discussed earlier, the following general axioms and specific recommendations are presented in an effort to gain an overall view of initial stabilization of the pregnant trauma patient. Protection of the airway is of utmost importance. The shouting patient obviously has an open airway. An unconscious patient requires a closer assessment and may need assistance in gaining an airway. Opening a trauma patient's airway requires a modified jaw thrust without extension of the neck, rather than the head tilt–chin lift method (Figure 20-1). The size of the uterus and elevation of the diaphragm late in pregnancy may lead to early compromise in respiration. Maintaining a patent airway and obtaining adequate oxygenation may require early endotracheal intubation in the pregnant patient (Mighty,

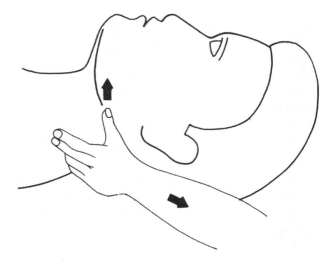

Figure 20-1. Modified jaw thrust.

1994). Cricoid pressure should be applied during intubation because the pregnant patient has delayed gastric emptying and is at an increased risk of gastroesophageal reflux and possible aspiration (Mighty, 1994).

Clearing the airway of vomitus, blood, teeth, or foreign matter may be accomplished with suction and/or forceps. In no instance should the trauma victim's head be turned while clearing the airway, as cervical spine injuries can be exacerbated and can result in iatrogenic cord injury. An important axiom in airway management for the trauma patient is to assume cervical spine injury until proved otherwise by radiographic exam of all cervical vertebrae, including the superior surface of the first thoracic vertebra.

The conscious patient who has suffered minimal damage to the face and neck will usually have no difficulty in maintaining an airway. If airway patency is in doubt, several methods may be utilized to assure this is achieved. A simple device, such as a nasopharyngeal or an oropharyngeal airway, may be all that is necessary. However, complete control of the airway may be required, necessitating endotracheal intubation. Nasal intubation should be avoided in the pregnant patient, because increased vascularity in the upper airway passages predisposes her to significant bleeding during this sometimes traumatic procedure. If endotracheal intubation is elected, care must be taken to manually stabilize and prevent extension of the cervical spine. A more drastic measure, surgical cricothyrotomy, may be required in rare cases to gain an adequate airway. Finally, pregnant women are at increased risk of aspiration. Insertion of a nasogastric tube and gastric decompression, along with vigilant assessment and rapid intervention in the event of vomiting, will decrease the incidence of this serious complication.

If turning a patient to the side is necessary in order to gain an adequate airway, this may be accomplished by turning her as a "whole-body" unit. Log rolling, while manually maintaining cervical alignment or tilting a patient who is fully secured to a spine board, will accomplish this objective (see Figure 20-2). The cervical spine may be immobilized at this point by application of a cervical collar or other stabilization device, if this has not already been accomplished by prehospital care personnel. Positioning of the pregnant patient is critical in promoting venous return. The supine position must be avoided, especially in women in their third trimester, because the gravid uterus may compress the iliac vessels, the inferior vena cava, and the abdominal aorta. This abdominal compression results in hypotension and a 25% reduction in cardiac output (American Heart Association, 1987). The

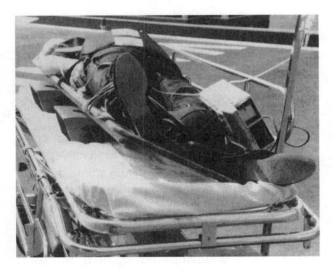

Figure 20-2. Tilting pregnant woman on spine board.

pregnant patient should be tilted to the left by approximately 15° using a wedge. A pillow wedge may be placed under the right abdominal flank and hip to displace the uterus to the left side of the abdomen. If the tilt is impossible, left lateral displacement of the uterus must be manually initiated to increase preload and thus cardiac output (Hill & Lense, 1996).

Aggressive ventilatory support is often demanded by the traumatized patient. Such a patient who is pregnant demands even greater attention to ventilation and oxygenation if fetal hypoxia is to be avoided. High-flow oxygen (12 l/min) should be administered via a nonrebreather face mask, even in the absence of respiratory distress, as the pregnant patient's oxygen requirement is 10–20% greater than normal (Campbell, 1985). Oxygen should never be withheld from any patient who is short of breath, has a head injury, or is in shock. Trauma victims with a respiratory rate of less than 12 or greater than 25 breaths/minute may need additional assistance. Mechanical ventilation should be guided by arterial blood gases, with an awareness that the pregnant woman is normally in a state of compensated respiratory alkalosis. Acidosis should not be exacerbated by allowing her pCO_2 to rise above 35–40 mm Hg.

Thoracic injuries demand immediate intervention to avoid catastrophe. Table 20-2 briefly describes each type of thoracic injury and its suggested initial management. When cardiopulmonary resuscitation is necessary, several issues associated with pregnancy should be considered. First, the thorax is less compliant, making mouth-to-mouth ventilation and chest compressions more difficult and less effective. Such alterations impede the success of standard closed-chest cardiopulmonary resuscitation (American Heart Association, 1987). Before 24 weeks gestation, the objective of cardiopulmonary resuscitation is maternal conservation. After 24 weeks gestation, fetal well-being may influence decision making. Prompt emergent delivery may enhance maternal resuscitation efforts. Regarding route of delivery, vaginal birth is preferable to cesarean section in most instances. The duration of continuous fetal and uterine monitoring remains a controversy in the literature. The time frame ranges in duration from 4 to 48 hours following trauma (Mighty, 1994; Pearlman et al., 1990). The degree and mechanism of maternal injury, evidence of maternal–fetal bleed, presence of contractions, abdominal pain, significant bruising, vaginal bleeding, rupture of membranes, or altered fetal heart rate patterns are factors that influence the duration of continuous monitoring (Hill & Lense, 1996). Because abruptio placentae can have a delayed onset, 24 hours of observation appears to be a reasonable time for fetal and uterine monitoring (Pearlman et al., 1990). The uterus can contain up to 2 liters of blood from a "concealed" abruption in the absence of vaginal bleeding (Hill & Lense, 1996). Uterine contraction activity should be a concern to the provider. Pearlman et al. (1990) demonstrated that patients with more than one contraction per 10 minutes had a 20% incidence of abruption; there were no cases of abruption in the trauma patients experiencing no uterine activity. It is recommended that an obstetrician and neonatologist be consulted in order that appropriate plans with the labor and delivery team for an emergency cesarean delivery be initiated. Many factors impact the decision of the physician to perform a cesarean section. The markedly hypertrophied and hypervascular gravid uterus presents a large, raw, bleeding surface, which may result in continued hemorrhage in the pregnant trauma patient with coagulopathy and acidosis (Chang, Chang, & Morris, 1994).

An organized and systematic approach in assessing the pregnant trauma patient will ensure that priorities of management and stabilization are met. Evaluation requires an understanding of the physiologic changes that are secondary to pregnancy. Assessment begins immediately upon encountering the patient and should follow a strict sequence, allowing life-threatening injuries to be corrected before more obvious, but non-life-threatening injuries, are managed.

Trauma is a precipitating event for cardiac arrest during pregnancy. Standard resuscitative measures and procedures should be taken without modification when cardiac arrest occurs in a pregnant woman (American Heart Association, 1987). The type and doses of medications and defibrillation are performed exact-ly as in the current ACLS guidelines. This is a change from previous guidelines, which recommended reduced doses and longer dosing intervals (American Heart Association, 1987). Attention should only be turned to the specific fetal needs after stabilizing and assessing the mother. Fetal survival is best achieved through maternal survival. Perimortem cesarean section should be considered when the pregnant woman experiences cardiac arrest. The viability of the fetus, the certainty of maternal death or poor outcome, and the duration of cardiac arrest should influence the physician's decision to perform this technique (Mighty, 1994). The limit for successful resuscitation in the presence of apnea and asystole of adults is 5–6 minutes (Lee & Mezzadri, 1990). Unless the pregnant woman shows a favorable response to resuscitation efforts within 4–5 minutes, bedside cesarean section or open-chest massage is recommended (Lee & Mezzadri, 1990; American Heart Association, 1987). Delivery effected within 4-5 minutes of the arrest will maximize the chances of both maternal and infant survival (Katz et al., 1986; Strong, Gocke, Levy, & Newel, 1987). The literature reports cases of "intact infant survival after more than 20 minutes of complete maternal arrest" (Katz et al., 1986).

Perimortem cesarean section procedure has been performed as much for religious as for medical benefit. Concern for the fetus of a dead mother has been mirrored in many cultures. For example, in Roman Catholic tradition, delivery was performed for the purpose of baptizing the unborn infant (Laverly & Staten-McCormick, 1995). It was only with improvement in surgical technique during the nineteenth century that postmortem cesarean section increased in numbers. Survival still remains less than 5% (Lee & Mezzadri, 1990). Perimortem cesarean delivery may be therapeutic for the mother if the cardiac arrest has resulted from a reversible cause. The gravid uterus has increased demands on oxygen consumption, thus delivery may benefit the woman by optimizing her oxygen transport (Laverly & Staten-McCormick, 1995).

Circulatory support is also critical for the pregnant trauma patient. Early resuscitation from hypovolemic or neurogenic shock will promote maternal well-being and adequate uteroplacental perfusion. It is particularly important to pay close attention to the gravid patient's hemodynamic status. As previously noted, significant hemorrhage may be masked by the hypervolemic state of pregnancy, and the fetus may be placed at extreme risk of hypoxic injury even in the face of apparent maternal stability. Compensatory responses occur in the pregnant woman as a result of blood loss. Vasoconstriction in the maternal kidneys, gastrointestinal tract, liver, and uterus occur, shunting blood from these areas to the brain and heart. The pregnant woman may maintain hemodynamic stability at the expense of the fetus (Huzel & Remsburg-Bell, 1996). One retrospective study of pregnant trauma victims associated an 80% fetal mortality with maternal shock (Rothenberger, Quattlebaum, Perry, Zabel, & Fischer, 1978). Astute assessment and timely intervention will avoid increased morbidity. Treatment for shock or suspected hemorrhage must begin immediately with vigorous intravenous (IV) hydration (Mighty, 1994). Placement of at least two large-bore intravenous catheters (14 or 16 gauge) with generous crystalloid and blood product administration should be initiated. In most instances, peripheral access is preferable to central access and is usually adequate for resuscitation (Mighty, 1994). In severe trauma, placement of a pulmonary artery catheter is recommended as soon as possible. Fluid resuscitation is best managed by central monitoring of maternal hemodynamics (Laverly & Staten-McCormick, 1995). Lactated Ringer's solution is the crystalloid of choice with a 3:1 replacement ratio (i.e., 3 cc lactated Ringer's solution per 1 cc of estimated blood loss). It provides a base from which to begin fluid resuscitation (Schwab & Shaikh, 1985; Hill & Lense, 1996; Mighty, 1994; Bremer & Cassata, 1986; Higgins, 1988). If maternal shock has not been reversed after a bolus of 3–4 liters of lactated Ringer's solution, or if the patient arrives in profound shock secondary to catastrophic hemorrhage, transfusion with O-negative packed red blood cells should begin immediately, followed by type-specific or cross-matched blood as soon as it is available. Blood pressure should be continuously monitored to evaluate the effectiveness of volume resuscitation. The pituitary gland increases in size by 30–50% during pregnancy. With increased blood flow to the organ, necrosis of the anterior pituitary gland (Sheehan's syndrome) may result from significant shock in the pregnant woman (Mighty, 1994).

The mainstay of therapy for hypovolemic shock is volume. If volume resuscitation is inadequate to maintain maternal blood pressure, vasoactive drugs are considered. Vasopressor drugs cause a significant reduction of blood flow to the uterus resulting in decreases in oxygen delivery to the fetus. Dopamine or ephedrine may be used and should be maintained at low enough levels to preserve uterine blood flow (Esposito, 1988; Mokriski & Malinow, 1990). Epinephrine and norepinephrine may be given if clinically indicated (American Heart Association, 1987).

Additional measures to combat hemorrhagic shock include use of Trendelenburg's position if ventilation is not impeded or manually holding the legs up and maintenance of the patient's warmth. Shock will be exacerbated in the pregnant trauma victim by the well-known supine hypotensive syndrome, which can be avoided by tilting the entire spine board 15° degrees laterally with pillows, blankets, or commercial wedges. Finally, continuous manual lateral displacement of the uterus by attending personnel may also be required (Higgins, 1988).

Blood pressure should be supported with vasopressor agents only as a last resort, because they do not specifically address the cause of the problem and they place the fetus at extreme risk for uteroplacental vasoconstriction (Huzel & Remsberg-Bell, 1996; Mighty, 1994; Daddario, 1989; Baker, 1982; Buchsbaum, 1986; Stauffer, 1986; Vander Veer, 1984). The single exception to this axiom is in the case of neurogenic shock, which occasionally results from high spinal cord transection or injury. Sympathetic tone is lost in this circumstance, and diffuse vasodilation causes venous pooling of the blood. Such a clinical picture includes profound hypotension accompanied by bradycardia rather than tachycardia. If no source of hemorrhage is found, neurogenic shock may be reversed through fluid bolus and low-dose dopamine infusion.

Pneumatic antishock garments (PASG) or military antishock trousers (MAST), whose primary mechanism of action involves an increase in peripheral vascular resistance, may have already been placed by prehospital personnel in an effort to control hemorrhage, stabilize pelvic fractures, or treat shock (Figure 20-3) (Laverly & Staten-McCormick, 1995; Schwab & Shaikh, 1985; Smith, 1988). It is important for the nurse to check to see if the antishock trousers are in place on admission to the emergency department. Their use is controversial because the inflation of the leg compartments may increase bleeding into already engorged and possibly torn pelvic veins (Esposito et al., 1989). The abdominal compartment of the trousers should not be inflated after 20 weeks gestation, as increased intraabdominal pressure may exacerbate caval compression and decrease cardiac return (Bremer & Cassata, 1986; Laverly & Staten-McCormick, 1995; Schwab & Shaikh, 1985). Inflation of the abdominal compartment forces the already elevated diaphram further into the chest and may precipitate or exacerbate respiratory compromise in the mother. The military antishock trousers are contraindicated in the presence of pulmonary edema and inflation over an impaled object (Laverly & Staten-McCormick,

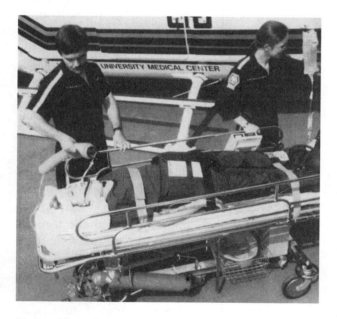

Figure 20-3. Pregnant woman in military antishock trousers.

1995). Continuous uterine displacement must be maintained. Clinical response of the mother is the key factor in determining efficacy of the military antishock trousers. Definitive surgical intervention will usually be required to achieve hemostasis for internal hemorrhage.

Finally, circulatory assessment and further support may be accomplished via invasive hemodynamic monitoring devices (e.g., intraarterial central venous or pulmonary artery catheters). These adjuncts are useful especially for long-term management but are sometimes employed quite early in the resuscitative phase. Early insertion of a urinary catheter will also aid in monitoring circulatory status, as renal perfusion is a function of blood flow and decreased urinary output is one of the earliest signs of shock (Bocka et al., 1988; Pearlman et al., 1990; Troiano, 1989).

Hematuria, either gross or microscopic, secondary to trauma should be followed with a standard workup (Levin & Edson, 1994). For example, after blunt urologic trauma, a cystogram may be ordered. If findings are normal, a computed tomography (CT) may be prompted by the significant blunt trauma of the head, abdomen, and pelvis. If the CT is normal, the hematuria may be attributed to a contusion of the bladder, and no further workup is recommended (Levin & Edson, 1994). The history, physical examination, and urinalysis will give the urologist a clinical impression. Adequate renal staging must be initiated in the presence of shock, gross hematuria, or any clinical indication of flank trauma. The single most accurate way to stage renal injuries is with CT. This technology is the standard for staging blunt trauma and allows the clinician the benefit of evaluating other visceral injuries (Levin & Edson, 1994). Ultrasonography may be used to determine the integrity of the renal parenchyma, status of the fetus, and the presence of a retroperitoneal hematoma or extravasation (Peters & Sagalowsky, 1993). Shearing forces and intimal tears resulting from blunt trauma may not show up on ultrasonography, necessitating either an angiogram or computed tomography (Federle, Kaiser, McAninch, Jeffrey, & Mall, 1981; McAninch & Dixon, 1994).

The potential risks of medications given during pregnancy must be weighed against expected therapeutic benefits. In the presence of cardiopulmonary arrest, the full range of cardiotonic and vasopressor agents may be utilized in an effort to resuscitate the mother. Under less urgent circumstances, care should be exercised in the selection and administration of medications. Tetanus toxoid or human tetanus immunoglobulin should be administered following any break in skin integrity if the patient has not been immunized in the last 10 years (Hill & Lense, 1996; Schwab & Shaikh, 1985; Smith, 1988). Antibiotics are commonly required for trauma victims with open injuries. With the notable exceptions of tetracycline and sulfa drugs, there is a wide variety of antibiotics that are considered relatively safe to administer during pregnancy. These include the penicillins (i.e., ampicillin, methicillin, and oxacillin), the cephalosporins (i.e., cephalothin, cefoxitin, and maxalactasm), erythromycin, and clindamycin. Sulfa-containing drugs may cause hyperbilirubinemia in the fetus if delivery occurs soon after their administration (Laverly & Staten-McCormick, 1995). Aminoglycosides (i.e., kanamycin, gentamicin, tobramycin, and amikacin) should be used with caution as childhood otologic and renal sequelae may result (Cesario, 1990; Laverly & Staten-McCormick, 1995). The use of chloramphenicol is contraindicated in the third trimester, especially near term (Cesario, 1990). Diuretics and antihypertensives may decrease uterine blood flow and should, therefore, be used with caution. When anticoagulation therapy is necessary, heparin is the drug of choice, as coumadin crosses the placenta (Laverly & Staten-McCormick 1995; Smith, 1988). Medications to avoid include dilantin, ergot agents, and warfarin derivatives.

Tocolytic therapy still remains a controversial issue in obstetrics. Many of the tocolytic agents used to treat preterm labor may have other consequences for the trauma patient and their use is disputed among trauma experts. Magnesium sulfate may disturb the sensorium, produce mild hypotension, decrease respiratory effort, and in high doses may lead to respiratory collapse or cardiac arrhythmias (Laverly & Staten-McCormick, 1995; Mighty, 1994). The betamimetic drugs, ritodrine and terbutaline, cause cardiac stimulation

resulting in maternal/fetal tachycardia, chest pain, increased cardiac oxygen consumption and workload, possible hypotension in high doses, and masked blood loss. Calcium channel blockers, such as nifedipine, may produce hypotension in the pregnant woman. Indomethacin may lead to platelet dysfunction, which can have adverse effects on the woman with a head injury or requiring surgery. Adverse effects of indomethacin on the fetus are premature closure of the ductus arteriosus and pulmonary hypertension (Laverly & Staten-McCormick, 1995; Mighty, 1994).

Many trauma victims require surgical intervention. If general anesthesia is required, avoidance of maternal hypotension and hypoxia is more important than the specific agents used. Succinylcholine chloride may not be employed, however, as the risk of hyperkalemia is increased. Instead, nondepolarizing agents, such as pancuronium bromide and vecuronium, are preferred (Deitch et al., 1985).

Treatment of the pregnant victim of a crush injury involves placement in the left lateral position, rapid volume infusion, oxygen administration, and introduction of a urinary catheter as soon as possible. Hyperkalemia and renal failure may be prevented by forced alkaline diuresis with mannitol. Hemorrhage may result from femur fractures or any open fracture. Hemostasis can usually be achieved through the use of pressure bandages and splinting.

Critical to the medical management of patients with severe head trauma is hyperventilation and mannitol. Hyperventilation decreases intracranial pressure by reducing cerebral blood flow and has little effect on the fetus. Mannitol causes osmotic diuresis by withdrawing free water from the brain and should only be used when brain herniation develops. In pregnancy, mannitol should be restricted because it results in the flow of free water from the fetus and amniotic fluid to the mother. Severe dehydration, contraction of blood volume, cyanosis, and bradycardia are potential fetal side effects (Jordan, 1994).

As noted previously, vasopressors should be employed as a last resort in the setting of trauma care of the pregnant woman and generally should be restricted to cardiopulmonary resuscitation efforts. A significant difference exists between such agents, relative to their effect on uterine blood flow. Peripheral vasoconstrictors will increase maternal mean arterial pressure, but decrease uterine blood flow. Central vasoconstrictors, however, will concomitantly increase uterine blood flow and mean arterial pressure (Patterson, 1984). Table 20-3 provides examples.

Blood should be drawn while venous access for fluid resuscitation is accomplished. The most significant laboratory studies to be obtained are complete blood count with hemoglobin and hematocrit levels; white blood count with the differential, platelet count, fibrinogen level, prothrombin, and partial thromboplastin time; fibrin degradation products; and type and cross-match. Clotting studies are indicated to provide a baseline in the event that the disseminated intravascular coagulation occurs. The fibrinogen level and factors VII, VIII, IX, and X are increased during pregnancy. This coupled with a decrease in circulating plasminogen activator will provide some benefit if hemorrhage occurs (Baker, 1982; Bocka et al., 1988; Smith, 1988). Conversely, these hematologic alterations will increase the risk of thromboembolic disease if prolonged immobilization secondary to trauma is enforced (Baker, 1982; Laverly & Staten-McCormick, 1995). Additional blood should be obtained for levels of electrolytes, glucose, blood urea nitrogen, creatinine, amylase, arterial blood gases, SGOT, SGPT, alkaline phosphatase, lactic acid dehydrogenase, and calcium. The Kleihauer-Betke stain diagnoses fetomaternal hemorrhage by detecting the presence and number of fetal erythrocytes in the maternal circulation. Also important is the indirect Coomb's test, which detects maternal Rh sensitization (Baker, 1982; Higgins, 1988; Laverly & Staten-McCormick 1995). A positive Kleihauer-Betke test should be an indication for prolonged fetal heart rate monitoring and administration of hyperimmune anti-D globulin to prevent sensitization. A single 300-mcg vial protects against 15 ml of fetal cells (Clark, et al., 1994; Laverly & Staten-McCormick, 1995). Blood and urine samples should be obtained for a urine analysis, toxicology screen for substance abuse and blood alcohol levels, and a screen for hepatitis B and HIV. It is not useful to collect blood and body fluids for culture and sensitivity during the initial resuscitation period unless the patient has a known history of an infectious process or sepsis.

Immediate assessment and treatment priorities for the pregnant woman with burn trauma remain the same as for any other traumatic injury, with particular attention paid to airway patency if inhalation injury is suspected. Estimation of the severity of the burn occurs during the secondary survey and is based on the depth of the burn, the total body surface area involved, the patient's age, the severity of associated injuries, and the victim's preinjury state of health (Bunkis & Waltong, 1984; Laverly & Staten-McCormick 1995). Blood gas determination would be ordered for any pulmonary problems as in smoke inhalation. The primary goals of initial stabilization and ongoing management are to maintain a normal intravascular volume and provide maximum oxygenation, as the fetus is especially vulnerable to maternal shock and hypoxia (Clark et al., 1994; Rozycki, 1990; Crosby, 1983; Deitch et al., 1985; Laverly & Staten-McCormick, 1995).

TABLE 20-3. Differences Associated with Vasopressors		
Vasopressor	Mean Arterial Pressure	Uterine Blood Flow
Norepinephrine	↑	↓ ↑
Dopamine 5 µg/kg/min	↑	↔
10 µg/kg/min	↑	↓
Ephedrine	↑	↑

Uterine blood flow may be sustained by adequate fluid resuscitation. Use of the Parkland formula will provide a guide for fluid administration (Shuck & Moncrief, 1986). Based on this formula, 4 ml of crystalloid solution per kilogram of maternal body weight per percent of body surface burn are administered over the first 24 hours postburn, with one half of this total infused during the first 8 hours. The Parkland formula may be written as follows:

(4 ml × Body weight (kg) × Percent body surface area (BSA) burned)

with one half of the total given over the first 8 hours and the remainder infused over the next 16 hours. For example, consider a 70-kg female with a 60% BSA second-degree burn. Calculate the Parkland formula as follows:

(4 × 70 × 60 – 16,800 ml over 24 hours)

with 8400 ml infused over the first 8 hours and 8400 ml over the next 16 hours. It is important to remember that the calculation of the time begins at the moment of the injury rather than at admission to the hospital. Therefore, the patient arriving 2 hours postburn would require the first 8400 ml of fluid over the next 6 hours postadmission. It is important to remember that this is only a guide. More vigorous fluid resuscitation may be required to maintain a urine output of at least 50 cc/hour, which is a more specific indicator of an adequate maternal intravascular volume.

Oxygen should be administered to the pregnant burn victim even in the absence of apparent hypoxia. The effects of decreased maternal oxygenation are magnified in the fetus, and fetal death may occur at pO_2 levels that are compatible with maternal survival (Crosby, 1983). Intubation and mechanical ventilation are warranted if hypoxemia persists following oxygen administration via a face mask.

Carbon monoxide intoxication, a frequent result of prolonged exposure to enclosed fires or suicide attempts, should be treated with 100% oxygen via a nonrebreathing mask. Levels of carboxyhemoglobin greater than 20%, the presence of neurologic changes, or obvious fetal distress would mandate consideration of hyperbaric oxygen therapy (Hollander, Nagey, Welch, & Pupkin, 1987; Van Hoesen, Camporesi, Moon, Hage, & Piantadosi, 1989).

All pregnant women should be instructed in the proper use of seat belts. Studies have demonstrated that maternal mortality would decrease if a properly placed lap belt in conjunction with a shoulder harness were worn by the mother (Wolf et al., 1993). (See Figure 20-4 for proper belt placement.) The lap belt should be secured low across the bony pelvis, avoiding the mid- or upper fundus (Laverly & Staten-McCormick, 1995).

In summary, pregnant trauma patients present a difficult management problem. There are competing concerns for maternal injuries and fetal well-being. Confusion and controversy exist because protocols and priorities for the pregnant trauma patient have not been well defined and it is still not clear who should have primary responsibility. Many experts report that the overall care of the pregnant trauma patient should be managed by the trauma service with the obstetrician an active participant (Towery, English, & Wisner, 1993). Initial efforts should be directed to the mother when there are severe or life-threatening injuries. It is only after the mother has been resuscitated and stabilized that evaluation of the patient by the obstetric team can proceed with ultrasound followed by electronic fetal

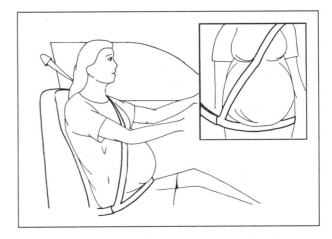

Figure 20-4. Proper seat belt use during pregnancy.

monitoring. Therapy would proceed according to the needs of the fetus. It is usually more convenient for continuous electronic fetal monitoring to be carried out in the labor and delivery area where the nursing personnel are experienced with monitoring and management of the obstetric patient. The most sensitive means of detecting nonreassuring fetal status is with external electronic fetal monitoring. Ultrasound assessments are of limited use in the acute setting but provide important information about the general status of the fetus following maternal trauma. Primary consideration is for the mother. Although fetal monitoring and obstetrical care are important aspects of treatment, fetal well-being remains ultimately dependent on maternal survival (Daddario & Johnson, 1992).

EXPECTED OUTCOMES IN MANAGEMENT OF THE PREGNANT TRAUMA PATIENT

Maternal Hemodynamic Stability

The patient will do the following:

1. Maintain vital signs within normal ranges.
2. Maintain a normovolemic state as evidenced by adequate hemodynamic parameters.
3. Avoid vena cava compression and hypotension by maintaining a lateral position.
4. Avoid coagulopathy by maintaining a normal coagulation profile.

Adequate Maternal Pulmonary Function

The patient will do the following:

1. Maintain a patent airway.
2. Maintain adequate gas exchange as evidenced by normal arterial blood gases.
3. Maintain adequate ventilation as evidenced by normal, nonlabored respirations.

Psychosocial Well-Being

The patient will do the following:

1. Demonstrate initial expression related to grief.
2. Verbalize decreased fear and increased understanding related to status of both herself and her fetus.
3. Verbalize understanding of assessment and intervention processes.
4. Demonstrate appropriate behaviors related to maternal–infant bonding.

Fetal Well-Being

The fetus will do the following:

1. Maintain reassuring fetal heart rate responses as evidenced by:
   a. Fetal heart rate between 110 to 160 beats per minute.
   b. Minimal or greater fetal heart rate variability (when applicable).
   c. Presence of reassuring accelerations.
   d. Absence of fetal heart rate decelerations.
2. Exhibit movement (appropriate for gestational age).

REFERENCES

Agran, P. F., Dunkle, D. E., Winn, D. G., & Kent, D. (1987). Fetal death in motor vehicle accidents. Annals of Emergency Medicine, 16(12), 1355–1358.

American College of Surgeons Committee on Trauma. (1993). Advanced trauma life support manual (pp. 285–292). Chicago: American College of Surgeons.

American Heart Association. (1987). Advanced cardiac life support. Dallas: AHA.

Auerbach, P. S. (1979). Trauma in the pregnant patient. Topics in Emergency Medicine, 1(1), 133–137.

Baker, D. P. (1982). Trauma in the pregnant patient. Surgical Clinics of North America, 62(2), 275–289.

Bocka, J., Courtney, J., & Pearlman, M., et al. (1988). Trauma in pregnancy. Annals of Emergency Medicine, 17(8), 829–834.

Boehm, F. H. (1990). Fetal distress. In R. D. Eden, & F. H. Boehm (Eds.), Assessment and care of the fetus. Norwalk, CT: Appleton & Lange.

Bondurant, S., Boehm, F. H., Fleischer, A. C., & Machin, J. E. (1984). Antepartum diagnosis of fetal intracranial hemorrhage by ultrasound. Obstetrics and Gynecology, 63, 25S–27S.

Bowdler, N., Faix, R. G., & Elkins, T. (1987). Fetal skull fracture and brain injury after a maternal automobile accident: A case report. Journal of Reproductive Medicine, 32(5), 375–378.

Bremer, C., & Cassata, L. (1986). Trauma in pregnancy. Nursing Clinics of North America, 21(4), 705–716.

Buchsbaum, H. J. (1986). Trauma in pregnancy. ACOG Update, 12(4), 1–10.

Bunkis, J., & Walton, R. I. (1984). Burns. In D. D. Trunkey & F. R. Lewis (Eds.), Current therapy of trauma. Philadelphia: B. D. Decker.

Campbell, J. C. (1995). Addressing battering during pregnancy: Reducing low birth weight and ongoing abuse. Seminars in Perinatology, 19(4), 301–306.

Campbell, J. E. (1985). Basic trauma life support: Advanced prehospital care. Bowie, MD Prentice-Hall.

Cesario, T. C. (1990). Antibiotic therapy in pregnancy. In U. Elkayam, & N. Gleicher (Eds.), Cardiac problems in pregnancy. NJ: Alan R. Liss.

Chang, S. S., Chang, M. C., Morris, J. A., Jr. (1994). Trauma in pregnancy: The maternal-fetal relationship. Journal of the Tennessee Medical Association, 87(7), 291–292.

Chez, R. A. (Interviewer), King, M. C., & Brown, J. (Guest Experts). (1997, Spring). Homing in on abuse: What to ask and how to listen. Contemporary Nurse Practitioner (pp. 20–28).

Christian, A. (1995). Home care of the battered pregnant woman: One battered woman's pregnancy. Journal of Obstetric, Gynecologic and Neonatal Nursing, 24(9), 836–842.

Civil, I. D., Talucci, R. C., & Schwab, C. W. (1988). Placental laceration and fetal death as a result of blunt abdominal trauma. Journal of Trauma, 28(5), 708–710.

Clark, S., Cotton, D., Hankins, G., & Phelan, J. (Eds.). (1994). Handbook of critical care obstetrics (pp. 269–278). Oxford: Blackwell Scientific.

Committee on Trauma of the American College of Surgeons. (1968). Hospital and prehospital resources for the optimal care of the injured patient. American College Surg Bull, 71, 4–40.

Crosby, W. M. (1983). Traumatic injuries during pregnancy. Clinical Obstetrics and Gynecology, 26(4), 902–912.

Cummings, P. H., & Cummings, S. P. (1984). Abdominal trauma. In J. D. Parker (Ed.), Emergency nursing: A guide to comprehensive care. New York: Wiley.

Daddario, J. B. (1989). Trauma in pregnancy. Journal of Perinatal and Neonatal Nursing, 3(2), 14–22.

Daddario, J. B., & Johnson, G. (1992). Trauma in pregnancy. In L. Mandeville, & N. Troiano (Eds.), High risk intrapartum nursing. Philadelphia: J. B. Lippincott.

Dees, G., & Fuller, M. (1989). Blunt trauma in the pregnant patient. Journal of Emergency Nursing, 15(6), 495–499.

Deitch, E. A., Rightmire, D. A., Clothier, J., & Blass, N. (1985). Management of burns in pregnant women. Surgery, Gynecology and Obstetrics, 161(1), 1–4.

Donn, S. M., Barr, M., & McLeary, R. D. (1984). Massive intracerebral hemorrhage in utero: Sonographic appearance and pathologic correlation. Obstetrics and Gynecology, 63, 28S–30S.

Dunn, P. A., Weiner, S., & Ludomirski, A. (1988). Percutaneous umbilical blood sampling. Journal of Obstetric, Gynecologic and Neonatal Nursing, 17(5), 308–313.

Esposito, T. (1988). Pitfalls in resuscitation and early management of the pregnant trauma patient. Trauma Quarterly, 5, 1–22.

Esposito, T. J. (1994). Trauma during pregnancy. Emergency Medicine Clinics of North America, 12(1), 167–199.

Esposito, T. J., Gens, D. R., Smith, L. G., & Scorpio, R. (1989). Evaluation of blunt abdominal trauma occurring during pregnancy. Journal of Trauma, 29(12), 1628–1632.

Federle, M. P., Kaiser, J. A., McAninch, J. W., Jeffrey, R. B., & Mall, J. C. (1981). The role of computed tomography in renal trauma. Radiology, 141(2), 455–460.

Fox, M. A., & Fabian, T. C. (1990). The pelvis. In E. E. Moore (Ed.), Early care of the injured patient. Philadelphia: B. C. Decker.

Fries, M. H., & Hankins, G. D. (1989). DV: Motor vehicle accident associated with minimal maternal trauma but subsequent fetal demise. Annals of Emergency Medicine, 18(3), 301–304.

Furniss, K. (1997). Battered women: How nurses can help. Lifelines, 12–14.

Gilson, G. J., Miller, A. C., Clevenger, F. W., & Curet, L. B. (1995). Acute spinal cord injury and neurogenic shock in pregnancy. Obstetrical and Gynecological Survey, 50(7), 556–560.

Goodwin, T. M., & Breen, M. T. (1990). Pregnancy outcome and fetomaternal hemorrhage after noncatastrophic trauma. American Journal of Obstetrics and Gynecology, 162(3), 665–671.

Greenberg, E. M., McFarlane, J., & Watson, M. G. (1997). Vaginal bleeding and abuse: Assessing pregnant women in the emergency department. MCN, 22, 182–186.

Grumbach, K., Mechlin, M. B., & Mintz, M. C. (1985). Computed tomography and ultrasound of the traumatized and acutely ill patient. Emergency Medical Clinics of North America, 3(3), 607–624.

Halpern, J. S. (1989). Mechanisms and patterns of trauma. Journal of Emergency Nursing, 15(5), 380–388.

Helton, A. (1986). Battering during pregnancy. American Journal of Nursing, 86(8), 910–913.

Hendey, G. W., & Votey, S. R. (1994). Injuries in restrained motor vehicle accident victims. Annals of Emergency Medicine, 24(1), 77–84.

Higgins, S. D. (1988). Perinatal protocol: Trauma in pregnancy. Journal of Perinatology, 8(3), 288–292.

Higgins, S. D., & Garite, T. J. (1984). Late abruptio placenta in trauma patients: Implications for monitoring. Obstetrics and Gynecology, 63(3), 10S–12S.

Hill, D. A., & Lense, J. J. (1996). Abdominal trauma in the pregnant patient. American Family Physician, 53(4), 1269–1274.

Hinkle, J., & Betz, S. (1995). Gunshot injuries. In Deborah G. Klein (Ed.), AACN Clinical Issues, 6(2), 175–186.

Hoff, W. S., D'Amelio, L. R., Tinkoff, G. H., Lucke, J. F., Rhodes, M., Diamond, D. L., & Indeck, M. (1991). Maternal predictors of fetal demise in trauma during pregnancy. Surgery of Gynecology and Obstetrics, 172(3), 175–180.

Hollander, D. I., Nagey, D. A., Welch, R., & Pupkin, M. (1987). Hyperbaric oxygen therapy for the treatment of acute carbon monoxide poisoning in pregnancy. Journal of Reproductive Medicine, 32(8), 615–617.

Huzel, P. S., & Remsburg-Bell, E. A. (1996). Fetal complications related to minor maternal trauma. Journal of Obstetric, Gynecologic and Neonatal Nursing, 25(2), 121–124.

Institute of Medicine. (1985). Preventing low birthweight. Washington, DC: National Academy Press.

Jordan, B. D. (1994). Maternal heat trauma during pregnancy. In O. Devinsky, E. Feldmann, & B. Hainline (Eds.), Neurological complications of pregnancy. New York: Raven Press

Katz, V. L., Dotters, D. J., & Droegemueller, W. (1986). Perimortem cesarean delivery. Obstetrics and Gynecology, 68(4), 571–576.

Kissinger, D. P., Rozycki, G. S., Morris, J. A., Jr., Knudson, M. M., Copes, W. S., Bass, S. M., Yates, H. K., & Champion, H. R. (1991). Trauma in pregnancy: Predicting pregnancy outcome. Archives of Surgery, 126(9), 1079–1086.

Kraus, J. F. (1991). Epidemiologic features of injuries to the central nervous system. In D. W. Anderson (Ed.), Neuroepidemiology: A tribute to Bruce Scholenberg (pp. 334–354). Boca Raton: CRC Press.

Landers, D. F., Newland, M., & Penney, L. L. (1989). Multiple uterine rupture and crushing injury of the fetal skull after blunt maternal trauma. Journal of Reproductive Medicine, 34(12), 988–993.

Laverly, J. P., & Staten-McCormick, M. (1995). Management of moderator to severe trauma in pregnancy. Obstetrics & Gynecology Clinics of North America, 22(1), 69–90.

Lavin, J. P., Jr., & Polsky, S. S. (1983). Abdominal trauma during pregnancy. Clinics in Perinatology, 10(2), 423–438.

Lee, R. V., & Mezzadri, F. C. (1990). Cardiopulmonary resuscitation of pregnant women. In U. Elkayam & N. Gleicher (Eds.), Cardiac problems in pregnancy. NJ: Alan R. Liss.

Levin, R. D., & Edson, M. (1994). A pregnant pause: Blunt urologic trauma in a young woman. Urology, 44(5), 764–767.

Lewis, F. R. (1984). Prehospital trauma care. In D. D. Trunkey, & F. R. Lewis (Eds.), Current therapy of trauma. Philadelphia: B. D. Becker.

McAnena, O. J., Moore, E. E., & Marx, J. A. (1990). Initial evaluation of the patient with blunt abdominal trauma. Surgical Clinics of North America, 70(3), 495–515.

McAninch, J. W., & Dixon, C. M. (1994). A practical approach for managing blunt renal trauma. Infection in Urology, 22.

McFarlane, J., Parker, B., & Soeken, K. (1996). Physical abuse, smoking, and substance use during pregnancy: Prevalance, interrelationships, and effects on birth weight. Journal of Obstetric, Gynecologic and Neonatal Nursing, 25(4), 313–320.

McLeer, S. V., Anwar, R. A., Herman, S., & Maquiling, K. (1989). Education is not enough: A system's failure in protecting battered women. Annals of Emergency Medicine, 18(6), 651–653.

McQuillan, K., & Wiles, C. E., III. (1988). Initial management of traumatic shock. In V. D. Cardona et. al. (Eds.), Trauma nursing: From resuscitation through rehabilitation. Philadelphia: W. B. Saunders.

Mighty, H. (1994). Trauma in pregnancy. Critical Care Clinics, 10(3), 623–634.

MMWR. (1993). Emergency department response to domestic violence—California, 1992. Morbidity & Mortality Weekly Report, 42, 617–620.

MMWR. (1994). Physical violence during 12 months preceding childbirth—Alaska, Maine, Oklahoma, and West Virginia, 1900–1991. Morbidity and Mortality Weekly Report, 132–136.

Mokriski, B., & Malinow, A. M. (1990). Anesthesia for the pregnant trauma patient. Problems in Anesthesia, 14, 530–540.

Neufeld, J. D. (1993). Trauma in pregnancy, what if . . . ? Emergency Medicine Clinics of North America, 11(1), 207–224.

Newberger, E. H., Barkan, S. E., Lieberman, E. S., McCormack, M. C., Yllo, K., Gary, L. T., & Schechter, S. (1992). Commentary: Abuse of pregnant women and adverse birth outcome. Journal of the American Medical Association, 267(17), 2370–2372.

Norton, L. B., Peipert, J. F., Zierler, S., Lima, B., & Hume, L. (1995). Battering in pregnancy: An assessment of two screening methods. Obstetrics and Gynecology, 85(3), 321–325.

Odeh, M. (1991). The role of reperfusion-induced injury in the pathogenesis of the crush

syndrome. New England Journal of Medicine, 86, 655–656.

Parker, B., McFarlane, J., & Soeken, K. (1994). Abuse during pregnancy: Effects on maternal complications and birth weight in adult and teenage women. Obstetrics and Gynecology, 84(3), 323–328.

Patterson, R. M. (1984). Trauma in pregnancy. Clinical Obstetrics and Gynecology, 27(1), 32–38.

Pearlman, M. D., Tintinalli, J. E., & Lorenz, R. P. (1990). A prospective controlled study of outcome after trauma during pregnancy. American Journal of Obstetrics and Gynecology, 162(6), 1502–1510.

Pearlman, M. D., Tintinalli, J. E., & Lorenz, R. P. (1990). Blunt trauma during pregnancy. New England Journal of Medicine, 323(23), 1609–1613.

Peters, P. C., & Sagalowsky, A. I. (1993). Genitourinary trauma. Campbell's urology (6th ed.). Philadelphia: W. B. Saunders.

Pimentel, L. (1991). Mother and child: Trauma in pregnancy. Emergency Medical Clinics of North America, 9(3), 549–563.

Roberts, G. L., Lawrence, J. M., Otoole, B. I., & Raphael, B. (1997). Domestic violence in the emergency department: I. Two case-control studies of victims; II: Detection by doctors and nurses. General Hospital Psychiatry, 19(1), 5–11, 12–15.

Rode, H., Millar, A. J., Cywes, S., Bloch, C. E., Boes, E. G., Theron, E. J., Lodder, J. V., van der Merwe, A. E., & deKock, M. (1990). Thermal injury in pregnancy: The neglected tragedy. South African Medical Journal, 77(7), 346–348.

Rothenberger, D., Quattlebaum, F. W., Perry, J. F., Jr., Zabel, J., & Fischer, R. P. (1978). Blunt maternal trauma: A review of 103 cases. Journal of Trauma, 18(3), 173–179.

Rozycki, G. S. (1990). Trauma in pregnancy. In E. E. Moore (Ed.), Early care of the injured patient. Philadelphia: B. C. Decker.

Sandy, E. A., & Koerner, M. (1989). Self-inflicted gunshot wound to the pregnant abdomen: Report of a case and review of the literature. American Journal of Perinatology, 6(1), 30–31.

Satin, A. J., Hemsell, D., Stone, I. C., Jr., Theriot, S., & Wendel, G. D., Jr. (1991). Sexual assault in pregnancy. Obstetrics and Gynecology, 77(5), 710–714.

Schoenfeld, A., Warchaizer, S., Royburt, M., Rosenblatt, M., Friedman, S., & Ovadia, J. (1995). Crush injury in pregnancy: An unusual experience in obstetrics. Obstetrics and Gynecology, 86, 655–665.

Schwab, C. W., & Shaikh, K. A. (1985). Shock in the pregnant patient. Emergency Care Quarterly, 1(2), 47–57.

Sherer, D. M., & Schenker, J. G. (1989). Accidental injury during pregnancy. Obstetrics and Gynecological Survey, 44(5), 330–338.

Shuck, J. M., & Moncrief, J. A. (1986). Thermal, electrical, and chemical injuries. In G. R. Schwartz, P. Safar, J. H. Stone, et al. (Eds.), Principles and practice of emergency medicine (2nd ed.). Philadelphia: W. B. Saunders.

Slutsker, L., Smith, R., Higginson, G., & Fleming, D. (1993). Recognizing illicit drug use by pregnant women: Reports from Oregon birth attendants. American Journal of Public Health, 83(1), 61–64.

Smith, L. G. (1988). The pregnant trauma patient. In V. D. Cardona, et al. (Eds.), Trauma nursing: From resuscitation through rehabilitation. Philadelphia: W. B. Saunders.

Smith, L. H. (1987). Surgical and gynecological complications. In K. R. Niswander (Ed.), Manual of obstetrics: Diagnoses and therapy (pp. 200–202). Boston: Little, Brown.

Sokal, M. M., Katz, M., Lell, M. E., & Fox, A. (1980). Neonatal survival after traumatic fetal subdural hematoma. Journal of Reproductive Medicine, 24(3), 131–133.

Stauffer, D. M. (1986). The trauma patient who is pregnant. Journal of Emergency Nursing, 12(2), 89–93.

Strong, T. H., Jr., Gocke, S. E., Levy, A. V., & Newel, G. J. (1987). Electrical shock in pregnancy: A case report. Journal of Emergency Medicine, 5(5), 381–383.

Stuart, G. C., Harding, P. G., & Davies, E. M. (1980). Blunt abdominal trauma in pregnancy. Canadian Medical Association Journal, 122(8), 901–905.

Taylor, J. W., Plunkett, G. D., McManus, W. F., & Pruitt, B. A. (1976). Thermal injury during pregnancy. Obstetrics and Gynecology, 47(4), 434–438.

Towery, R., English, P. T., & Wisner, D. (1993). Evaluation of pregnant women after blunt injury. The Journal of Trauma, 35(5), 731–736.

Troiano, N. H. (1989). Cardiopulmonary resuscitation of the pregnant woman. Journal of Perinatal and Neonatal Nursing, 3(2), 1–13.

Trunkey, D. D. (1984). Thoractic trauma. In D. D. Trunkey, & F. R. Lewis (Eds.), Current therapy of trauma. Philadelphia: B. D. Decker.

Trunkey, D. D. (1990). Trauma: A public health problem. In E. E. Moore (Ed.), Early care of the injured patient. Philadelphia: B. C. Decker.

U.S. Department of Health and Human Services. (1991). Healthy people 2000: National health promotion and disease prevention objectives. DHHS Publication PHS 91-50212. Washington, DC: Author.

Vaizey, C. J., Jacobson, M. J., & Cross, F. W. (1994). Trauma in pregnancy. British Journal of Surgery, 8(10), 1406–1415.

Van Hoesen, K. B., Camporesi, E. M., Moon, R. E., Hage, M. L., & Piantadosi, C. A. (1989). Should hyperbaric oxygen be used to treat the pregnant patient for acute carbon monoxide poisoning? A case report and literature review. Journal of the American Medical Association, 261(7), 1039–1043.

Vander Veer, J. B., Jr. (1984). Trauma during pregnancy. Topics in Emergency Medicine, 6(1), 72–77.

Wolf, M. E., Alexander, B. H., Rivera, F. P., Hickok, D. E., Maier, R. V., & Starzyk, P. M. (1993). A retrospective cohort study of seatbelt use and pregnancy outcome after a motor vehicle crash. The Journal of Trauma, 34(1), 116–119.

Cardiopulmonary Resuscitation in Pregnancy

Carol Jean Luppi

Cardiopulmonary resuscitation (CPR) in pregnancy is a procedure few health-care providers have had the occasion to perform in their professional careers. Many nurses and physicians will never experience the challenge of resuscitating two patients at once; notwithstanding, the opportunity may present itself at any moment. This opportunity is not defined by clinical setting or patient population. Nurses working at free-standing birthing centers as well as nurses at "high-risk" tertiary care centers may be faced with the challenge of resuscitating a pregnant patient. The physiologic adaptations to pregnancy complicate cardiopulmonary resuscitation. The fact that cardiopulmonary arrest in pregnancy is so extremely rare limits the scientific data available to create treatment guidelines and provides little or no opportunity for practitioners to develop expertise in these treatment guidelines.

The nursing profession has accepted the formidable task of providing a therapeutic milieu for patient care as an integral part of the provision of nursing care. The nursing care of a pregnant patient in cardiopulmonary arrest consists of the manual tasks of resuscitation together with control of the environment of the resuscitation efforts. This chapter addresses the known causes of cardiopulmonary arrest in pregnancy, the physiologic adaptations to pregnancy that affect CPR, and the manual tasks of maternal resuscitation, as well as the issues surrounding the environment of resuscitation efforts.

CAUSES OF CARDIOPULMONARY ARREST IN PREGNANCY

The causes of cardiopulmonary arrest in pregnancy are varied but can be divided into three categories: (1) preexisting medical conditions; (2) obstetric complications; and (3) random, catastrophic events. Lists of these causes can be found in Table 21-1. The current leading cause of cardiopulmonary arrest in all pregnancies is hemorrhage (Pritchard, MacDonald, & Gant, 1985); however, the results change when the data are analyzed by trimesters. The current leading cause of arrest in late pregnancy is embolism (Berg, Atrash, Koonin, & Tucker, 1996; Bouvier-Colle, Varnoux, Costes, & Hatton, 1991), followed by hemorrhage and hypertension. These prominent causes of maternal death have changed over time and, no doubt, will continue to change in the future. Case reports of puerperal sepsis (Stevenson, 1969) have decreased with the advent of more effective antibiotics, yet group A beta-hemolytic *Streptococcus* (Slowey & Piacquadio, 1994), unrecognized sepsis (Morgan, 1995), disseminated herpes simplex virus (Gelven, Gruber, Swiger, Cina, & Harley, 1996), and pneumococcal

TABLE 21-1. Causes of Cardiopulmonary Arrest in Pregnancy

1. Hemorrhage	Uterine Atony Placental Abruption Placenta Previa/Accreta/Increta/Percreta DIC
2. Ventilation/Perfusion Mismatch	Hypovolemia Pulmonary Embolism—Thrombus, Amniotic Fluid, Air, Fat Pulmonary Pathology Pulmonary Aspiration Pneumothorax Bronchospasm
3. Severe Pregnancy-Induced Hypertension	
4. Drug Related	Illicit Drug Abuse Drug Error Anaphylaxis Drug Overdose Hypermagnesemia
5. Infection	
6. Trauma	
7. Cerebral Pathology	Subarachnoid Hemorrhage Herniation (Cerebral Edema)
8. Inadequate Ventilation	Failed Intubation Esophageal Intubation Pulmonary Aspiration
9. Anesthetic Related	Intravascular Local Anesthetic Overdose Total Spinal Drug Allergy (Rare) Regional Anesthetic Associated Sympathectomy
10. Preexisting Heart Disease	Congenital Heart Disease Acquired Valvular Disease Arrhythmia Myocardial Infarction
11. Recent Onset Heart Disease	Idiopathic Peripartum Cardiomyopathy Arrhythmia Traumatic Myocardial Contusion Myocardial Infarction
12. Malignant Hyperthermia	

Adapted from Johnson, M. D., Luppi, C. J., & Over, D. (In press). Cardiac Arrest and Resuscitation in the Parturient. In Gambling, D., & Douglas, J. Obstetric Anesthesia and Uncommon Disorders. Philadelphia: W. B. Saunders.

meningitis (Vives et al., 1996) are cited in 1995–1996 literature. Moreover, because the vast majority of women infected with the human immunodeficiency virus (HIV) are of reproductive age (DeFerrari, Paine, Gregor, Summers, & Anderson, 1993), it is possible that infection may escalate as a cause of cardiopulmonary arrest in pregnancy (Bongain, Fuzibet, & Gillet, 1992; Kell et al., 1991).

The causes of arrest in pregnancy may vary according to geographical location and clinical situation. A 1995 report of the causes of maternal death in New York City attributed 39% of maternal deaths to injury (homicide (63%), suicide (13%), motor vehicle crashes (12%), and drug overdoses (7%)) (Dannenberg et al., 1995). A 1992 report from Cook County also revealed trauma as the leading cause (46.3%) of maternal death (Fildes, Reed, Jones, Martin, & Barrett, 1992). Three recent reports have cited cocaine abuse as a prevalent cause of cardiopulmonary arrest in pregnancy (Burkett, Bandstra, Cohen, Steele, & Palow, 1990; Collins, Davis, & Lantz, 1994; Iriye, Asrat, Adashek, & Carr, 1995) Amniotic fluid embolism has also been cited as a significant cause of maternal mortality (Davies & Harrison, 1992; Lau, 1994). Recent review of the literature has further cited previous cesarean delivery (Catanzarite, Foster, Robinette, Cousins, & Schneider, 1992), acute myocarditis (Chen et al., 1994), pregnancy-induced-hypertension (Neuman, Ron-El, Langer, Bukovsky, & Caspi, 1990), terbutaline sulfate administration (Hadi, 1994), and anesthetic complications (Myint, Bailey, & Milne, 1993) as causes of cardiopulmonary arrest.

It is tempting to assign degrees of risk based on these statistics; however, catastrophic events can occur without any risk factors. Inaccurate reporting of maternal death may have also skewed statistics. It has been suggested that official statistics of the causes of death may be inaccurate because of (1) failure to realize that the patient was pregnant at the time of certification and (2) the complexity of the pathological states (Bouvier-Colle et al., 1991). Obstetric care providers should have a general level of preparedness for this event despite perceived risk factors.

PHYSIOLOGIC ADAPTATIONS TO PREGNANCY PERTINENT TO CARDIOPULMONARY RESUSCITATION

The many physiologic adaptations to pregnancy (Table 21-2) limit the effectiveness of every aspect of the standard cardiopulmonary resuscitation framework. The respiratory and cardiovascular physiologic adaptations to pregnancy are the most consequential factors and increase the probability of maternal and fetal morbidity/mortality following cardiopulmonary arrest. The American Heart Association (AHA) has provided expert guidance to professionals and lay persons for the organization of resuscitative efforts. Despite the need for modification of the AHA framework, the "A,B,Cs" of resuscitation are an excellent foundation for resuscitation in pregnancy.

Airway

Airway anatomy is altered in normal pregnancy. The larynx is more anterior and cephalad. The laryngeal and pharyngeal mucosa is edematous and friable. Pregnancy complicated by diabetes (Wallace & Gilstrap, 1996) or pregnancy-induced hypertension (Cheek & Samuels, 1996) may contribute to even greater difficulty in airway maintenance. The incidence of failed intubation in the pregnant population compared to the general surgical population is 1:500 versus 1:2000 (Wallace & Gilstrap, 1996).

The pregnant patient is at increased risk of airway injury and pulmonary aspiration of stomach contents during cardiopulmonary resuscitation. The stomach is displaced cephalad by the gravid uterus, the pH of stomach contents is decreased, the cardiac sphincter is relaxed, the patient has no protective gag reflex, and external chest compressions are squeezing the thorax.

Breathing

Pregnancy is associated with significant changes in respiratory anatomy and physiology. The diaphragm is displaced 4–7 centimeters by the gravid uterus, which causes a decreased functional residual capacity and decreased chest

TABLE 21-2. Physiologic Adaptations to Pregnancy Pertinent to Cardiopulmonary Resuscitation

Cardiovascular System

Total Blood Volume	Increased 35%	
Plasma Volume	Increased 45%	
Red Cell Volume	Increased 20%	
Cardiac Output	Increased 40%	
Heart Rate	Increased 15%	
Systolic Blood Pressure	Unchanged	
Systemic Vascular Resistance	Decreased 15%	
Central Venous Pressure	Unchanged	
Pulmonary Capillary Wedge Pressure	Unchanged	
Ejection Fraction	Unchanged	
Femoral Venous Pressure	Increased 15%	
Uterine Blood Flow	Increased 20–40%	

Respiratory System

Minute Ventilation	Increased 50%	
Alveolar Ventilation	Increased 70%	
Tidal Volume	Increased 40%	
Respiratory Rate	Increased 10–15%	
Functional Residual Capacity	Decreased 20%	
Residual Volume	Decreased 20%	
Oxygen Consumption	Increased 20%	
Arterial pH	Slightly Increased	Average 7.40–7.45
PaO_2 (mm Hg)	Increased	104–108 mm Hg
$PaCO_2$ (mm Hg)	Decreased	27–31 mm Hg

Renal System

Renal Blood Flow	Increased 50%	(by 4th month)
Glomerular Filtration Rate	Increased 50%	(by 4th month)
Upper Limit of Blood Urea Nitrogen	Decreased 50%	
Upper Limit of Serum Creatinine	Decreased 50%	

Hepatic System

Total Plasma Protein Concentration	Decreased 20%
Pseudocholinesterase Concentration	Decreased
Coagulation Factors	Mainly Increased

Gastrointestinal System

Gastric Emptying	Delayed
Gastric Fluid Volume/Acidity	Increased
Gastroesophageal Sphincter Tone	Variable Changes

Adapted from Johnson, M. D., Luppi, C. J., & Over, D. (In press). Cardiac Arrest and Resuscitation in the Parturient. In Gambling, D., & Douglas, J. Obstetric Anesthesia and Uncommon Disorders. Philadelphia: W. B. Saunders.

compliance (Longo, Hill, & Powe, 1972). Breast hypertrophy further decreases chest compliance.

Maternal oxygen consumption, carbon dioxide production, and basal metabolic rate are increased by 20% secondary to the demands of the feto-placental unit and maternal metabolic activity (Lee, Rodgers, White, & Harvey, 1994). To meet these oxygen demands, the pregnant woman must hyperventilate to markedly (50%) increase minute ventilation (Weinberger et al., 1980). The increase in minute ventilation is achieved by a minimal increase in respiratory rate and a significant increase in tidal volume, which is stimulated by progesterone (Troiano, 1989). This requisite oxygenation and ventilation of the pregnant patient during cardiopulmonary resuscitation is complicated by the previously mentioned decrease in chest compliance and the physiologic anemia of pregnancy.

The "hyperventilation of pregnancy" causes a chronic respiratory alkalosis related to the excess loss of carbon dioxide. This loss of carbon dioxide, in turn, stimulates an excess excretion of bicarbonate by the maternal kidneys, which produces a low serum bicarbonate level. These changes are reflected in arterial blood gas samples obtained from healthy pregnant women (deSwiet, 1994) (Display 21-1). It is normal for a woman to be in a state of compensated respiratory alkalosis throughout her pregnancy. However, the renal excretion of bicarbonate does render the pregnant woman exceptionally intolerant of any level of hypoxia, because her buffering capacity has been significantly compromised.

Circulation

Pregnancy also produces dramatic changes in cardiovascular anatomy and physiology (AHA, 1992). Blood volume increases (Monga & Creasey, 1994) 45%, which translates into approximately 1500 cc for a singleton pregnancy and greater than 2000 cc in multiple gestations. The increase in red cell volume is proportionally smaller than plasma volume and results in a state of physiologic anemia (Monga & Creasey, 1994).

Maternal cardiac output increases 30–50% because of increased stroke volume and heart rate. The first trimester increase in cardiac output

DISPLAY 21-1

Normal Arterial Blood Gas Levels

pH	7.43–7.45
PO_2	100–105
PCO_2	28–31
HCO_3	18–22

Source:

is primarily caused by an increase in stroke volume. Stroke volume declines toward term and the increase in cardiac output is primarily achieved by a 15–20 bpm increase in heart rate (Monga & Creasey, 1994). Cardiac output is also affected in labor when uterine contractions can further increase output by 20%. Maternal cardiac output changes are positional and may decrease 30% in the supine patient by the 36th gestational week. A small percentage of pregnant women (8–10%) will become symptomatic with this drop in cardiac output and experience "supine hypotensive syndrome" (hypotension, bradycardia, & syncope) (Monga & Creasey, 1994). These symptoms are explained by the mechanical effect of the gravid uterus. Maternal positioning defines the degree of these mechanical effects of the gravid uterus on the cardiovascular system.

By 20 weeks gestation the gravid uterus can cause significant compression of the pelvic vessels. Compression of the inferior vena cava and major pelvic veins may sequester up to 30% of the circulating blood volume and seriously compromise venous return to the heart, thereby severely limiting cardiac output. What does not get returned to the heart cannot be pumped out by the heart. Compression of the abdominal aorta causes considerable aortic outflow obstruction with subsequent decreases in renal and uterine blood flow (Lee, Rodgers, White, & Harvey, 1986). Perfusion during cardiopulmonary resuscitation is dependent upon both venous return and forward flow. The mechanical effects of the gravid uterus will significantly impede successful cardiopulmonary resuscitation.

Perfusion during cardiopulmonary resuscitation is also affected by alterations in systemic vascular resistance (SVR). SVR is decreased in pregnancy because of vasodilation and utero-placental blood flow. Progesterone, prostaglandins, and atrial natriuretic factors cause relaxation of tubular structures, which reduces peripheral vascular resistance (Lee et al., 1986). A large portion of the cardiac output (20–30%) is directed to the uterus and placenta. The vessels in the uterus and placenta are maximally dilated and provide an extremely low-pressure system for perfusion. Placental perfusion will be decreased during periods of maternal hypoxia or hypotension.

The unique alterations in the physiology and anatomy of the pregnant woman challenge every healthcare provider during cardiopulmonary resuscitation. The obstetric code team must be organized and prepared for CPR to be successful. The team should follow an uncomplicated protocol that addresses the unique needs of pregnancy.

OBSTETRIC CARDIOPULMONARY RESUSCITATION PROTOCOLS

In the past 10 years, three different protocols for cardiopulmonary resuscitation in pregnancy can be found in the literature: (1) Lee, Rodgers, White, and Harvey Protocol (1986) (Tables 21-3, 21-4); (2) Advanced Cardiac Life Support (ACLS)/ American Heart Association (AHA, 1987) (Displays 21-2–7); and (3) Johnson, Luppi and Over Protocol (Displays 21-8–10) (Johnson, Luppi, & Over, in press). The American Heart Association's ACLS protocols are an undisputed guide to resuscitation. The most recent edition of the ACLS manual provides the following guidelines to adapt the protocols to the pregnant patient:

> If 5–10 minutes of standard CPR, leftward displacement of the gravid uterus, airway management, fluid volume restoration, and defibrillation (if indicated) fail to restore effective circulatory function, an attempt to evaluate fetal viability via external monitoring or real-time ultrasound, though difficult, may be useful in deciding if and when open-chest heart massage and/or cesarean section is required. . . . If standard measures are not

successful within 15 minutes of the onset of arrest, thoracotomy and open-chest massage should be performed if the fetus is still viable. If there is no return of spontaneous effective maternal circulation or there is evidence of fetal distress after 15 minutes of CPR with open-chest cardiac massage, some have recommended that cesarean section be performed immediately. (AHA, 1992).

The more recent report from the 1992 National Conference on Cardiopulmonary Resuscitation (CPR) and Emergency Cardiac Care (ECC) advocates a more aggressive approach than the previous protocols. This report dictates that delivery take place within 4–5 minutes of cardiac arrest (AHA, 1992). Each protocol shares a basic framework of early perimortem delivery and open-chest cardiac massage. The Johnson, Luppi, and Over protocol is the most recent and diverse.

The Johnson, Luppi, and Over protocol was developed based on the existing protocols, the current literature, and the authors' clinical experience. The protocol is intended as a user-friendly guideline for the obstetric staff who rarely if ever confront this emergency. The protocol focuses on the use of an aggressive and organized approach to cardiopulmonary resuscitation of the pregnant woman. The authors considered multiple issues to modify the existing protocols.

The most apparent difference is the lack of fetal monitoring. This decision was based upon the following factors:

1. The effectiveness and accuracy of electronic fetal monitoring (EFM) during maternal resuscitation is controversial. EFM as a tool of assessing intrapartum fetal well-being is also controversial. Assessment of EFM data takes time away from other resuscitative efforts. There is also a danger of electrical fire in the fetal monitor if the monitor is connected during maximal defibrillation. Many fetal monitors are not grounded for that energy.
2. Both the mother and the fetus are at increased risk during periods of maternal apnea. The apneic pregnant patient becomes acidotic much faster than her nonpregnant counterpart. Maternal oxygen reserves are limited and brain dam-

TABLE 21-3. Lee, Rodgers, White, and Harvey Protocol—1		
Less Than 25 Weeks	25 to 32 Weeks	32 Weeks or More
Continue CPR until appropriate endpoint	Position patient to decrease aortocaval compression by the uterus	Position patient to decrease aortocaval compression by the uterus
Consider open-chest cardiac massage after 15 minutes of continuous CPR; sooner if maternal hypoxia or inadequate circulation uncorrected by closed-chest CPR	Special attention to fetal status, especially with Defibrillation Lidocaine, verapamil Epinephrine	Special attention to fetal status, especially with Defibrillation Lidocaine, verapamil beta-blockers Epinephrine
	Consider open-chest massage when decision to perform emergency cesarean section is made	Emergency cesarean section after 15 minutes continuous CPR; sooner if maternal hypoxia or inadequate circulation uncorrected by CPR or fetal distress
	Emergency cesarean section after 15 minutes continuous CPR; sooner if maternal hypoxia or inadequate circulation uncorrected by CPR or fetal distress	Continue CPR during and after delivery
	Continue CPR during and after delivery	Consider open-chest massage if maternal condition after delivery warrants

Adapted from Johnson, M. D., Luppi, C. J., & Over, D. (In press). Cardiac Arrest and Resuscitation in the Parturient. In Gambling, D., & Douglas, J. <u>Obstetric Anesthesia and Uncommon Disorders</u>. Philadelphia: W. B. Saunders.

age is likely after 4–6 minutes of sustained cardiac arrest (AHA, 1987; Archer, & Marx, 1974). Irreversible maternal brain damage may be caused by a delay of even 6–9 minutes (Weber, 1971). Fetal oxygen reserve is approximately 2 minutes (Longo et al., 1972). Katz, Dotters, & Droegemueller (1986) published a retrospective analysis of perimortem delivery time and neonatal outcome (Table 21-5). This report illustrates that the fetus may survive for longer than the 2-minute oxygen reserve; however, the greatest chance of intact survival is when the per-

imortem *delivery* occurs within 5 minutes of the maternal arrest (Katz et al., 1986). Effective maternal resuscitation offers the only chance of survival for both mother and baby. If the mother's condition is poor, the baby's condition will be worse; therefore, what is good for the mother is good for the baby.

3. The gravid uterus mechanically inhibits successful resuscitation, consumes maternal oxygen stores, and generates carbon dioxide and hydrogen ions. There are data from animal and human studies that indicate that effective resuscitation is unlikely

TABLE 21-4. Lee, Rodgers, White, and Harvey Protocol—2

Time	Resuscitative Action	Diagnostic Action	Pharmacologic Agents
0	Chest thump Ventilation (mouth to mouth) External cardiac massage Defibrillate Intravenous access: central line	Electrocardiography for rhythm Check for pulses and perfusion Determine gestational age	Intravenous fluids Ventricular fibrillation—lidocaine Supraventricular tachyarrhythmia— digitalis/beta-blocker as appropriate
1 to 2 minutes	Endotracheal intubation plus ventilation with oxygen	Measure arterial blood gases Check for pulses and perfusion Check fetal heart, sonography	pH less than 7.3—sodium bicarbonate Asystole/bradyarrhythmia—atropine Pulmonary edema—furosemide
2 to 5 minutes	Defibrillate as needed Position to move uterus to left	Electrocardiography for rhythm Electrocardiography for rhythm Quick measure of blood pressure, pulses, perfusion Portable chest radiography Measure arterial blood gases	Ventricular fibrillation—lidocaine Ventricular fibrillation—bretylium Electromechanical dissociation— calcium chloride, epinephrine (one time only), isoproterenol
5 to 10 minutes	Continue ventilation plus external massage Begin preparation for operative procedure as appropriate Arterial line Defibrillate as needed	Check fetal heart, sonography Check for tension pneumothorax, cardiac tamponade, hypovolemia Measure arterial blood gases	pH less than 7.3—sodium bicarbonate
15 minutes	Open-chest cardiac massage and/or emergency cesarean section as appropriate	Continue as above	Continue as above

Adapted from Johnson. M.D., Luppi, C. J., & Over, D. (In press). Cardiac Arrest and Resuscitation in the Parturient. In Gambling, D., & Douglas. J. Obstetric Anesthesia and Uncommon Disorders. Philadelphia: W. B. Saunders.

DISPLAY 21-2

ACLS Approach to Emergency Cardiac Care

Primary Survey = CPR and defibrillation

- Airway
  - Open the airway
- Breathing
  - Provide positive-pressure ventilation
- Circulation
  - Perform chest compressions
- Defibrillation
  - Shock ventricular fibrillation/pulseless ventricular tachycardia

Secondary Survey = Intubation, IV access, rhythms, drugs, and etiology

- Airway
  - Establish advanced airway control
  - Perform endotracheal intubation
- Breathing
  - Assess adequacy of ventilation via endotracheal tube
  - Provide positive-pressure ventilations
- Circulation
  - Obtain IV access to administer fluids and medications
  - Continue CPR, defibrillate as needed
  - Provide rhythm-appropriate cardio-vascular pharmacology
- Defibrillation
  - Consider possible reasons for the arrest
  - Identify possible reversible causes that have a specific therapy

Adapted from Aehlert, Barbara. (1994). <u>ACLS Quick Review Study Guide</u> (pp. 252–255). St. Louis: Mosby-Year Bock.

when the vena cava is occluded (Kasten & Martin, 1986; Rees & Willis, 1988). The mother and fetus both stand to gain significant benefit from perimortem delivery if the procedure is completed within the first 5 minutes of maternal arrest. Time is a tremendous factor. These modifications were made to decrease the time between maternal arrest and delivery to 5 minutes.

4. Blood is shunted away from the uterus during periods of maternal hypoxia, hypotension, and lactic acidosis by utero-placental vasoconstriction. Any maternal blood supply the fetus does appreciate will be hypoxic and acidotic.
5. Closed-chest cardiac massage becomes less effective with time and is virtually ineffective in the pregnant patient after 15 minutes.

The Johnson, Luppi, and Over protocol also identified only two perimortem cesarean delivery treatment groups defined by uterine size of (1) greater than or equal to 20 weeks and (2) less than 20 weeks. Gestational age determination may be difficult. The protocol specifies uterine *size*. A uterus of 20-week size is universally defined by palpation of the fundus at the level of the umbilicus. Delivery of the fetus and placenta decreases maternal oxygen requirements, allows return of vena cava function, relieves aortic outflow obstruction, and permits independent resuscitation of the mother and fetus. The viability gap between 20 and 24 weeks was not ignored. As discussed previously, the gravid uterus can dangerously inhibit vena cava function as early as 20-week size. If a mother of a preterm, nonviable fetus cannot be resuscitated, the fetus will perish with the mother. This ethical dilemma will need to be addressed at every institution providing obstetrical care.

The protocol also emphasized the following issues:

1. Early intubation, to protect the high-risk airway;
2. Manual uterine displacement to limit aorto-caval compression rather than the use of tilt or wedging. Rees and Willis studied the effectiveness of external chest massage

DISPLAY 21-3

ACLS Ventricular Fibrillation/Pulseless Ventricular Tachycardia

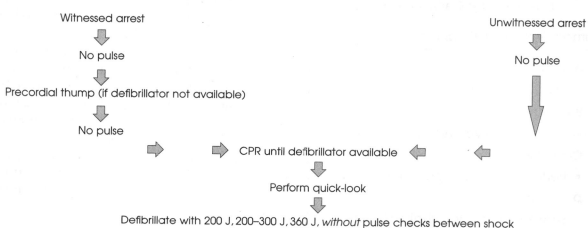

Witnessed arrest

⬇

No pulse

⬇

Precordial thump (if defibrillator not available)

⬇

No pulse

Unwitnessed arrest

⬇

No pulse

⬇

➡   ➡   CPR until defibrillator available   ⬅   ⬅

⬇

Perform quick-look

⬇

Defibrillate with 200 J, 200–300 J, 360 J, *without* pulse checks between shock
Leave the paddles in place on the chest between shocks
(or use adhesive defibrillation pads for remote defibrillation)
Visually reconfirm rhythm between defibrillations

⬇

Continue CPR
Intubate at once
(Confirm tube placement)

⬇

IV access
Large-bore IV
Antecubital or external jugular vein if no IV in place at time of arrest
Normal saline or lactated Ringer's solution

⬇

Epinephrine 1 mg IV q 3–5 min
(or, after initial dose, appropriate alternative)**
If IV access delayed, endotracheal (ET) dose is 2–2.5 mg
diluted in 10 ml of normal saline or distilled water

⬇

Defibrillate with 360 J within 30–60 sec

**IV Dosing Alternatives
Recommended: 1 mg every 3–5 minutes
Intermediate: 2–5 mg IV push, every 3–5 min
Escalating: 1 mg–3 mg–5 mg (IV 3 min apart)
High: 0.1 mg/kg IV push every 3–5 min
ET dose: 2–2.5 mg diluted in 10 ml of normal saline or distilled water

Adapted from Aehlert, Barbara. (1994). ACLS Quick Review Study Guide (pp. 252–255). St. Louis: Mosby–Year Book.

DISPLAY 21-4

ACLS Refractory Ventricular Fibrillation

Lidocaine 1–1.5 mg/kg IV push
May repeat in 3–5 min for maximum dose of 3 mg/kg

Defibrillate with 360 J within 30–60 sec

Bretylium 5 mg/kg
May repeat with 10 mg/kg every 5 min as needed to
a maximum dose of 30–35 mg/kg

Defibrillate with 360 J within 30–60 sec

Magnesium sulfate 1–2 grams IV (2–4 ml of a 50% solution) diluted in 10 ml over 1–2 min

Defibrillate with 360 J within 30–60 sec

Procainamide 30 mg/min
Maximum dose 17 mg/kg

Defibrillate with 360 J within 30–60 sec

Consider sodium bicarbonate 1 mEq/kg

Adapted from Aehlert, Barbara. (1994). <u>ACLS Quick Review Study Guide</u> (pp. 252–255). St. Louis: Mosby-Year Book.

when the patient is tilted/wedged. The force of compression is limited by the angle of inclination (Rees & Willis, 1983).

3. Central venous access as soon as possible for volume resuscitation and drug administration. Kuhn et al. published a study in 1981 that medication administered in a peripheral vein during CPR does not reach a central artery for 300 seconds (Kuhn et al., 1981).

4. Use of open-chest cardiac massage if perimortem cesarean delivery while utilizing

closed-chest cardiac massage does not produce a maternal pulse or generate a maternal blood pressure. Open-chest cardiac massage can be successful when closed-chest cardiac massage has failed (Bayne & Josing, 1984; Brunette et al., 1992; Cooper, 1964; Linton & Ledingham, 1966; Russell, 1962; Shocket & Rosenblum, 1967; Stewart, Stewart, & Gillles, 1962; Sykes & Ahmed, 1963). Open-chest cardiac massage increases cardiac output (Alimoff, Safar, & Bircher, 1980; Babbs, 1987; Cohen et al., 1993;

DISPLAY 21-5

ACLS Asytole

CPR

Confirm rhythm in another lead
Change lead-selector on the monitor
If using paddles in quick-look mode, rotate paddles 90 degrees

Intubate
(Confirm tube placement)
Assess breath sounds
Observe chest rise

Establish IV access
Large bore IV
Normal saline or lactated Ringer's
Antecubital or external jugular

Consider possible causes:
H(x4)AD
Hypoxia
Hypokalemia
Hyperkalemia
Hypothermia
Acidosis
Drug Overdose

Consider immediate transcutaneous pacing

Epinephrine 1 mg IV every 3–5 min
(or, after initial dose, appropriate alternative**)

Atropine 1 mg IV every 3–5 min to maximum 3 mg
ET dose 2–2.5 mg diluted in 10 ml of normal saline or distilled water

Consider sodium bicarbonate 1 mEq/kg

Consider termination of efforts

**IV Dosing Alternatives
Recommended: 1 mg every 3–5 minutes
Intermediate: 2–5 mg IV push, every 3–5 min
Escalating: I mg–3 mg–5 mg (IV 3 min apart)
High: 0.1 mg/kg IV push every 3–5 min
ET dose: 2–2.5 mg diluted in 10 ml of normal saline or distilled water

Adapted from Aehlert, Barbara. (1994). ACLS Quick Review Study Guide (pp. 252–255). St. Louis: Mosby-Year Book.

DISPLAY 21-6

ACLS Pulseless Electrical Activity

CPR

Intubate (confirm tube placement)
Assess breath sounds
Observe chest rise

Establish IV access
Large-bore IV
Normal saline or lactated Ringer's
Antecubital or external jugular
500 ml fluid challenge

Assess blood flow using Doppler

Consider underlying causes

MATCHED (x 4) ED
Myocardial infarction (massive acute)
Acidosis (severe)
Tension pneumothorax
Pericardial tamponade
Hypoxia (severe)
Hypothermia
Hypovolemia
Hyperkalemia
Pulmonary embolism (massive)
Drug overdose

Epinephrine 1 mg IV every 3–5 min
(or after initial dose, appropriate alternative**)

If bradycardic, atropine 1 mg IV every 3–5 min to maximum 3 mg

Consider sodium bicarbonate 1 mEq/kg

**IV Dosing Alternatives
Recommended: 1 mg every 3–5 minutes
Intermediate: 2–5 mg IV push, every 3–5 min
Escalating: 1 mg–3 mg–5 mg (IV 3 min apart)
High: 0.1 mg/kg IV push every 3–5 min
ET dose: 2–2.5 mg diluted in 10 ml of normal saline or distilled water

Adapted from Aehlert, Barbara. (1994). ACLS Quick Review Study Guide (pp. 252–255). St. Louis: Mosby-Year Book.

DISPLAY 21-7

Sodium Bicarbonate Use

Class I (definitely helpful) if known preexisting hyperkalemia

Class IIa (probably helpful)

- If known preexisting bicarbonate-responsive acidosis
- If overdose with cyclic antidepressants
- To alkalinize the urine in drug overdoses (phenobarbital, aspirin)

Class IIb (possibly helpful)

- If intubated and long arrest interval
- Upon return of spontaneous circulation after long arrest interval

Class III (not indicated, may be harmful)

- Hypoxic lactic acidosis

Adapted from Aehlert, Barbara. (1994). ACLS Quick Review Study Guide (pp. 252–255). St. Louis: Mosby-Year Book.

Weiser, Adler, & Kuhn, 1962) and does not hinder cerebral or coronary blood flow (Barnett et al., 1986; Bircher & Safar, 1980; Del Guercio et al., 1965; Robertson, 1991). Open-chest cardiac massage may be the only effective method of resuscitation in arrests caused or complicated by chest trauma, tension pneumothorax, massive pulmonary embolism, cardiac tamponade, profound hypovolemia, and hypothermia.

5. Timely differential diagnosis is emphasized. Their simplified approach to diagnosing the cause of arrest is illustrated in Display 21-11. The initial approach to every cardiopulmonary resuscitation scenario will follow the protocol as described; however, ultimate interventions vary depending upon the precipitating or primary cause.

6. Limited indications for cardiopulmonary bypass. Cardiopulmonary bypass is not indicated in every arrest situation, nor is it universally available as a treatment modal-

ity. Indications for cardiopulmonary bypass include ventilation/perfusion mismatch, local anesthetic toxicity, profound hypovolemia, and hypothermia-related dysrhythmias. If cardiopulmonary bypass is available as a treatment option, all disciplines involved should be consulted in devising an emergency plan to access the equipment and personnel required for cardiopulmonary bypass during a maternal code. Cardiopulmonary bypass is an exceptionally sophisticated treatment option that cannot be considered a standard of care.

7. Evaluation of iatrogenic cause for cardiopulmonary arrest. This protocol suggests early discontinuation of intravenous and epidural fluids that were infusing at the time of the arrest. All solutions and tubing can then be assessed for any substance that could potentially cause cardiopulmonary arrest.

8. Maternal stabilization to ensure fetal well-being. As previously discussed, the Johnson, Luppi, and Over protocol recommends discontinuation of electronic fetal monitoring and delivery of the fetus (20-week size or greater) if resuscitation efforts are unsuccessful after 5 minutes.

PERIMORTEM CESAREAN DELIVERY DISCUSSION

Each protocol recommends perimortem cesarean delivery. There are issues associated with perimortem cesarean delivery beyond the physiological and ethical issues previously discussed. Common practical issues that arise are speed, hemostasis, infection, and liability.

Speed

Each protocol has stressed the importance of the timing of the cesarean delivery. To ensure delivery within 5 minutes of a cardiac arrest is a logistical challenge. The multidisciplinary consultation for planning of protocols, efficient lines of communication, and the rehearsal of protocols cannot be stressed enough and will be discussed in the next section. Personnel and equipment must be imme-

DISPLAY 21-8

Johnson, Luppi, and Over Protocol

1. **A**irway	ntubate as soon as possible
2. **B**reathing	Control ventilation
3. **C**irculation	Central venous access ASAP
	Closed-chest massage
4. **D**isplacement	Manual left uterine displacement ASAP
5. **D**efibrillate	As per ACLS protocol
6. **D**rugs	As per ACLS protocol
7. **D**elivery	Deliver fetus and placenta within 5 minutes if standard resuscitation techniques are not successful
8. **D**ocument	
Consider	
9. **O**pen-Chest Cardiac Massage	Within 15 minutes if standard resuscitation techniques are not successful
10. **C**ardiopulmonary Bypass	Where indicated

Adapted from Johnson, M. D., Luppi, C. J., & Over, D. (In press). Cardiac Arrest and Resuscitation in the Parturient. In Gambling, D., & Douglas, J. <u>Obstetric Anesthesia and Uncommon Disorders.</u> Philadelphia: W. B Saunders.

diately accessible for successful resuscitation. An efficient communication system should be available to summon the entire team immediately. Proper equipment beyond the routine resuscitation requirements should be readily available for obstetrical intubation and perimortem cesarean delivery. Maternal cardiopulmonary arrest can occur in many institutional locations. The Joint Commission for Accreditation of Hospitals Organization (1996) has stressed that the care available for a patient population in one area of an institution should be available for that patient population in every area of the institution. This JCAHO guideline and the requisite timing of the perimortem cesarean delivery dictate that equipment should be readily portable. Examples of portable obstetrical intubation kits and perimortem cesarean section kits are found in Displays 21-12 and 21-13. Once this equipment is available, the logistics of performing a perimortem cesarean delivery are left to the skill of the obstetrician; nevertheless, it is usually most effectively performed via vertical abdominal and uterine incisions.

Hemostasis

During the perimortem cesarean delivery, there may be remarkably little bleeding noted, because during periods of profound maternal hypoxia and hypotension, blood will be shunted away from nonessential organs to vital organs. This limited blood flow decreases the amount of oxytocin available for uterine contraction after delivery of the placenta. Any uterine atony after delivery of the placenta may be treated with direct intramuscular dilute pitocin (10 units in 9 cc of normal saline) administration at multiple sites. Pitocin vials (10 units), normal saline vials (10 cc), 10-cc sterile syringe, and an intramuscular needle should be available for the perimortem cesarean kit. Severe uterine atony and hemorrhage can refill the uterus and cause recurrent aortocaval compression and severe

DISPLAY 21-9

Johnson, Luppi, and Over Antepartum Guidelines

1. **CALL CODE BLUE,** OB CODE TEAM, CODE LOCATION
2. CLOSED CHEST CPR WITH **MANUAL LEFT UTERINE DISPLACEMENT**
3. **ENDOTRACHEAL INTUBATION** AS SOON AS POSSIBLE
   - Consider use of transtracheal medications
4. **RAPID CENTRAL ACCESS** FOR LARGE VOLUME REPLACEMENT
   - Consider subclavian approach
   - Send labs for: Venous arterial blood gases
                           Electrolytes
                           Hemoglobin and hematocrit/Coagulation studies

   - Avoid Hypothermia
5. MONITORING
   - Pulse oximeter
   - ECG
   - Early use of arterial monitoring
   - Consider aortic arterial line
6. ASSESS FOR HEMORRHAGE
   - Control site of bleeding
   - Consider manual aortic tamponade
   - Consider ligation of hypogastric arteries
7. **BY 4 MINUTES**
   - CONSIDER **PERIMORTEM CESAREAN SECTION** IF MATERNAL RESUSCITATION IS FAILING AND UTERINE SIZE IS **20 WEEKS** OR MORE (FUNDUS AT LEVEL OF UMBILICUS OR ABOVE)
8. **BY 5 MINUTES**
   - ENSURE DELIVERY OF BABY
   - DELAY ABDOMINAL CLOSURE UNTIL HEMODYNAMIC STABILITY ENSURED
9. **BY 15 MINUTES**
   - If maternal resuscitation remains inadequate consider **direct cardiac massage** via transabdominal, left thoracotomy, or median sternotomy
10. EVALUATE NEED FOR **CARDIOPULMONARY BYPASS**:
    - POOR V/Q MATCHING
      - Pulmonary embolus/Amniotic fluid embolus
    - MASSIVE HEMORRHAGE
      - Electromechanical dissociation/DIC
    - DRUG/ANESTHESIA OVERDOSE
      - Bupivacaine toxicity
    - HYPOTHERMIA RELATED DYSRHYTHMIA

ALSO
   - REMOVE EXISTING IV AND EPIDURAL INFUSION FLUIDS
     - KEEP FOR ANALYSIS
     - DIAGNOSE THE CAUSE OF THE ARREST

Adapted from Johnson, M. D., Luppi, C. J., & Over, D. (In press). Cardiac Arrest and Resuscitation in the Parturient, In Gambling, D., & Douglas, J. Obstetric Anesthesia and Uncommon Disorders. Philadelphia: W. B. Saunders.

DISPLAY 21-10

Johnson, Luppi, and Over Postpartum Guidelines

1. **CALL CODE BLUE,** OB CODE TEAM, CODE LOCATION
2. CLOSED CHEST CPR WITH **MANUAL LEFT UTERINE DISPLACEMENT**
   - Uterus may be blood filled
3. **ENDOTRACHEAL INTUBATION** AS SOON AS POSSIBLE
   - Consider use of transtracheal medications
4. **RAPID CENTRAL ACCESS** FOR LARGE VOLUME REPLACEMENT
   - Consider subclavian approach
   - Send labs for:　　　　　　　Venous ABGs
   　　　　　　　　　　　　　　Electrolytes
   　　　　　　　　　　　　　　HB and HCT
   　　　　　　　　　　　　　　Coagulation studies

   - Avoid hypothermia
5. MONITORING
   - Pulse oximeter
   - ECG
   - Early use of arterial monitoring
   - Consider aortic arterial line
6. ASSESS FOR HEMORRHAGE
   - Control site of bleeding
   - Consider opening/re-opening the abdomen
   - Delay abdominal closure until hemodynamic stability ensured
   - Consider manual aortic tamponade
   - Consider ligation of hypogastric arteries
7. **BY 15 MINUTES**
   - IF MATERNAL RESUSCITATION REMAINS INADEQUATE CONSIDER **DIRECT CARDIAC MASSAGE** VIA TRANSABDOMINAL, LEFT THORACOTOMY, OR MEDIAN STERNOTOMY
8. EVALUATE NEED FOR **CARDIOPULMONARY BYPASS**
   - POOR V/Q MATCHING
     - Pulmonary embolus/Amniotic fluid embolus
   - MASSIVE HEMORRHAGE
     - Electromechanical dissociation/DIC
   - DRUG/ANESTHESIA OVERDOSE
     - Bupivacaine toxicity
   - HYPOTHERMIA RELATED DYSRHYTHMIA

ALSO
- REMOVE EXISTING IV AND EPIDURAL INFUSION FLUIDS
  - KEEP FOR ANALYSIS
  - DIAGNOSE THE CAUSE OF THE ARREST

Adapted from Johnson, M. D., Luppi, C. J., & Over, D. (In press). Cardiac Arrest and Resuscitation in the Parturient. In Gambling, D., & Douglas, J. <u>Obstetric Anesthesia and Uncommon Disorders.</u> Philadelphia: W. B. Saunders.

TABLE 21-5. Postmortem Cesarean Deliveries with Surviving Infants with Reports of Time of Death of the Mother Until Delivery (from 1900–1986)

Time (mins)	Number of patients	Outcome	Percentage
0–5	42	Normal infants	70
6–10	7	Normal infants	13
	1	Mild neurological sequelae	
11–15	6	Normal infants	12
	1	Severe neurological sequelae	
16–20	1	Severe neurological sequelae	1.7
21+	2	Severe neurological sequelae	
	1	Normal infant	3.3
Total	61		100

Reprinted from Katz, V. L., Dotters, D. J., & Droegemueller, W. (1986). Perimortem cesarean delivery. Obstetrics and Gynecology, 68(4), 571–576.

hypotension. Careful monitoring of the postoperative uterus is essential.

The lack of blood flow to the uterus during perimortem cesarean delivery also limits the effective closure of the surgical site. Final closure of the uterus and the abdominal cavity may need to be delayed until restoration of maternal pulse and blood pressure. Packing the abdomen with wet lap packs and covering the wound with a clear plastic drape allow the surgeons to delay closure until successful resuscitation has restored perfusion and bleeding sites are identified. The clear drape allows the surgeons to assess the surgical site during continued resuscitative efforts and intervene when appropriate.

Infection

As with any surgery, infection is a risk. Delivery of the fetus within 5 minutes of maternal arrest does not allow for moving the patient to the operating room or usual operative standards of care. Customary surgical preparation, draping, and routine operating room procedures are not performed. When the resuscitation efforts are successful, broad spectrum antibiotic coverage can be considered.

Liability

Issues related to liability in obstetrics are always a controversy. Civil and criminal liability relate specifically to cardiopulmonary resuscitation

during pregnancy. For a perimortem cesarean delivery to be a criminal offense, wrongful dissection and or wrongful intent would have to be established (LaFave & Scott, 1972). The intent of a perimortem delivery is to save the life of the mother and baby; therefore (whether the operation was successful or unsuccessful), the intent

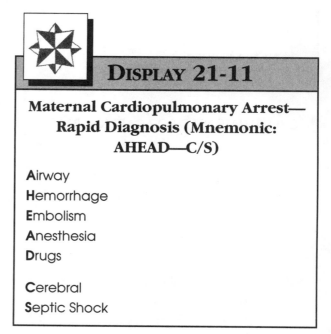

DISPLAY 21-11

Maternal Cardiopulmonary Arrest— Rapid Diagnosis (Mnemonic: AHEAD—C/S)

Airway
Hemorrhage
Embolism
Anesthesia
Drugs

Cerebral
Septic Shock

Adapted from Johnson, M. D., Luppi, C. J. & Over, D. (In press). Cardiac Arrest and Resuscitation in the Parturient. In Gambling, D., & Douglas, J. Obstetric Anesthesia and Uncommon Disorders. Philadelphia: W. B. Saunders.

DISPLAY 21-12

Obstetric Intubation Kit

- Datta handle laryngoscope (1)
  - MAC 3 blade (1)
  - Miller 2 blade (1)
- #7 and #6.5 endotracheal tube with stylette and syringe in place (1 each)
- Laryngeal mask airway, size 3 and 4 (1 each)
- Sheridan combitube (1)
- Knife handle (1) with #10 blade (2)
- Skin hook (1)
- 10 cc/100 mg Lidocaine prefilled syringe (1)
- 10 cc vial of 10 mg/cc succinylcholine chloride (1)
- 500 mg sodium pentothal (1)

Adapted from Johnson, M.D., Luppi, C.J. & Over, D. (In press). Cardiac Arrest and Resuscitation in the Parturient. In Gambling, D., & Douglas. J. *Obstetric Anesthesia and Uncommon Disorders* Philadelphia: W. B. Saunders.

DISPLAY 21-13

Perimortem Cesarean Section Kit

- Knife handle (1) with #10 blade (2)
- Kelly clamps (4)
- Mayo scissors (1)
- Bandage scissors (1)
- Tooth forceps (2)
- Needle holders (2)
- Uterine closure sutures (4)
- Laparotomy sponges (2 packs of 5 each)
- Adhesive clear plastic abdominal drape (1)
- 1 cc/10 units pitocin vials (2)
- 10 cc normal saline vials (2)
- 10 cc syringe with intramuscular needle

Adapted from Johnson, M. D., Luppi, C. J. & Over, D. (In press). Cardiac Arrest and Resuscitation in the Parturient. In Gambling, D., & Douglas, J. *Obstetric Anesthesia and Uncommon Disorders.* Philadelphia: W. B. Saunders.

is not wrongful. The issue of battery has also been considered when surgery is performed without the patient's consent. Surgical consent in a life-threatening emergency is unnecessary because consent is implied. In October 1986, Katz et al. wrote, "No physician has ever been found liable in performing a postmortem section" (1986). One hopes that legal risk for physicians when performing perimortem cesarean delivery will continue to be minimal.

STAFF ROLES AND RESPONSIBILITIES

Obstetrical care providers are proficient at instituting many emergency protocols. Every staff member is aware of his or her role during typical obstetrical emergencies such as uterine rupture, eclampsia, umbilical cord prolapse, or postpartum hemorrhage. The staff roles and responsibilities during cardiopulmonary resuscitation in pregnancy should mirror those of common obstetrical emergencies. Each member of every discipline should be well aware of his or her function. Examples of staff role and responsibilities from Brigham and Women's Hospital, Boston, Massachusetts are included in Table 21-6. It is essential that all disciplines involved create a mutually agreeable maternal resuscitation protocol and all staff roles and responsibilities are remarkably clear. During maternal resuscitation, there is no time for duplication of efforts or clarification of protocols.

Prior planning is one key to success in cardiopulmonary resuscitation in pregnancy. Practice is another. Repeated rehearsal of the maternal resuscitation protocol promotes the development of an efficient code team and detects any logistical issues that may limit the efficacy of the team. Frequent mock codes on an obstetrical unit provide safe learning opportunities for the entire staff as well as increase staff exposure to code protocols. Most experts recom-

TABLE 21-6. Staff Roles and Responsibilities

Primary Nurse	• Ascertains cardiopulmonary arrest and notes time
	• **Unresponsive**
	• Calls for help
	• **A**mbu bag
	• **B**ack Board
	• **C**ode Team
	• **D**efibrillator
	• Positions patient with head of bed flat, left uterine displacement
	• **Airway**
	• Opens airway with jaw-thrust/head-tilt maneuver
	• Assesses for airway obstruction
	• **Breathing**
	• Looks, listens, and feels for breathing
	• Obtains mask-valve device (at bedside)
	• Provides two rescue breaths
	• **Circulation**
	• Assesses carotid pulse
	• Begins chest compressions
	• Initiates one-person CPR (if alone) *or* two-person CPR if other personnel in room
	• 1 (One) person CPR—15:2 ratio
	• 2 (Two) person CPR—5:1 ratio
	• Provides report to code team personnel
	• **Disconnects electronic fetal monitor prior to defibrillation**
Secretary	• Calls hospital code operator
	• States "Code Blue, OB code team, location"
	• Operator activates alphanumeric OB code team beepers
	• Private physician's patient: Also calls "Code Blue, Dr. X, location"
	• Calls blood bank to report code status
	• Code secretary identified by Nurse-In-Charge (NIC)
	• Second secretary called to nursing station to help
	• Identifies code phone—Not main extension
	• Prepares extra patient labels and lab slips
	• Code status written on lab slips
	• Communicates all lab results and phone messages to the NIC
	• Notifies Cardiac Surgery Service per Surgical Service Senior Resident
	• Calls main operating room for support personnel/equipment

Adapted from Johnson, M. D., Luppi, C. J. & Over, D. (In press). Cardiac Arrest and Resuscitation in the Parturient. In Gambling, D., & Douglas, J. Obstetric Anesthesia and Uncommon Disorders. Philadelphia: W. B. Saunders.

TABLE 21-6 continued	

Second Nurse	• Brings code cart OUTSIDE of room
	  • Obtains oral airway and ambu bag
	  • Obtains back board from code cart and assists primary nurse in placing board under the patient, maintaining LEFT UTERINE DISPLACEMENT
	• Connects ambu bag to wall oxygen at full flow
	• Calls for defibrillator
	• Assists with 2 (two)-person CPR
	  • Provides ventilations
	  • Compression to ventilation ratio 5:1
	• Becomes **Recorder** when anesthesia personnel arrive to perform endotracheal intubation and ventilation

Third Nurse	• **MANUAL LEFT UTERINE DISPLACEMENT**

Fourth Nurse	• Prepares drugs/ABG syringes/IVs at the code cart
	  • Lidocaine
	  • Epinephrine
	  • Atropine
	  • Narcan
	  • Dopamine—Never IV push, always as a drip
	• **Recorder** until Anesthesia Arrives
	• Encourages universal precautions—Face shields/goggles/gloves

Obstetrical Anesthesia Fellow	• Calls for anesthesia code cart to be brought OUTSIDE of room
	• Brings transport monitoring device to room
	  • Portable pulse oximetry/NIBP Monitoring
	• Performs endotracheal intubation ASAP
	  • Intubation kit on nursing code cart
	  • OB code intubation kit (Display 21-12) on defibrillator cart
	    • Cricothyrotomy kit
	    • Combitube
	• Provides large-volume central access
	  • Central access tray, cordis, single and triple lumen catheters on nursing code cart

Obstetrical Anesthesia Attending	**CODE TEAM LEADER**

Defibrillator Nurse	• Applies defibrillator pads and connects cable
	  • Position: to the right of the sternum below the clavicle and at the fourth intercostal space on the mid-axillary line
	  • NEVER over bone
	  • Heart is dextroverted due to pregnancy

TABLE 21-6 continued	
	• Defibrillator to be maintained with defibrillator pads and cable assembled
	• Provides rhythm strip and defibrillation capability in one step
	• Turns defibrillator ON
	• Ascertains that the machine is in the correct mode
	• Charges the defibrillator according to team leader order
	• Assists in clearing all personnel from the bed PRIOR to defibrillation
Obstetrical Attending/ Physician of Record	• Upon entry to room, ascertains time of maternal arrest
	• Dons gloves, surgical gowns
	• Opens perimortem cesarean kit and loads blades into handle
	• Calls for perimortem cesarean section at 4 (four) minutes from maternal arrest to effect delivery within 5 (five) minutes from maternal arrest (when uterine *size* is greater than or equal to 20 (twenty) weeks gestation = at umbilicus)
	• Perimortem cesarean section kit on defibrillator cart
	• Delays closure of abdomen until maternal pulse/BP is restored to ensure hemostasis
	• Saline packs
	• Clear plastic, adhesive abdominal drape
	• Continues to monitor the postpartum uterus to avoid aortocaval compression and excessive blood loss
Obstetrical Chief Resident	Same as Obstetrical Attending/Physician of Record
Neonatal ICU Attending/NICU Triage Nurse	• Provides NICU code cart, neonatal resuscitation personnel, and transport isolette
Labor and Delivery Nurse-In-Charge	• Delegates nursing responsibilities
	• Assigns nursing roles, considering critical care obstetric team resources
	• Assigns "code" unit secretary
	• Facilitates code logistics
	• Removes support person(s) and obtains personnel to assist them
	• Designates neonatal resuscitation location
	• **Provides crowd control**
	• **Provides volume control**
	• **Encourages personnel to respond to code team leader only**

TABLE 21-6 continued	
Surgical Service Senior Resident On-call & Cardiac Surgery Service	• Consider thoracotomy for direct cardiac massage per protocol • Thoracotomy kit and bypass kit on defibrillator cart • Surgical Service Resident to carry code beeper for immediate availability to perform thoracotomy • Notify Cardiac Surgery Service ASAP • Ask for call to be made to the main operating room for support personnel/equipment • Consider cardiopulmonary bypass if indicated per cardiac surgery/protocol • Sternotomy saw and nitrogen tank next to defibrillator cart

mend regular practice performance of resuscitation skills because competence decreases when skills are not used regularly (Kaye, Mancini, Rallis, & Hanel, 1989; Stross, 1983). Staff members who are unfamiliar with advanced cardiac life-support techniques are naturally apprehensive, and repeated exposure tends to demystify the events.

NURSING EDUCATION COMPONENTS/COMPETENCIES

Cardiopulmonary resuscitation (CPR) training for all nurses is required by the Joint Commission for Accreditation of Hospitals Organization; however, Advanced Cardiac Life Support (ACLS) training is not required for obstetric nurses (AWHONN, 1993). Each facility providing obstetric care should have some method of documenting regular CPR training for the staff. An example for maternal resuscitation competency validation is provided in Display 21-14.

Training should include traditional cognitive and psychomotor objectives as well as affective objectives (AHA, 1994). Didactic content may vary between institutions but should include

1. Routine American Heart Association (AHA) basic life support (BLS) content;
2. Physiologic adaptations to pregnancy pertinent to maternal resuscitation;
3. Requisite adaptations to BLS for the pregnant woman;
4. Equipment review (e.g., code cart,

defibrillator);
5. Pharmacology review of first-line resuscitation drugs;
6. Maternal resuscitation protocol review; and
7. Documentation.

Psychomotor objectives should evaluate American Heart Association recommended skills. The equipment used during practice sessions should be the same equipment used during the real emergencies (e.g., mask valve devices, ambu bags, back boards, etc.). Affective objectives should clarify the staff member's feelings and attitudes toward performing CPR. Promoting staff confidence in performing maternal resuscitation is a crucial objective during CPR training. A confident, well-trained nursing staff is essential to a successful maternal code team.

INSTITUTIONAL APPLICATION LOGISTICS

Creating a successful maternal code team begins and ends with efficient communication. All disciplines involved must be consulted from the inception. Obstetrics, Anesthesia, Nursing, Neonatology, Cardiology, Thoracic Surgery, Emergency Department, Pharmacy, Blood Bank, Communications, Chaplain, Social Service, and Security departments all have a unique expertise to contribute to the successful creation of an institution's protocol. One of the most important decisions that needs to be made by this multi-

DISPLAY 21-14

Nursing Competency Validation Form

Name _____   Date _____

Performance Guidelines	Met	Not Met

1. Ascertains cardiopulmonary arrest and notes time
2. Calls for help specifying
   - Ambu bag
   - Back board
   - Code team
   - Defibrillator
3. Positions patient with head of bed flat and maintains left uterine displacement
4. Opens airway with jaw-thrust/head tilt maneuver
5. Assesses for obvious airway obstruction
6. Looks, listens, and feels for breathing
7. Obtains mask–valve device
8. If no breathing, provides two rescue breaths
9. Assesses carotid pulse
10. If no pulse, begins chest compressions
    - 1-person CPR—15:2 ratio
    - 2-person CPR—5:1 ratio
11. After 1 minute of rescue support, check pulse
12. Verbalizes mock report to code team personnel
13. Disconnects electronic fetal monitor prior to defibrillation
14. Verbalizes code protocol
15. Verbalizes commonly used code drugs and their locations
    - Epinephrine
    - Lidocaine
    - Atropine
    - Narcan
    - Dopamine
16. Demonstrates defibrillation competency
    - Per hospital standard
17. Verbalizes location and content of documentation
    - Per hospital standard

Comments _____
_____
_____

Instructor Signature _____

disciplinary group is the identification of a consistent code team leader. Leadership skills should be practiced and perfected during training. During the resuscitation, all communication and instructions should originate with the team leader to minimize noise and confusion.

Each medical discipline will have preferences for familiar equipment that will enhance the efficiency of its team member. The importance of an efficient communication system cannot be over emphasized. The Blood Bank should be consulted to ensure rapid response for blood component replacement, and should be aware that the most common cause of maternal cardiopulmonary arrest is hemorrhage. The institution's chaplain and social workers are extremely valuable resources for the patient's family as well as the staff. The pregnant woman's family/support person(s) require careful and thoughtful support during and after the maternal code. Maternal cardiopulmonary arrest is an extremely emotional and difficult time for the entire staff, regardless of the outcome. The members of the maternal code team should be offered a private meeting to review the events of the code and to discuss the emotional impact The chaplains and social workers can be exceptionally helpful as a support group for the staff.

Once the protocol is created, it should be well disseminated to every area of the institution. Educational sessions should emphasize the unique physiologic state of the pregnant woman that mandates alternative resuscitation protocols.

CONCLUSION

Cardiopulmonary resuscitation in pregnancy is profoundly challenging for every discipline involved in the efforts to save a mother and her unborn child. The resources that are necessary to attempt resuscitation of a pregnant patient are impressive. Fortunately, we rarely have to call upon these valuable resources to help our most viable and precious patients. The rare nature of the event and the physiologic challenge of the pregnant woman require exceptional teamwork and communication, combined with a simple protocol that is well prepared and practiced.

REFERENCES

AHA. (1987). American Heart Association: Textbook of advanced cardiac life support. Dallas, TX: AHA.

AHA. (1992). American Heart Association Subcommittee on Emergency Cardiac Care: Standards and guidelines for cardiopulmonary resuscitation and emergency cardiac care. Journal of the American Medical Association. 268, 2172, 2249.

AHA. (1994). American Heart Association, Instructor Manual for Basic Life Support. Dallas, TX: American Heart Association.

Alimoff, J. K., Safar, P., & Bircher, N. (1980). Cardiac resuscitability and cerebral recovery after closed-chest, MAST augmented and open chest CPR. Anesthesiology, 53, 147–151.

Archer, G. W., & Marx, G. F. (1974). Arterial oxygen tension during apnoea in parturient women. British Journal of Anaesthesia, 46, 358–360.

AWHONN. (1993). AWHONN Position Statement, Postanesthesia Nursing for Obstetric Patients.

Babbs, C. F. (1987). Hemodynamic mechanisms in CPR: A theoretical rationale for resuscitative thoracotomy in non-traumatic cardiac arrest. Resuscitation, 15, 37–50.

Barnett, W. M., Alimoff, J. K., Paris, P.M., et al. (1986). Comparison of open-chest cardiac massage techniques in dogs. Ann Emergency Med, 15, 408.

Bayne, C. G., & Josing, W. (1984). Reversal of inadequate cardiac output and perfusion during CPR by open-chest cardiac massage. American Journal of Emergency Medicine, 1, 138.

Berg, C., Atrash, H., Koonin, L., & Tucker, M. (1996). Pregnancy-related mortality in the United States, 1987–1990. Obstetrics and Gynecology, 88(2), 161–167.

Bircher, N., & Safar, P. (1980). Comparison of standard and "new" closed-chest CPR and open-chest CPR in dogs. Critical Care Medicine, 8, 147–152.

Bouvier-Colle, M. H., Varnoux, H., Costes, P., & Hatton, F. (1991). Maternal mortality in France. Frequency and reasons for its underestimation in the statistics of medical cause of death. Group of experts on Maternal Mortality. J Gynecol Obstet Biol Reprod (Paris), 20(7), 985–991.

Bongain, A., Fuzibet, J. G., & Gillet, J. Y. (1992). Pneumocystis carinni. Two cases responsible for maternal death during pregnancy (letter). Presse Med, 21(20), 950.

Brunette, D. D., Biros, M., Mlinek, E. J., et al. (1992). American Journal of Emergency Medicine, 10, 32–33.

Burkett, G., Bandstra, E. S., Cohen, J., Steele, E., & Palow, D. (1990). Cocaine-related maternal death. American Journal of Obstetrics & Gynecology, 163,(1, Pt. 1), 40–41.

Catanzarite, V. A., Foster, E., Robinette, P., Cousins, L. M., & Schneider, J. M. (1992). Maternal death due to rupture of a low transverse cesarean section incision during labor at home. West J Med, 157(4), 454–455.

Cheek, T. C., & Samuels, P. (1996). Pregnancy-induced hypertension. In Datta, S. (Ed.), Anesthetic and obstetric management of the high-risk patient. St. Louis, MO: Mosby-Yearbook.

Chen, H. F., Lee, C. N., Huang, G. D., Hsieh, F. J., Huand, S. C., & Chen, H. Y. (1994). Delayed maternal death after perimortem cesarean section. Acta Obstetrica Gynaecoligica Scandinavica, 73(10), 839–841.

Cohen, et al. (1993). A comparison of active compression-decompression cardiopulmonary resuscitation with standard cardiopulmonary resuscitation for cardiac arrests occurring in the hospital. New England Journal of Medicine, 329, 1916–1922.

Collins, K. A., Davis, G. J., Lantz, P. E. (1994). An unusual case of maternal-fetal death due to vaginal insufflation of cocaine. American Journal of Forensic Medicine, 15(4), 335–339.

Cooper, D. R. (1964). Cardiac arrest on the myelographic tilt table. Journal of the American Medical Association, 187, 674.

Dannenberg, A. L., Carter, D. M., Lawson, H. W., Ashton, D. M., Dorfman, S. F., & Graham, E. W. (1995). Homicide and other injuries as causes of maternal death in New York City. 1987 through 1991. American Journal of Obstetrics & Gynecology, 172(5), 1557–1564.

Davies, M. G., & Harrison, J. C. (1992). Amniotic fluid embolism: Maternal mortality revisited. British Journal of Hospital Medicine, 47(10), 775–776.

De Ferrari, E., Paine, L., Gregor, C., Summers, L. & Anderson, J. (1993). Midwifery care for women with human immunodeficiency virus disease in pregnancy. Journal of Nurse-Midwifery, 38(2), 97–109.

DelGuercio, L. R. M., Feins, N. R., Cohn, J. D., et al. (1965). Comparison of blood flow during external and internal cardiac massage in man. Circulation, 32(Suppl.), 171–180.

deSwiet, M. (1994). Pulmonary disorders. In Creasy, R. K., & Resnik, R. (Eds.), Maternal-fetal medicine: Principles and practice. Philadelphia: W. B. Saunders.

Fildes, J., Reed, L., Jones, N., Martin, M., & Barrett, J. (1992). Trauma: The leading cause of maternal death. J Trauma, 32(5), 643–645.

Gelven, P. L., Gruber, K. K., Swiger, F. K., Cina, S. J., & Harley, R. A. (1996). Fatal disseminated herpes simplex in pregnancy with maternal and neonatal death. Southern Medical Journal, 89(7), 732–734.

Hadi, H. A. (1994). Maternal death after terbutraline administration (letter; comment). American Journal of Obstetrics & Gynecology, 170(4), 1208–1209.

Iriye, B. K., Asrat, T., Adashek, J. A., & Carr, M. H. (1995). Intraventricular haemorrhage and maternal brain death associated with antepartum cocaine abuse. British Journal of Obstetrics and Gynaecology, 102(1), 68–69.

Johnson, M. D., Luppi, C. J., & Over, D. (in press). Cardiopulmonary resuscitation in pregnancy. In Gambling, D. (Ed.), Obstetric anesthesia and uncommon disorders.

Joint Commission for Accreditation of Hospitals Organization. (1996). 1996 Comprehensive accreditation manual for hospitals, Standard LD.1.6, p. 293.

Kasten, G. W., & Martin, S. T. (1986). Resuscitation from bupivacaine-induced cardiovascular toxicity during partial inferior vena cava occlusion. Anesthesia and Analgesia, 65, 341–344.

Katz, V. L., Dotters, D. J., & Droegemueller, W. (1986). Perimortem cesarean delivery. Obstetrics and Gynecology, 68, 571–576.

Kaye, W., Mancini, M. F., Rallis, S. & Hanel, L. P. (1989). Education aspects: Resuscitation training and evaluation. In Kaye, W., & Bircher, N. G. (Eds.), Cardiopulmonary resuscitation. New York: Churchill Livingstone.

Kell, P. D., Barton, S. E., Smith, D. E., Nelson, M., Marwood, R. P., & Gassard, B. (1991). A maternal death caused by AIDS. Case report. British Journal of Obstetrics and Gynaecology, 98(7), 725–727.

Kuhn et al. (1981). Peripheral vs. central circulation times during CPR: A pilot study. Ann Emerg Med., 10, 417–419.

LaFave, W. R., & Scott, A. W., Jr. (1972). Criminal law (S27), St. Paul, MN: West.

Lau, G. (1994). Amniotic fluid embolism as a cause of sudden maternal death. Medical Science Law, 34(3), 213–220.

Lee, R. V., Rodgers, B. D., White, L. M., & Harvey, R. C. (1986). Cardiopulmonary resuscitation of pregnant women. American Journal of Medicine, 81, 311–318.

Linton, A. L., & Ledingham, I. M. (1966). Severe hypothermia with barbiturate intoxication. Lancet, 1, 24–26.

Longo, L. D., Hill, E. P., & Powe, G. C. (1972). Factors affecting placental oxygen transfer. In Longo, L. D., Bartels, H. (Eds.), Respiratory gas exchange and blood flow in the placenta. Bethesda, MD: Public Health Service. 345–391k (DHEW (NIH) 73-761) as quoted in Greenberger, P. A., & Patterson, R. (1985). Management of asthma in pregnancy. New England Journal of Medicine, 312, 897.

Monga, M., & Creasey, R. K. (1994). Cardiovascular and renal adaptation to pregnancy. In Creasy, R. K., & Resnik, R. (Eds.), Maternal–fetal medicine: Principles and practice. Philadephia: W. B. Saunders.

Morgan, P. J. (1995). Maternal death following epidural anesthesia for cesarean section delivery in a patient with unsuspected sepsis. Canadian Journal of Anaesthesia, 42(4), 330–334.

Myint, Y., Bailey, P. W., & Milne, E. R. (1993). Cardiorespiratory arrest following combined spinal epidural anaesthesia for cesarean section. Anaesthesia, 48(8), 684–686.

Neuman, M., Ron-El, R., Langer, R., Bukovsky, I., & Caspi, E. (1990). Maternal death caused by HELLP syndrome (with hypoglycemia) complicating mild pregnancy-induced hypertension in a twin gestation. American Journal of Obstetrics & Gynecology, 162(2), 372–373.

Pritchard, J. A., MacDonald, P. C., & Gant, N. F. (1985). Obstetrics in broad perspective. In Pritchard, J. A., et al. (Eds.), Williams obstetrics (17th ed., p. 3). New York: Appleton-Century-Crofts.

Robertson, C. (1991). The value of open chest CPR for non-traumatic cardiac arrest. Resuscitation, 22, 203–208.

Russell, E. S. (1962). Cardiac arrest: (A) Survival after two and one-half hours of open-chest cardiac massage and (B) survival after closed chest cardiac massage. Canadian Medical Association Journal, 87, 512.

Shocket, E., & Rosenblum, R. (1967). Successful open cardiac massage after 75 minutes of closed massage. Journal of the American Medical Association, 200, 333–335.

Slowey, M. J., & Piacquadio, K. M. (1994). Generalized Shwartzman reaction caused by group A beta-hemolytic streptococcus, resulting in maternal death. A case report. Journal of Reproductive Medicine, 39(7), 553–56.

Stevenson, C. S. (1969). Maternal death from puerperal sepsis following vaginal delivery. A 17-year study in Michigan, 1950–1966. American Journal of Obstetrics & Gynecology, 104(5), 699–712.

Stewart, J. S. S., Stewart, W. K., & Gillies, H. G. (1962). Cardiac arrest and acidosis. Lancet, 2, 964.

Stross, J. K. (1983). Maintaining competency in advanced cardiac life support skills. Journal of the American Medical Association, 249, 3339–3341.

Sykes, M. K., & Ahmed, N. (1963). Emergency treatment for cardiac arrest. Lancet, 2, 347–349.

Troiano, N. H. (1989). Cardiopulmonary resuscitation of the pregnant woman. Journal of Perinatal and Neonatal Nursing, 3(2), 1–13.

Vives, A., Carmona, F., Zabala, E., Fernnandez, C., Cararach, V., & Iglesias, X. (1996). Maternal brain death during pregnancy. International Journal of Gynaecology and Obstetrics, 52(1), 67–69.

Wallace, D. H., Gilstrap III, L. C. (1996). Endocrine disorders. In Datta, S. (Ed.), Anesthetic and obstetric management of the high-risk patient. St. Louis, MO: Mosby-Yearbook.

Weber, C. E. (1971). Postmortem cesarean section: Review of the literature and case reports. American Journal of Obstetrics & Gynecology, 110, 158–165.

Weinberger, S. E., Weiss, S. I., Cohen, W. R., et al. (1980). Pregnancy and the lung. American Review of Respiratory Disease, 121, 559–581.

Weiser, F. M., Adler, L. N., & Kuhn, L. A. (1962). Hemodynamic effects of closed and open chest cardiac resuscitation in normal dogs and those with acute myocardial infarction. American Journal of Cardiology, 10, 555–561.

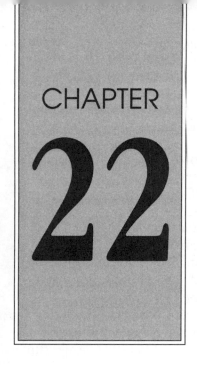

CHAPTER 22

The Chemically Dependent Pregnant Woman

Diane M. Shannon and Marykay Hill

SUPPORTIVE DATA

Incidence

Chemical substance use, abuse, and dependence among women of child-bearing age is a growing problem that presents many challenges in perinatal health care. In 1996, approximately 13 million people in the United States were using illicit drugs, meaning they had used an illicit drug in the month prior to interview (SAMHSA, 1997). In 1993, the U.S. Department of Health and Human Services reported results of the National Household Survey on Drug Abuse. Over 38 million women between the ages of 12 and 35 admitted trying illicit drugs, of which nearly 10 million admitted use in the past year (Jessup, 1997).

Rarely today do pregnant patients use only one substance. The drugs most frequently used by pregnant women are alcohol, cigarettes, marijuana, cocaine, and heroin. Although polysubstance use is a prevalent phenomenon, most studies focus on one specific substance. The Drug Abuse Warning Network reports heroin-related emergency room visits have increased substantially from 1993 to 1995. A National Household Survey on Drug Abuse proclaims a fourfold increase in heroin use between 1990 and 1995 (Kaltenbach, Berghella, & Finnegan, 1998). The 1993 survey estimated over one million women had used crack cocaine, of which over 200,000 had used it in the past year. Alcohol-related problems have been identified in

an estimated 10–50% of all individuals admitted to hospitals in the United States (Jessup, 1997).

A 36-hospital survey conducted by the National Association of Perinatal Addiction Research and Education revealed an 11% incidence of illicit "substance abuse" during pregnancy. Reported hospital rates of chemical dependence during pregnancy varied from 0.4–27% and were directly related to the thoroughness of the substance use assessment. An estimated 375,000 babies had been prenatally exposed to illegal substances, although current figures do not account for exposure to alcohol, cigarettes, over-the-counter drugs, and prescribed medications (VanBreman, 1991).

Lack of formal training in chemical dependence for perinatal healthcare providers can impede the identification process. Without a working knowledge of the addictive process and good assessment skills, healthcare professionals may lack the tools for proper identification of chemically dependent pregnant women. When these factors are taken into account, the number of pregnant women who use alcohol and other drugs is probably greater than estimated. It is important to remember that chemical dependence affects women of all ages, races, ethnic backgrounds, and socioeconomic strata.

Significance

Maternal chemical dependence has been associated with numerous medical and obstetric complications. Alcohol and other drugs used during pregnancy have adverse effects on the mother, fetus, and neonate. Maternal morbidity and mortality have been directly related to the type of drug used, timing of drug use, and the route of administration.

Alcohol

Women (and men with chronic alcoholism) have less alcohol dehydrogenase activity in the gastric mucosa than men without alcoholism. This enzyme detoxifies alcohol, so deficiency results in higher bioavailability of alcohol. Women, therefore, suffer the effects of alcohol intake at much lower doses in a shorter time span than men (Schenker & Speeg, 1990).

Alcohol is a mood-elevating, central nervous system depressant that affects every organ in the body, but the most profound effects are on the central nervous system. Areas of the brain associated with highly integrated functions are depressed, causing loss of control, disorganized thought processes, and decreased coordination. Alcohol is a respiratory depressant and also affects temperature-regulating mechanisms. Polyneuropathy, Wernicke's disease, and Korsakoff's psychosis with memory loss are potential long-term complications of alcoholism. Wernicke's syndrome consists of neurologic problems such as ataxia, nystagmus, and paralysis of certain ocular muscles. Korsakoff's syndrome consists of psychological symptoms such as severe recent memory loss, confusion, and confabulation (made-up stories to fill in gaps in memory loss).

Alcohol alters hormonal balance and carbohydrate metabolism, sometimes resulting in glucose intolerance. It also interferes with adrenocortical, adrenomedullary, thyroid, gonadal, and pituitary functioning. Hematologic abnormalities include anemia, thrombocytopenia, and sequestration of white cells in the spleen. Anemia is caused by folate deficiency and granulocytopenia from toxic effects of ethanol on bone marrow. In addition, alcoholics are vulnerable to infectious diseases and have difficulty combating them.

Cardiomyopathy may occur in patients with long-standing alcohol intake. Symptoms include shortness of breath, fatigue, palpitations, anorexia, and dependent edema. Hypertension, coronary artery disease, and cardiac dysrhythmias are also prevalent.

There is an increased incidence of esophageal cancer, and cancer of the mouth, pharynx, larynx, and liver, as well as esophageal and gastric varices, peptic ulcer disease, duodenitis, esophagitis, pancreatitis, and other pancreatic conditions. Malabsorption and alteration in intestinal motility, structural changes in the upper gastrointestinal tract, and impaired transport of glucose, amino acids, electrolytes, thiamine, vitamin B_{12}, and calcium also frequently occur.

Alcohol use is fundamentally related to nutritional status, because alcohol decreases intake of food with nutritional value. In addition, alcohol affects organ systems involved in the digestion and absorption of nutrients and produces deficiencies of folic acid, pyridoxine, thiamine, iron, zinc, and vitamins A, D, and K. Pregnant women with a zinc-deficient diet who drink alcohol have substantially impaired ability to metabolize alcohol. Therefore, for these women the risks of fetal alcohol syndrome or fetal alcohol effects may be increased (Cefalo & Moos, 1988).

Tremors resulting from alcohol withdrawal occur about 4–6 hours after the last drink ingested. Tremors may be accompanied by irritability, retching, nausea, vomiting, diaphoresis, and increased body temperature, heart rate, respirations, and blood pressure. The peak effects of minor withdrawal occur 12–24 hours after the last drink. Alcoholic hallucinosis involving a confused state in which the person misinterprets existing stimuli can occur in up to 25% of those withdrawing from alcohol. Visual or tactile misinterpretation and disorientation give rise to restlessness and sometimes fearfulness with paranoia.

Some patients may experience hallucinations with alcohol withdrawal. Auditory hallucinations usually involve voices familiar to the patient and may often be threatening and guilt producing. The patient believes the voices are real and often acts on the hallucination, which can lead to self-injury or harm to others. Although auditory hallucinations occur with alcohol withdrawal, they are more commonly associated with cocaine and benzodiazepine withdrawal. Alcoholics are more prone to visual and tactile hallucinations during withdrawal. Seizures can also accompany alcohol withdrawal and usually occur within 48 hours of the last drink. Delirium tremens is the most serious form of alcohol withdrawal. Delirium refers to heightened autonomic nervous system activity, which produces tremors, agitation, rapid pulse, and fever. DTs may occur as early as 1 or 2 days or as late as 14 days after the last drink.

Cigarettes and Marijuana

Approximately one out of every four women smoke cigarettes. Among pregnant women, the percentage who smoke ranges from 20–50% depending upon income, race, age, and educational level. Spontaneous quit rates are highest among pregnant women, with a range of 20–41% who quit smoking upon pregnancy confirmation. However, most women who smoke before pregnancy continue to smoke during and after pregnancy (Scheibmeir & O'Connell, 1997).

Smoking cigarettes decreases maternal calcium, zinc, and B vitamins and is associated with low birth weight, premature birth, placenta previa, and sudden infant death syndrome. Smoking also doubles the effects of alcohol on infant birth weight so that the patient who drinks 10 alcoholic beverages per week and does not smoke can be compared with the patient who smokes cigarettes and drinks 5 drinks per week.

Marijuana is lipophilic, readily crosses the placenta, and can be detected for up to 30 days in maternal urine. Marijuana increases maternal heart rate and blood pressure, impairs lung function, and may cause fetal hypoxia (Zuckerman, Frank, & Hingson, 1989). Marijuana smoke contains more tar than high-tar tobacco cigarettes. A psychoactive ingredient in marijuana, tetrahydrocannabinol, impairs specific intellectual and psychomotor tasks. It interferes with transfer of data to long-term memory, which impedes acquisition of knowledge. Impairment of driving ability occurs, as well as anxiety, paranoia, and loss of perspective. Local irritation of the bronchial mucous membranes leads to increased secretions, chronic bronchitis, lung inflammation, and possible degeneration. Shortening of the luteal phase of the menstrual cycle occurs, which may decrease fertility. When marijuana is discontinued, mild abstinence symptoms may include anorexia, tremors, perspiration, irritability, cramps, diarrhea, nausea, and sleep disturbances.

Cocaine

Cocaine, a powerful stimulant, is often classified as the most addicting substance. It stimulates rapid release of norepinephrine, dopamine, and epinephrine in the brain, causing a "rush." Tolerance and craving occur quickly after initial use, and dependence can occur within a few weeks. Cocaine causes vasoconstriction and activates the sympathetic nervous system, which controls numerous functions of the brain and other organs, including blood pressure, heart rate, heart muscle contractility, blood glucose level, mood, and appetite. Blood pressure increases with use, as do temperature, physical activity, and mental alertness. Tachycardia and ventricular fibrillation may occur. Rapidly increasing blood pressure may lead to aneurysms with resulting hemorrhage that is often fatal. Cocaine also precipitates grand mal seizures at relatively low doses. Long-term use can sensitize the individual to seizures at lower doses (known as "kindling"), occasionally resulting in status epilepticus. Cocaine decreases lung functioning and the ability to transport oxygen into the blood because of its powerful vasoconstrictive effects. Free-basing cocaine may lead to serious lung dysfunction after only 3 months exposure (Weiss & Mirin, 1987). Cocaine suppresses appetite and may cause weight loss and vitamin deficiency, particularly water soluble B and C vitamins, leading to malnutrition, anemia, and metabolic abnormalities. Other problems are skin infections, edema and redness related to vaginally administered cocaine, hepatitis, infection from human immunodeficiency virus, endocarditis, and burns caused by free-basing. An overdose is evidenced by irregular heart rate, ventricular tachycardia or fibrillation, cerebral hemorrhage, seizures, heat stroke, and respiratory failure. Symptoms of chronic use include nasal problems such as congestion and cold symptoms, frequent nosebleeds, ulcerations of the nose, and perforated nasal septum.

Opiates

Opiates (narcotics), such as morphine, heroin, codeine, hydromorphone (Dilaudid), oxycodone (Percodan), meperidine (Demerol), methadone (Dolophine), and propoxyphene (Darvon), produce analgesia, drowsiness, euphoria, and respiratory depression. Opiates can cause dysphoria, consisting of mild anxiety, fear, nausea, vomiting, inability to concentrate, apathy, decreased physical activity, and diminished visual acuity.

Chronic effects of narcotic dependence include decreased socialization and increased isolation, diminished libido, menstrual irregularities, and constipation. Because of ingredients frequently used to dilute narcotics for intravenous nonmedical administration, foreign substances may enter the lungs and cause acute embolic phenomenon or chronic granuloma formation. In addition, injection by unsterile methods may lead to infectious complications such as abscesses and cellulitis at the injection site, septic thrombophlebitis, hepatitis, septic arthritis, and, less commonly, tetanus, bacterial endocarditis, meningitis, and brain or spinal epidural abscesses. Acute intoxication includes varying degrees of unresponsiveness, shallow and slow respirations, miosis, bradycardia, and hypothermia. Unless treated, pupils dilate from severe cerebral hypoxia, skin becomes cyanotic, and circulation fails. Death may occur from respiratory depression and apnea.

Withdrawal syndrome is characterized by increased respiratory rate, diaphoresis, lacrimation, yawning, rhinorrhea, piloerection, tremors, anorexia, irritability, anxiety, and dilated pupils. These symptoms occur approximately 8–12 hours after the last dose is taken. Later signs occurring 24–48 hours after the last dose include insomnia, nausea, vomiting, diarrhea, weakness, abdominal cramps, tachycardia, hypertension, involuntary muscle spasms, back pain, arthralgias, and chills alternating with sweating and flushing. Symptoms gradually subside over 7–10 days. However, methadone withdrawal symptoms may last as long as 3 weeks.

Medical and obstetrical complications that occur frequently among opioid-dependent women are listed in Display 22-1.

Tranquilizers

Minor tranquilizers ("antianxiety" agents) are more similar in action to sedative hypnotics than to major tranquilizers or neuroleptics. They suppress anxiety and easily produce dependence. The two major classes of minor tranquilizers are propranedial and benzodiazepines. Meprobamate (Equanil), a propranedial, is a central nervous system depressant that sedates and tranquilizes. Effects include drowsiness, ataxia, slurred speech, weakness, fatigue, visual disturbances, syncope, and euphoria. Long-term effects include hematologic disorders, rapid eye movement suppression, and cardiac abnormalities. Acute intoxication or overdose produces stupor, coma, convulsions, and circulatory and respiratory collapse. Withdrawal can produce delirium, convulsions, tremors, ataxia, headache, and insomnia. Because of these complications, withdrawal should be medically supervised.

Diazepam (Valium) and alprazolam (Xanax) are two of the most widely prescribed and misused benzodiazepines. They are prescribed for insomnia, acute reactive anxiety, chronic anxiety, seizures, neuromuscular disorders, as a preanesthetic, and for alcohol withdrawal syndrome. Benzodiazepines increase the seizure threshold and are used as anticonvulsants. Side effects include drowsiness, ataxia, fatigue, slurred speech, and other indicators of central nervous system depression. Depending on the specific benzodiazepines abused, withdrawal symptoms begin to appear from 12–24 hours after cessation and peak within 5–8 days. If the patient is physiologically addicted, withdrawal must be initiated cautiously and under medical supervision, as respiratory arrest can occur. Overdose causes respiratory depression and stupor.

Inhalants

Inhalants such as paint thinners (toluene) and aerosols cause neurotoxicity and brain damage after chronic, long-term use (Filey, Heaton, & Rosenberg, 1990). Patients will often appear mentally slow or exhibit depressed reaction time. Inhalants are most often used in conjunction with other illicit drugs.

DISPLAY 22-1

Medical and Obstetrical Complications that Occur Frequently Among Opioid-Dependent Women

Medical Complications

Anemia	STDs
Bacteremia/septicemia	Chlamydia
Cardiac disease, especially endocarditis	Condylomata acuminatum
Cellulitis	Gonorrhea
Depression and other psychiatric disorders	Herpes
Diabetes mellitus	HIV
Edema	Syphilis
Hepatitis, acute and chronic	Tetanus
Hypertension	Tuberculosis
Phlebitis	Urinary tract infection
Pneumonia	Pyelonephritis
Poor dental hygiene	Urethritis

Obstetrical Complications

Spontaneous abortion	Placental insufficiency
Intrauterine growth restriction	Preeclampsia
Premature labor/delivery	Premature rupture of membranes
Chorioamnionitis	Abruptio placentae
Intrauterine death	Intrauterine passage of meconium
Low apgar scores	Postpartum hemorrhage
Septic thrombophlebitis	

Source: Kaltenbach, Berghella, & Finnegan (1998).

RISKS

Substance use increases maternal morbidity and mortality. The major contributing factor to death is drug overdose with cardiac or respiratory arrest. Status epilepticus may also lead to respiratory arrest and fatal cardiac arrhythmias. Acute hypertension can cause cerebral infarction and hemorrhage. Because alcohol and drugs impair fine motor coordination as well as judgment, the incidence of trauma increases substantially. It is estimated that approximately one half of all traffic accident fatalities and between 20% and 40% of all trauma treated in hospital emergency rooms are alcohol related (Roizen, 1988). This includes falls, motor vehicle accidents, gunshot wounds, blunt trauma, and other violence.

Exposure to hepatitis and human immunodeficiency virus (HIV) is greater among substance-dependent patients, especially among women who use drugs intravenously and who prostitute to buy drugs. The pregnant patient may not engage in these behaviors but may be involved or living with a partner who uses drugs and who, therefore, substantially increases her risk for exposure. Hepatitis B and hepatitis C are transmitted by parenteral and sexual contact. Hepatitis B is more prevalent in pregnancy and poses a serious risk to neonates of infected mothers. Perinatal transmission occurs commonly with hepatitis B virus in the absence of neonatal prophylaxis. Up to 90% of neonates born to chronic carrier mothers will acquire infection without such measures (ACOG, 1992). Therefore, hepatitis B immune globulin (HBIG) and hepatitis B vaccine are given to prevent hepatitis B infection and the chronic carrier state in neonates. Perinatal transmission of hepatitis C has been documented, although the risk is estimated at no more than 6% (NIH, 1997). The risk is increased if the mother is also infected with HIV. Immunoprophylaxis is currently not available for neonates of mothers with hepatitis C. In women with HIV, intravenous AZT therapy is recommended during the antepartum and intrapartum periods to reduce the risk of perinatal transmission. AZT prophylaxis antepartum (200 mg orally tid) and intrapartum (2 mg/kg IV bolus over 1 hour, then 1 mg/kg IV every hour) has shown to decreased perinatal transmission from 25 to 8% (Sperling, Shapiro, & Coombs, 1996).

In this high-risk population, routine screening is recommended for hepatitis C and HIV as well as hepatitis B. Diagnosis of hepatitis C is confirmed by identification of antibody to the virus. Hepatitis B surface antigen (HBsAg) is the first antigen to appear after infection with hepatitis B virus. HBsAg is positive in patients with acute or chronic hepatitis and indicates the ability to transmit hepatitis B to others. A person who continues to test positive for HBsAg for over six months is considered a hepatitis B carrier. Acute hepatitis B is confirmed by HBsAg and IgM antibody to the core antigen. The presence of HBeAg (e antigen) indicates a highly infectious state (ACOG, 1992).

The medical and obstetrical complications associated with drug dependence are often further complicated by financial, social, and psychological problems. These include single parenthood, poverty, homelessness or inadequate housing, lack of education, domestic violence, and sexual abuse. Many opioid-dependent women have less than a high school education and are progeny of substance-abusing parents. A majority also suffer from depression, have poor self-esteem, and have difficulty with interpersonal relationships (Kaltenbach et al., 1998).

Fetal and Neonatal Effects

Fetal dependence on drugs such as opiates can develop, leading to fetal withdrawal coinciding with maternal withdrawal. Fetal withdrawal may lead to intrauterine growth restriction, fetal demise, or preterm delivery.

The fetus of a woman using alcohol and other drugs is also at higher risk for congenital anomalies. It has been estimated that fetal alcohol syndrome affects at least 50,000 neonates each year, and 10% suffer irreversible birth defects. This preventable disorder is associated with maternal consumption of more than 4 drinks per day. However, the Seventh Special Report to the United States by the Congress on Alcohol and Health stated that no safe threshold has been identified (1990). Criteria for the diagnosis of fetal alcohol syndrome (FAS) include abnormal growth, central nervous system dysfunction, craniofacial abnormalities, and major organ system malformation. When only some of these criteria are met, a diagnosis of fetal alcohol effects (FAE) can be made.

Researchers hypothesize that the vasoconstrictive action of cocaine may cause defects in the genitourinary system, gastrointestinal tract, and neural tube, as well as cause limb reduction (VanBreman, 1991). The following malformations are most commonly seen:

Prune belly syndrome
First-degree hypospadias
Second-degree hypospadias
Hydronephrosis
Ileal atresia
Anal atresia
Neural tube defects
Missing digit three on left hand
Missing digit four on left hand

Cocaine increases the frequency of spontaneous abortions, uterine contractions, preterm labor, precipitous delivery, and abruptio placentae (Peters & Theorell, 1991). Cocaine increases blood catecholamine levels, which causes generalized vasoconstriction, decreased uteroplacental blood flow, and reduced oxygen delivery to the fetus. Cocaine exposure in utero at any time during pregnancy places the neonate at risk for permanent neurobehavioral abnormalities and impaired motor development due to effects on the developing central nervous system (Plessinger & Woods, 1993).

Infants exposed to drugs during pregnancy will experience varying degrees of withdrawal, or neonatal abstinence syndrome (NAS). The most severe reactions appear to be related to cocaine and opiates. NAS symptoms usually occur within the first 2 weeks of life, most frequently within 24–72 hours of birth. Neonatal opiate withdrawal generally peaks at 3 or 4 days of age and may last several weeks, with some symptoms persisting for up to 6 months. The signs and symptoms of NAS are listed in Display 22-2 (Finnegan & Kaltenbach, 1992).

These conditions impact the infant's ability to grow and thrive, as well as to interact and bond with family or care givers. Infants experiencing NAS related to opiate exposure who are managed with the appropriate pharmacotherapy can be maintained and detoxified within a relatively short period of time without any untoward neonatal effects (Kaltenbach, 1996). However, maternal opiate and cocaine dependence increases the risk of sudden infant death syndrome by 5–10% over the general population. (See Appendix 22-1.)

Etiology

Existing theories of the etiology of substance abuse and dependence proliferate. As early as 1942, Jellinek suggested hereditary as well as environmental causes of alcoholism (Jellinek, 1942). He observed that alcoholics with a family history of alcoholism had a poorer prognosis than alcoholics with no family history of alcoholism. The National Council on Alcoholism and the American Medical Society on Addiction Medicine in 1990 stated, "Alcoholism is a primary, chronic disease with genetic, psychosocial and environmental factors influencing its development and manifestations" (National Council, 1990). In the 1970s and 1980s, hormonal neurotransmitters were first implicated in the etiology of alcoholism, and other data suggested a deficiency of naturally produced enkephalins in the brains of alcoholics (Blum & Frachtenberg 1987; Cohen, 1988).

Personality factors have been implicated in the development of alcoholism; however, treatment research has not substantiated these theories. Nevertheless, there is evidence to indicate that personality does play an important role in chemical dependence. Three central behaviors identified among the chemically dependent population were impulsivity, failing to inhibit behavior that leads to negative consequences, and placing more value on immediate drug effects (e.g., intoxication) than on long-term consequences (e.g., liver damage). In addition, genetic factors have been implicated in certain personality traits preceding the onset of alcohol and drug problems. Many alcohol and drug

DISPLAY 22-2

Symptoms of Neonatal Abstinence Syndrome

High-pitched cry	Irritability	Inconsolability
Exaggerated reflexes	Hypertonicity	Tremors
Seizures	Elevated temperature	Mottling
Rapid heart and respiratory rates	Respiratory difficulties	Nasal stuffiness
Sneezing	Sporadic sleep patterns	Poor feeding
Excessive noneffective sucking	Gastrointestinal irritation	Regurgitation
Loose or watery stools	Skin excoriation	Sweating

treatment researchers, however, believe the behaviors are most often identifiable after the onset of dependence (Flores, 1988).

The evolution of chemical dependence in a given individual is probably a combination of biological and psychological factors, as well as environmental and social factors that serve either to increase or decrease the likelihood for alcohol and other drug dependency. Biologic influences include individual responses to drugs (i.e., sensitivity and qualitative effects). Some individuals may have inherently higher tolerance, thus placing the person at greater risk for dependence. Some of the environmental and social factors include drug availability, family and peer influences, culture, and initial experimentation or exposure.

FRAMEWORK FOR ACCEPTED THEORY

Pregnant women who use alcohol and other drugs are at high risk because of the many potential complications of alcohol and drug use. Drug abuse may include over-the-counter medications, prescription medications, alcohol, tobacco, illicit drugs, hallucinogens, inhalants and solvents. All of these substances produce mood-altering effects that impede the ability to make sound decisions and use good judgment.

Traditionally, substance abuse is defined as the use of alcohol and other drugs in a way that differs from approved medical or social practices. Addiction or dependence infers a physiologic or psychological need for the drugs, but not necessarily both. There is also an inability to stop using drugs without help. A diagnosis of chemical dependence can be made even in the absence of physiologic withdrawal symptoms.

Psychologic dependence is characterized by mental preoccupation with a drug's effects and persistent cravings for the drug. In physical dependence the body adjusts to the presence of the drug, such that uncomfortable or painful symptoms occur when the drug is no longer present (Flagler, Hughes, & Kovalesky, 1997). *Tolerance* is the body's need for higher and higher doses to achieve the same effects. *Withdrawal* is the appearance of physiological symptoms

when the drug is stopped too quickly. In the late stages of dependence, the individual may exhibit decreased tolerance or the need for lower dosages of alcohol and other drugs because of the liver's inability to clear toxins as readily. Thus, the patient has already passed the point of tolerance (i.e., needing higher and higher doses to achieve the same effects; see Figure 22-1). Characteristics of chemical dependence are directly proportional to the severity of the disease and include denial, minimizing, rationalizing, and blaming. The dependent person typically feels guilt and shame and may try to hide drug use, which leads to difficulty in obtaining an accurate history.

Physical symptoms of the disease include blackouts (i.e., periods when the individual cannot remember what happened while using drugs or alcohol), tremors, hallucinations, seizures, weight loss, poor concentration, and sometimes physical illness directly related to use (i.e., malnutrition and hepatitis). Behavioral symptoms include preoccupation with use, attempts to cut down use, and feelings of guilt about use. The user frequently becomes annoyed when others mention that dependence may be a problem, often uses drugs or alcohol when awakening just to feel normal, and has irresponsible behaviors and difficulties with authority figures (e.g., police, courts, and financial institutions). Problems with school, job, family members, relationships with significant others, and decreased spirituality usually occur.

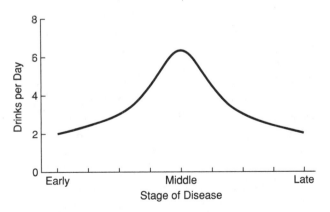

Figure 22-1. Tolerance occurs with alcohol and other drugs. It is the body's need for higher and higher doses to achieve the same effects.

Numerous myths have flourished surrounding dependence to alcohol and other drugs, which must be dispelled if the disease is to be clearly understood. Initially, these patients do not have to want help to receive help and they do not have to hit bottom before beginning recovery. A common misconception is that people dependent on alcohol and other drugs lack willpower; however, an effect of dependence is the loss of ability to abstain. With chemical dependence, one continues to use alcohol and drugs despite the negative consequences it creates. Therefore, intervening for these very needy and severely compromised patients is as appropriate as any other medical decision by the healthcare team.

Treatment

There are varied approaches for treatment of substance dependence during pregnancy. Chemical dependency programs may be designed for inpatient or outpatient treatment, with admission based on individual needs. Treatment ranges from 5 days of nonmedical detoxification in a freestanding facility, to 28–30 days of hospital-based inpatient treatment, to a comprehensive outpatient program. Inpatient treatment is usually the treatment of choice for women with no support systems, a home environment not conducive to recovery, or medical requirements that necessitate hospitalization. After treatment, referral is sometimes made to a halfway house to continue treatment in a less-structured environment but with provisions for support during recovery.

A multidisciplinary team of nurses, social workers, physicians, dieticians, spiritual counselors, and chemical dependence therapists should be available in the treatment setting. The goal of the model is to meet the physiologic, psychosocial, and chemical dependence treatment needs of the pregnant patient. Referral sites are located in major medical centers, social service agencies, and university hospital settings.

Most widely recognized treatment programs are based on the 12-step philosophy of Alcoholics Anonymous (see Table 22-1). The 12-step philosophy is based on the 12 traditions (see Table 22-2). The overall goal is to provide an intensive setting that encourages abstinence in pregnancy and supports the patient's long-

term recovery. Treatment assists the patient in understanding the disease of addiction and the impact of alcohol and other drugs on pregnancy, and explores the developmental tasks of pregnancy. The use of alcohol and other drugs interferes with the ability of the chemically dependent pregnant woman to understand the impact of substance abuse on herself and her unborn fetus. It also interferes with the developmental tasks of pregnancy, which can be described as follows:

1. Acceptance of the pregnancy.
2. Differentiation of herself from her fetus.
3. Adjustment to changes in her self-image.
4. Reflection and evaluation of her relationship with her own mother and working through these feelings.
5. Coming to terms with her dependency on others and the loss of certain freedoms.

Treatment for pregnant women will explore these tasks and help the patient understand which tasks she has accomplished and how chemical dependence has interfered in this process.

At some point, patients must realize the critical nature of their disease and become committed to recovery and to "working the program." Those who are unable to do so are usually asked to leave. Once an educational basis for participation is established and motivation is observed, patients participate in individual and group therapy. Individual therapy provides a nurturing, nonjudgmental relationship in which the patient can focus on drug use, recovery, and underlying psychopathology. Group psychotherapy provides peer support and an opportunity to work on interpersonal relationships and decreases the patient's isolation. Feedback is given in an atmosphere of caring and concern and is facilitated by a professional counselor. It is hoped that behavioral changes evolve as a result. Mandatory attendance at Alcoholics Anonymous, Narcotics Anonymous, or other 12-step meetings is required.

Group education classes provide a structured environment for understanding the impact of drug use on pregnancy, the fetus, and the newborn and acquiring parenting skills. An integral part of recovery are classes that focus on assertive-

TABLE 22-1. The Twelve Steps of Alcoholics Anonymous
1. We admitted we were powerless over alcohol—that our lives had become unmanageable.
2. Came to believe that a Power greater than ourselves could restore us to sanity.
3. Made a decision to turn our will and our lives over to the care of God as we understood Him.
4. Made a searching and fearless moral inventory of ourselves.
5. Admitted to God, ourselves, and to another human being the exact nature of our wrongs.
6. Were entirely ready to have God remove all these defects of character.
7. Humbly asked Him to remove our shortcomings.
8. Made a list of all persons we had harmed, and became willing to make amends to them all.
9. Made direct amends to such people whenever possible, except when to do so would injure them or others.
10. Continued to take personal inventory and when we were wrong, promptly admitted it.
11. Sought through prayer and meditation to improve our conscious contact with God as we understood Him, praying only for knowledge of His will for us and the power to carry that out.
12. Having had a spiritual awakening as the result of these steps, we tried to carry this message to alcoholics, and to practice these principles in all our affairs.

Source: Alcoholics Anonymous (1939). The Story of How Many Thousands of Men and Women Have Recovered from Alcoholism ("The Big Book") (3rd ed.). New York: Alcoholics Anonymous World Services, Inc.

ness, coping skills, problem solving, and conflict management.

Family therapy is also a crucial component of chemical dependence services. The family can potentially support the patient's recovery or they can interfere with her efforts to maintain abstinence. Addiction affects each family member, and therapy can help individuals to understand their roles and recognize unhealthy patterns of communication. A spiritual focus emphasizes balanced lifestyle and integration of concepts such as wholeness into daily life.

The comprehensive outpatient model provides a full range of medical and psychosocial support, the benefits of which are numerous. The model provides an integration of the patient's needs, decreases fragmentation of care, increases communication between service providers, and increases patient compliance because all services are centrally located.

Continuing chemical dependence services, also known as aftercare services, are critical because mothers dependent on alcohol and other drugs are at high risk for relapse after delivery. The return to drug use can be precipitated by the delivery, postpartum depression, adjustment to motherhood, and poor maternal–infant interactions.

Methadone Therapy

In the case of opiate dependency in pregnancy, methadone therapy is an additional facet to comprehensive service programs. It has been established that withdrawal is dangerous to the fetus and may cause distress or demise. Even medically monitored withdrawal involves risk. Therefore, it is recommended that a pregnant opiate-dependent woman be placed in the hospital for 3–4 days while stabilizing her on an appropriate methadone dose (Kaltenbach, Silverman, &

TABLE 22-2. The Twelve Traditions

One—Our common unity should come first; personal recovery depends upon AA unity.

Two— For our group purpose there is but one ultimate authority—a loving God as He may express Himself in our group conscience. Our leaders are trusted servants; they do not govern.

Three—The only requirement for AA membership is a desire to stop drinking.

Four—Each group should be autonomous except in matters affecting other groups of AA as a whole.

Five—Each group has but one primary purpose—to carry its message to the alcoholic who still suffers.

Six—An AA group ought never endorse, finance or lend the AA name to any related facility or outside enterprise, lest problems of money, power and prestige divert us from our primary purpose.

Seven—Every AA group ought to be fully self-supporting, declining outside contributions.

Eight—Alcoholics Anonymous. should remain forever nonprofessional, but our service centers may employ special workers.

Nine—Alcoholics Anonymous as such, ought never be organized; but we may create service boards or committees directly responsible to those they serve.

Ten—Alcoholics Anonymous has no opinion on outside issues; hence the AA name ought never be drawn into public controversy.

Eleven—Our public relations policy is based on attraction rather than promotion; we need always maintain personal anonymity at the level of press, radio and films.

Twelve—Anonymity is the spiritual foundation of all our Traditions, ever reminding us to place principles before personalities.

Source: Alcoholics Anonymous (1939). The Story of How Many Thousands of Men and Women Have Recovered from Alcoholism ("The Big Book") (3rd ed.). New York: Alcoholics Anonymous World Services, Inc.

Wapner, 1992). The stabilizing dose eliminates withdrawal symptoms, diminishes physiologic drug craving, and subsequently blocks the euphoric effects of illicit self-administered narcotics. A widely accepted protocol is to give an initial oral dose of 10–20 mg/day, followed by dosage adjustments based on patient responses. Additional doses of 5 mg should be given every 4–6 hours if withdrawal symptoms occur. On Day 2, the previous day's total methadone dose should be administered as the new maintenance dose (Kaltenbach et al., 1998). After stabilization and discharge from the hospital, the woman should be maintained on daily methadone to avoid withdrawal. Methadone therapy should be managed by her obstetrical team as an adjunct to prenatal care, and in cooperation with a comprehensive drug treatment program. As the pregnancy progresses, it may be necessary to increase the dosage to eliminate withdrawal due to drug dilution in an increasing fluid space and enlarging tissue reservoir, especially in the third trimester (Kaltenbach & Finnegan, 1992).

The administration of an adjustable stabilizing dose of methadone is a practice that meets with some controversy. There is concern that the amount of methadone and degree of neonatal abstinence syndrome may be related; however, this has not been established. It is clear that methadone therapy has the potential to decrease poor maternal health behaviors, decrease the incidence of obstetrical and fetal complications, prolong the pregnancy, reduce the incidence of neonatal morbidity and mortality, and creates no consequential long-term sequelae in health and development of the infant (Kaltenbach et al., 1998; Kaltenbach, 1996; Myers, Carmichael-Olson, & Kaltenbach, 1992). Therefore, in cooperation with a healthcare facility proficient in managing neonatal abstinence syndrome, and with medical and psychosocial follow-up, the infants born addicted to methadone can be safely detoxified and discharged to their families within a relatively short period of time (Kaltenbach, 1998). The ultimate goals after discharge are to facilitate and promote maintenance of maternal abstinence, enhance parenting skills and maternal–infant bonding, and consequently establish a healthier family.

Assessment

It is difficult to obtain accurate histories from patients using alcohol and other drugs because of the sensitive social nature of chemical dependence. If patients suspect reprisal from answering questions honestly, they will be less likely to respond accurately. Patients with defensive postures brought on by accusatory perinatal staff may be anxious and attempt to mask substance use. Also, recall may be inaccurate due to denial, minimizing, level of alertness, or decreased memory retention. In order to elicit the most accurate and complete information, care providers should be aware of these factors and present questions in a therapeutic, non-judgmental manner.

Some states now have reactive laws pertaining to reports of maternal drug use and the rights of unborn children that impede obtainment of accurate histories. Women may fear reprisal and conceal drug use even when they are aware their urine toxicology is being tested. Assessing the patient's compliance with other recommendations made by the healthcare team in the past may be helpful in assessing present compliance or inability to comply. If obtaining information from the patient is difficult, other resources can be utilized, such as family members who accompany the patient and phone calls to previously used healthcare agencies (with the permission of the patient).

Sources of Information for the History
Patient

Family members
Physical exam and laboratory results
Past medical history
Previously utilized healthcare agencies

Assessment of the patient begins with a medical and obstetric history. Factors associated with drug and alcohol use should alert the nurse to obtain comprehensive screening. Historical and psychosocial characteristics associated with chemical dependence are listed.

Major depressive episodes
History of marked emotional deprivation
Poor relationships with family members
Family history of alcohol or drug use
Self-induced social isolation
Reference to drug-using partner
Minimal coping and communication skills
Secrecy or vagueness
Low self-esteem
Self-destructive behavior
Mistrust of authority figures or other
   professionals
Short attention span
Excessively talkative
Late prenatal care

Factors associated with chemical dependence that may be revealed in the medical history are as follows:

Cellulitis
Hepatitis
Bacterial endocarditis
Pancreatitis
Pneumonia
Multiple drug allergies
Cirrhosis
Depression
Suicide attempt
Acute hypertension
Acquired immunodeficiency syndrome
Sexually transmitted disease
Insomnia
Anorexia
Irregular menstrual cycles or periods of
   amennorhea
Multiple physical injuries
Rape

The following factors may be exposed when taking the obstetric history and can signal chemical dependence:

Abruptio placentae
Fetal death
Low-birth-weight infant
Meconium-stained amniotic fluid
Premature labor
Premature rupture of membranes
Spontaneous abortion
Amnionitis
Preeclampsia, eclampsia
Gestational diabetes
Placental insufficiency
Septic thrombophlebitis
Sexually transmitted disease
Sudden infant death syndrome

Physical assessment is integral with the history and should begin with an assessment of the following aspects of the patient's physical appearance, which may be associated with chemical dependence:

Patient looks physically exhausted
Pupils are extremely dilated or constricted
Appearance of pregnancy fails to coincide with stated gestational age
Track marks, abscesses, or edema are visible in upper or lower extremities
Nasal mucosae are inflamed or indurated
Jaundice, pallor, or dusky skin
Lethargy, nodding, or agitation
Patient is not well oriented

The skin is examined for integrity, bruises, cellulitis, open sores, and lesions. Physical findings consistent with substance use may lead the practitioner to consider further screening for those patients who deny use. For example, the pregnant patient with middle-to-late-stage alcoholism may have facial angiomata and other skin lesions, increased blood pressure, and an enlarged liver. Past or present drug users may have thrombophlebitis or sclerosed veins on hands, arms, legs, ankles, or feet. Changes in pupillary size may be noted, or complaints of sleep difficulty, early morning awakenings, and associated feelings of anxiety and depression may be present. Lethargy, fatigue, weight loss,

perforated nasal septum (as a result of insufflated cocaine), rhinitis, congested lungs, or decreased breath sounds may be noted. In addition, cardiac arrhythmias, tender abdomen or abnormal liver size, and vaginal redness or edema (related to vaginally administered cocaine) may be observed. The following are obstetric factors related to substance use: contractions, spotting or vaginal bleeding, inactive or hyperactive fetus, poor weight gain, sexually transmitted disease, no prenatal or late prenatal care.

Elevations in liver function studies (e.g., GGTP, SGOT/AST, SGPT/ALT, LDH, MCV, and triglycerides) and decreased levels of white and red blood cell counts and platelet count may be indicative of chronic alcohol or drug use. See Display 22-3 for recommended laboratory tests for pregnant, opioid-dependent women.

To encourage patient compliance, explain that an accurate intake history of alcohol and other drug use is necessary for a clear picture of all factors affecting the pregnancy. Teaching the patient first about the damaging effects of alcohol and other drugs on the unborn child only increases the patient's sense of guilt and shame, and she may be less likely to answer honestly. Feelings of low self-esteem, guilt, and shame occur with chemical dependence. Therefore, education about drug effects on the fetus is helpful only after rapport has been established and the patient has been open about her drug use.

The educational focus should be placed on the maternal effects of drug and alcohol use. This accomplishes several goals. It encourages the patient to take care of herself and establishes the nurse's primary interest in the patient. It acknowledges her as an individual separate from her unborn child. This is important because acceptance of the unborn fetus may or may not have been consciously established.

A caring, nonjudgmental attitude should be maintained while questioning patients about substance use to facilitate rapport and increase the patient's responsiveness and honesty. Symptoms of the disease are denial, minimizing, rationalizing, and blaming; thus, open, honest answers cannot be expected immediately. Often, information must be pieced together to give a clearer picture of chemical dependence. All

DISPLAY 22-3

Recommended Laboratory Tests for Pregnant, Opioid-Dependent Women

Blood type, Rh, and indirect Coombs

Complete blood count with differential and platelets

SMA-12

Rubella titer

Serology (VDRL or RPR)

Hepatitis B surface antigen (full panel if positive)

Hepatitis C antibody

Sickle cell prep (if appropriate)

Varicella (if unsure history)

HIV (with counseling)

Blood alcohol level

Liver function tests (hepatic panel)

Tuberculin skin test (Mantoux)

Pap smear

Cervical culture for *Neisseria gonorrhoeae* and *Chlamydia*

Group B Strep vaginal–rectal culture at 35–37 weeks gestation

Urine:
    Urinalysis and microscopic
    Culture and sensitivity
    Urine toxicology

Triple screen between 15 and 21 weeks gestation (optimal 16–18 weeks)

One hour 50 gm glucose test at 24–28 weeks (at initial visit if risk factors)

Source: Kaltenbach, Berghella, & Finnegan (1998).

potential substances must be discussed during the assessment (see Table 22-3). The same question format is repeated for each chemical, and it is important to be as accurate as possible regarding amount, method, and frequency of drug use.

Ask the least invasive questions first to lower the patient's defenses and increase her comfort. It is also helpful to imply that drug use is expected. For example: "When was the last time you used a narcotic?" For many patients this would be the last time they had surgery or severe pain and used a prescription according to the physician's instructions. With this type of questioning, no judgments about substance use are made. Because cigarettes, over-the-counter drugs, prescription medications, and alcohol use are legal and socially acceptable, it is helpful to begin questioning about these substances and then proceed to illicit drugs.

Obtain information about past use first and then ask about present use. This can be accomplished by inquiring about each month of gestation beginning with the month before the last menstrual period.

1. When did you first start smoking?
2. How many cigarettes a day did you smoke at that time?
3. When did you notice an increase in your smoking?
4. At present, how many cigarettes a day do you smoke? Has this changed throughout your pregnancy?
5. Are there times when you smoke more?

Next, proceed to questions concerning over-the-counter medications. In an effort to obtain medications, "doctor shopping" occurs when the patient consults more than one physician for the same complaint. The following questions assist in identifying the practice of doctor shopping, as well as in assessing patient compliance to prescribed health practices. The same questions may be used for prescription medicines.

1. When was the last time you used an over-the-counter medication in this pregnancy?
2. Why did you use the medication?
3. Did you take it as directed or did you find taking an extra dose helped?
4. How many tablets (doses) did you take daily, weekly, and monthly?
5. What over-the-counter medications are you now taking?
6. How many different physicians are prescribing these medications for you?
7. Were these medications prescribed for you specifically?

In obtaining a history about alcohol use, the nurse must be very specific and definitive about what constitutes alcohol (e.g., beer, malt, wine, champagne, coolers, liqueurs such as Kahlua or schnapps, spirits, or mixed drinks containing hard alcohol).

1. How many drinks does it take to make you high?
2. When did you first start drinking alcohol?
3. How much did you drink at that time?
4. What alcoholic beverages did you drink then?
5. How often did you drink at that time: weekly, daily, monthly?
6. Were there times when you drank more?
7. How much are you now drinking?
8. Is this more or less than you used to drink?
9. Has anyone in your family ever had a problem with alcohol or drugs? If so, who?

Questions 1 and 8 may help determine tolerance. Most women will reply with two or fewer drinks. If they respond with more than two drinks, a higher tolerance to alcohol is indicated. If alcohol use increases over time, there is tolerance (i.e., more and more of the same is required to achieve the same effects). Patients who once were able to drink a certain amount of alcohol, but find they now tolerate less, may be experiencing progression to late-stage alcoholism.

Once alcohol use is discussed, illicit drug use should be the next topic (see Table 22-3). If the patient denies use of one drug, questioning should proceed to the next drug. Examiners must remember to be nonjudgmental and matter of fact. Because illicit drugs vary in different areas of the country, it is helpful to be familiar with the drugs particular to that community. Questioning can proceed as follows:

1. When was the first time you used cocaine?
2. Did you snort it, free-base, or use it intravenously—"shoot it"?
3. How much did you use in one day?
4. How many days of the week did you use it?
5. In this pregnancy, has your use remained the same as we have talked about?

6. If it is different, what amount are you now taking? How often? What route?

With cocaine you may have to interpret the amount used based on cost, as some women cannot tell you the amount or sometimes even the cost.

After all drugs are discussed, it is a good idea to ask, "Have you used any other drug we have not talked about?" The following four questions are helpful in determining a problem with substance use. Called the CAGE, it consists of the following:

1. **C** Have you ever tried to **C**ut down on your use?
2. **A** Have you ever been **A**nnoyed when someone mentioned that your alcohol or drug use was a problem?
3. **G** Do you ever feel **G**uilty about your use?
4. **E** Do you ever use an **E**ye opener in the morning to feel better after using the night before?

One of four positive answers indicates there might be a problem. Two of four positive is indicative of chemical dependence. The test is up to 62% reliable with all populations and, although first used to determine alcohol misuse and dependence, is also applicable to other drug use (Hays & Spickard, 1987).

A similar but longer instrument, the Michigan Alcoholism Screening Test, has been studied and applied extensively. It is a 24-item questionnaire requiring yes-no responses that correctly identifies 87–95% of the population (see Table 22-4) (Hays & Spickard, 1987).

Nursing Diagnoses

- Potential for sensory-perceptual alterations related to intoxication or withdrawal manifested by maternal drug dependence (e.g., alcohol, cocaine, opiates, and sedative-hypnotics)
- Anxiety related to indefinite outcome of newborn
- Potential for impaired skin and tissue integrity related to maternal intravenous drug dependence as manifested by

TABLE 22-3. Potential Substances of Abuse

Psychoactive Substances *with* Known-Dependence Liability

Central Nervous System Depressants

Alcohol

Minor tranquilizers

Atarax	Serax
Ativan	Softran
Donnatol	Valium
Equanil (meprobamate, Miltown, Milpath)	Vistaril
Librax	Xanax
Librium	

Hypnotic sedatives and barbiturates

Ambar	Nytol
Amytal	Paraldehyde
Chloral hydrate	Pentothal
Compoz	Phenobarbital
Dalmane	Placidyl
Doriden	Quaalude (Sopor)
Luminal	Seconal
Mebaral	Sleep-Ez
Nembutal	Sominex
Noludar	Tuinal

Cough medicine and other alcohol-based medication

Antihistamines—cold medications

Central Nervous System Stimulants

Benzedrine (Bennies)	Dexamyl	Nicotine
Caffeine	Dexaspan	Preludin
Cocaine (crack, snow, blow, free-base)	Dexedrine	Ritalin
	Methamphetamine (crystal meth, ice, crank)	Tenuate
Desbutal		
Desoxyn	Methedrine	

Analgesics

Narcotic		*Nonnarcotic*	
Codeine	Nisentil	Aspirin	Mydol
Demerol	Pantopon	Cope	Phenaphen
Dilaudid	Paregoric	Darvon	Ponstel
Heroin	Princdol	Emperin compound	Soma
Levo-Dromoran	Talwin	Equagesic	Vanquish
Lomotil		Excedrin	
Methadone		Florinal	
Morphine			

TABLE 22-3. continued

Hallucinogens

DMT—Dimethyltryptamine
Ecstasy
LSD—Lysergic acid diethylamide
MDA—Methylenedioxyamphetamine
Mescaline
Morning glory seeds
Peyote
Psilocin
Psilocybin
STP (DOM)—2,5-Dimethoxy-4-methylamphetamine

THC-Tetrahydrocannabinol

Marijuana
Hashish

Muscle Relaxants

Psychoactive Substances *without* Known-Dependence Liability

Major Tranquilizers

Compazine	Stelazine
Haldol	Taractan
Mellaril	Thorazine
Pacatal	Trilafon
Sparine	Vesprin

Antidepressants

Aventyl	Parnate
Elavil	Sinequan
Lithium	Tofranil
Morpramin	Triavil
Nardil	Vivactil

---

evidence of cellulitis and thrombosis of veins

- Potential for altered health maintenance related to maternal drug dependence is manifested by spontaneous abortion, abruptio placentae, precipitous delivery, nonreassuring fetal heart pattern, gestational diabetes, preeclampsia, and other medical complications
- Potential for infections related to maternal intravenous drug use and multiple sexual contacts as manifested by sexually transmitted diseases, human immunodeficiency virus, and premature rupture of membranes

- Pain related to maternal tolerance to narcotics secondary to chemical dependence
- Potential for ineffective coping related to guilt regarding maternal drug use as manifested by increased anxiety and defensive behaviors
- Knowledge deficit regarding impact of drug use during pregnancy related to lack of knowledge regarding drug use in pregnancy
- Poor prenatal care related to noncompliance
- Potential for impaired parenting ability

TABLE 22-4. Michigan Alcoholism Screening Test		

Carefully read each statement and decide whether your answer is yes or no. Please give the best answer or the answer that is right most of the time. Circle the appropriate response.

Circle Yes or No

1. Do you feel you are a normal drinker? (By normal we mean you drink less than or as much as most other people.) — Yes No
2. Have you ever awakened the morning after some drinking the night before and found that you could not remember a part of the evening? — Yes No
3. Does your wife, husband, a parent, or other relative ever worry or complain about your drinking? — Yes No
4. Can you stop drinking without a struggle after one or two drinks? — Yes No
5. Do you ever feel guilty about your drinking? — Yes No
6. Do friends or relatives think you are a normal drinker? — Yes No
7. Are you able to stop drinking when you want to? — Yes No
8. Have you ever attended a meeting of Alcoholics Anonymous? — Yes No
9. Have you ever gotten into physical fights when drinking? — Yes No
10. Has drinking ever created problems between you and your wife, husband, a parent, or other near relative? — Yes No
11. Has your wife, husband, a parent, or other near relative ever gone to anyone for help about your drinking? — Yes No
12. Have you ever lost friends because of your drinking? — Yes No
13. Have you ever been in trouble at work because of your drinking? — Yes No
14. Have you ever lost a job because of drinking? — Yes No
15. Have you ever neglected your obligations, your family or work for two or more days in a row because you were drinking? — Yes No
16. Do you drink before noon fairly often? — Yes No
17. Have you ever been told you have liver trouble? (Cirrhosis?) — Yes No
18. After heavy drinking have you ever had delirium tremens (DTs) or severe shaking or heard or seen things that weren't really there? — Yes No
19. Have you ever gone to anyone for help about your drinking? — Yes No
20. Have you ever been in a hospital because of drinking? — Yes No
21. Have you ever been a patient in a psychiatric hospital or on a psychiatric ward of a general hospital where drinking was part of the problem that resulted in hospitalization? — Yes No
22. Have you ever been seen at a psychiatric or mental health clinic or gone to any doctor, social worker, or clergyman or help with any emotional problem, where drinking was part of the problem? — Yes No
23. Have you ever been arrested for drunken driving under the influence of alcoholic beverages? — Yes No
24. Have you ever been arrested, even for a few hours, because of other drunken behaviors? — Yes No

---

TABLE 22-4. continued

MAST Scoring Key

Item

1.	Yes—0	No—2	13.	Yes—2	No—0
2.	Yes—2	No—0	14.	Yes—2	No—0
3.	Yes—1	No—0	15.	Yes—2	No—0
4.	Yes—0	No—2	16.	Yes—1	No—0
5.	Yes—1	No—2	17.	Yes—2	No—0
6.	Yes—0	No—2	18.	Yes—2	No—0
7.	Yes—0	No—2	19.	Yes—5	No—0
8.	Yes—5	No—0	20.	Yes—5	No—0
9.	Yes—1	No—0	21.	Yes—2	No—0
10.	Yes—2	No—0	22.	Yes—2	No—0
11.	Yes—2	No—0	23.	Yes—2	No—0
12.	Yes—2	No—0	24.	Yes—2	No—0

Total possible: 53 points

Score: 0–4 nonalcoholic; 5–6 suggestive of alcoholism; 7 or more definite alcoholism.

Positive response to 8, 19, or 20 considered diagnostic.

THEORETICAL BASIS FOR THE PLAN OF NURSING CARE AND INTERVENTION

The patient who is both pregnant and chemically dependent often experiences a heightened sense of anxiety as labor begins and often fears that analgesia or anesthesia will be withheld. This fear of potential pain and increased anxiety may lead to self-medication with alcohol or drugs at the time of labor. The use of illicit drugs at the onset of labor may prolong the latent phase until the drugs are cleared, and progression into active labor may then occur. Pain medications should never be withheld because a pregnant patient is chemically dependent; instead regional anesthetics (epidural or pudendal block) are generally recommended. It is important to obtain blood alcohol and urine toxicology on all patients suspected of chemical use to assess level of intoxication and rule out the presence of other drugs.

Alcohol

The intoxicated intrapartum patient with a history of heavy alcohol use will be likely to have established tolerance and should be closely monitored for withdrawal symptoms. Vital signs are monitored regularly. Injury during intoxication (e.g., falls, burns, and other accidents) is possible, thus patient safety is an important nursing activity. Symptoms of alcohol intoxication include slurred speech, increased blood pressure, rapid pulse, increased respirations, constricted pupils, and lethargy or hyperactivity.

Alcohol overdose is characterized by various levels of anesthesia and decreased central nervous system, cardiac, and respiratory functioning. Pupils may be slowly reactive and at midpoint with depressed tendon and pain reflexes. Cardiac arrhythmias may be present, and lungs may be congested. Nursing management includes establishing an airway, assessing frequent vital signs, evaluating cardiovascular status, controlling shock, establishing a means of measuring urinary output, frequently making neurologic assessments, and maintaining adequate intravenous intake. If the patient is alert, oriented, and can take oral fluids, electrolyte solutions such as Gatorade should be encouraged, unless the patient is on a sodium-restricted diet. In addition, vitamin and thiamine supplements are usually administered to patients with chronic alcoholism.

The patient experiencing alcohol withdrawal may have any of the following symptoms: anxiety; increased blood pressure, pulse, respirations, temperature; tremors; nausea; vomiting; diarrhea; decreased appetite; sleep disturbance; poor proprioception; auditory, visual, or tactile hallucinations; and a decreased ability to distinguish reality from fantasy. The patient in withdrawal should be assessed at least hourly until vital signs are stable and symptoms have subsided (see Table 22-5). The usual drug of choice for alcohol withdrawal is diazepam. Maternal vital signs and fetal heart rate are assessed each hour prior to administration of additional doses of diazepam. If the patient is stuporous or if the fetal heart rate is nonreassuring, diazepam is withheld. Diazepam loading is effective because of its long half-life (20–50 hours), which provides tapering of blood levels and ensures smooth withdrawal, increased patient comfort, and decreased anxiety. Patients should be restrained only if absolutely necessary.

Opiates

Nursing management of the opiate-addicted woman should include thorough assessment of vital signs, neurological status, level of intoxication or withdrawal, illicit drug use, and medication history within the past 24 hours; symptoms or history of recent physical or sexual abuse, injury, or infection; assessment and assistance with psychosocial support; and assessment of fetal well-being by activity history and fetal heart rate monitoring.

The patient experiencing opiate intoxication may have constricted pupils and lethargy. Withdrawal symptoms include dilated pupils, rhinorrhea, lacrimation, piloerection, nausea and vomiting, diarrhea, yawning, abdominal cramps, and restlessness. Sclerotic veins may necessitate insertion of a central intravenous line for vascular access. Extreme caution should be taken in handling blood and body fluids because of the increased risk of human immunodeficiency virus and hepatitis in these patients.

The patient experiencing opiate withdrawal may require methadone. If the patient is already receiving methadone maintenance, the last administered dose must be confirmed. If the mother experiences withdrawal, the fetus may become hyperactive and also experience withdrawal. A urine toxicology will confirm opiate use as well as the presence of polydrug use. With opiate-dependent patients, it is important to avoid administration of butorphanol (Stadol), pentazocine (Talwin), and other narcotic antagonists for pain management as these drugs will precipitate withdrawal and increase risk of harm to mother and fetus.

Methadone Therapy

For women receiving methadone therapy, it should be established that the usual daily dose has been administered; or the dose should be given during the intrapartum period to avoid the onset of withdrawal (Kaltenbach et al., 1998). Signs and symptoms of opiate withdrawal include various degrees and combinations of the following: musculoskeletal pain, especially leg and back cramps; abdominal pain, anorexia, nausea, vomiting or diarrhea; agitation and aggression; dilated pupils, lacrimation, rhinorrhea, and yawning; nonreassuring fetal heart pattern. Because many of these symptoms also occur with labor, patient history and subjective statements must be seriously considered and lab evaluations obtained as soon as possible. If the patient is not on methadone or the dose cannot be verified, and the patient appears to be withdrawing from opiates, a methadone dose of 10–20 mg can be given orally or intramuscularly. Analgesia and anesthesia can be administered in conjunction with methadone and are managed as in nonaddicted women, with the exception of narcotic antagonists (such as Stadol and Talwin) and narcotics with mixed agonist–antagonist properties (Kaltenbach et al., 1998). Patients who have used illicit drugs intravenously may have sclerotic veins, abscesses, or cellulitis, creating difficulty in obtaining venous access. A central intravenous line may be required for emergency or intrapartal care.

Cocaine

The patient experiencing cocaine intoxication may have increased blood pressure, rapid pulse, increased respirations, dilated pupils, elevated

TABLE 22-5. Clinical Institute Withdrawal Scale for Alcohol

Temperature (per axilla)
1. 98.7–99-5
2. 99.5–100.4
3. Greater than 100.4

Pulse (beats per minute)
1. 90–95
2. 95–100
3. 100–105
4. 105–110
5. 110–120
6. Greater than 120

Respiration Rate (inspirations per minute)
1. 20–24
2. Greater than 24

Blood Pressure (diastolic)
1. 95–100 mm Hg
2. 100–103 mm Hg
3. 103–106 mm Hg
4. 106–109 mm Hg
5. 109–112 mm Hg
6. Greater than 112 mm Hg

Nausea and Vomiting: Ask "Do you feel sick to your stomach? Have you vomited?" (Observation)
0. No nausea and no vomiting
2. Mild nausea with no vomiting
4. Intermittent nausea with dry heaves
6. Constant nausea, dry heaves and vomiting

Tremor: Arms extended and fingers spread apart. (Observation)
0. No tremor
2. Not visible, but can be felt fingertip to fingertip
4. Moderate with patient's arms extended
6. Severe, even with arms not extended

Paroxysmal Sweats (Observation)
0. No sweat visible
2. Barely perceptible sweating, palms moist
4. Beads of sweat obvious on forehead
6. Drenching sweats

Tactile Disturbances: Ask "Have you any itching, pins and needles sensations, any burning, any numbness, or do you feel bugs crawling on or under your skin?" (Observation)
0. None
2. Mild itching, pins and needles, burning, or numbness
4. Intermittent tactile hallucinations (i.e., bugs crawling)
6. Continuous tactile hallucinations

TABLE 22-5. continued

Auditory Disturbances: Ask "Are you more aware of sounds around you? Are they harsh? Do they frighten you? Are you hearing anything that is disturbing to you? Are you hearing things you know are not there?" (Observation)
0. Not present
2. Mild harshness or ability to frighten (increased sensitivity)
4. Intermittent auditory hallucinations (appears to hear things you cannot)
6. Continues auditory hallucinations (shouting, talking to unseen persons)

Visual Disturbance: Ask "Does the light appear to be too bright? Is its color different? Does it hurt your eyes? Are you seeing anything that is disturbing to you? Are you seeing things you know are not there?" (Observation)
0. Not present
2. Mild sensitivity (bothered by lights)
4. Intermittent visual hallucinations (occasionally sees things you cannot)
6. Continuous visual hallucinations (seeing things constantly)

Hallucinations: Ask "Are you hallucinating?" (Observation)
0. None
1. Auditory, tactile or visual only
2. Nonfused auditory and visual
3. Fused auditory and visual

Clouding of Sensorium: Ask "What day is this?" "Where are you?" "Who am I?"
0. Oriented
2. Disoriented for date by no more than 2 calendar days
3. Disoriented for date by more than 2 calendar days
4. Disoriented for place and/or person. Reorient to time, place, and person, if necessary

Quality of Contact (Observation)
0. In contact with examiner
2. Seems in contact, but is unaware or oblivious to environment
4. Periodically appears to become detached
6. Makes no contact with examiner

Anxiety: Ask "Do you feel nervous?" (Observation)
0. No anxiety. At ease
2. Appears anxious
4. Moderately anxious, or guarded
6. Overt anxiety (equal to panic)

Agitation (Observation)
0. Normal activity
2. Somewhat more than normal activity
4. Moderately fidgety and restless
6. Paces back and forth during most of the interview, or constantly thrashes about

Thought Disturbances (Flight of Ideas) (Observation)
0. No disturbance
2. Does not have much control over nature of thoughts
4. Plagued by unpleasant thoughts continuously
6. Thoughts come quickly and in disconnected fashion

Convulsion (Observation) In progress notes, note duration, extent, and type.
0. No   6.   Yes

TABLE 22-5. continued

Headache, Fullness in Head: Ask "Does your head feel different?" "Does it feel like there is a band around your head?" Do not rate for dizziness or light-headedness. Otherwise, rate severity.
   0. Not present
   2. Mild
   4. Moderately severe
   6. Severe

Flushing of Face (Observation)
   0. None
   1. Mild to moderate
   2. Severe

Total CIWA Score _____

Rater _____

Clinical Observations Related to Detox (i.e., evaluate mental status including mood, thought processes, perceptions, cognitive functions.)

Treatment Protocol

Assessments will be done on admission and every 4 hours (while awake) by the nurse for the first 48 hours. If the CIWA score at any time is greater than 10, the assessment will be done every 2 hours and if greater than 15, assessments will be done every hour. Treatment will be instituted if the CIWA score is greater than 15 on two consecutive occasions or above 20 once. The treatment will be diazepam 20 mg p.o. × 1, then 10 mg every hour until the score falls to 10 or less on two occasions. (The physician may instead elect to administer hourly doses of 20 mg until the CIWA score falls to 10 or less if clinically indicated.)

Source: Sellers, E. The Addiction Research Foundation, Toronto, Canada.

temperature, hyperactivity, and tremors. Cocaine acts as a central nervous stimulant and causes stimulation of the pregnant uterus and vasoconstriction of placental and uterine vessels. The complications seen in the intrapartum period are abruptio placentae, precipitous delivery, preterm labor, and premature rupture of membranes. There may be fetal hyperactivity, meconium-stained amniotic fluid, and fetal intolerance to labor as evident by nonreassuring fetal heart patterns. Medications are not usually given to assist in detoxification of cocaine.

Tranquilizers and Barbiturates

Use of benzodiazepines such as diazepam, alprazolam (Xanax), and oxazepam (Serax) and barbiturates such as thiopental (Pentothal), pentobarbital (Nembutal), along with other barbiturate-like drugs such as methaqualone (Quaalude), ethchlorvynol (Placidyl), and chloral hydrate (Noctec), cause central nervous system depressive symptoms in the intoxicated patient. These drugs are frequently used in combination with other substances. The patient may have slurred speech, drowsiness, ataxia, weakness, fatigue, visual disturbances, syncope, and euphoria. Occasionally in withdrawal, hallucinations may be present.

Many women also use hypnotics or antianxiety drugs, and complications include accidental or deliberate overdose. The toxic reaction develops over a period of several hours, and the patient may or may not have evidence of recent drug ingestion. This usually occurs when the patient mixes depressants together (such as alcohol and hypnotics). A confused organic state may occur, and more of the same drugs may be inadvertently taken. Heart rates of the mother and fetus should be monitored closely. The patient should also be closely observed to prevent injury or accidents and should be restrained only if necessary. Evidence of withdrawal includes hyperactivity, anxiety, seizure activity, confusion, disorientation, and hallucinations. If the patient exhibits any seizure activity, behavior that would require restraint, or becomes disoriented, phenobarbital is generally administered (see Table 22-6). This drug is highly effective in the management of withdrawal from barbiturates and other hyposedatives and is practical and safe. Loading involves hourly administration of 120 mg of phenobarbital to accomplish several goals, including patient comfort and sedation; prevention of seizures or respiratory arrest; and patient's orientation to time, place, and person. It is similar to the diazepam load described earlier for alcohol withdrawal and is equally efficient as it produces smooth withdrawal because of a long drug half-life. Often chemically dependent patients require high doses of drugs for detoxification as a result of tolerance and a phenomenon known as "cross-tolerance." Cross-tolerance is exhibited when the pregnant patient who is dependent on one substance can ingest other drugs in unusually high doses without appearing to be overdosed.

Toxic overdose, withdrawal, and temporary psychosis are the most common acute problems seen in patients who use central nervous system depressants. Naloxone (Narcan), a narcotic antagonist, is not effective in the treatment of central nervous system depressant overdose. Symptoms of overdose include abnormal vital signs, confusion, impaired memory, disorientation, and potentially, coma. The patient should be closely observed, and drug administration should be avoided.

COMMON EMERGENCIES RELATED TO SUBSTANCE USE

Acute physical symptoms may obscure immediate identification of the patient who is either in withdrawal or overdosed from drugs and alcohol. Table 22-6 lists some acute emergencies where substance use may be suspected.

When a patient has an acute emergency, a urine drug screen and blood alcohol level should be ordered immediately. If the patient is alert and oriented, an attempt to obtain an alcohol and drug history should be made. The potential for acute life-threatening illness mandates that care be managed on a unit that provides intensive perinatal nursing. For all emergency admissions where overdose or severe withdrawal is present, an intravenous line should be established and the patient placed on cardiorespiratory and fetal monitoring.

Treatment and Follow-Up

All efforts should be made to address alcohol and drug use while the patient is still in the hospital. Consultation with an alcohol and drug treatment professional is warranted, and hospitals with an inpatient alcohol and drug treatment facility can usually provide in-house consultations. If there is no hospital-based treatment program for chemical dependency, consultation may be sought from a local treatment facility while the patient is still hospitalized. The patient should be assessed by a chemical dependency counselor who will conduct a thorough history and recommend referral resources or treatment depending on the patient's medical and psychosocial situation.

If admission on the inpatient antepartum unit is planned, education of the patient regarding effects of substance use on her health and that of the fetus should be implemented. Once delivered, treatment options become limited because of child care issues and many patients will be less compliant with treatment suggestions. If inpatient or outpatient treatment is recommended but the patient declines, other resources for assessment, referral, and home health care should be planned.

A proactive approach to the chemically dependent woman using alcohol and other drugs is more effective than a reactive approach and will facilitate better communication and an understanding by the patient that the healthcare team is most concerned about her welfare.

EXPECTED OUTCOMES

Maternal Stability

The patient will do the following:

1. Demonstrate decreased signs of intoxication from polydrug use as evidenced by stable vital signs and mental status

---

TABLE 22-6. Phenobarbital Loading Guidelines

Use for hypnosedatives, short-acting benzodiazepines (Halcion, Xanax) or barbiturate withdrawal. Individualize for each patient. Draw blood levels and urine drug screen on admission to establish baseline.

Withdrawal symptoms (subjective):
1. anxiety, apprehension
2. insomnia
3. visual hallucinations (severe)
4. tactile hallucinations (severe) (sense of insects on skin)

Withdrawal Symptoms (objective):
1. course tremor (mainly hands and fingers)
2. anorexia, nausea cnd vomiting
3. tachycardia
4. increased B.P. and orthostasis on standing
5. diaphoresis
6. increased temperature
7. hyperreflexia
8. fasiculations (muscle twitching)

Patients in suspected withdrawal should be assessed and vital signs obtained hourly for the above symptoms.

At the first sign of **two or more signs or symptoms** (one must be objective) physician should be notified and phenobarbital load should be instituted:

120–240 mg p.o. first cose (1.8–2.4 mg/kg) **then** 120 mg p.o. q 1 hr is given until patient is intoxicated and displays at least **two** of the following symptoms:
1. patient is asleep and arousable
2. ataxic
3. dysarthric
4. nystagmus and constricted pupils
5. labile mood

Patient should continue to be observed and vital signs recorded hourly during phenobarbital load. Hold for pulse <60, systolic blood pressure <90, or diastolic blood pressure <60, respirations <12. Phenobarbital blood level should be measured exactly 8 hours after the load has been stopped.

---

2. Avoid opiate withdrawal after methadone administration as evidenced by absence of signs and symptoms of withdrawal
3. Identify anxiety and verbalize concerns for well-being of the newborn
4. Identify causes of obstetric complications and the need for drug abstinence
5. Demonstrate knowledge of risk factors associated with potential for infection (e.g., human immunodeficiency virus, sexually transmitted diseases, and hepatitis)
6. Verbalize that others validate existence of pain and will relate a decrease in pain after relief measures have been initiated
7. Verbalize guilt feelings regarding alcohol or drug use and demonstrate a decrease in anxiety and defensive behaviors
8. Verbalize a need for abstinence and chemical dependence treatment

Fetal Well-Being

The fetus will do the following:

- Remain stable as evidenced by normal fetal activity, baseline heart rate within normal limits (i.e., 110–160 beats per minute) and reassuring fetal heart patterns

REFERENCES

ACOG. (1992). Hepatitis in pregnancy. Technical Bulletin 174.

Alcoholics Anonymous. (1939). The story of how many thousands of men and women have recovered from alcoholism ("The Big Book") (3rd ed.). New York: Alcoholics Anonymous World Services.

Blum, K., & Frachtenberg, M. (1987). New insight into the causes of alcoholism. Profess Couns, 433.

Cefalo, R. C., & Moos, M. K. (1988). Preconceptional health promotion. Rockville, MD: Aspen.

Chasnoff, I. J. (1989). Drugs and women: Establishing a standard of care. Ann NY Acad Sci, 562, 203.

Cohen, S. (1988). The chemical brain: The neurochemistry of addictive disorders. MN: CompCare Publishers.

Denber, H. C. (1979). Clinical psychopharmacology. New York: Stratton Intercontinental Medical Book.

Filey, C. M., Heaton, R. K., & Rosenberg, N. L. (1990). White matter dementia in chronic toluene abuse. Neurology, 40, 532.

Finnegan, L. P., & Kaltenbach, K. (1992). Neonatal abstinence syndrome. In R. Hoekelman & N. Nelson (Eds.), Primary pediatrics care (2nd ed., pp. 1367–1378). St. Louis, MO: Mosby Yearbook.

Finnegan, L. P. (1978). Drug dependence in pregnancy: Clinical management of mother and child. National Institute of Drug Abuse, Service Research Monograph Series. Rockville, MD: U.S. Government Printing Office.

Flagler, S., Hughes, T., & Kovalesky, A. (1997). Toward an understanding of addiction. JOGNN, 26(4), 441–448.

Flores, P. (1988). Group psychotherapy with addicted populations. New York: Haworth Press.

Hays, J. T., & Spickard, W. A. (1987). Alcoholism: Early diagnosis and intervention. J Gen Intern Med, 2, 424.

Jellinek, E. M. (1942). Alcohol addiction and chronic alcoholism. Research Council on Problems of Alcohol, Scientific Committee. New Haven: Yale University Press.

Jessup, M. (1997). Addiction in women: Prevalence, profiles, and meaning JOGNN, 26(4).

Kaltenbach, K., Berghella, V., & Finnegan, L. (1998). Opioid dependence during pregnancy: Effects and management. OB/GYN Clinics of North America, 25(1), 139–151.

Kaltenbach, K., Silverman, N. & Wapner, R. (1992). Methadone maintenance during pregnancy. State Methadone Maintenance Treatment Guidelines. Center for Substance Abuse Treatment, U.S. Department of Health and Human Services, Public Health Service, S.A.M.S.H.A.

Kaltenbach, K. (1996). Exposure to opiates: Behavioral outcomes in preschool and school aged children. NIDA Research Monograph, 164.

Kaltenbach, K., & Finnegan, L. P. (1992). Methadone maintenance during pregnancy: Implications of perinatal and developmental outcome. In T. Sonderegger (Ed.), Perinatal substance abuse: Research findings and clinical implications (pp. 239–253). Baltimore: Johns Hopkins University Press.

Kaltenbach, K., & Finnegan, L. P. (1992). Prenatal opiate exposure: Physical, neurobehavioral, and developmental effects. In M. Miller (Ed.), Development of the central nervous system: Effects of alcohol and opiates (pp. 37–46). New York: Wiley-Liss.

Martin, P. R., Bhushaw, K. M., Whiteside, E. A., & Sellers, E. M. (1979). Intravenous phenobarbital therapy in barbiturate and other hyposedative reactions: A kinetic approach. Clin Pharmacol Therapeut, 26, 256.

Myers, B., Carmichael-Olson, H., & Kaltenbach, K. (1992). Cocaine exposed infants: Myths and misunderstandings. Zero-to-Three. National Center for Clinical Infant Programs, 13(1).

National Council on Alcoholism and the American Medical Society on Addiction Medicine Editorial. (1990). The disease of alcoholism. Part VIII: Is alcoholism really a disease? Med/Scientif Advis, 5(4), 7.

NIH. (1997). NIH Consensus Statement. Management of Hepatitis C. Bethesda, MD: National Institutes of Health.

Pastorek, J. (1993). The ABCs of hepatitis in pregnancy. Clinical Obstetrics and Gynecology, 36(4), 843–853.

Pasquale, P., (1993). Pregnancy and smoking: The unrecognized addiction. Journal of Perinatal Education, 2(2), 15–19.

Peters, H., & Theorell, C. (1991). Fetal and neonatal effects of maternal cocaine use. JOGNN, 20(2), 121–126.

Plessinger, M., & Woods, J. (1993). Maternal, placental, and fetal pathophysiology of cocaine exposure during pregnancy. Clinical Obstetrics and Gynecology, 36(2), 267–276.

Roizen, J. (1988). Alcohol and trauma. In N. Giesbrecht, R. Gonzales, M. Grant, et al. (Eds.), Drinking and casualties: Accidents, poisonings and violence in an international perspective. London: Routledge.

SAMHSA (Substance Abuse and Mental Health Services Administration) Dept. of Health and Human Services (1997). Preliminary results from the 1996 National Household Survey on Drug Abuse. Rockville, MD: SAMHSA.

Scheibmeir, M., & O'Connell, K. (1997). In harm's way: Childbearing women and nicotine. JOGNN, 26(4), 477–483.

Schenker, S., & Speeg, K. V. (1990). The risk of alcohol intake in men and women: All may not be equal. New England Journal of Medicine, 322(2), 127.

Silverman, N. (1997). Current recommendations on hepatitis C in pregnancy. Contemporary Obstetrics and Gynecology, 42, 106–122.

Sperling, R., Shapiro, D., & Coombs, W. (1996). Maternal viral load, zidovudine treatment and the risk of transmission of human immunodeficiency virus type I from mother to infant. New England Journal of Medicine, 335(22), 1621–1629.

VanBremen, J. (1991). A first national hospital incidence study. Perinat Addict Res Ed Update, 4.

Weiss, R. D., & Mirin, S. M. (1987). Cocaine. Washington, DC: Psychiatric Press.

Zuckerman, B., Frank, D. A., Hingson, R., et al. (1989). Effects of maternal marijuana and cocaine use on fetal growth. New England Journal of Medicine, 320, 762.

Appendix 22-1

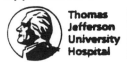

Thomas Jefferson University Hospital

Neonatal Abstinence Score

Evaluator should place a number next to each sign or symptom observed at various time intervals, then add scores for total score.

Complete or imprint with Address-O-Plate

	Date:			Daily Weight						
System	Signs and Symptoms	Score	AM			PM				Comments
Central Nervous System Disturbances	Excessive High Pitched (other) Cry	2								
	Continuous High Pitched (other) Cry	3								
	Sleeps < 1 hour after feeding	3								
	Sleeps < 2 hours after feeding	2								
	Sleeps < 3 hours after feeding	1								
	Hyperactive Moro reflex	2								
	Markedly Hyperactive Moro reflex	3								
	Mild Tremors Disturbed	1								
	Moderate-Severe Tremors Disturbed	2								
	Mild Tremors Undisturbed	3								
	Moderate-Severe Tremors Undisturbed	4								
	Increased Muscle Tone	2								
	Excoriation (specific areas)	1								
	Myoclonic Jerks	3								
	Generalized Convulsions	5								
Metabolic/Vasomotor/Respiratory Disturbances	Sweating	1								
	Fever < 101 (99–100.8F/37.2–38.2C)	1								
	Fever > 101 (38.4C and higher)	2								
	Frequent Yawning (> 3–4 times/interval)	1								
	Mottling	1								
	Nasal Stuffiness	1								
	Sneezing (> 3–4 times/interval)	1								
	Nasal Flaring	2								
	Respiratory Rate > 60/min.	1								
	RR > 60/min. with Retractions	2								
Gastro-Intestinal Disturbances	Excessive Sucking	1								
	Poor Feeding	2								
	Regurgitation	2								
	Projectile Vomiting	3								
	Loose Stools	2								
	Watery Stools	3								
	Total Score									
	Initials of Scorer									

Initials	Signature		Initials	Signature

*Finnegan, L. P. "Neonatal Abstinence Syndrome: Assessment and Pharmacotherapy," Neonatal Therapy: An Update, Rubatelli, F. F. and Granati, B. (eds.) Excerpta Medica, Amsterdam–New York–Oxford, 1986.

Thomas Jefferson
UNIVERSITY HOSPITAL
Department of Nursing
Neonatal Abstinence Syndrome Protocol

Objective: To assess for and quantify neonatal narcotic withdrawal. To be used in determining appropriate treatment and response to that treatment.

Equipment Available: NAS score sheet

Steps in Procedure

1. Determine if there is a history of maternal drug abuse.

2. Obtain results of infant's admission urine drug screen.

3. Assess infant for signs of withdrawal 2 hours after birth and then every 4 hours. Use NAS score sheet as assessment tool.

4. If score is 8 or greater, scoring should be performed every 2 hours and continued at least 24 hours. A physician should be alerted if pharmacotherapy is indicated.

5. NAS scoring may be discontinued if infant does not require pharmacotherapy by 72 hours of age.

6. For the infant on pharmacotherapy: monitor for control and/or overtreatment.

7. Assist physician in obtaining any lab specimens required as NAS can mimic other medical conditions such as hypoglycemia, hypocalcemia, sepsis.

Points to be Emphasized

1. To aid in early recognition of NAS.

2. Cocaine and heroin metabolites are recoverable in urine two to seven days after last maternal drug use.

3. NAS score sheet provides objective tool to measure extent of neonatal withdrawal symptoms.

4. If score is 8 or greater three consecutive times, or the average of three consecutive scores is 8, pharmacotherapy may be started by the physician.

6. When control or over treatment is achieved, detoxification can begin.

Pharmacotherapy

1. Administer prescribed medications as ordered by physician.

   a. Phenobarbital: most effective against multiple substance abuse.

      Loading dose—20 mg/kg/dose: increase 10 mg/kg/dose until control achieved.

      Maintenance—5–8 mg/kg/day × 3–4 days

      Detox by—3 mg/kg/day until level is less than 15 and discontinue

   b. Paregoric

      Loading dose—.8 ml/kg/day in 6 divided doses. If symptoms continue, increase dose by .4 ml/kg/day until control is achieved.

      Maintenance—same dose for 72 hours

      Detox—by decreasing dose 10% daily

      Discontinue when dose reaches 0.5 mg/kg/day.

1a. To control symptomatology of withdrawal.

Phenobarbital level may be indicated.

PART

IV

Clinical Care Guidelines

Guidelines for the Initial Assessment and Triage of Obstetric Patients

I. **Policy**—Qualified personnel collaboratively provide care for patients during the initial assessment/triage of obstetric patients.

II. **Generic Guidelines**—Assessment of all patients arriving on the Perinatal Service will include:
- Maternal physical status
- Fetal status
- Labor status
- Psychosocial needs
- Review of prenatal records
- Patient interview
  - Further assessment parameters will be directed by patient's chief complaint and information gathered during the generic data collection. Triage guidelines for frequently seen chief complaints are outlined following the generic guidelines.

A. Maternal Status
   1. Patient's chief complaint or description of symptoms
   2. Date and time of arrival
   3. Gravida and parity (gravida, term, preterm, abortions, living)
   4. Vital signs
   5. Estimated date of delivery (EDD) determined by dates, ultrasound
   6. Estimated gestational age
   7. Vaginal bleeding including date, time, duration, associated events
   8. Pregnancy risk factors
   9. Current medications
   10. Allergies

B. Fetal Status
   1. Fetal movement (as applicable)
   2. Fetal heart rate obtained by auscultation or electronic fetal monitor (as applicable)

C. Labor Status
   1. Uterine contractions including date and time of onset
   2. Membrane status including date and time of rupture, color of amniotic fluid

D. Psychosocial Needs
   Assessment may include but is not limited to:
   1. Significant stress
   2. Relationship problems
   3. Economic problems
   4. Education level and needs
   5. Support systems
   6. Cultural and religious needs
   7. Substance use

III. **Guidelines for the Evaluation of Labor**

A. Maternal Physical Status—see generic guidelines

B. Fetal Status
   1. Obtain a 20-minute fetal monitor strip to evaluate baseline and presence or absence of periodic patterns (see *Guidelines for Fetal Monitoring*).
   2. Assess fetal presentation.

C. Labor Status
   1. Review prenatal record for information regarding last cervical exam.
   2. Palpate abdomen for tenderness, uterine contractions, and resting tone.

3. If no history of prematurity, rupture of membranes, vaginal bleeding, or placenta previa proceed with digital cervical examination to include dilation, effacement, position, and consistency.
4. Encourage patient to ambulate following reassuring monitor strip.
5. Repeat cervical exam (e.g., in approximately 1 hour) to assess for change.

D. Patient/Family Teaching
1. Signs/symptoms of labor
2. Fetal movement awareness
3. Follow-up appointment with care provider

IV. **Guidelines for the Evaluation of Preterm Labor**

A. Maternal Physical Status
Further information to be obtained during patient interview includes:
1. Change in vaginal discharge
2. Backache
3. Symptoms of urinary tract infection
4. Precipitating events
5. Symptoms of dehydration

B. Fetal Status
1. If gestational age is < 24 weeks gestation, auscultate fetal heart rate.
2. If gestational age is ≥ 24 weeks gestation, obtain 20-minute fetal monitor strip to evaluate baseline rate and periodic patterns (see *Guidelines for Fetal Heart Rate Monitoring*).
3. Assess fetal presentation.

C. Labor Status
1. Review prenatal history for information regarding previous cervical exams and prescribed measures for preterm labor.
2. Palpate abdomen for tenderness, uterine resting tone, and uterine contractions.
3. Obtain monitor strip for uterine contraction assessment.

D. Patient/Family Teaching
1. Signs and symptoms of preterm labor
2. Precipitating events
3. Interventions
4. Fetal movement awareness
5. Follow-up appointment with care provider

V. **Guidelines for the Evaluation of Vaginal Bleeding**

A. Maternal Physical Status

1. Further information to be obtained in patient interview includes:
   a. onset and amount of bleeding
   b. previous episodes of bleeding
   c. precipitating events
2. Review prenatal record to obtain information regarding most recent ultrasound report (location of placenta) and previous cervical exam.
3. Assist physician with sterile speculum exam to determine origin of bleeding.

B. Fetal Status
1. If gestational age is < 24 weeks, auscultate fetal heart rate.
2. If gestational age is ≥ 24 weeks, obtain 20-minute fetal monitor strip to evaluate for baseline rate and periodic patterns (see *Guidelines for Fetal Heart Rate Monitoring*).

C. Labor Status
1. Palpate abdomen for tenderness, uterine contractions, and resting tone.

D. Patient/Family Teaching (may include but is not limited to)
1. Signs and symptoms of preterm/term labor
2. Fetal movement awareness

VI. **Guidelines for the Evaluation of Ruptured Membranes**

A. Maternal Physical Status
1. Interview patient regarding:
   a. time of suspected rupture of membranes
   b. description of fluid (color, odor)
   c. volume of fluid

B. Fetal Status
1. If low risk, not ruptured, reporting normal fetal movement, auscultate fetal heart rate.
2. If high risk and/or reporting decreased fetal movement, obtain 20-minute fetal monitor strip to assess baseline and periodic patterns.

C. Labor Status
1. Palpate abdomen for tenderness, uterine contractions, and resting tone.
2. Refer to labor guidelines if applicable.

D. Patient/Family Teaching
1. Signs/symptoms of preterm/term labor
2. Fetal movement awareness
3. Signs of ruptured membranes
4. Follow-up appointment with care provider

VII. **Guidelines for the Evaluation of Decreased Fetal Movement**

A. Maternal Physical Status
  *See generic guidelines for assessment of maternal physical status.

B. Fetal Status
  1. If gestational age < 24 weeks, auscultate fetal heart rate.
  2. If gestational age ≥ 24 weeks, assess for fetal reassurance (see *Guidelines for Fetal Monitoring*).

C. Labor Status
  *Refer to labor guidelines if applicable.

D. Patient/Family Teaching
  1. Fetal movement awareness
  2. Follow-up appointment with care provider

VIII. **Guidelines for the Evaluation of Pre-eclampsia**

A. Maternal Physical Status
  1. Interview patient regarding:
    a. previous blood pressure problems
    b. presence of subjective symptoms including headache, vision changes, right upper quadrant pain, nausea, heartburn
  2. Review medical record for the following information:
    a. initial blood pressure (first trimester)
    b. previously ordered interventions to manage blood pressure
  3. Assess patient for edema and proteinuria

B. Fetal Status
  1. If gestational age is < 24 weeks gestation, auscultate fetal heart rate.
  2. If gestational age is ≥ 24 weeks gestation, obtain 20-minute monitor strip to evaluate baseline and periodic patterns.

C. Labor Status
  *Refer to labor guidelines if applicable.

D. Patient/Family Teaching
  1. Signs/symptoms of labor
  2. Fetal movement awareness
  3. Sign/symptoms of preeclampsia
  4. Interventions
  5. Follow-up appointment with care provider

IX. **Guidelines for the Evaluation of Urinary Tract Infections**

A. Maternal Physical Status

  1. Interview patient regarding:
    a. onset of symptoms
    b. type of symptoms
  2. Review prenatal record for:
    a. history of UTIs
    b. suppression therapy
  3. Assess for suprapubic discomfort, abdominal tenderness, CVA tenderness

B. Fetal Status
  *See generic guidelines

C. Labor Status
  *Refer to labor guidelines as indicated.

D. Patient/Family Teaching
  1. Interventions
  2. Medications
  3. Fetal movement awareness
  4. Follow-up appointment with care provider

X. **Guidelines for the Evaluation of Nausea, Vomiting, Diarrhea**

A. Maternal Physical Status
  1. Interview patient regarding:
    a. onset of symptoms
    b. type of symptoms
    c. nutritional intake
    d. precipitating events
    e. characteristics of stools if complaint includes diarrhea
  2. Assess for signs/symptoms of dehydration including:
    a. dry mucous membranes
    b. urine volume, color, and clarity
    c. maternal temperature
    d. maternal tachycardia
  3. Administer clear liquid diet
  4. If unable to tolerate clear liquid diet, consider antiemetic and/or antidiarrheal agent

B. Fetal Status
  1. If gestational age is < 24 weeks, auscultate fetal heart rate.
  2. If gestational age is ≥ 24 weeks, obtain 20-minute fetal monitor strip to evaluate baseline rate and periodic patterns. Fetal tachycardia may be related to maternal dehydration.
  3. Refer to *Guidelines for Fetal Heart Rate Monitoring*.

C. Labor Status
  *Obtain a 20-minute monitor strip to assess for uterine contractions

D. Patient/Family Teaching
1. Symptoms of dehydration
2. Clear liquid diet advancing as tolerated
3. Medications
4. Fetal movement awareness

XI. **Documentation**

A. Nursing assessment findings, interventions, and plan of care.

B. Obstetrical Triage/Admission Record should include parameters assessed.

XII. **Nursing Implications**
Notify physician for the following:

- Significant system assessment findings
- BP > 140/90 or < 80/40
- Sustained maternal heart rate > 120 or < 60
- Respiratory rate > 26 or < 14
- Temperature > 100.4
- Fetal heart rate abnormalities
- Labor status

XIII. **References**

AWHONN. (1998). Standards for Professional Nursing Practice in the Care of Women and Newborns (5th ed.).

American Academy of Pediatrics and the American College of Obstetricians and Gynecologists. (1997). Guidelines for Perinatal Care (4th ed.).

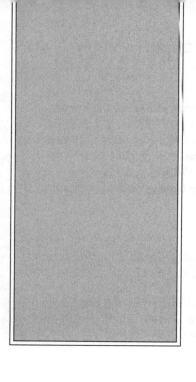

Guidelines for Fetal Heart Rate Monitoring

I. **Methods of Assessment**

A. Auscultation—generally involves intermittent assessment of the fetal heart rate (FHR), and may be accomplished by doppler ultrasound (US) transducer, or fetascope. The FHR is auscultated for a full 60 seconds and the rate is counted in beats per minute (BPM). If the patient is in labor, the FHR is auscultated before, during, and after a uterine contraction at the appropriate time intervals.

B. Electronic Fetal Monitoring (EFM) may be accomplished by the following two methods:
1. External appliances
   a. Ultrasound transducer permits evaluation of baseline FHR and the presence or absence of periodic patterns.
   b. Tocodynamometer permits evaluation of uterine contraction (UC) frequency and approximate duration. Intensity of the UC and resting tone must be estimated by abdominal palpation.
2. Internal appliances
   a. Fetal ECG electrode (FECG) permits evaluation of FHR baseline, fetal heart rate variability (FHRV), and presence or absence of periodic patterns.
   b. Intrauterine pressure catheter (IUPC) permits evaluation of contraction frequency, intensity, duration, and uterine resting tone. Uterine activity can be quantified by calculation of Montevideo units (MVU). See Glossary. Research

indicates that 180–240 MVUs produce normal progression along labor curves.

II. **Assessment Parameters**

A. Auscultation
1. FHR assessment includes the following:
   a. Rate in beats per minute
   b. Presence/Absence of audible decelerations or accelerations
2. Uterine activity assessment may be completed at the time of FHR assessment and includes palpation of frequency, duration, and intensity of uterine contractions, along with palpation of uterine resting tone.

B. EFM—during intermittent or continuous EFM, the following parameters are assessed:
1. FHR
   a. Baseline rate expressed as a range
   b. Baseline variability
   c. Presence/Absence or periodic patterns (accelerations or decelerations)
2. Uterine activity
   a. Frequency, duration, and intensity of uterine contractions
   b. Uterine resting tone

III. **Interpretation of Data**

A. Auscultation
1. Reassuring FHR responses include a normal baseline between 110 and 160 bpm, presence of audible accelerations, and absence of audible decelerations.

2. Nonreassuring FHR responses include either of the following:
   a. Abnormal baseline rate
   b. Audible decelerations

B. EFM
1. Reassuring FHR responses include:
   a. External US transducer
      – baseline rate between 110–160 bpm
      – accelerations along the baseline (accelerations defined by gestational age—see Glossary)
   b. Internal FECG electrode
      – baseline rate between 110–160 bpm
      – minimal or greater baseline variability
2. Reassuring FHR responses with need for follow-up include:
   a. External US transducer
      – accelerations along the baseline with an abnormal baseline rate or presence of variable or late decelerations
   b. Internal FECG electrode
      – minimal or greater baseline variability with an abnormal baseline rate or presence of variable or late decelerations
3. Nonreassuring FHR responses include:
   a. External US transducer
      – absence of accelerations along the baseline with evidence suggestive of decreased baseline variability, presence of decelerations, or abnormal baseline rate
   b. Internal FECG electrode
      – absent FHRV with abnormal baseline rate and/or presence of decelerations

IV. **Interventions**

A. Auscultation
1. Reassuring FHR responses—continue assessment at appropriate intervals.
2. Nonreassuring FHR responses—initiate EFM. Further interventions are dependent upon subsequent assessment, diagnosis, gestational age of the fetus, and maternal status.

B. EFM
1. Reassuring FHR responses—continue assessment at appropriate intervals.
2. Reassuring FHR responses with need for follow-up: initiate interventions as described below and notify the physician.

a. Late decelerations with minimal or greater baseline variability
   – lateral positioning
   – oxygen administration by face mask at 10 L/minute
   – 500 cc intravenous crystalloid bolus may be ordered
   – decrease or discontinue oxytocin if hypertonus is suspected
b. Variable decelerations with minimal or greater baseline variability
   – assessment for prolapsed umbilical cord
   – amnioinfusion may be ordered
3. Nonreassuring FHR responses—initiate interventions as described below and notify physician.
   a. Late and variable decelerations with absent baseline variability
      – lateral positioning
      – oxygen administration by face mask at 10 L/minute
      – 500 cc intravenous crystalloid bolus may be ordered
      – discontinue oxytocin infusion
      – fetal stimulation may be performed to elicit an acceleration by fetal scalp stimulation (see Glossary) or fetal acoustic stimulation (see Appendix)
   b. Prolonged decelerations—result from a variety of maternal and fetal conditions. Care should be taken to identify the causative factor leading to the prolonged deceleration in order to initiate appropriate treatment. Possible causes include:

   Maternal hypotension
   – assess maternal blood pressure every 2–3 minutes until stable
   – place patient in lateral recumbent position
   – administer oxygen by tight face mask at 10 L/minute
   – notify physician
   – prep for delivery as indicated

   Cord prolapse, rapid cervical change, sudden fetal descent
   – perform cervical examination for cord prolapse, rapid cervical change, or sudden fetal descent

– notify anesthesia and obstetric MD for imminent delivery if indicated
– prep for delivery as indicated

Uterine hypertonus
– assess uterine tone for evidence of abruption
– decrease or discontinue oxytocin if hypertonus is present
– Terbutaline .25 mg IV to bedside
– prep for delivery as indicated

V. **Procedure for Antepartum Testing**

A. Nonstress Test (NST)
1. "Reactive" implies at least two accelerations of the FHR are seen within a 20-minute period. The accelerations must increase in rate by at least 15 bpm and last 15 seconds from increase to return to baseline.
2. "Nonreactive" implies the above criteria have not been met.

B. Contraction Stress Test (CST)
1. "Negative" implies no late decelerations are seen and contractions lasting between 40–60 seconds are occurring at least every 3 minutes over a 10-minute period.
2. "Suspicious" implies at least one late deceleration occurs.
3. "Positive" implies late decelerations are present with 50% or more contractions.

VI. **Nursing Implications**

Notify physician for the following:
– Significant system findings
– BP > 140/90 or < 80/40
– Sustained maternal heart rate > 120 or < 60
– Maternal temperature > 100.4
– Imminent delivery
– Cord prolapse
– Nonreassuring fetal status

VII. **Patient/Family Education**

– Plan of care
– Unit routine
– Method of fetal monitoring

VIII. **References**

ACOG Technical Bulletin. (1994). Antipartum fetal surveillance (No. 188).

ACOG Technical Bulletin. (1995, July). FHR patterns: Monitoring, interpretation and management (No. 207).

AWHONN. (1991). Nursing practice competencies and educational guidelines: Antepartum fetal surveillance and intrapartum fetal heart monitoring (2nd ed.).

AWHONN. (1998). Standards for the nursing care of women and newborns (4th ed.).

NAACOG. (1992). Nursing responsibilities in implementing intrapartum fetal monitoring. Position Statement.

NICHD. (1997). Electronic Fetal Heart Rate Monitoring: Research Guidelines for Interpretation. JOGNN, 26(6), 635–640.

VIV. **Glossary**

Acceleration (accel): a visually apparent abrupt increase (defined as onset of acceleration to peak in < 30 seconds) in FHR above the baseline. The increase is calculated from the most recently determined portion of the baseline. The acme is ≥ 15 bpm above the baseline, and the acceleration lasts ≥ 15 seconds and < 2 minutes from the onset to return to baseline. Before 32 weeks of gestation, accelerations are defined as having an acme ≥ 10 bpm above baseline, and a duration of ≥ 10 seconds. Prolonged acceleration is of duration ≥ 2 minutes and < 10 minutes. Accelerations of ≥ 10 minutes in duration is a baseline change.

Artifact: false fetal or maternal data printed on the tracing.

Baseline (FHRB): the approximate range of FHR rounded to increments of 5 bpm during a 10-minute segment, excluding periodic or episodic changes, periods of marked FHR variability or segments of the baseline that differ by > 25 bpm. In any 10-minute window the minimum baseline duration must be at least 2 minutes, otherwise the baseline for that period is indeterminate.

Baseline Fetal Heart Rate Variability (FHRV): fluctuations in the baseline FHR of two cycles per minute or greater. The fluctuations are irregular in amplitude and frequency, and are visually quantitated as the amplitude of the peak-to-trough in bpm as follows:
• Amplitude range undetectable
– absent FHR variability
• Amplitude range > undetectable ≤ 5 bpm

- minimal FHR variability
- Amplitude range 6–25 bpm
  - moderate FHR variability
- Amplitude range > 25 bpm
  - marked FHR variability

Bradycardia: fetal heart rate baseline less than 110 bpm for at least 10 minutes (some fetuses have a normal baseline rate of 100–110 bpm).

Contraction Stress Test (CST): antepartum surveillance method using induced or spontaneous contractions to evaluate fetal response. A negative test implies no late decelerations are seen. A suspicious test implies at least one late deceleration is seen. A positive test implies that lates are seen with 50% or more contractions occurring in a 10-minute period.

Early Deceleration (early): a visually apparent gradual decrease (defined as onset of deceleration to nadir ≥ 30 seconds) with return to baseline FHR by the end of a uterine contraction. The decrease is determined from the most recently determined portion of the baseline. The nadir of the deceleration occurs at the same time as the peak of the contraction.

Electronic Fetal Monitoring (EFM): instrument used to show graphically and continuously the relationship between maternal uterine activity and FHR.

Fetal ECG Electrode (FECG): a bipolar terminal that detects the difference in voltage between the fetal presenting part and vaginal wall of the mother.

Fetal Heart Rate (FHR): generally refers to the rate in beats per minute.

Intrauterine Pressure Catheter (IUPC): a fluid-filled or transducer-tipped catheter inserted transvaginally into the uterus. Intrauterine pressure is conducted through the catheter, exerted on a diaphragm and transformed to an electronic signal, then printed on the tracing.

Late Deceleration (late): a visually apparent gradual decrease (defined as onset of deceleration to nadir ≥ 30 seconds) and return to baseline FHR after a uterine contraction. The decrease is determined from the most recently determined portion of the baseline. The deceleration is delayed in timing, with the nadir of the decel-eration usually occurring after the peak of the contraction.

Montevideo Units (MVUs): the sum total in mm Hg of the strength of all contractions occurring during a 10-minute period, excluding uterine resting tone. IUPC is required. The strength of each uterine contraction in mm Hg is totaled over 10 minutes then resting tone between each contraction is subtracted.

Non-Stress Test (NST): antepartum surveillance method used to evaluate fetal condition and placental function in a stable state. A reactive result implies that at least two accelerations of the FHR are seen within a 20-minute period. A nonreactive (NR) test does not meet the above criteria.

Overshoots: accelerations occurring immediately after the deceleration. The acceleration has a smooth, blunted, and more prolonged increase and return to baseline and is usually accompanied by absent baseline variability.

Oxytocin Challenge Test (OCT): a CST that is conducted by stimulation of uterine contractions with intravenous oxytocin. Sometimes used symon with the term "Contraction Stress Test."

Periodic Pattern: FHR changes, either accelerations or decelerations, from the baseline lasting less than 10 minutes.

Prolonged Deceleration: a visually apparent decrease in FHR at least 15 bpm below the baseline, lasting ≥ 2 minutes but usually < 10 minutes from onset to return to baseline.

Shoulders: accelerations occurring immediately before or after the deceleration, the accelerations have a rapid increase and return to baseline and are associated with selective compression of the umbilical vein.

Tachycardia: baseline FHR greater than 160 bpm lasting for 10 minutes or longer.

Tocotransducer (toco): an external device used to measure uterine activity.

Transducer: various devices that convert mechanical energy into electrical energy.

Uterine Contractions (UC): periodic increase in intrauterine pressure. When externally palpated, uterine contractions may be classified as mild, moderate, or strong.

Uterine Resting Tone: baseline intrauterine pressure measured via an IUPC between UC's. Average resting tone is 5–15 mm Hg. When externally palpated, uterine resting tone may be classified as relaxed or nonrelaxed.

Variable Deceleration (variable): visually apparent abrupt decrease (defined as onset of deceleration to beginning of nadir < 30 seconds) in FHR below the baseline. The decrease in FHR (below the baseline) is at least 15 bpm below the baseline, lasting ≥ 15 seconds and ≤ 2 minutes from onset to return to baseline. The timing of onset and return to baseline in relation to the contraction is variable.

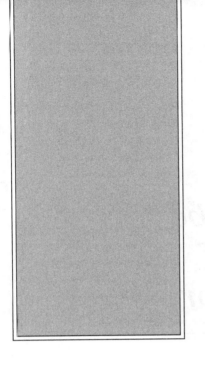

Guidelines for Use of Fetal Acoustic Stimulation

Fetal acoustic stimulation (FAS) used as an adjunct for the assessment of fetal condition in both the antepartum and intrapartum periods has received much attention in the obstetric literature. Available data clearly suggest clinical utility. Listed below are guidelines for use of FAS.

I. **Fetal Acoustic Stimulation May Be Applied in the Following Situations:**

    A. Antepartum Testing

        1. Acoustic stimulation is accomplished after 10 minutes of established FHR baseline and only if the test is not reactive.

        2. The NST is read as reactive if two FHR accelerations occur in a 20-minute window. The NST may also be read as reactive if a single prolonged acceleration occurs following acoustic stimulation. Additionally, the test can end on a prolonged acceleration without return to baseline as long as the baseline can be determined from the preceding test segment.

        3. Expected benefits include:

           a. decreased testing time

           b. a decrease in false nonreactive tests and fewer follow-up tests (biophysical profile, contraction stress test) required.

    B. Intrapartum Fetal Surveillance

        1. Nonreassuring FHR patterns are not uniformly associated with fetal acidemia, but further clarification of fetal condition is warranted.

        2. Spontaneous or stimulus-evoked FHR accelerations, such as those stimulated by FAS, are considered to be a reliable indicator of fetal well-being. Fetal acoustic stimulation provides a rapid, easily performed, noninvasive means for eliciting FHR accelerations.

        3. Current data suggest that a reactive response to FAS (FHR acceleration) is associated with a fetal pH > 7.20. Approximately 50% of fetuses who do not exhibit accelerations will be associated with fetal acidemia.

        4. Expected benefits:

           a. rapid, easily performed, noninvasive yet effective adjunctive method of determining intrapartum fetal well-being

           b. decrease in number of scalp pH assessments and cervical exams for the purpose of scalp stimulation

II. **Equipment and Technique**

    A. Acoustic stimulation may be accomplished with an AT&T fetal acoustic stimulator.

    B. The acoustic stimulator is to be placed on the maternal abdomen over the fetal vertex and stimulus applied for < 3 seconds. The stimulus may be repeated at 1-minute intervals for a maximum of three attempts.

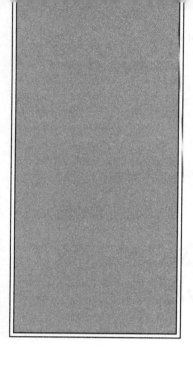

Guidelines for the Management of Patients in Labor

I. **Initial Assessment—See** *Guidelines for the Initial Assessment and Triage of Obstetric Patients*

II. **Maternal Physical Status**

A. Vital Signs
1. Low-Risk Patients—Blood pressure, pulse, and respirations are assessed and recorded every 1 hour during the first stage of labor and every 30 minutes during the second stage of labor.
2. High-Risk Patients—Blood pressure, pulse, and respirations are assessed and recorded every 30 minutes during the first stage of labor and every 15 minutes during the second stage of labor.
3. Temperature is taken every 4 hours if membranes are intact, every 2 hours if membranes are ruptured.

B. Nutrition
1. Patients in early labor may have clear liquids. Patients in active labor are restricted to ice chips and small sips of water.
2. Measure and record intake and output following placement of intravenous catheter.
3. IV access may be initiated with an 18–20 gauge heparin lock or IV fluids such as D5LR or LR infused.
4. The nurse may initiate a 500–1000 cc bolus of crystalloid fluid immediately prior to anticipated epidural anesthesia.

C. Elimination
1. Assess urinary output.
2. Encourage voiding every 2–3 hours.
3. Assess for bladder distention every 2 hours following fluid bolus or after epidural anesthesia.
4. Patients with bladder distention or who are unable to void may be catheterized.
5. Enema prn or per patient request.

D. Hygiene
1. Oral hygiene prn.
2. Personal hygiene—bed, bath, or self care performed prn and at least every 24 hours.
3. Perineal care prn.

E. Activity
1. Following initial assessment, low risk patients with reassuring fetal status may ambulate. Patients in active labor should be instructed to return every 30 minutes to assess and document fetal heart rate (see *Guidelines for Fetal Heart Rate Monitoring*).
2. Laboring patients receiving $MgSO_4$, have neuromuscular blockaid from epidural anesthesia, have received narcotic analgesics, or have altered level of consciousness should be on strict bed rest.
3. All patients should be instructed and encouraged to avoid supine positioning to prevent venal caval syndrome when in bed.

F. Lab Data
 1. Hematocrit and type and screen should be obtained on all laboring patients.
 2. Consider CBC with differential, Beta-Strep test, and urinalysis with culture and sensitivity on patients with preterm labor and premature rupture of membranes.

III. **Labor Status**

A. Uterine Activity
 1. Assess and document the frequency, duration, and intensity of contractions every 30 minutes for low-risk patients and every 15 minutes for high-risk patients.
 2. Palpate maternal abdomen for uterine resting tone and uterine contraction intensity with the use of external toco-transducer monitoring device.
 3. Quantify uterine resting tone and uterine contraction intensity in mm Hg with the use of an internal uterine pressure catheter (IUPC).
 4. When inducing or augmenting labor with pitocin or cytotec refer to the *Guidelines for the Management of Patients Requiring Induction/Augmentation of Labor.*
 5. Refer to the *Guidelines for Fetal Heart Rate Monitoring* for guidelines for the interpretation of the electronic fetal monitor tracing and nursing intervention related to uterine activity.

B. Amniotic Membranes
 1. Assess the patient for rupture of membranes (ROM).
 2. If ROM occurs, document amount, nature (clear, bloody, meconium, malodorous), and fetal heart rate at time of rupture.

C. Cervical Status
 1. The registered nurse may perform a cervical exam to check dilation, effacement, consistency as well as fetal station and fetal presentation except in the presence of abnormal vaginal bleeding or a known placenta previa.
 2. Assess for vaginal bleeding. Note time, amount, and characteristics when applicable.
 3. Limit number of cervical exams when membranes are ruptured unless delivery is imminent to decrease possibility of infection.

D. Precipitous Delivery—In the event of precipitous delivery, the registered nurse will call for assistance then provide supportive measures during delivery of the infant and reduce trauma to the infant and mother until the arrival of a physician.

IV. **Fetal Status**

A. Low-Risk Patients—Assess fetal status every 30 minutes in the first stage of labor and every 15 minutes in the second stage of labor. See *Guidelines for Fetal Heart Rate Monitoring.*

B. High-Risk Patients—Assess fetal status every 15 minutes during the first stage of labor and every 5 minutes during the second stage of labor.

V. **Pain Management**

A. Pain management during parturition involves continuous assessment of the patient's response to labor. The nurse may explain procedures for pain management options, including breathing and relaxation techniques, intravenous narcotics, or epidural anesthesia. Combinations of techniques may be required to minimize discomfort and meet individualized patient needs and requests.

B. Nursing care for the patient receiving narcotics involves understanding of the pharmacology of the specific medication including actions, contraindications, and maternal and fetal side effects.

C. Nursing care for the patient receiving epidural anesthesia involves assessing for side effects including maternal hypotension, nonreassuring fetal heart rate findings, and rising epidural levels with respiratory compromise.

D. Support of the laboring patient requires knowledge and understanding of the physical and emotional changes during the various stages of labor. The nurse may be required to assist in coaching, teach various breathing and relaxation techniques, and offer nonpharmacologic comfort measures to decrease pain. The patient must be frequently assessed during labor and appropriate techniques used to individualize care for the patient.

E. Breathing Techniques
   1. Cleansing Breath—Begin and end each uterine contraction with a deep breath expelled in a heavy sigh to promote relaxation and counteract possible hyperventilation.
   2. Slow Breathing—Deep even breaths in through the nose and out through the mouth throughout the contraction. The rate of breathing may gradually increase with the peak of the contraction and subside with the easing of the contraction.
   3. Abdominal Breathing—Shallow breathing (preferably in a patterned technique) offers both a psychological distraction and lifts the abdominal wall off the uterus relieving pressure and subsequently pain.
   4. Panting—A form of rapid, shallow breathing helpful to prevent pushing.
   5. Closed Glottis Pushing—The patient takes a cleansing breath followed by a deep breath which is held during a valsalva maneuver.
   6. Open Glottis Pushing—The patient is instructed to take 1–2 cleansing breaths followed by controlled exhalation during valsalva maneuver.

F. Relaxation, Support, and Comfort Measures
   1. Controlled Relaxation—Focused relaxation of all muscle groups except the uterus during contractions, especially the neck, face, and upper body. Focusing on breathing may facilitate this process.
   2. Physical comfort measures include frequent position changes, the use of positioning supports, massage, effleurage, and the use of heat or cold to back or abdomen.
   3. Environmental control measures to promote rest and relaxation include control of lighting, temperature, external noise,

and number of visitors according to the individual needs of the woman.
   4. The nurse should attempt to assure privacy and prevent exposure, explain processes and procedures, and cluster care to promote relaxation.
   5. Facilitation of comfort measures should incorporate the use of family and support people.

VI.   **Nursing Implications**

Notify physician for any of the following:
- Spontaneous rupture of membranes, unsure status of amniotic membranes, meconium or bloodstained amniotic fluid
- Vaginal bleeding beyond normal bloody show
- Analgesia or anesthesia needs of the patient
- Vital signs
   – Repeated BP > 140/90 or < 80/40
   – Temp > 100.4
   – Sustained maternal heart rate > 120 or < 60
   – Respirations > 26 or < 14
- Imminent delivery
- Nonreassuring FHR tracing
- Significant system assessment findings
- Failure to make adequate cervical change

VII.   **Patient/Family Teaching**
- Plan of care
- Unit routine
- Electronic fetal monitoring
- Pain management options
- Treatments

VIII.   **References**

American Academy of Pediatrics and the American College of Obstetricians and Gynecologists. (1992). Guidelines for perinatal care (4th ed.).

May, K. A., & Mahlmeister, L. R. (1990). Comprehensive maternity nursing. Philadelphia: J.B. Lippincott.

AWHONN. (1998). Standards for Professional Nursing Practice in the Care of Women and Infants (5th ed.).

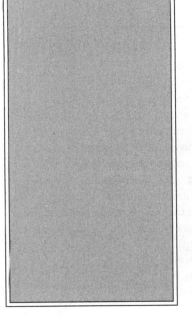

Guidelines for the Management of Patients With Preterm Labor Requiring Tocolytic Therapy

I. **Protocol**

A. Initial Assessment
1. History—Special attention should be directed toward risk factors that may increase the likelihood of preterm delivery.
    a. prior preterm labor or preterm delivery
    b. multiple gestation
    c. one or more second trimester abortions
    d. uterine anomaly
    e. low socioeconomic status
    f. maternal smoking
    g. substance abuse
    h. symptoms of vaginal or urinary tract infection
    i. preterm rupture of membranes
    j. prior obstetric or gynecologic procedure (diethylstilbestrol exposure in utero, cervical biopsy)
    k. poly- or oligohydramnios
    l. physical abuse/battery
2. Physical Examination and Evaluation
    a. Obtain initial cervical exam on admission and 1 hour after admission, preferably by the same examiner. Extreme prematurity, significant cervical dilation, excessive uterine contractions, or previous history may preclude documented cervical change and require immediate intervention with tocolytic therapy.
    b. Avoid unnecessary cervical examination that may increase prostaglandin release and increase the risk of infection.
    c. Assist with sterile speculum examination if necessary to diagnose premature rupture of membranes. Obtain fluid for nitrazine and fern test.
    d. Laboratory:
        – assist with cervical, vaginal, and rectal samples for Group B Strep cultures
        – consider CBC with differential
        – consider urinalysis and culture
        – consider toxicology screen
    e. Medications:
        – consider antibiotic therapy pending culture results
        – consider corticosteroid therapy— Betamethasone 12 mg IM (2 doses 12–24 hours apart)
        – consider mild sedation for anxious patients experiencing preterm contractions to decrease endogenous catecholamine production
    f. Assess for signs and symptoms of uterine infection:
        – palpate for uterine tenderness
        – maternal temperature
        – inspect perineum for vaginal discharge or inflammation
    g. Assess for signs and symptoms of maternal dehydration:
        – elevated maternal temperature
        – decreased blood pressure
        – maternal and/or fetal tachycardia
        If symptoms present, consider 500 cc intravenous crystalloid infusion bolus over 30 minutes.

h. Auscultate breath sounds and heart sounds

B. Stabilization of Patients Requiring Tocolytic Therapy
1. Vital Signs
   a. Assess blood pressure every 15 minutes during the administration of magnesium sulfate ($MgSO_4$) loading dose.
   b. Assess blood pressure, pulse, respirations every 30 minutes while on intravenous (IV) tocolytic infusion.
   c. Temperature every 4 hours if membranes are intact. Increase frequency to every 2 hours if membranes are ruptured.
   d. Discontinue terbutaline (if applicable), apply continuous ECG monitor and notify physician with sustained maternal heart rate > 120 bpm.
2. Intake and Output
   a. Obtain IV access with an 18-gauge intravenous catheter.
   b. All IV fluids should be administered via infusion pump.
   c. Patients receiving intravenous tocolytics may have restricted PO intake.
   d. Measure urine output with each void.
   e. Measure and record intake and output hourly.
3. Respiratory
   a. Auscultate breath sounds every 2 hours.
   b. Monitor SaO_2 every hour.
   c. Monitor for signs and symptoms of pulmonary edema including c/o chest tightness, SaO_2 < 95%, cough, shortness of breath, tachypnea, tachycardia, or adventitious breath sounds.
4. Neurologic
   a. Assess DTRs every hour during continuous $MgSO_4$ infusion.
   b. Assess level of consciousness (LOC) every 1 to 2 hours during $MgSO_4$ infusion.
5. Gastrointestinal
   a. Assess patient for evidence of abdominal tenderness.
   b. Interview patient daily regarding bowel function—consistency, constipation, nausea, or diarrhea.
6. Activity
   a. Strict bed rest with side rails up during $MgSO_4$ infusion.

   b. Instruct patient to rest in a position to optimize cardiac output and prevent vena cava syndrome.
7. Fetal Status and Uterine Contractions
   a. Continuous electronic fetal monitoring during $MgSO_4$ infusion.
   b. Assess and document fetal heart rate baseline and periodic patterns every 15 minutes until stable then every 30 minutes during IV tocolytic therapy.
   c. Assess and document uterine contraction frequency, duration, intensity and resting tone every 15 minutes until stable then every 30 minutes during IV tocolytic therapy.

II. **Procedure for Tocolysis**

A. Magnesium Sulfate Administration

Magnesium sulfate acts by decreasing the release of acetylcholine at the neuromuscular junction. This decreases the availability of acetylcholine, causing a decrease in the amplitude of electrical signals in myometrial cells. Maternal side effects include nausea, vomiting, and vasodilation during loading dose. Overdose of $MgSO_4$ may lead to both central nervous system and respiratory depression/arrest. Neonatal side effects include hypermagnesemia and hypocalcemia, which may lead to central nervous system and/or respiratory depression/arrest and hypotonia.

1. After receiving physician's order to start infusion of $MgSO_4$, obtain from pharmacy the prepared solution. One method of preparation is 40 grams $MgSO_4$ in 1000 cc crystalloid solution (yields 1 gram/25 cc).
2. $MgSO_4$ solution is piggybacked into main intravenous line and the infusion is controlled via infusion pump.
3. Loading dose: Infuse 4–6 gram bolus over 15–30 minutes.
4. Maintenance dose: Infuse at 2–3 grams per hour (50–75 cc/hr).
5. Assess for signs and symptoms of $MgSO_4$ toxicity such as absent DTRs, decreasing LOC or decreasing respiratory rate. If toxicity is suspected, discontinue $MgSO_4$ infusion, provide respiratory support if indicated, notify physician. Consider obtaining order for $MgSO_4$ serum level.

Monitor blood pressure, pulse, respirations, LOC, and DTRs every 5 minutes until stable

6. Antidote: For reversal of $MgSO_4$ effect, the physician may order calcium gluconate. The usual dose is 10 ml of a 10% solution to be given over 1–2 minutes IV push.

B. Terbutaline (Brethine) Administration

Terbutaline is a beta sympathomimetic agent that acts to decrease gap junction formation in uterine muscle. Terbutaline may be administered by oral, subcutaneous, or intravenous dosing. Maternal side effects include anxiety, tachycardia, hypotension, hyperglycemia, hypokalemia, and pulmonary edema. Fetal side effects include tachycardia and hyperinsulinemia. Neonatal side effects include hypoglycemia and hypotension.

1. Oral dose: 2.5–5.0 mg every 4–6 hours
2. Initial subcutaneous dose: 0.25 mg every 15 minutes, up to three doses or 0.25 mg every 30–60 minutes up to 1 mg.
3. Transitional dose: 0.25 mg every 4–6 hours

C. Indomethacin Administration

Indomethacin is a prostaglandin synthetase inhibitor with potential benefit as a tocolytic agent through its inhibition of prostaglandin formation. Prostaglandins promote uterine contractions and cervical ripening associated with labor by increasing gap junction formation. Maternal side effects include gastrointestinal distress, gastrointestinal bleeding, and increased vaginal bleeding during all stages of labor. The most common fetal side effect is oligohydramnios.

1. Initial dose: 50 mg PO or PR
2. Maintenance dose: 25 mg PO or PR every 6 hours for 72 hours.
3. When administering indomethacin by mouth, simultaneous administration of food may decrease gastrointestinal irritation.

D. Nifedepine (Procardia) Administration

Nifedepine is a calcium channel blocker that inhibits myometrial activity by blocking the influx of calcium through membranes of myometrial cells. The primary tocolytic effect of nifedepine may result from a decrease in the strength of contractions rather than the frequency. Maternal side effects may include headache, hypotension, tachycardia, facial flushing, nausea, and palpitations. Fetal side effects may include tachycardia.

1. Loading dose: 10 mg sublingually every 20 minutes up to three doses.
2. Maintenance dose: 10–20 mg PO every 6 hours.
3. Assess blood pressure, pulse, and respirations every 15 minutes (x2 following loading dose administration and prior to subsequent doses).
4. Hold dose and notify physician for BP < 100/60 and sustained maternal tachycardia > 120 bpm.

E. Weaning Tocolytics
1. Assess vital signs, FHR baseline and periodic changes, uterine activity, and maternal respiratory status.
2. Administer PO or PR tocolytic.
3. If intravenous $MgSO_4$ has been utilized, continue current infusion for 60 minutes following administration of initial oral tocolytic agent, unless otherwise ordered.
4. Reassess maternal uterine activity and FHR baseline and periodic changes every 30 minutes x2.
5. During oral tocolytic therapy, vital signs and respiratory status are assessed every 4 hours, or immediately prior to administration.

III. **Nursing Implications**

Notify physician for any of the following:
- sustained systolic blood pressure > 140 mm Hg or < 90 mm Hg
- sustained diastolic blood pressure > 90 mm Hg or < 50 mm Hg
- sustained tachycardia > 120 bpm
- respirations < 14 or > 26
- absent DTRs
- urine output < 30 cc/hour or < 240 cc in 8 hours
- symptoms of pulmonary edema
- SaO_2 < 95%
- change in neurologic status
- suspected $MgSO_4$ toxicity
- symptoms of placental abruption

- significant systems assessment changes
- nonreassurring fetal status
- imminent delivery

IV.   **Patient/Family Education**

- Plan of care
- Unit routine
- Electronic fetal monitoring
- Signs and symptoms of preterm labor
- Bed rest and physical activity restrictions
- Diversional activities
- Indication for basic mechanism of action and side effects of medications

- Indication for special testing—ultrasound or lab work

V.   **References**

American College of Obstetricians and Gynecologists and American Academy of Pediatrics. (1997). Guidelines for perinatal care. (4th) ed.

American College of Obstetricians and Gynecologists. (1995, June). Preterm labor. ACOG Technical Bulletin NO. 206.

AWHONN. (1991). Standards for the Professional Nursing Practice in the Care of Women and Newborns (5th ed.). Washington, DC.

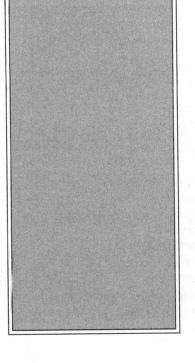

Guidelines for the Management of Patients With Diagnosed or Suspected Placenta Previa During the Peripartum Period

I. **Initial Assessment**

    1. See *Guidelines for the Initial Assessment and Triage of Obstetric Patients.*

    2. Interview patient for additional history of onset of bleeding, amount, color and character of blood, onset of uterine contractions in relation to bleeding (if present), and presence or absence of pain associated with bleeding.

    3. Physical assessment should include current vaginal bleeding, hematocrit, and signs or symptoms of excessive blood loss.

II. **Maternal Physical Status**

    A. Vital Signs

        1. Pulse, respirations, and blood pressure every 5–15 minutes with active bleeding or if patient is unstable. Following stabilization, vital signs may be taken every 30–60 minutes and every 4 hours during expectant management phase.

        2. Temperature every 4 hours if membranes are intact. Increase frequency to every 2 hours if membranes are ruptured or more frequently with hypothermia or hyperthermia.

    B. Vaginal Bleeding

        1. Inspect perineum every 1–2 hours when stable and more frequently as indicated.

        2. Note character, color, and estimate amount of all vaginal bleeding.

    C. Laboratory Tests

        1. On admission, obtain hematocrit, type and screen/cross as ordered.

        2. Repeat type and screen every 72 hours while hospitalized depending upon patient condition.

        3. Consider obtaining the following labs when profuse bleeding occurs or delivery is scheduled: CBC, platelets, PT/PTT, fibrinogen, and type and cross for 4 units of PRBCs.

III. **Fetal Surveillance**

    A. Electronic Fetal Monitoring (EFM)

        1. Continuous EFM is used during the initial and subsequent episodes of vaginal bleeding in accordance with the *Guidelines for Fetal Heart Rate Monitoring.*

        2. Evaluate EFM tracing every 15 minutes in the presence of active vaginal bleeding or if the patient is otherwise unstable. When stable without vaginal bleeding, EFM evaluation can occur every 30–60 minutes.

    B. Obstetrical Ultrasound—OB ultrasound is obtained to confirm placental position, gestational age, and fetal position.

    C. Biophysical Profile (BPP)—BPP may be done when determination of fetal reassurance is not possible by EFM.

IV. **Patient Care Management**

    A. Consultation and Consent

        1. Informed consent is obtained by the physician for cesarean delivery and potential need for hysterectomy if intraoperative bleeding cannot be controlled by conservative measures or fetal distress occurs.

2. An OB anesthesia consult is obtained and consent forms signed prior to transport to the antepartum unit.
3. Neonatal personnel should be informed of potential delivery, estimated gestational age, and need for consultation as appropriate.

B. Vaginal Exams
1. Vaginal exams are never to be performed by nurses or students in this patient population.
2. A vaginal exam may be performed by the physician of the patient who has a stable marginal previa and who is a candidate for vaginal delivery. However, this is generally accomplished with availability for an emergency cesarean section should profuse bleeding occur.
3. Sterile speculum exams may be performed in order to evaluate cervical dilation and obtain cervical cultures.

C. Intake and Output
1. Intravenous access is obtained with a large bore IV catheter (18 gauge or larger) on admission. Consider the use of blood tubing according to patient status.
2. When profuse bleeding continues or delivery is anticipated a second large bore IV may be placed.
3. In extreme hemorrhage a central line (usually in the right internal jugular vein) and placement of a pulmonary artery catheter to guide blood and fluid replacement should be considered.
4. A urinary catheter should be placed in the presence of active bleeding.
5. Document estimated blood loss in cc's.
6. Maintain hourly and 24-hour intake and output totals.

D. Uterine Contractions
1. In the presence of uterine contractions, tocolysis with magnesium sulfate or indocin may be considered.
2. Beta-agonist (Ritodrine, Terbutaline) are contraindicated in the presence of active bleeding.

E. Activity
1. Maintain strict bed rest in the lateral recumbent position.
2. Stable patients may be allowed bed rest with bathroom privileges.

F. Recurrence of Acute Vaginal Bleeding
1. Notify physician.
2. Evaluate color, character, and amount of vaginal bleeding.
3. Ensure patent, large bore IV catheter.
4. Apply pulse oximeter and evaluate SaO_2 every 15 minutes.
5. Vital signs (pulse, respirations, blood pressure) every 15 minutes until stable.
6. Begin oxygen at 10 L face mask.
7. Observe for signs of hypovolemic shock: tachycardia, hypotension, tachypnea, dizziness, pallor, and decreasing level of consciousness.

V. **Nursing Implications**

Notify physician for any of the following:
A. Onset or increase of vaginal bleeding
B. BP < 90/60
C. Pulse > 120 or < 60
D. Respirations > 26 or < 14
E. Temperature > 100.4
F. Urine output < 30 cc/hour
G. SaO_2 < 95%
H. Decreasing level of consciousness
I. Onset or increase in uterine contractions
J. Nonreassuring fetal status

VI. **Patient/Family Teaching**

A. Unit routine
B. Placenta previa
C. Treatments and procedures
D. EFM and antepartum testing
E. Plan of care
F. Cesarean delivery

VII. **References**

Varner, M. W., and Clark, S. L. (1993, December). Antepartum bleeding. Contemporary OB/GYN, 11–24.

Guidelines for the Management of Patients With Diabetes Mellitus During the Peripartum Period

I. **Protocol**

A. Initial Assessment

1. Maternal History—Patient's diabetic history, classification of diabetes, currently prescribed insulin regimen, type of self blood glucose monitoring utilized, daily total caloric intake, recent trends in serum blood glucose levels, recent history of nausea, vomiting or diarrhea, recent history of infection, other medications.

2. Maternal Physical Status:

a. current blood glucose value.

b. signs and symptoms of diabetic ketoacidosis (DKA) including nausea, vomiting, abdominal pain, Kussmaul breathing, acetone breath, ketonuria, glucosuria, decreased level of consciousness (LOC), decreased serum pH and bicarbonate levels.

c. signs and symptoms of hypoglycemia (serum glucose level < 40 mg/dl) including shaking; headache, severe hunger, anxiety, diaphoresis, cool and clammy skin, pallor, or confusion.

B. Management of the Patient With Type I Diabetes During Labor

1. Hemodynamics

a. First Stage Labor—Blood pressure. pulse, and respirations every 30 minutes.

b. Second Stage Labor—Blood pressure, pulse, and respirations every 15 minutes.

c. Temperature every 4 hours with intact membranes and every 2 hours for ruptured membranes or elevated temperature.

2. Intake and Output

a. Obtain intravenous access.

b. Administer mainline intravenous fluids of D51/4 NS or D51/2 NS via infusion pump at prescribed rate.

c. Bolus with 500–1000 cc .9% NS solution prior to epidural placement, hypotension, or for fetal indications.

d. Measure and record all intake and output. Calculate and document hourly and 24-hour totals.

e. Dipstick urine for ketones and glucose every void or every 4 hours.

3. Metabolic

a. Continually assess patient for evidence of hypoglycemia, hyperglycemia, and/or DKA.

b. Monitor serum glucose every 1–2 hours.

c. Maintain serum blood glucose between 80–120 mg/dl.

C. Nursing Management of Patient in DKA

1. Assess patient for signs and symptoms of DKA—Polyuria, polyphagia, polydypsia, dehydration, nausea, vomiting, abdominal pain, gastric stasis, ileus, increased respiratory rate, Kussmaul breathing, acetone breath, drowsiness, coma, high levels of ketonuria, glucosuria, decreased blood pH and serum bicarbonate.

2. Hemodynamics

a. Monitor blood pressure, pulse, respirations every 30–60 minutes.

b. Apply ECG and monitor for dysrhythmias.

c. Consider placement of arterial line for continuous blood pressure monitoring, frequent laboratory analysis, and blood gas values.

3. Respiratory
   a. Maintain patient airway.
   b. Administer oxygen via tight face mask at 10 L/minute.
   c. Consider need for mechanical ventilation.
   d. Auscultate breath sounds every 2 hours.

4. Intake and Output
   a. Insert urinary catheter.
   b. Measure and record all intake and output. Calculate hourly and 24-hour totals.
   c. Assess urine ketones every hour until clear then every 4 hours.

5. Hydration per MD Order
   a. Administer 1–2 L of .9% NS over the first hour.
   b. Consider need for second intravenous line.
   c. Begin glucose containing solutions (D51/2 NS or D51/2 NS) when serum glucose levels fall to 200 mg/dl.
   d. Administer 1 L of IV fluid per hour until 4–6 liters have been replaced.

6. Insulin Replacement per MD Order
   a. Insulin replacement may be administered IV push and/or IV infusion pump.
   b. Usual dose of regular insulin IV push is 0.1 units/kg.
   c. May begin regular insulin infusion of 5 to 10 units/hour. May double infusion rate if serum glucose has not decreased by 25% in 2 hours.
   d. May decrease infusion rate to 1–2 units per hour if serum glucose levels fall below 150 mg/dl.

7. Correction of Electrolyte Imbalances per MD Order
   a. Assess serum pH and bicarbonate levels.
   b. Assess arterial blood gases.
   c. Initial laboratory orders may include: CBC, SMA6, ketones, BUN, and creatinine.
   d. Consider adding KCL 20–40 meq/liter to maintenance IV fluids after adequate urine output is established.

e. Consider administration of sodium bicarbonate 44 meq IV in 1000 ml 1/2 NS for arterial pH < 7.10.

II. **Procedure for the Administration of Intravenous Insulin Infusion**

A. After receiving order for intravenous insulin infusion, have pharmacy prepare .9% NS solution with regular insulin so that 1 cc = 1 unit regular insulin.

B. Administer insulin solution via infusion pump, through most proximal port of main intravenous line at prescribed rate.

C. Monitor patient serum glucose levels at least every hour during intravenous insulin infusion. Titrate insulin drip to serum glucose levels as prescribed.

D. Hypoglycemic episodes:
   1. Notify MD.
   2. Discontinue IV insulin infusion for serum glucose levels < 60 mg/dl.
   3. Administer 300 cc 5% dextrose IV solution over 15–30 minutes for serum glucose of 20–40 mg/dl in the conscious patient.
   4. If serum blood glucose < 20 mg/dl and/or unconsciousness occurs, administer 10 cc 50% dextrose IV push over 5 minutes. Monitor pulse, respirations, and blood pressure every 5 minutes until stable. Repeat blood glucose testing every 15 minutes until stable.

E. Hyperglycemic episodes:
   1. Notify MD.
   2. Administer insulin as prescribed.
   3. Repeat blood glucose in 30 minutes.
   4. Monitor for signs and symptoms DKA.

III. **Nursing Implications**

Notify physician for the following:
- Sustained systolic blood pressure > 140 mm Hg or < 90 mm Hg
- Sustained diastolic blood pressure > 90 mm Hg or < 50 mm Hg
- Sustained tachycardia > 120 bpm
- Respirations < 14 or > 26
- Abnormal blood glucose values
- Signs or symptoms of hypoglycemia
- Urine output < 30 cc/hour
- Urine ketones

- Change in neurologic status
- Significant system changes
- Nonreassuring fetal status
- Imminent delivery

IV. **Patient/Family Education**
- Plan of care
- Unit routine
- Electronic fetal monitoring
- Signs and symptoms of hypoglycemia, hyperglycemia, DKA

- Self care practices including home glucose monitoring, insulin and dietary regimes

V. **References**

Clark, S. L., Cotton, D. B., Hankins, G. D. V., & Phelan, J. P. (1997). Critical care obstetrics. Boston: Blackwell Scientific.

Mandeville, L. (1992). Diabetes mellitus in pregnancy. In L. K. Mandeville & N. H. Troiano (Eds.). High risk intrapartum nursing. Philadelphia: Lippincott.

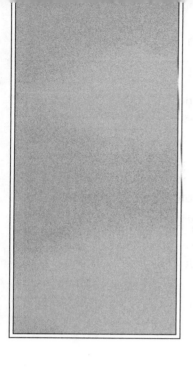

Guidelines for the Management of Patients Experiencing Fetal Loss

I. **Protocol**

A. Maternal Physical Status
1. Vital Signs—Assess vital signs according to medication administered for induction of labor.
    a. Prostaglandin E_2—Blood pressure, pulse, and respirations are assessed and recorded every 30 minutes (x2 following insertion followed by Q I hour if stable).
    b. Cytotec/Hypertonic saline/Laminaria—Blood pressure, pulse, and respirations are assessed and recorded every 4 hours.
    c. High Dose Pitocin—Blood pressure, pulse, and respirations are assessed and recorded every hour.
    d. Temperature every 4 hours if membranes intact. Increase frequency to every 2 hours if membranes ruptured or if temperature greater than 100.4.

B. Respiratory
1. Auscultate breath sounds every shift. Increase frequency if tachypnea or tachycardia present.
2. Assess SaO_2 every 30 minutes if IV sedation is used for pain management.

C. Intake
1. Patients may have clear liquids as tolerated until active labor or epidural placement.
2. Measure and record all intake. Document hourly and 24-hour totals.

3. Intravenous access may be initiated with an 18–20 gauge catheter using a mainline infusion of D5LR at 125 cc/hour unless otherwise ordered.
4. The nurse may initiate a 500–1000 cc bolus of crystalloid fluid immediately prior to anticipated placement of an epidural.

D. Elimination
1. Assess urinary output. Document 24-hour totals.
2. Assess for bladder distention every 2 hours after epidural placement.
3. Patients with bladder distention and unable to void may be catheterized (in and out).
4. A 500–1000 cc tap water enema may be administered prior to insertion of prostaglandin E_2 suppository if patient desires.

E. Activity
1. Patients should remain on bed rest for 30 minutes following placement of prostaglandin E_2 and at least 2 hours following Cytotec administration.
2. Patients may ambulate following hypertonic saline administration or during the administration of pitocin.

F. Labor Status—Assessment of uterine activity may be accomplished by palpation, patient report, or external/internal appliances.

G. Lab Data—Obtain type and screen and hematocrit upon admission.

H. Psychosocial Needs
1. Assess patient's understanding regarding procedure, action, and side effects of medication, labor, and delivery process.
2. Explain grief process.
3. Patients should be offered a memory packet including items such as lock of hair, baby bracelets, crib label, footprints, handprints, measurements, pictures, etc.
4. Patients and family members should be encouraged to see, touch, and hold newborn if possible.

I. Pain Management—Pain management options may include IV sedation, epidural anesthesia, or PCA pain pump per physician order and patient request.

J. Patient Informed Consent
1. Informed consent must be obtained by the physician prior to initiation of procedure.
2. Options for disposition of fetal remains should be discussed with the patient prior to procedure or IV sedation. Appropriate forms will be determined by the state and institution.

II. **Procedures**

A. Procedure for Prostaglandin E$_2$ Suppository Administration
1. Obtain 20 mg prostaglandin E$_2$ suppository (PGE2) after receiving physician's order.
2. Pre-medicate patient with antipyretic, antiemetic, and antidiarrheal as ordered.
3. Assist physician with insertion of vaginal suppository by placing patient in lithotomy position.
4. Assess patient for side effects including nausea, vomiting, diarrhea, headache, fever, chills, tachycardia, hypertension, and bronchoconstriction.
5. Assess and record blood pressure, pulse, and respirations every 30 minutes (x2 then every 1 hour if stable).

B. Procedure for Laminaria Cervical Insert Placement
1. Obtain specific size and number of laminaria cervical inserts per physician's order.
2. Assist physician with insertion of laminaria by placing patient in lithotomy position.
3. Assess maternal vital signs every 4 hours.

C. Procedure for High Dose Pitocin Administration
1. Obtain 100 units pitocin in 100 cc NS after receiving physician's order.
2. The infusion is placed on an infusion pump to run IV piggyback into the mainline IV at the port most proximal to the patient.
3. Infuse pitocin at 17 units/hour (17 cc/hour) for 3 hours, then turn off pitocin for 1 hour.
4. Resume infusion following 1 hour at 33 units/hour (33 cc/hour) for 3 hours then turn pitocin off for 1 hour.
5. Resume infusion following 1 hour at 50 units/hour (50 cc/hour) for 3 hours.
6. Assess and record vital signs every hour.
7. With inadequate progression of labor, consider other medications.

D. Procedure for Administration of Hypertonic Saline
1. Obtain 23.4% saline solution (amount of saline administration varies with physician) after receiving physician's order.
2. Assist physician with abdominal prep and set-up of equipment, including amniocentesis tray and ultrasound.
3. Side effects may include hypernatremia, dehydration, tachycardia, facial flushing, and headache.
4. Assess vital signs every 4 hours.

E. Procedure for Cytotec Administration
1. Obtain cytotec tablets after receiving physician's order (usual dosage is 200–300 mcg every 12 hours).
2. Assist physician with intravaginal placement of cytotec by placing patient in lithotomy position.
3. Assess vital signs every 4 hours.

III. **Nursing Implications**

Notify physician for the following:

- Spontaneous rupture of membranes, unsure status of membranes
- Vaginal bleeding in excess of normal bloody show
- Analgesia or anesthesia needs of patient
- Vital signs
  - BP > 140/90 or < 90/60
  - Temp > 100.4
  - Sustained pulse > 120 or < 60 bpm

– Respirations > 26 or < 14
- Imminent delivery
- Significant system assessment findings

IV. Patient/Family Education

- Plan of care
- Unit routine
- Pain management options
- Medications and associated side effects
- Expected length of stay
- Components of grief process and support groups
- Disposition of fetal remains

V. References

Bugalho, A., Bique, C., Machungo, F., & Faundes, A. (1994). Induction of labor with intravaginal misoprostol in intrauterine fetal death. American Journal of Gynecology & Obstetrics, 171(2), 538–551.

Mueller, L. (1991). Second trimester termination of pregnancy: Nursing care. JOGNN, 20(4), 284–289.

Winkler, C. L., Gray, S. E., Hanth, J. C., Owen J., & Tucker, J. M. (1991). Mid-second trimester labor induction: Concentrated oxytocin compared with prostaglandin E2 vaginal suppositories. OBGYN, 77(2), 297–300.

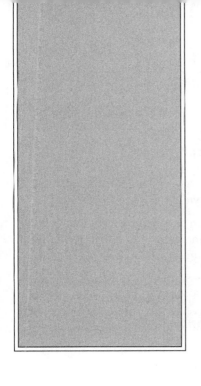

Guidelines for the Management of Patients With Preeclampsia

I. **Protocol**

A. Initial Assessment

Special attention should be directed toward the admission history and physical examination to include:

1. History of: preeclampsia, eclampsia, chronic hypertension, neurological irritability (headache, visual disturbances), or hepatic involvement (epigastric pain, nausea, vomiting, excessive heartburn).
2. Physical assessment: deep tendon reflexes (DTRs), presence of clonus, protenuria, level of consciousness (LOC), edema (amount and location), and breath sounds.

B. Maternal Physical Status

1. Hemodynamics
   a. Assess blood pressure every 15 minutes during the administration of $MgSO_4$ loading dose.
   b. Assess blood pressure, pulse, respirations every 30 minutes during maintenance $MgSO_4$ infusion during the antepartum and intrapartum periods.
   e. Assess blood pressure, pulse, respirations every hour following delivery and if stable.
   d. Assess blood pressure every 5–15 minutes during severe hypertensive episodes and with IV antihypertensive medication use.
   e. Assess edema every shift.
   f. Assess temperature every 4 hours if membranes intact. Increase frequency to every 2 hours if membranes are ruptured.

2. Intake
   a. Obtain intravenous access with an 18-gauge catheter.
   b. Patients receiving intravenous $MgSO_4$ may have restricted PO intake.
   c. Measure and record all intake. Calculate and document hourly and 24-hour totals.
   d. All IV fluids must be maintained on an infusion pump.

3. Renal
   a. Insert urinary catheter to gravity drain.
   b. Measure and record all output. Calculate and document hourly and 24-hour totals.

4. Respiratory
   a. Auscultate breath sounds every 2 hours.
   b. Assess SaO_2 every 30 minutes.
   c. Assess for signs of pulmonary edema including c/o chest tightness, $SaO_2 <$ 95%, cough, shortness of breath, tachypnea, tachycardia, or adventitious breath sounds.

5. Neurologic
   a. Assess DTRs and presence or absence of clonus every hour during continuous $MgSO_4$ infusion.
   b. Assess level of consciousness every hour during continuous $MgSO_4$ infusion.
   c. Assess for headache and visual disturbances every shift and prn.

6. Activity

a. Strict bed rest with side rails up during MgSO$_4$ infusion.

b. Instruct patients to rest in a position to optimize cardiac output and prevent vena caval syndrome.

7. Labs

a. "PIH labs" ordered by the physician may include but are not limited to Hct, type and screen, platelets, creatinine, uric acid, SGOT, and LDH.

C. Fetal Status—Continuous electronic fetal monitoring is recommended during MgSO$_4$ infusion. All parameters of fetal monitoring interpretation are assessed and documented every 30 minutes on the nonlaboring patient and increased to every 15 minutes during the first stage of labor and every 5 minutes during the second stage.

D. Eclamptic Seizure

1. Turn patient on her side.

2. Protect patient from physical harm.

3. Insert oral airway if possible. Do not force jaw open.

4. Notify physician and call for help.

5. Administer MgSO$_4$ IV bolus as ordered.

• Seizure dose: Administer 4–6 grams IV over 10–15 minutes and return to maintenance dose of 2–3 grams per hour. If seizure activity recurs, administration of 2 grams over 3–5 minutes may be ordered. With continued seizure activity, prepare patient for paralyzation, intubation, sedation, and mechanical ventilation.

6. Once seizure activity stops:

a. administer O$_2$ at 10 L per minute by face mask. (If not intubated and on mechanical ventilation).

b. suction nose and mouth as necessary.

c. assess blood pressure, pulse, respirations, and fetal heart rate parameters every 5 minutes until stable.

7. Note characteristics of seizure:

a. presence or absence of aura

b. duration of seizure

c. tonic, clonic phases

d. duration of postictal phase

e. length of unconsciousness

f. maternal and fetal responses

8. Assess for evidence of placental abruption and/or imminent delivery.

II. **Procedure for Magnesium Sulfate Administration**

A. After receiving physician's order to start infusion of MgSO$_4$, obtain prepared solution. One method is to mix 40 grams of MgSO$_4$ in 1000 cc D5LR yielding 1 gram per 25 cc.

B. MgSO$_4$ solution is piggybacked into main intravenous line and the infusion should always be controlled via infusion pump.

C. Loading Dose: Infuse 4–6 grams loading dose over 15–30 minutes. Consider a decreased dosage in the presence of decreased urine output.

D. Maintenance Dose: Infuse at 1–3 grams per hour via infusion pump.

E. Assess for signs and symptoms of MgSO$_4$ toxicity such as absent DTRs, decreasing LOC or decreasing respiratory rate. If toxicity is suspected, discontinue MgSO$_4$ infusion, provide respiratory support (if indicated), notify physician and consider obtaining order for MgSO$_4$ level. Monitor blood pressure, pulse, respirations, LOC, and DTRs every 5 minutes until stable.

F. Antidote: For reversal of MgSO$_4$ effect, the physician may order calcium gluconate. The usual dose is 10 ccs of a of 10% solution to be given over 1 to 2 minutes IV push.

III. **Nursing Implications**

Notify physician for any of the following:
• Systolic blood pressure > 160 mm Hg
• Diastolic blood pressure ≥ 110 mm Hg
• Respirations < 14 or > 26
• DTRs absent
• Urine output < 30 cc/hour
• Symptoms of pulmonary edema
• Seizure activity
• Suspected MgSO$_4$ toxicity
• SaO$_2$ < 95%
• Symptoms of placental abruption
• Change in neurologic status or development of visual disturbances or headache
• Complaints of nausea, vomiting, epigastric pain, or heartburn
• Significant system changes
• Increasing weight gain or edema
• Nonreassuring fetal status
• Imminent delivery

IV.   **Patient/Family Education**

Plan of care
Unit routine
Electronic fetal monitoring
Signs and symptoms of preeclampsia
Preeclampsia disease process
Diversional activities
$MgSO_4$
Special testing—BPP, ultrasound, lab work

V.   **References**

ACOG Technical Bulletin. (1996, January). Hypertension in pregnancy (No. 219).

Clark, S. L., Cotton, D. B., Hankins, G. D. V., & Phelan, J. P. (1997). Critical care obstetrics. Boston: Blackwell Scientific.

Harvey, C. J., & Burke, M. E. (1992). Hypertensive disorders of pregnancy. In L .K. Mandeville & N. H. Troiano (Eds.). High risk intrapartum nursing. Philadelphia: Lippincott.

Surrat, N. (1993). Severe preeclampsia: Implications for critical care obstetrical nursing. JOGNN, 22(6), 500–507.

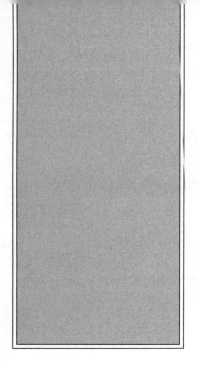

Guidelines for the Management of Patients Requiring Induction, Augmentation, or Active Management of Labor

I. **Guidelines for Outpatient Cervical Ripening**

A. Patient Selection
1. Patients at term gestation that have a Bishop Score less than or equal to 6 and who are scheduled for induction of labor the following morning may be considered for outpatient cervical ripening.
2. High-risk patients such as those with preeclampsia, insulin dependent diabetes mellitus, maternal cardiac disease, or chronic hypertension may be excluded from outpatient cervical ripening.

B. Procedure
1. Initiate continuous electronic fetal monitoring to establish fetal reassurance.
2. Assist physician with prostaglandin application.
3. Patient should remain at bed rest with continuous fetal monitoring for 2 hours after insertion of prostaglandin agent.
4. Patient may have a clear liquid diet.
5. No intravenous access is required.

C. Discharge Criteria
1. Cervical exam to rule out labor by a consistent examiner.
2. Stable maternal status.
3. Fetal reassurance by reactive nonstress test or negative contraction stress test (refer to Guidelines for Fetal Heart Rate Monitoring).

D. Patient/Family Teaching
1. Labor and rupture of membranes precautions.

2. Regular diet until AM.
3. Return to Labor and Delivery for scheduled induction.

II. **Guidelines for Prostaglandin Cervical Ripening**

A. Vital Signs
1. Assessment and documentation of the patient's vital signs (BP, pulse, respirations) will be obtained on admission and every 30 minutes (x2 following application of a prostaglandin preparation.
2. If vital signs are stable prior to and following application, the assessment and documentation of vital signs may be done every 4 hours.
3. Temperature should be obtained on admission and every 4 hours. Increase frequency to every 2 hours if rupture of membranes occurs.

B. Electronic Fetal Monitoring
1. EFM and uterine activity is initiated prior to application of prostaglandin preparations. Continuous EFM and uterine activity monitoring should continue for 2 hours following prostaglandin administration and may then be discontinued with a reassuring EFM tracing (refer to the *Guidelines for Fetal Heart Rate Monitoring*) and in the absence of regular uterine contractions (every 5 minutes).
2. If uterine contractions become regular or more frequent than every 5 minutes, the patient is reassessed and the physician notified.

3. If the patient is in labor, refer to the *Guidelines for Management of Patients in Labor.*

4. Hypertonicity (increased uterine resting tone) is the most common side effect of prostaglandin gel preparations.

C. Activity—The patient is maintained on bed rest for at least 30 minutes following prostaglandin gel application and then may ambulate as risk status allows.

D. Intake and Output

1. Obtain intravenous access prior to prostaglandin gel application using infusion or heplock as ordered.

2. Measure and record hourly and 24-hour intake and output totals.

3. Patients should be restricted to "sips and chips" prior to and 2 hours following prostaglandin gel application. Patients may then have clear liquids as risk status allows.

III. **Guidelines for Induction of Labor**

A. Procedure for Oxytocin Infusion

Obtain prepared oxytocin solution from the pharmacy. One method of preparation is to mix 15 units oxytocin in 250 cc D51/4 NS. With this preparation 1 ml/hr is equivalent to 1 mu/min when infusing through an infusion pump.

The infusion is placed on an infusion pump to run IV piggyback into the mainline IV at the port most proximal to the patient. Other IV bolus medications may be administered through the distal port of the main IV line without altering oxytocin delivery.

Induction of Labor

1. Begin oxytocin infusion at 1–2 mu/min.

2. Dosage may he increased every 15 minutes in increments of I mu/min unless otherwise ordered.

3. Maintain continuous infusion once adequate uterine activity is achieved.

Augmentation of Labor

1. Begin oxytocin infusion at 0.5–1 mu/min.

2. Dosage may be increased 1–2 mu/min every 40–60 minutes unless otherwise ordered.

3. Maintain continuous infusion once adequate uterine activity is achieved.

B. Procedure for Cytotec Administration

1. Obtain cytotec from the pharmacy per physician's order.

2. Usual dosage is 25–50 mcg every 4–6 hours.

3. Cytotec is placed by the physician in the posterior fornix of the vagina. Limit the use of K-Y jelly when placing cytotec as it may inhibit the absorption.

C. Vital Signs

1. Assess and document blood pressure, pulse, and respirations with every increase in pitocin.

2. Assess and document blood pressure, pulse, and respirations every 60 minutes if stable and when not increasing pitocin or when using cytotec.

3. Assess temperature every 4 hours if membranes intact, every 2 hours if membranes ruptured.

D. Uterine Activity

1. Assess and document uterine activity every 15 minutes.

2. Observe for signs and/or symptoms of uterine rupture: uterine hypertonus, fetal distress, vascular collapse, hypotension, tachycardia, maternal shock, respiratory distress, vaginal bleeding, marked abdominal tenderness, rigidity, or severe pain.

3. Decrease or discontinue oxytocin infusion for uterine hypertonus or hyperstimulation.

4. Patients who are stable may have uterine activity documented every 30 minutes if pitocin not being increased.

5. Once consistent uterine activity has been established with cytotec administration, uterine activity should be documented every 30 minutes.

E. Fetal Status

1. Fetal monitoring is used in accordance with the *Guidelines for Fetal Heart Rate Monitoring.*

2. Evaluate and document fetal heart rate every 15 minutes.

3. Discontinue oxytocin administration for nonreassuring fetal status.

4. Patients who are stable and have a reassuring fetal status, FHR may be documented every 30 minutes if pitocin is not increased.

IV. **Guidelines for Active Management of Labor**

A. Active Management of Labor (AML) Criteria

1. Nulliparous, greater than or equal to 37 weeks gestation

2. Single gestation in vertex presentation

3. Spontaneous, painful uterine contractions occurring at least every 5 minutes

4. 90–100% cervical effacement

5. Cervical dilation greater than or equal to 2 cm

B. Physician Responsibilities

1. Identification of appropriate AML candidate.

2. Time of initiation of AML is documented in the progress notes.

3. Evaluation 1 hour following initiation of AML for cervical change with AROM if not previously ruptured.

4. Physician order to initiate pitocin infusion if cervical dilation does not occur at the rate of 1 cm/hour.

C. Oxytocin Titration

1. Titration of oxytocin infusion is based upon frequency of uterine contractions as well as cervical change.

2. Begin oxytocin infusion at 6 mu/minute.

3. Dosage is increased by 6 mu increments every 15 minutes until uterine contraction frequency equals seven uterine contractions in 15 minutes or until expected cervical change is noted.

4. Maximum infusion rate is 36 mu/min.

5. If uterine contractions exceed seven in 15 minutes or are closer than every 2 minutes, decrease oxytocin infusion in 6 mu increments until acceptable pattern is achieved as stated above.

6. If pitocin augmentation becomes necessary during the second stage of labor to achieve descent of the fetal head, the infusion should be initiated at 1 mu/min then increased by 2 mu/min every 15 minutes.

V. **Nursing Implications**

Notify physician for any of the following:

• Spontaneous rupture of membranes, unsure status of amniotic membranes, meconium or blood-stained amniotic fluid

• Vaginal bleeding beyond normal bloody show

• Analgesia or anesthesia needs of the patient

• Vital Signs

1. BP > 140/90 or BP < 90/60

2. Temperature > 100.4

3. Pulse > 120 or < 60

4. Respirations > 26 or < 14/min

• Imminent delivery

• Nonreassuring FHR tracing

• Significant system assessment findings

• Inadequate uterine response at oxytocin dose of 20 mu/min

• Suspected uterine rupture

• Uterine hypertonus unresponsive to nursing management

VI. **Patient/Family Education (may include but not limited to)**

A. Plan of care

B. Unit routine

C. Fetal monitoring

D. Pain management options

E. Treatment

F. Risk/benefits of induction/augmentation procedure

VII. **References**

ACOG & AAP. (1997). Guidelines for perinatal care (4th ed.).

ACOG Technical Bulletin. (1991). Induction and augmentation of labor. ACOG Committee Opinion (No. 123).

AWHONN Practice Resource. (1993). Cervical ripening and induction of labor.

Adoury, H., Brodie, G., Caddick, R., McLaughin, V., & Pugh, P. (1988). Active management of labor and operative delivery in nulliparous women. American Journal of Obstetrics and Gynecology, 158(2), 255–258.

Boylan, P., Frankowski, R., Roundtree, R., Selwyn, B., & Parrish, K. (1991). Effect of active management of labor on the incidence of cesarean section for dystocia in nulliparas. American Journal of Perinatology, 8, 375.

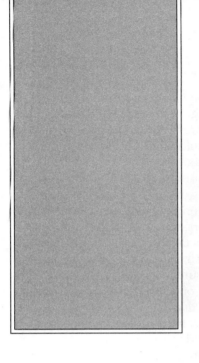

Guidelines for the Management of Critically Ill Obstetric Patients (CCOB)

I. **Cardiovascular Assessment**

  A. General Assessment—A complete cardiovascular assessment should be performed and abnormal findings documented every 8 hours, or more frequently with adverse change in patient status. A graphic recording of heart rate, rhythm, P-R interval, and QRS width, labeled with patient name, date, and time, should be evaluated every 8 hours.

  B. Hemodynamic Monitoring
    1. During pulmonary artery (PA) catheter insertion, a graphic recording of central venous pressure (CVP), right ventricular pressure, pulmonary artery pressure (PAP), and pulmonary artery occlusion pressure (PAOP) should be obtained (if possible).
    2. All waveforms should appear continuously on the digital display and be inspected frequently for configuration changes. Situations may occur that warrant intermittent interruptions in CVP waveform reading (e.g. volume resuscitation, cardiac output measurement, or medication administration).

  C. Central Pressure Assessment
    1. Assessments may be performed from the digital display if waveform configurations are appropriate. All assessments should be performed from the graphic recording for patients receiving artificial mechanical ventilation with PEEP > 10 cm H_2O.

    2. Routine assessment frequency may be as follows:
      a. Patients who are undelivered or ≤ 12 hours post delivery—CVP and PAP every hour and PAOP every 2 hours.
      b. Patients who are > 12 hours post delivery—CVP and PAP every hour and PAOP every 4 hours.
    3. Assessments may be performed more frequently in the following situations:
      a. The patient is hemodynamically unstable (abnormal central or arterial blood pressures).
      b. The patient is receiving intravenous vasoactive medications.
    4. PA catheter placement may be verified daily by chest x-ray.
    5. PA catheters are usually repositioned and discontinued by a physician or designated advanced practice nurses. PA catheters displaying a spontaneous occlusion waveform may be repositioned by the physician or CCOB nurse by withdrawing the catheter slowly with the balloon deflated until an appropriate PAP waveform returns.

  D. Derived Hemodynamic Assessment
    1. The following derived hemodynamic and oxygen transport parameters should be obtained for all patients with a fiberoptic PA catheter:
      a. Cardiac Index (CI)
      b. Systemic vascular resistance (SVR)
      c. Pulmonary vascular resistance (PVR)

d. Left ventricular stroke work index (LVSWI)

e. Arterial oxygen content (CaO_2)

f. Venous oxygen content (CvO_2)

g. Oxygen delivery (DO_2)

h. Oxygen consumption (VO_2)

i. Oxygen extraction ratio (O_2ER)

j. Shunt fraction (Qs/Qt)

2. Routine assessment frequency of derived hemodynamic and oxygen transport parameters may be as follows:

a. Patients who are undelivered or ≤ 12 hours post delivery—every 2 hours.

b. Patients who are > 12 hours post delivery—every 4 hours.

3. Assessments may be performed more frequently if patient is hemodynamically unstable.

E. Instrumentation

1. Pulmonary Artery Catheter Line Set-up

a. Obtain from pharmacy prepared heparin flush solution (2500 units heparin to 500 cc bag 0.9% normal saline).

b. Place solution in pressure bag.

c. Prepare pressure lines for central venous pressure and pulmonary artery ports. Flush tubing and transducer with heparin solution using gravity to remove air.

d. Replace all stopcock ports with non-vented caps. Ensure that system is free of air.

e. Inflate pressure bag to 300 mm Hg. Pressure is maintained at 300 mm Hg to ensure an infusion rate to each pressure line of 3–5 cc/hour.

f. Zero each pressure line to the patient's phlebostatic axis.

g. Calibrate the transducer.

h. Ensure that informed patient consent has been obtained by the physician.

i. Initiate continuous electrocardiographic monitoring to detect ventricular ectopy which may occur when the catheter enters the right ventricle. Have available at the bedside lidocaine 1 mg/kg for suppression as needed.

j. Test balloon for patency.

2. Hemodynamic Monitoring

a. Hemodynamic pressure readings may be taken with the patient in a position that allows for adequate cardiac out-put maintenance and patient comfort. Following patient position change and prior to pressure readings, all pressure lines should be re-zeroed at the phlebostatic axis.

b. For consistency, all pulmonary artery pressures should be taken at the patient's end-expiration.

c. Pulmonary artery occlusion pressure (PAOP) is taken as a mean pressure.

d. In mechanically ventilated patients, all pressure measurements will be obtained on the ventilator unless otherwise ordered.

e. The pulmonary artery catheter should be secured to the patient.

f. Pressure bags should be maintained at 300 mm Hg pressure.

g. All ports on the pressure line will be protected with occlusive port covers.

h. Stopcocks used for blood sampling should be flushed prior to replacing the nonvented cap.

i. No fluids except the flush solution will be infused into the distal port of the patient.

3. Cardiac Output—Thermodilution cardiac output (CO) assessment may be routinely performed and documented as follows:

a. Patients who are undelivered or ≤ 12 hours post delivery—every 2 hours.

b. Patients who are delivered or > 12 hours post delivery—every 4 hours.

c. Assessment of cardiac output may be performed more frequently if patient is hemodynamically unstable.

d. All cardiac output assessments should be performed using 10 ml iced injectate (0.9 sodium chloride) at a temperature between 6 degrees and 12 degrees C.

e. The computation constant for cardiac output measurement is PA catheter specific and should be determined prior to the procedure.

f. Cardiac output injectate should be recorded as intake.

g. Thermodilution technique is used for measuring cardiac output by injecting 10 cc of iced saline into the CVP port. Positioning for the obstetric patient to allow optimization of cardiac output includes right side-lying, left side-lying, sitting, and knee chest.

4. Fiberoptic (SvO_2) PA Catheter
   a. An in-vitro calibration should be performed prior to insertion of a fiberoptic catheter.
   b. An in-vivo calibration should be performed by obtaining a mixed venous gas sample from the PA port:
      – as soon as possible after insertion if an in-vitro calibration is not performed
      – every 24 hours for all patients with AM labs
   c. If interruption of monitoring is necessary, the cable should be disconnected at the input jack. If disconnection occurs at the optical module or continues beyond 4 hours, an in-vivo calibration should be performed.
   d. An adequate signal quality index should be verified (according to manufacture's recommendations) prior to documentation of SvO_2.
5. Arterial Blood Pressure (ABP) Monitoring
   a. ABP and MAP may be assessed every 4 hours for all patients.
   b. The catheter insertion site should serve as the zero-reference point for intraarterial BP monitoring.
   c. The extremity containing the intraarterial catheter should be assessed every 2 hours.
   d. If unexplained direct ABP changes by > 20 mm Hg, an indirect assessment should be performed for comparison.
   e. An indirect ABP should be obtained and documented each shift for patients with an intraarterial catheter.
6. Deep Vein Thrombus (DVT) Prophylaxis
   a. All CCOB patients > 24 hours should be evaluated for the use of sequential compression/decompression (SCD) hose.
   b. If SCD hose are in use. they should be removed for 1 hour every 8 hours.

II. **Respiratory Assessment**

A. General Assessment—A complete respiratory assessment should be performed and abnormal findings documented each shift, or more frequently if evidence of respiratory compromise exists.

B. Ongoing Assessment—Routine assessment of respiratory status should be performed as follows:

1. Respiratory rate and arterial oxygen saturation (SaO_2) every hour.
2. Venous oxygen saturation (SvO_2) every hour for patients with a fiberoptic PA catheter.
3. Auscultate breath sounds every 2 hours.

C. Mechanical Ventilation
1. Following intubation, the following should be assessed and documented: Endotracheal tube (ETT) size and position at teeth, date of placement, and breath sounds.
2. Placement of ETT should be verified by a chest x-ray as soon as possible after intubation.
3. Routine assessment should be performed as follows:
   a. Ventilator settings (mode, rate, FiO_2, Vt, PEEP, PSV, Peak Inspiratory Pressure)—every 2 hours and after any ventilator change.
   b. Arterial blood gases—every 24 hours and after any change in ventilator settings, or more frequently as indicated by patient respiratory status.
4. Ventilator setting changes should be made according to hospital protocol. In a STAT or emergency situation, when neither a physician nor respiratory care practitioner is immediately available, a CCOB nurse should initiate changes necessary to meet a patient's ventilatory needs.
5. A nasogastric (NG) tube should be inserted in patients requiring mechanical ventilation > 4 hours and connected to low wall suction.
6. Suctioning of the patient via ETT or tracheotomy tube should be as follows:
   a. Performed when indicated by respiratory assessment (increasing PIP, visible secretions, patient coughing or decreasing SaO_2).
   b. Preceded and followed by hyperoxygenation with FiO_2 of 1.0 as necessary to maintain adequate SaO_2 ($\geq$ 95%).
   c. Preceded by hyperventilation if open suction technique is used.
   d. Stabilization of ETT by additional personnel may be required during open suction procedure.
   e. Limit each suction episode to maximum of two catheter passes.

f. Suction containers should be changed every 24 hours and emptied every shift.

7. A manual resuscitation bag, capable of delivering PEEP and connected to an oxygen source providing 1.0 FiO_2 should be immediately accessible at all times.

8. When the patient is intubated and on a ventilator, restraints may be applied to patient's extremities to decrease the risk of extubation. Application and removal should be documented. The need for and expected time of restraint should be explained to the patient and family. A physician's order should be obtained.

D. ETT and Tracheotomy Care
1. ETT tape should be assessed every 8 hours. When tape is soiled or no longer secure, it should be changed with the assistance of another staff person as follows:
    a. Old tape should be removed with ETT stabilization at specified centimeter mark at the patient's teeth.
    b. New adhesive tape should be secured around patient's head and above upper lip.
    c. Tube placement should be verified by assessing breath sounds.
    d. Tape should not be wrapped around the head of a patient with documented or suspected neurologic injury.
2. An extra ETT or tracheotomy tube, identical to patient's, should be immediately accessible at all times.
3. Respiratory therapy should be consulted when the ETT requires repositioning or alteration of length in needed. No more than 5 cm of tube should protrude from the patient's mouth.

III. **Neurological Assessment**

A complete neurological assessment will be performed and abnormal findings documented every 8 hours, or more frequently when neurological instability exists.

IV. **Gastrointestinal/Genitourinary Assessment**

A. General Assessment—A GI/GU assessment will be performed and abnormal findings documented every 8 hours, or more frequently if instability exists.

B. Nasogastric Tube (NG)
1. Position of NG tube should be documented.
2. Gastric pH should be assessed and documented every 4 hours.
3. Correct placement should be verified by auscultation prior to each irrigation or administration of medication.
4. Tape should be positioned to avoid pressure on the flares.
5. Tape should be changed prn when soiled.

C. Feeding/Drainage Tubes
1. Feeding bag and tubing should be changed every 24 hours.
2. Location of enteral feeding tube should be verified every 24 hours.
3. No more than 4 hours of feeding solution will be hung to prevent risk of bacterial contamination.
4. Feeding tubes should be irrigated with 20 ml warm water before and after feeding or every 4 hours.
5. Gastric residuals should be assessed every 4 hours. If residuals are greater than the hourly rate, feedings should be held and the physician notified.

D. Bowel Function
1. Passage of stool should be documented in medical record.
2. If a rectal tube is in place, the balloon should be deflated for 10 minutes every 2 hours. Balloons should be inflated with normal saline.
3. Rectal bags should be changed every 48 hours or prn. The rectal area should be cleaned and dried following bag change.

E. Urinary Output
1. An indwelling urinary catheter should be inserted in all CCOB patients unless otherwise ordered by the physician.
2. Indwelling urinary catheters should be connected to a graduated urimeter and bedside drainage bag.
3. Urine output should be assessed and documented every hour. Twenty-four-hour total urine output should be calculated and documented.

V. **Integument Assessment**

A. General Assessment—A skin assessment will be performed and abnormal findings documented every 8 hours.

B. Therapeutic Mattress/Bed—Therapeutic beds should be considered for patients with special skin care needs. Use of these beds usually requires a physician order.

C. Skin Care

1. All patients should be repositioned/turned at least every 2 hours unless contraindicated. Position changes should be documented.

2. Additional skin care protection (e.g., heel, elbow pads, and decubitus care) may be ordered by the nurse as needed.

3. A protective blanket should be applied between the skin and hyper/hypothermia blanket when in use.

4. If the corneal reflex is absent, a saline sponge should be placed over the patient's eyes each shift or eyes may be taped closed.

5. Patients should be bathed each day as tolerated. Hair care (combing and shampooing) should be done prn.

6. Perineal care prn.

D. Mouth Care

1. Mouth care prn.

2. Intubated patients should receive mouth care every 8 hours and supplemented with swabbing with sponge and mouth wash every 4 hours and prn. Oral airways should be removed during mouth care.

VI. **Uterine Activity and Fetal Monitoring**

All critically ill undelivered patients should have uterine activity and fetal assessments should be performed and documented according to the high-risk criteria in the *Guidelines for Care of Patients in Labor* and *Guidelines for Fetal Heart Rate Monitoring*.

VII. **Metabolic Assessment**

A. Temperature Assessment—Temperature should be assessed and documented every 4 hours. Assessment should be performed and documented every 2 hours in the following situations:

1. temperature is > 100 degrees F

2. temperature is < 97 degrees F

3. amniotic membranes are ruptured

B. If a cooling or warming adjunct is in place, the patient's temperature should be assessed and documented every hour.

VIII. **Vascular Line Care**

A. General Assessment

1. Peripheral and central vascular line access sites should be assessed every 2 hours for integrity and documented.

2. All vascular infusion lines should be assessed every 8 hours.

3. Infusion pumps should be used for all venous infusions unless rapid volume expansion is in progress.

B. Tubing Changes

1. All pressure tubing and IV tubing should be changed every 72 hours.

2. TPN and lipid tubing should be changed every 24 hours.

3. Cardiac output Co-Set tubing should be changed every 72 hours.

C. Dressing Changes—Transparent (e.g., Opsite) dressings should be changed every 5 days or more frequently if integrity warrants.

D. Blood Sampling

1. From intraarterial line, withdraw and discard 3 ml blood prior to obtaining sample.

2. From PA or triple lumen central catheters:

a. Turn off all infusions via catheter ports prior to blood sampling.

b. Withdraw and discard 10 ml blood if sampling port has been in use for an active infusion.

c. Withdraw and discard 5 ml blood if sampling port has been capped off or used for a pressure line.

E. Vascular Access

1. All critically ill patients should have venous access at all times. Peripheral access should be obtained prior to discontinuation of central venous access.

2. All vasoactive medications should be administered via a central line except in STAT situations or when the medication to be administered is for a short period of time.

F. Transport—Patients with PA catheter or requiring mechanical ventilation should be attended by a CCOB nurse and physician during transport.

IX. **Rest and Activity**

A. Every effort should be made to optimize the patient's opportunity for rest and sleep.

B. Patients with a PA catheter may be out of bed to a chair with assistance when stable with physician's order.

X. **Psychosocial**

A. Philosophy—It is the philosophy of nursing that all patients and their family/support system be viewed in a holistic way: mind, body, and spirit. All care should adhere to this model.

B. Visitation—Insofar as is reasonably possible, open visitation should be implemented for critically ill patients. Every effort should be made to facilitate access between patient/family and their newborn, when applicable. If it is not possible for the newborn to leave the nursery setting, every effort should be made to provide information to patient regarding newborn status.

XI. **Nursing Implications**

Notify physician for any of the following:
A. Systolic blood pressure > 160 mm Hg
B. Diastolic blood pressure ≥ 110 mm Hg
C. Respirations < 14 or > 26
D. DTRs absent
E. Urine output < 30 cc/hour or < 240 cc in 8 hours

F. Symptoms of pulmonary edema
G. SaO_2 < 95%
H. Seizure activity
I. Significant system changes
J. Imminent delivery

XII. **Patient/Family Education**

A. Plan of care
B. Unit routine
C. Electronic fetal monitoring
D. Disease process
E. Bed rest and physical activity restrictions
F. Diversional activities
G. Expected length of stay
H. Special testing/equipment
I. Arterial and PA catheter placement
J. Delivery method

XIII. **References**

ACOG Technical Bulletin. (1996, January). Hypertension in pregnancy. (No. 219). <u>American College of Obstetricians and Gynecologists</u>. Washington, DC.

Clark, S. L., Cotton, D. B., Hankins, G. D. V., & Phelan, J. P. (1991). <u>Critical care obstetrics</u>. Boston; Blackwell Scientific.

Troiano, N. H., & Harvey, C. (Eds.). (1992). <u>NAACOG's clinical issues in perinatal and women's health nursing</u>, <u>3</u>(3), Critical Care Obstetrics. Philadelphia: Lippincott.

Guidelines for the Care of the Obstetric Trauma Patient

I. **Primary Survey**

A. Airway
1. Assess airway for patency; look, listen, and feel for air movement.
2. Use modified jaw thrust maneuver to open airway and assess for obstruction or foreign matter.
3. Do not turn patient's head to assess or open airway.
4. Assume potential for cervical spine injury until proven otherwise.

B. Breathing
1. Assess ventilatory and respiratory function noting the following:
   a. rate and quality of respirations
   b. signs and symptoms of respiratory distress
      - inability to move air despite presence of open airway
      - asymmetric chest excursion
      - shallow or painful respirations
      - dyspnea
      - use of accessory muscles
      - tachypnea
      - bradycardia
2. Assess trachea noting the following:
   a. position
   b. deviation from midline (indication of possible pneumothorax or massive hemothorax)
3. Visually inspect chest noting the following:
   a. contusions
   b. asymmetric excursion
   c. paradoxical breathing (indication of possible flail chest)
   d. open sucking wounds (indicative of possible open pneumothorax)
4. Auscultate breath sounds bilaterally noting the following:
   a. hyperresonance (indicative of possible pneumothorax)
   b. dullness (indicative of possible hemothorax), if decreased or absent breath sounds noted, percuss thorax
5. Palpate thorax noting the following:
   a. presence of pain
   b. rib instability
   c. subcutaneous emphysema (indicative of possible flail chest)
6. Auscultate heart sounds noting the following:
   a. distant heart sounds
   b. muffled heart sounds (indicative of possible cardiac tamponade)

C. Circulation
1. Assess cardiac output
   a. palpate pulses to estimate blood pressure
      - carotid: systolic $\geq$ 60 mm Hg
      - femoral: systolic $\geq$ 70 mm Hg
      - radial: systolic $\geq$ 80 mm Hg
   b. assess neck veins for flatness or distention
      - flatness may indicate hypotension secondary to hypovolemia
      - distension may indicate tension pneumothorax or cardiac tamponade

c. assess capillary bed refill

d. note skin color and temperature

2. Assess for bleeding

a. external

b. evidence of internal

D. Neurologic Status

1. Assess level of consciousness

2. Determine Glasgow coma score

Eye opening

Spontaneously	4
To verbal command	3
To pain	2
None	1

Best verbal response

Oriented	5
Confused	4
Inappropriate words	3
Incomprehensible sounds	2
None	1

Best motor response

Follows commands	6
Localizes pain	5
Withdraws from pain	4
Flexor posturing	3
(decorticate)	2
Extensor posturing	1
(decerebrate)	
None	
	Total 3–15

II. **Interventions**

A. Airway Access and Maintenance

1. Maintain cervical alignment at all times.

2. Immobilize cervical spine with collar or other device.

3. Clear airway of foreign matter.

4. Use nasopharyngeal or oropharyngeal airway to maintain airway patency.

5. Anticipate and assist with endotracheal intubation as necessary.

6. Place nasogastric tube to prevent aspiration and relieve abdominal distention.

7. Use "log rolling" or tilting of spine board to turn patient for airway management.

B. Respiratory Interventions

1. Administer oxygen at 12 L/minute by tight nonrebreather mask.

2. Anticipate need for mechanical ventilation if respiratory rate is > 25 or < 12 per minute.

3. Obtain arterial blood gases as ordered.

4. Apply petrolatum gauze or airtight dressing to any open sucking chest wound.

C. Circulatory Interventions

1. Initiate cardiopulmonary resuscitation as indicated, with lateral uterine displacement.

2. Apply direct pressure or pressure bandages to control external bleeding.

3. Obtain peripheral intravenous access using large bore catheter(s). Two lines may be necessary.

4. Obtain appropriate blood specimens as ordered.

5. Apply pneumatic antishock garment as indicated. Abdominal compartment may be left uninflated.

III. **Secondary Survey**

A. Reassess Neurologic Status Noting the Following

1. Level of consciousness

a. A—alert and oriented

b. V—responds to verbal stimulus

c. P—responds only to pain

d. U—unresponsive

2. Sensorimotor function

a. response to painful stimuli

b. presence of flaccid paralysis

c. Glasgow coma scale

B. Examine Head Noting the Following

1. Contusions, lacerations, and bony deformities

2. Signs and symptoms of basilar skull fracture

a. check for bleeding from ear or nose

b. cheek for Battle's sign: postauricular swelling and discoloration

c. check for "raccoon eyes": periorbital edema and ecchymosis

d. anticipate order for portable x-ray for evaluation of cervical spine

C. Reassess Chest and Circulation

D. Anticipate Order for X-ray of Thorax

E. Make Abdominal Assessment Noting the Following

1. Pain and tenderness

2. Distention

F. Assess Musculoskeletal Status Noting the Following
   1. Soft tissue injury
   2. Skeletal injury
   3. Neuromuscular function of affected extremity
      a. sensation
      b. movement
      c. color
      d. swelling
      e. capillary refill
      f. distal pulses

IV. **Uterine Assessment**

A. Assess Uterine Activity
   1. Contraction frequency, intensity, and duration
   2. Resting tone

B. Assess Fundal Height for Approximation of Gestational Age (fundus at level of umbilucis equals to approximately 20 week gestation)

C. Inspect Perineum for Presence of Bleeding or Leakage of Amniotic Fluid

D. Perform Cervical Exam (in the absence of vaginal bleeding or prematurity)
   1. Cervical dilation, effacement, position, and consistency
   2. Status of amniotic membranes
   3. Fetal station, lie, presentation

E. Assess for Signs and Symptoms of Placental Abruption
   1. Presence of frequent uterine contractions
   2. Vaginal bleeding or increasing fundal height
   3. Evidence of fetal hypoxemia
   4. Maternal hemodynamic instability
   5. Abdominal tenderness
   6. Increased resting tone

V. **Fetal Assessment and Interventions**

A. Assess Fetal Heart Rate According to the *Guidelines for Fetal Heart Rate Monitoring*.

B. Promote Uteroplacental Perfusion
   1. Displace uterus laterally and avoid supine position.
   2. Correct hypovolemia with fluid resuscitation.
   3. Administer oxygen as indicated.

VI. **Psychosocial Assessment and Interventions**

A. Identify patient's support persons. Allow for contact as soon as acute resuscitative measures are completed.

B. Inform patient and family of status of baby and mother.

C. Allow expression of fear and anxiety.

D. Provide support and reassurance.

VII. **Documentation**

A. Maternal and Fetal Assessment

B. Initiation of Protocols Used in Patient Care

C. All Medical and Nursing Intervention and Patient's Response

D. Resuscitation Measures

E. Physician Notification Including Indication and Response

VIII. **References**

ACOG Technical Bulletin. (1991, November). Trauma during pregnancy (No. 161).

Astarita, D. C., & Feldman, B. (1997, April). Seat belt placement resulting in uterine rupture. Journal of Trauma, 42(4), 738–740.

Chang, S. S., Chang, M. C., & Morris, J. A. (1992, July). Trauma in pregnancy—the maternal-fetal relationship. Journal of the Tennessee Medical Association, 87(7), 291–292.

Esposito, T. J. (1994, February). Trauma during pregnancy. Emergency Medicine Clinics of North America, 12(1), 167–199.

Goldman, S. M., & Wagner, L. K. (1996, April). Radiologic management of abdominal trauma in pregnancy. American Journal of Roentgenology, 166(4), 763–767.

Huzel, P. S., & Remsburg-Bell, E. A. (1996, February). Fetal complications related to minor maternal trauma. Journal of Obstetric, Gynecologic, and Neonatal Nursing, 25(2), 121–124.

Lavery, J. P., & Staten-McCormick, M. (1995, March). Management of moderate to severe trauma in pregnancy. Obstetrics and Gynecology Clinics of North America, 22(1), 69–90.

Mighty, H. (1994, July). Trauma in pregnancy. Critical Care Clinics, 10(3), 623–634.

Protocol for the Nursing Management of the Obstetric Patient Requiring Transport

I. **Nursing Care Immediately Prior to Transport**

   A. General Assessment
      1. Reason for transport
      2. Respiratory function including the following:
         a. patency of airway
         b. rate and quality of respirations
         c. signs and symptoms of respiratory compromise
      3. Hemodynamic function including the following:
         a. blood pressure
         b. heart rate and rhythm
         c. intake and output
         d. signs and symptoms of hemodynamic compromise
      4. Change in maternal condition

   B. Labor Assessment
      1. Note estimation of gestational age
      2. Note labor status
         a. contraction frequency, duration, and intensity
         b. uterine resting tone
         c. cervical status
         d. fetal station and presentation
         e. note presence or absence of vaginal bleeding
         f. status of membranes, if ruptured note the following:
            – date and time of rupture
            – color of amniotic fluid

   C. Fetal Assessment
      1. Assess fetal heart rate according to the *Guidelines for Fetal Heart Rate Monitoring.*
      2. Document the following:
         a. baseline rate expressed as a range
         b. baseline variability (if applicable)
         c. presence/absence of periodic patterns

   D. Nursing Interventions
      1. Assure functioning intravenous access with appropriate gauge catheter.
      2. Anticipate need for indwelling urinary catheter.
      3. Measure and record all intake and output.
      4. Initiate guidelines for care related to specific maternal diagnosis.
      5. Obtain alternative orders from primary physician for complications that may arise during transport:
         a. treatment of seizures
         b. additional or alternative medications
      6. Assign transport personnel as appropriate for patient's level of care.
      7. Assure that all necessary equipment is available and in proper working condition including the following:
         a. airway management kit, bag-valve ventilation unit, and portable suction equipment
         b. medications including intravenous fluids and supplies
         c. infusion pumps for intravenous fluid administration
         d. electrocardiographic monitor

450

e. blood pressure cuff, sphygmo-manometer, and thermometer

f. fetoscope or doppler

g. oxygen with manual control, adjustable flow meter with gauge, and humidification attachment

h. obstetric delivery kit and isolette with oxygen

E. Psychosocial Assessment and Interventions

1. Explain to patient and support persons reasons for transport and transport process.

2. Allow for expression of anxiety concerning transport and answer all questions.

3. Frequently update patient and family on maternal and fetal status.

4. Anticipate need for directions, transportation, and contact persons for patient's family at arrival to receiving hospital.

F. Documentation

1. Obtain copy of prenatal records including name, phone number, and address of prenatal caregiver if different from referring physician.

2. Obtain copies of obstetric information including:

a. pertinent clinical information including admission history and physical

b. treatments

c. laboratory tests and results

d. ultrasound or other diagnostic tests and results

e. medications administered

f. fetal status

g. labor status

h. intake and output

II. **Nursing Care During Transport**

A. Maternal Care

1. Assess blood pressure, pulse, respirations, and temperature every 30 minutes unless otherwise indicated.

2. Measure and record intake and output hourly.

3. Assess deep tendon reflexes, if patient receiving $MgSO_4$, every hour.

4. Assess contractions by palpation noting frequency, duration, and intensity every 15–30 minutes.

5. Assess for vaginal bleeding or leaking of amniotic fluid.

6. Assess fetal heart rate using fetoscope or doppler according to *Guidelines for Fetal Heart Rate Monitoring*.

B. Nursing Interventions

1. Position patient

a. allow for clear view and access to patient at all times during transport

b. avoid supine position which decreases maternal cardiac output

c. utilize approved safety restraints during transport

d. administer oxygen via face mask as indicated

e. continue care by utilizing patient care guidelines initiated prior to transport

f. initiate all patient care guidelines as patient's condition dictates

C. Psychosocial Assessment and Interventions

1. Continue to update patient regarding status.

2. Explain all procedures and answer questions.

3. Allow for expression of anxiety during transport and give reassurance.

4. Support and encourage relaxation and controlled breathing techniques.

D. Documentation

1. Maternal and fetal assessments

2. Initiation of guidelines used in patient care

3. Nursing and medical interventions and patient's response

4. Initial and subsequent medication dosages as well as time of dosage changes

5. Completed follow-up status report sent to referring physician and hospital

III. **References**

American College of Obstetricians and Gynecologists & American Academy of Pediatrics. Guidelines for perinatal care. (1997).

AWHONN. (1998). Standards for the Professional Nursing Practice in the Care of Women and Newborns (5th ed.). Washington, DC.

Strobino, D. M., et al. (1993, January–March). Development of an index of maternal transport. Medical decision making, 13(1), 64–73.

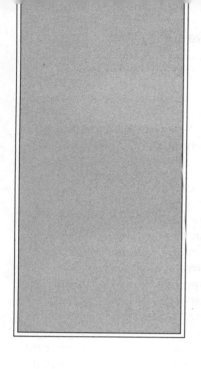

Critical (Collaborative) Pathway: Asthma in Pregnancy

Goals
1. Maintain patient's normal PEFR and/or FEV1
2. Prevention of acute attack by avoiding environmental and medication triggers
3. Prompt intervention for symptoms of exacerbation

Nursing Diagnoses
1. Potential alteration in oxygenation related to acute attack
2. Potential knowledge deficit related to treatment regime and medications used during labor and delivery

	Labor	Delivery	Acute Attack
Nutrition	po/IV to maintain hydration	IV to maintain hydration	IV to maintain hydration
Tests/Labs	PEFR/FEV1 q12 hr or with symptoms consider CBC, CXR sputum culture	PEFR/FEV1 prn	PEFR/FEV1 prn
Treatments	O_2 prn remove asthma triggers Epidural prn	O_2 prn	O_2 to maintain SaO_2 at 95% or greater Mech vent for PEFR < 25% or CO_2 > 35
Meds	routine asthma meds Hydrocortisone IV prn Fentanyl prn pain Pitocin prn	cont. routine meds po to IV meds avoid prostin F2 alpha	inhaled beta agonists systemic cortico-steroids
Consults	Anesthesia Perinatology prn		Anesthesia, Pulmonary Neonatology, Perinat.
Assessments	History & Physical EFM, attack symptoms	SaO_2, EFM attack symptoms	attack symptoms PEFR/FEV, EFM
Teaching	Assessment strategy treatment regime meds		treatment regime meds

REFERENCES

Clark, S. L., & the National Asthma Education Working Group on Asthma in Pregnancy. (1993). Obstetrics and Gynecology, 82(6), 1036–1040.

Heart, Lung, and Blood Institute. (1993). Management of Asthma During Pregnancy. U. S. Department of Health and Human Services.

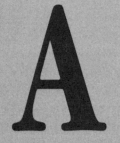

APPENDIX

A

Forms and Flowsheets

APPENDIX A: Forms and Flowsheets

Date: Pathway:				ANTEPARTUM/ INTRAPARTUM FLOWSHEET								
Signature & Title				√ = no significant findings								
Signature & Title				* = significant finding see narrative note								
Signature & Title				→ = no change from last significant finding								
Signature & Title												
Time												
Temperature												
Blood Pressure												
Pulse												
Respiration												
SaO₂												
O₂ (L/min)												
Breath Sounds												
DTRs/Clonus												
Maternal Pos.												
Mon. Mode												
FHR												
Variability												
Accelerations												
Decelerations												
Mon. Mode												
UC Freq. (min)												
Duration (sec)												
Intensity												
MVU's												
Resting Tone												
Pitocin mu/min												
MgSO₄ gm/hr												
Insulin u/hr												
Cardiac												
Respiratory												
Neuro												
GU												
GI												
Skin												
Musculoskel.												
Psychosocial												
Safety												
Comfort												
Pt. Hygiene												
Vag. Discharge												
VE												
VE Examiner												
Initials												

Vanderbilt University Medical Center
Significant Findings

Date: Pathway:			COLLABORATIVE PATHWAY FLOWSHEET			

√ In Indicated Column = desired goal for patient

Initials = Goal Met

*in **Met** column = goal not (see narrative notes)

Signature	
Signature	
Signature	
Signature	

GOALS	I	MET			DONE		DONE	DONE
Pt/Family Understand Plan of Care			C	Anesthesia			T&S	
Appropriate Consent Forms Signed			O	NICU		L	PCV	
Obtains Pain Relief Option			N	Social Work		A	CBC c diff	
Adequate Progression of Labor			S	Dietary		B	Platelets	
No Indications of Fetal Distress			U	Lactation		S	Creatinine	
Vaginal Delivery of Infant			L				Uric Acid	
Term Infant with Apgar >7 at 5 min			T				SGOT/LDH	
Placenta Del. wo Surg. Intervention			P	Ster. Spec.			SMA-6	
Ambulate with Assistance			R	Abd. Prep			PT/PTT	
Transfer to PP in < 2 hours			O	Enema			Fibrinogen	
Hemodynamically Stable			C	Amnioinfus.			Cx Culture	
Patient without Seizures			E				B-Strep	
Tx Started within 1 hr of Diagnosis			D				UA/C&S	
PTL Patients without Cx Change			T	US			24 hr Urine	
PTL Pts to 4E if no Cx Change or			E	BPP			ABG	
IV tocolysis			S	Doppler Flow				
Specimens to Appr. Destination			T	Amniocent.				
Fetal Remains to Appr. Destination			S					
Grief Packet Completed								
Verbalize Home Care Instructions								
			T	Unit Routine		A	Bedrest	
			E	Plan of care		C	BR w BRP	
			A	Meds		T	Up Ad Lib	
			C	Ante. Tests				
			H	S/S PTL				
			I	S/S PIH		E	IMED (1)	
			N	S/S Infection		Q	IMED (2)	
			G	Self Care		U	IMED Tube	
				PTL Stimul.		I	Epid. Pump	
				Induction		P	Epid. Tube	
				EFM		M	Epid. Tray	
						E	Foley	
						N	IUPC	
						T	FSE	
							Aminf. Kit	
							Amnio Tray	
			D	NPO				
			I	Ice Chips				
			E	Clear Liquids				
			T	Adv. as Tol.		O		
				Regular		T		
						H		
						E		
						R		

COLLABORATIVE PATHWAY FLOWSHEET

DONE: Caregiver's initials in each category indicate this service/activity has been completed. Date and time included when appropriate.

CONSULTS: Appropriate consult completed.

PROCEDURE: Procedure appropriate for patient and administered in a timely manner.

TESTS: Prescribed test was ordered and administrated by appropriate person.

TEACHING: Appropriate teaching given to patient/family.

DIET: Patient is tolerating prescribed diet.

LABS: Prescribed lab ordered. Drawn and sent to lab in a timely manner.

ACTIVITY: Patient is tolerating prescribed activity.

EQUIPMENT: The piece of equipment or supply is in use at the bedside.

ASSESSMENT PARAMETERS

The RN will perform a complete assessment on admission and every shift. Appropriate system assessment/s will be performed with any significant change in patient status or as applicable for indicated collaborative pathway.

The following parameters will be considered a negative assessment and constitute the use of a "√."

CARDIAC: No cyanosis or chest pain is noted/reported. Pulse is < 120 bpm. Regular rate and rhythm. Dependent edema < 1+ in feet and ankles.

RESPIRATORY: Respirations regular. Rate 14–24. Vesicular breath sounds are present bilaterally by auscultation. Patient is not short of breath. SaO_2 above 95% if pulse oximeter in use.

NEURO: Alert and oriented to person, place, time, and event. When applicable, denies HA or visual disturbance. DTR's 2–3+, no clonus. Level of Consciousness 1 = Asleep 2 = Alert/Oriented 3 = Disoriented.

GU/BLADDER: Bladder is not palpable. UOP >/= 30 cc/hr. Urine clear. Foley catheter, if present, is patent to bedside bag and draining clear yellow urine. PP: Large amounts of blood-tinged fluid may be normal. Burning on urination possible if episiotomy or perineal laceration present.

GI/UTERUS: Bowel sounds present in all 4 quadrants (generally not assessed in intrapartum patient). Denies diarrhea, N/V, constipation, or RUQ pain. Tolerating prescribed diet. Abdomen without excessive tenderness in absence of uterine contractions. PP: Fundus firm to palpation, located in midline. Fundal height is at or below umbilicus.

SKIN: Skin warm and dry with pink mucous membranes. No wounds, lesions, or breakdown noted.

MUSCULOSKELETAL: Moves all extremities equal bilaterally. Normal ROM. No abnormal muscle weakness. After epidural placement expect lower extremity deficit.

PSYCHOSOCIAL: Affect and emotional status is appropriate for patient situation and consistent with stage of pregnancy. Support system available.

SAFETY: ID band present. Call light within reach. Side rails up when appropriate. Caregiver has checked on patient and found patient in no apparent distress. Safety equipment to bedside (ambubag, airway, mask, O_2).

COMFORT: 1 = Asleep 2 = Comfortable 3 = Mild discomfort 4 = Pain 5 = Severe pain. PRN meds administered as ordered and the expected result is anticipated.

VAGINAL DISCHARGE: If ROM fluid clear and without foul odor. No bleeding except for normal bloody show. PP: Rubra lochia present in small to moderate amounts. A few 1–2 cm clots may be present. Lochia has the fleshy odor of normal menses.

INCISION/PERINEUM: PP: Edges of wound well approximated. No increase from initial amount of erythema, ecchymosis, edema, drainage, or discomfort. Hemorrhoids are not bleeding and are without excessive swelling or pain. Abdominal dressing, if present, is dry and intact.

LOWER EXTREMITIES: PP: 1 = Unable to move without assistance 2 = Some movement of either or both legs without assistance 3 = Able to extend and raise both legs without assistance.

LEGENDS /ABBREVIATIONS

MATERNAL POSITION	FHR CHANGES	VARIABILITY	DTR'S
left lateral tilt	Accel. = acceleration	A = absent (0–2 bpm)	0 = absent
right lateral tilt	E = early deceleration	Min = minimal (3–5 bpm)	1+ = present with hammer
supine	L = late deceleration	Mod. = moderate (6–25 bpm)	2+ = present with fingertips
? = knee chest	V = variable deceleration	Mkd = marked (25+ bpm)	3+ = brisk with fingertips
? = rendelenberg	P = prolonged deceleration		4+ = clonus present
? = semi-fowlers			
? = high fowlers	UC INTENSITY	BREATH SOUNDS	UTERINE TONE
	m = mild	C = clear	rlx = relaxed
MONITOR MODE	mod = moderate	Cr = crackles	nr = nonrelaxed
? = external	str = strong	Wh = wheezes	
? = internal			

APPENDIX A: Forms and Flowsheets

VANDERBILT UNIVERSITY MEDICAL CENTER
PERINATAL TEACHING RECORD

Signature & Title	IN	Signature & Title	IN	

Patient/Family demonstrates or verbalizes understanding of:	Date/ Initial	Date/ Initial	Date/ Initial	Patient/Family demonstrates or verbalizes understanding of:	Date/ Initial	Date/ Initial	Date/ Initial
Prenatal Visit Schedule & Content				Infant Hospital Security Procedures			
Warning/Danger Signs				Use of Bulb Syringe			
When and Who to Call				Breastfeeding Techniques			
Fetal Growth & Development				Formula Prep & Bottle Feeding			
Maternal Physical Changes				Infant Feeding Issues			
Maternal Emotional Changes				Cord & Genitalia Care			
Family Adjustments				Infant Bath & Skin Care			
Activity, Exercise, & Rest				Thermometer Use and Temp Taking			
Common Discomforts of Pregnancy				Warning Signs of Infant Illness			
Nutrition				Infant Elimination Pattern			
Employment, Travel				Infant's PKU/Thyroid Test			
Prenatal Classes Available				Car Seat Information & TN law			
Signs of Labor				Infant Safety in the Home			
				Normal Newborn Characteristics			
				Crying/Sleeping Patterns			
Unit Routine in Labor and Delivery				Well Baby Visits/Immunizations			
Plan of Care in Labor and Delivery							
Analgesia/Anesthesia				**Packets or Information Given**			
Delivery Method Vag/VBAC/C/S				VUH Perinatal Info Book			
EFM				Car Seat Information			
Prostin Gel				Postpartum Packet			
Induction/Augmentation				NBN Breastfeeding Packet			
Tocolytics				NBN Packet			
Antepartum Testing				NICU Breastfeeding Packet			
PTL Stimulating Activities				NICU Information			
S/S Infection/Amnionitis				Grief Packet/Empty Arms			
Postpartum Unit Routine				**PP Discharge Planning**			
Postpartum Plan of Care				Pt Transportation Available ☐ Yes ☐ No			
Antepartum Plan of Care				PP WIC ☐ Yes ☐ No Done			
Antepartum Home Care Instructions				PP Follow-up Appointment on			
Care of Breast/Breast exam				Family Planning Method Chosen			
Expected Lochia Changes				☐ BTL Done ☐ DepoProvera Given ☐ OCP Given			
Care of the Perineum				Home Health Care Evaluation ☐ Yes ☐ No ☐ Done			
Care of the Abdominal Incision				Breast Pump Rental ☐ Yes ☐ No ☐ Done			
PP Sexual Activity/Birth Control				Other Referrals:			
PP Exercise and Rest							
PP Diet and Elimination							
PP Danger Signs							
PP Family Adjustments							
Immunizations/Rhogam							
Use of Breast Pump							

458

CRITICAL CARE OBSTETRICS FLOWSHEET

DATE _____ TIME									
CARDIOVASCULAR									
Temp (O R A C)									
SBP/DBP									
Art Line SBP/DBP									
MAP									
Heart Rate									
Rhythm									
PA Sys/Dia									
CVP									
PAOP									
PVR/SVR									
CO/CI									
RESPIRATORY									
Breath Sounds R/L									
FiO2 NC FM Vent)									
SaO_2 / SvO_2									
CaO_2 / CvO_2									
DO2 / VO2									
O2ER / Qs/Qt									
ABG pH / CO_2									
pO_2 / B.E.									
Mode: PSV AC SIMV									
TV (Spon / Set)									
Rate (Total / Set)									
PSV / PEEP / CPAP									
Peak Inspir. Pres.									
Suction									
FETAL/UC ASSESS									
Maternal Position									
Monitor Mode									
FHR									
Variability									
Accelerations									
Decelerations									
Monitor Mode									
UC Freq. (min)									
Duration (sec)									
Intensity									
MVU's									
Resting Tone									
Vaginal Exam									
Membranes/Fluid									
Medications									
Pitocin (init/min)									
$MgSO_4$ (gm/hr)									
Insulin									
Initials									

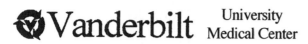

Vanderbilt University Medical Center

CRITICAL CARE OBSTETRIC
ASSESSMENT FORM

DATE	SIGNATURE & TITLE	INITIALS

ASSESSMENT PARAMETERS	PT. SPECIFIC ASSESSMENT	TIME								
√ Meets assessment parameter → No significant change from last finding * See narrative notes	(for pt diagnosis and condition)									
Neurological: When awake is alert, oriented × 3. Obeys commands, responds appropriately. DTR's 1–3+. Pupil reaction brisk. PERRL. Denies HA or visual changes	☐ IV Sedation ☐ Paralyzing agents									
Cardiovascular: HR < 120 bpm at rest; Sinus rhythm. Pulse regular. SI, S2 noted without murmur. No cyanosis or chest pain; Capillary refill < 2 sec; No jugular venous distention; Radial, Dorsalis Pedis, Post Tibial pulses palpable, equal bilaterally. Edema < 1+ Waveforms appropriate.	☐ PAC Type _____ Placement _____ Position _____ cm at introducer ☐ Arterial Line Placement _____									
Pulmonary: Vesicular breath sounds in all lung fields; Pt denies dyspnea or SOB. Sputum, if present, is clear. SaO2 > 95%. ET tube dry and secure.	☐ Airway Type _____ Position _____									
Musculoskeletal: Functional ROM all joints; no muscle weakness; extremity strength equal bilaterally.	☐ Epidural—expect lower extremity deficit.									
GI: Abdomen soft, nondistended, appropriately tender. No nausea, vomiting or diarrhea. Tolerating prescribed diet. If enteric tube present, well secured and patent. Placement checked.	Bowel Sounds ☐ Absent ☐ Hypotonic ☐ Present 4 quad. ☐ Enteric Tube ☐ ILWS ☐ CLWS ☐ Other _____									
Genitourinary: Clear, yellow/amber urine. Neg ketones, < 1+ proteinuria	☐ Foley to BSB ☐ Other _____									
Integument: Skin warm and dry, CVC site and IV site(s) wifliout redness, swelling, or tenderness. Dressing(s) dry and intact.	IV Site _____ IV Site _____ Other _____									
Incision/Perineum: Sutures, staples or steristrips if present are intact. Wound edges well approximated, without redness, drainage or induration, if visible. Hemorrhoids without bleeding, swelling or pain.										
Drains: Patent, activated and well secured. Dressing dry and intact.	☐ Bloody ☐ Serosanguinous ☐ Minimal drainage									
Psychosocial: Affect and emotional status appropriate for patient, consistent with diagnosis and condition. Support system available. Denies spiritual/cultural needs.										
Safety: Call light within reach, bed in low position, siderails up when appropriate, ID band present, ambubag at bedside or on emergency cart.	☐ Monitor alarms on. ☐ Restraints—Upper/Lower.									
Comfort: 1 = asleep, 2 = comfortable, 3 = mild discomfort, 4 = pain, 5 = severe pain. If PP, comfort level is adequate to allow movement following delivery.	☐ PCA Pump. ☐ PRN meds administered as ordered. Expected result is anticipated.									
Uterus: Abdomen w/o excessive tenderness in the absence of uterine contractions. PP- fundus firm, midline at or below umbilicus.	☐ PP -rubra lochia present in sm-mod amts. A few 1–2 cm clots may be present. Decreasing to moderate or less rubra or serosa after PP day 2.									
Breast/Nipples: 1st 24 hrs PP soft, non-tender w/o fissures or cracking. 25–48 hrs PP feel firm & may be tender and warm to touch.										
Personal Hygiene: Bath/shower and mouth care q 24 hrs. If bedrest assisted with care. Pericare done prn. Linens ▲'d daily or prn	☐ Foley Care q 8 hrs. ☐ Mouth care q 4 hrs if ETT.									
Initials										

Competency Validation Checklist for Critical Care OB

VANDERBILT UNIVERSITY MEDICAL CENTER
OBSTETRIC INTENSIVE CARE UNIT
COMPETENCY VALIDATION
SKILLS CHECKLIST

SKILL: **Pressure Line Set-Up, Calibration, Zero-Referencing**

NAME: _____

Behavior/Skill   **Completed/Date**   **APN Initials**

1. Identifies appropriate amount of NS flush solution
    (500 ml) and heparin (2500 u)

2. Identifies components of pressure line (compliant tubing,
    pressure transducer/cable noncompliant tubing, and
    pressure bag)

3. Primes/flushes pressure line correctly (tightens all connections,
    removes air from tubing using stopcocks correctly and replaces
    vented with nonvented caps)

4. Connects pressure line cable to monitor

5. Calibrates pressure transducer correctly (zeroes line, opens
    stopcock to air, raises stopcock 27 cm and observes digital reading
    of 20 mm Hg ± 1)

6. Zero-references transducer correctly (locates patient phlebostatic
    axis, marks on chest wall, opens stopcock proximal to patient to air,
    depresses zero button, closes stopcock to air)

7. Inflates pressure bag to 300 mm Hg

8. Demonstrates infection control principles during above
    procedures

VANDERBILT UNIVERSITY MEDICAL CENTER
OBSTETRIC INTENSIVE CARE UNIT
COMPETENCY VALIDATION
SKILLS CHECKLIST

SKILL: **Assisting with PA and Intraarterial Catheter Insertion**

NAME: _____

Behavior/Skill	**Completed/Date**	**APN Initials**
1. Identifies ports correctly (CVP, PA, balloon, VIP/paceport, thermistor and fiberoptic), flushes each, checks balloon patency and connects to monitor		
2. Explains procedure to client and offers support during procedure		
3. Assists physician appropriately during insertion of introducer and PA catheter		
4. Identifies normal characteristics of CVP, PA, PAOP, and ASP waveforms then obtains a reading from graphic recording		
5. Stabilizes catheter with appropriate dressing and tape (transparent opsite without antiseptic ointment)		
6. Verbalizes normal values during pregnancy for CVP, PAP, PAOP, CO, and SvO_2		
7. Demonstrates infection control principles during above procedures		

VANDERBILT UNIVERSITY MEDICAL CENTER
OBSTETRIC INTENSIVE CARE UNIT
COMPETENCY VALIDATION
SKILLS CHECKLIST

SKILL: **Fiberoptic (SvO_2) PA Catheter Use/Maintenance**

NAME: _____

Behavior/Skill	**Completed/Date**	**APN Initials**

1. Connects SvO_2 cable to monitor prior to insertion

2. Performs in-vitro calibration prior to insertion (enters hemoglobin value)

3. Performs in-vivo calibration appropriately (obtains mixed venous blood sample from PA port, identifies need for adjustments based on values)

4. Identifies appropriate disconnection point for patient transport situations

5. Verbalizes normal SvO_2 range during pregnancy

VANDERBILT UNIVERSITY MEDICAL CENTER
OBSTETRIC INTENSIVE CARE UNIT
COMPETENCY VALIDATION
SKILLS CHECKLIST

SKILL: **Thermodilution Cardiac Output**

NAME: _____

Behavior/Skill	**Completed/Date**	**APN Initials**

1. Sets up Co-set correctly (spikes 1 liter bag of NS, places coil in ice bath, connects syringe to tubing and flushes air from line)

2. Connects cables correctly (injectate temperature, thermistor)

3. Identifies and correctly enters/confirms computation constant

4. Connects injectate syringe to CVP port

5. Identifies correct iced injectate temperature

6. Performs three injections, edits curves, and stores data appropriately

7. Demonstrates infection control principles during above procedures

VANDERBILT UNIVERSITY MEDICAL CENTER
OBSTETRIC INTENSIVE CARE UNIT
COMPETENCY VALIDATION
SKILLS CHECKLIST

SKILL: **Artificial Mechanical Ventilation**

NAME: _____

Behavior/Skill	**Completed/Date**	**APN Initials**

1. Explains the difference in selected modes of artificial mechanical ventilation (control, assist control, IMV/SIMV, CPAP) and adjuncts (PEEP pressure support)

2. Locates selected settings on the ventilator (FiO$_2$, tidal volume, mode, PEEP, rate and pressure support)

3. Describes correct cause of and response to selected ventilator alarms (high pressure, low pressure, humidity/heater)

4. Provides appropriate care measures for the patient with an ETT (securely tapes tube, notes tube size and location, assesses for cuff leak, provides oral hygiene prn)

5. Assures that manual ventilation bag (with PEEP capability) is connected and delivering FiO$_2$ of 1.0 and is immediately accessible

VANDERBILT UNIVERSITY MEDICAL CENTER
OBSTETRIC INTENSIVE CARE UNIT
COMPETENCY VALIDATION
SKILLS CHECKLIST

SKILL: **Suctioning the Patient with an Endotracheal Tube**

NAME: _____

Behavior/Skill	**Completed/Date**	**APN Initials**

1. Verbalizes indications for ETT suctioning (increasing PIP, visible secretions, increased patient coughing efforts)

2. Demonstrates proper technique for both open and closed ETT suctioning
   - explains procedure to patient
   - hyperventilates/hyperoxygenates as indicated by patient status
   - stabilizes ETT
   - limits suction episode to maximum of two catheter passes
   - observes patient response (SaO_2, SvO_2, heart rate, ECG rhythm changes)

3. Demonstrates infection control principles during above procedures

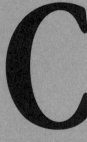

APPENDIX C

Blood and Component Therapy

Hemodynamics	Normal Values During Pregnancy
CVP (right preload)	1–7 mm Hg
PAOP (left preload)	6–10 mm Hg
P.A.P. (reflects right afterload)	systolic 18–30 mm Hg
	diastolic 6–10 mm Hg
	mean 11–15 mm Hg
P.V.R. (right afterload) [(M.P.A.P. – P.A.O.P.) ÷ C.O.] × 80	78 ± 22
S.V.R. (left afterload) [(M.A.P. – C.V.P.) ÷ C.O.] × 80	1210 ± 266
C.O.	6–7 L/min
C.I.	3.2 ± 0.7 L/min
S.V. [(C.O. ÷ H.R.) × 1000]	70 ml
L.V.S.W.I. [(M.A.P. × S.V. × .0136) ÷ B.S.A.]	45 ± 9

* C.V.P. = Central Venous Pressure
* P.A.O.P. = Pulmonary Artery Occlusion Pressure
* P.A.P. = Pulmonary Artery Pressure
* P.V.R. = Pulmonary Vascular Resistance
* S.V.R. = Systemic Vascular Resistance
* C.O. = Cardiac Output
* C.I. = Cardiac Index
* S.V. = Stroke Volume
* L.V.S.W.I. = Left Ventricular Stroke Work Index
* B.S.A. = Body Surface Area
* M.A.P. = Mean Arterial Pressure
* M.P.A.P. = Mean Pulmonary Artery Pressure

Critical Care Obstetrics
Medication Reference

Drug	Actions/Indications	Dosage	Precautions/Side Effects
Amrinone (Inocor)	Inotrope –increases LVSWI –increases CO –decreases SVR	–IV bolus of 0.75 to 1.5 mg/kg given over 3–5 minutes, and follow with infusion of 5–10 mcg/kg/min –Second bolus of 0.75 mg/kg can be given 15–30 minutes after the initial bolus	–1/2 life is 3 hours –thrombocytopenia (2–4%) –may increase myocardial ischemia –may accumulate in pts. with renal and hepatic failure
Bretylium Tosylate	antifibrillatory and antiarrhythmic-ventricular fibrillation	–5 mg/kg undiluted IVP- increase to 10 mg/kg and repeat prn if v-fib persists –24 hour dosage should not exceed 30 mg/kg	hypotension
Dobutamine Hydrochloride (Dobutrex)	Inotrope –increases LVSWI and SV resulting in increased CO	250 mg/250 cc 2.5–10 mcg/kg/min titrate to desired effect	–tachycardia –hypertension –ventricular ectopy –reduce dose gradually to prevent hypotension –Hypovolemia should be corrected prior to start
Dopamine Hydrochloride (Intropin)	**–Low dose** for decreased urinary output causes renal and mesenteric vasodilatation (2–5 mcg/kg/min) **–Low to medium dose** for decreased BP, CO (5–30 mcg/kg/min) **–High dose** for severe hypotension—increases PVR and renal vasoconstriction (30 mcg/kg/min)	Titrate to desired effect	–nausea, headache –ectopy, tachycardia –decreased urinary output secondary to vasoconstriction in high dose
Esmolol (Brevibloc)	Beta blocker-cardioselective –decreases HR, LVSWI, CO, and conduction velocity within the heart –consider administration with tachycardia from Dobutamine administration	Titrate to decrease HR and increase filling time to enhance CO IV: 50 mcg/kg/min	–correct preload prior to administration –delayed AV node conduction
Nicardipine (Cardene)	Calcium Channel Blocker –peripheral vasodilatation, decreases BP	–start at 10 mcg/kg/min –decrease to 1–3 mcg/kg/min with desired blood pressure Alternative dose: –start at 1–20 mg/hr –decrease to 3–5 mg/hr (5 mg/hr is = 1.2 mcg/kg/min in a 70 kg patient)	–tachycardia – vasodilation (flushing, edema, hypotension, headache)
Epinephrine (Adrenalin)	Cardiac stimulant –increases LVSWI –increases HR –vasoconstriction Bronchodilator	IV Bolus– 1:10,000 0.5–1 mg diluted in 10 ml NS	–anxiety headaches –palpitations –tachycardia –hypertension –ventricular fibrillation
Norepinephrine Bitartrate (Levophed)	Alpha –vasoconstriction—use for severe hypotension Beta –inotropic stimulation of the heart and dilation of coronary arteries	4 mg/250 ml 2–4 mcg/min by continuous central line infusion *rate is titrated to maintain BP	CV: –reflex bradycardia –hypertension –severe peripheral and renal vasoconstriction Ischemic injury due to potent vasoconstriction and tissue hypoxia **Must not be given to patients who are hypotensive from blood volume deficits except as an emergency measure to maintain coronary and cerebral artery perfusion until blood volume replacement therapy can be completed

Drug	Actions/Indications	Dosage	Precautions/Side Effects
Nitroglycerin (Tridil)	Venous dilation –promotes peripheral dilation/pooling –decreases venous return –decreases preload Arterial dilation –especially in coronary vessels which reduces myocardial ischemia –decreases SVR –decreases myocardial oxygen consumption	50 mg/250 cc = 200 mcg/ml Initial dose should be 5 mcg/min then titrate by 5 mcg/min increases every 3–5 min to desired effect *Infuse via central line *Use only glass bottle-migrates into plastic	CV: –tachycardia-reflex response to BP CNS: –headache, dizziness GI: –nausea, vomiting *monitor CVP, PAP, and PCOP *hypovolemia must be corrected prior to use
Phenylephrine (Neosynephrine)	Adrenomimetec amines –vasoconstriction—increasing systolic and diastolic BP	start at 15 mcg/min IV, titrate up	– Sinus bradycardia due to vagal reflex; blocked with atropine
Sodium Nitroprusside (Nipride)	Vasodilation by direct effect on arterial and venous smooth muscle with no effect on uterine or duodenal smooth muscle or myocardial contractility	50 mg/250 cc Average dose is 3 mcg/kg/min Range of 0.5–10 mcg/kg/min The rate should be titrated to achieve desired effect by 0.5 mcg/kg/min increments	–Hypotension may occur rapidly –Metabolizes into cyanide-metabolic acidosis is earliest sign of cyanide toxicity –Crosses placenta –nausea, vomiting, headache, bradycardia. ECG changes, tachycardia, increases ICP

INDEX

Page numbers in italics represent figures; those followed by a d represent displays; those followed by a t represent tables.

A

Abdominal trauma, 323, 324
  assessment of, 336, 337
Abortion
  previous, risk for preterm labor and delivery in, 105
Abruption of placenta, 106
  disseminated intravascular coagulation in, 216–217, 218
  intrauterine fetal demise in, 214, 217
  in trauma, 323, 325, 339, 342
Abstinence
  from alcohol, 388
  neonatal syndrome, 386, 386d, 390–391
    assessment of, 407–408
Abuse
  in domestic violence, 326–331
  of drugs, 380–404. *See also* Substance abuse
Acid secretion, gastric, 20
  in heartburn, 22
Acid-base balance
  fetal, 44
  maternal, 13, 13t
Acidosis, 13
  diabetic ketoacidosis, 226, 228, 248–252, 429–430
  fetal, 44
  in renal failure, 264
  in trauma, 341
Acoustic stimulation
  fetal, 419
Adaptation to at-risk childbearing, 53
  assessment of, 57–58
  and crisis management, 55–56
  interventions promoting, 58–62
  and shifting expectations, 54–55
β-Adrenergic receptors
  stimulation in preterm labor, 109, 110–112
Afterload, 67
  assessment of, 81
  factors affecting, 179
  in hypertension, pregnancy-induced, 169
  management of, 179
AIDS. *See* HIV infection and AIDS
Airway management
  in cardiopulmonary resuscitation, 355
  physiologic changes in pregnancy affecting, 355
  suctioning in, 96–97, 97t, 197–198
    competency validation skills checklist on, 467
  in trauma, 333, 335t, 340, *340*, 341
    guidelines on, 447, 448
    positioning of patient in, 341, *341*
  in ventilatory support, 96–97, 97t
Alanine aminotransferase serum levels
  in fatty liver of pregnancy, 279, 280, 280d
Albumin
  serum levels of, 8, 24–25
Alcohol use, 380, 381–382

assessment of, 392, 393, 394
  screening test in, 394, 397t–398t
  etiology of, 386–397
  fetal effects of, 381, 385
  follow-up in, 403
  myths concerning, 388
  nursing care and interventions in, 398–399
  overdose in, 398
  and smoking, 382
  tolerance in, 387, *387*, 398
  trauma in, 384, 398
  treatment of, 388, 389t, 390t
  withdrawal from, 381–382, 398, 399
    symptoms in, 399, 400t–402t
Alcoholics Anonymous, 388, 389t, 390t
Aldosterone
  and renin activity, 19, 37
Alkaline phosphatase serum levels, 24
  in fatty liver of pregnancy, 280, 280d
Alveoli
  physiology of gas exchange in, 185–186
American Heart Association
  advanced cardiac life support protocols, 358, 361d, 362d–365d, 366d
Amino acid metabolism
  liver in, 278
  normal changes in pregnancy, 20
Ammonia levels, 278
  in fatty liver of pregnancy, 280, 280d, 283
Amnioinfusion, 41, 135
Amniotic fluid
  embolism from, 191, 194
    disseminated intravascular coagulation in, 191, 218
  lecithin to sphingomyelin ratio in, 108
  meconium stained, 41
    in prolonged pregnancy, 129, 135
  pH of, 108
  volume in prolonged pregnancy, 130–131
Amniotic membrane
  premature rupture of, 102–118
    in antiphospholipid syndrome, 292–293
    assessment procedures in, 108, 411–412
    etiology of, 107
    initial management of, 109d
    nursing care and interventions in, 116–118
    nursing diagnosis in, 115–116
    risk factors for, 105, 106, 107
    in trauma, 323, 326
    treatment of, 114–115
    stripping in labor induction or augmentation, 131–132, 146
Amniotomy
  in labor induction or augmentation, 145–146, 149
Ampicillin
  in endocarditis prophylaxis, 181t
Amrinone
  in critical care obstetrics, 469
Anabolism
  facilitated, 21
Anaphylactoid syndrome of pregnancy, 191
Anemia, 5, 14
  iron deficiency, 15, 24
  oxygen delivery to fetus in, 39
Anesthesia
  in cardiac disorders, 180

cardiopulmonary arrest in, 354t, 355
Angioma
  spider, 24
Angiotensin
  and renin activity, 19
  fetal, 37
  in pregnancy-induced hypertension, 162
Angiotensin-converting enzyme inhibitors
  in pregnancy-induced hypertension, 168
Antacids
  in heartburn, 22
Antepartum care
  cardiopulmonary resuscitation in, 368d
  fetal surveillance in, 41–45, 416
    in prolonged pregnancy, 129–131, 132
  forms and flowsheets in, 454
  in HIV infection and AIDS, 315d
  in prolonged pregnancy, 132
    fetal surveillance in, 129–131, 132
Antianxiety drugs, 383, 402–403
Antibiotics
  in cardiac disorders, 181, 181t
  in pneumonia, 189–190
  in risk of preterm labor, 115
  in sepsis, 210
  in trauma, 345
Anticardiolipin antibody, 289, 291, 292, 297d
Anticonvulsant therapy, 166–167
Antidiuretic hormone secretion
  in fetal response to hypoxemia, 36
  in ventilatory support, 92
Antihypertensive agents, 167d, 167–168
Antinuclear antibodies
  in lupus erythematosus, 289, 290, 297d
Antioxidants, 204
Antiphospholipid antibody, 289, 291, 292
Antiphospholipid syndrome, 291–293
  assessment procedures in, 291, 295, 296
    laboratory tests in, 292, 297d
  and lupus erythematosus, 289, 291
  management of, 293, 298
Antiprogestins
  in cervical ripening, 145
Antiretroviral therapy
  in HIV infection and AIDS, 313–314
Antishock garments
  in trauma, 344
Antithrombin III, 215–216
  in disseminated intravascular coagulation, 218, 218t, 220
Anuria
  in renal failure, 260
Anxiety, 52–53
  and antianxiety drugs, 383, 402–403
  interventions in, 60
Aortic coarctation, 176
Aortic stenosis, 177–178, 181
Arachidonic acid, 204–205
  in spontaneous labor, 104
Arrhythmias
  in atrial septal defect, 175
  in betamimetic therapy for preterm labor, 111–112, 117
  fetal, 37–38
    bradycardia in, 34, 38
    in preterm labor, 112, 118
    in prolonged pregnancy, 128
    tachycardia in, 34, 37–38, 118, 128
  in hyperthyroidism, 270

in hypertension, pregnancy-induced, 163
and HELLP syndrome, 164, 164d
in neonate, 294, 295
normal changes in pregnancy, 15
Pleural effusions, 193
Pneumatic antishock garments
in trauma, 344
Pneumonia, 189–190
aspiration, 93, 189, 190
assessment of, 193–194
bacterial, 93, 189–190
in HIV infection and AIDS, 190
in ventilatory support, 92–93
and suctioning, 97, 97t
viral, 190
Pneumothorax
assessment of, 193
signs and symptoms in, 92, 92t
in trauma, 333, 334, 335t
in ventilatory support, 92
Polymerase chain reaction technique
in HIV infection and AIDS, 309
Polyuria
in renal failure, 260
Positioning and posture
in aortic stenosis, 181
blood pressure in, 7, 40, 357
cardiac output in, 5–6, 39
and oxygen delivery to fetus, 39, 40
edema in, 9
in induction of labor, 150
in mitral stenosis, 181
renal function in, 17, 19
in trauma
for airway management, 341, *341*
and hemorrhagic shock, 343
Positive airway pressure
continuous, 89, 196
Positive end-expiratory pressure (PEEP), 89, 94t, 196
complications of, 91, 92
Positive pressure ventilation, 85–86
high-frequency, 90
Postmaturity syndrome, 124, 125, 128–129
care of neonate in, 136
characteristic appearance in, 128, *128, 129, 130*
stages of, 128–129
Postpartum period
cardiopulmonary resuscitation in, 369d
in diabetes mellitus, 242–248
hemodynamic changes in, 9–10
hemorrhage in. *See* Hemorrhage, postpartum
in HIV infection and AIDS
disease transmission to neonate in, 315, 316
lupus erythematosus in, 289
in prolonged pregnancy, 135–136
renal failure in, 259
respiratory changes in, 12, *12*
thyroid disorders in, 268
Posture. *See* Positioning and posture
Potassium serum levels
in betamimetic therapy for preterm labor, 112
in diabetic ketoacidosis, 252
in renal failure, 264

Preconception care
in diabetes mellitus, 228–230
Prednisone
in autoimmune thrombocytopenia, 295
in lupus erythematosus, 259, 290
Preeclampsia, 159–160, 161
aspirin therapy in, 170
calcium supplementation in, 170
cardiovascular disorders in, 162
disseminated intravascular coagulation in, 217, 218
evaluation of, 412
and fatty liver of pregnancy, 276–277
hemodynamic monitoring in, 168
in hyperthyroidism, 270
and lupus erythematosus, 290
management guidelines on, 435–437
neurologic disorders in, 163, 166
renal disorders in, 163
severe, 160, 161d
Preload, 67
assessment of, 81
factors affecting, 179
management of, 179
Pressure cycled ventilation, 86
Pressure support ventilation, 89
Preterm labor and delivery, 102–118
in antiphospholipid syndrome, 292–293
assessment procedures in, 108–109, 411
birth weight in, 103
in diabetes mellitus, 112, 252
etiologies of, 103–105
history of patient in, 105
in lupus erythematosus, 290
nursing care and interventions in, 116–118
guidelines on, 423–426
nursing diagnosis in, 115–116
in premature rupture of membranes, 114–115
respiratory distress syndrome of neonate in, 103
risk factors for, 105d, 105–107
in substance abuse, 106, 107, 385
tocolytic therapy in. *See* Tocolytic therapy
in trauma, 337, 345
in burn injuries, 325
Progesterone
in spontaneous labor, 104, 142
Prolactin serum levels
in systemic inflammatory response syndrome, 206
Prolonged pregnancy, 123–136
antepartum care in, 132
cervical ripening in, 131, 132, 133
common findings in, 125
complications of, 124, 125–129
definition of, 123–124
etiologies of, 125
fetal surveillance in, 129–131, 132, 133, 135
incidence of, 124
intrapartum care in, 126, 133–135
macrosomia in, 124, 125–126, *126, 127d*
management options in, 131–132
membrane stripping or sweeping in, 131–132, 133

placental insufficiency in, 124, 126–128, *127*
postmaturity syndrome in, 124, 125, 128–129
postpartum care in, 135–136
Propranolol
in thyroid crisis or storm, 270–271, 272t
Propylthiouracil
in hyperthyroidism, 270, 272, 272t
Prostacyclin
in pregnancy-induced hypertension, 162, 170
Prostaglandins
in cervical ripening, 143–145, 150
guidelines on, 438–439
side effects of, 145
in fetal loss, 433
inhibitors of, 113–114
in preterm labor, 106
inhibitors of, 113–114
in prolonged pregnancy, 133
in spontaneous labor, 104, 142
Proteases, 204
Protein
metabolism of, 278
in fatty liver of pregnancy, 283
normal changes in pregnancy, 20
serum levels of, 24–25
urine levels of, 20, 161–162
in hypertension, 159, 161–162, 163
Protein C, 215, 216
normal changes in pregnancy, 216, 216d
Proteinuria, 159
diagnosis of, 161–162
renal function in, 163
Prothrombin time, 15
in disseminated intravascular coagulation, 218t, 219
Pruritus
in cholestasis of pregnancy, 25–26
Psychosocial factors, 51–62
in adaptation to at-risk childbearing, 53
assessment of, 57–58
in crisis situations, 55–56, 61
in critical illness, 446
in diabetes mellitus, 229, 248
in disseminated intravascular coagulation, 222
documentation on, 58
in emergent stress, 60–61
family-centered care in, 61
in fatty liver of pregnancy, 283
in fear of intrapartum loss, 56–57, 60
in induction or augmentation of labor, 150, 153
interventions in, 58–62
in intrauterine resuscitation, 41
in parent-fetal/infant attachment, 53–54, 58
in preexisting stress, 52
in preterm labor and delivery, 107, 116
in prolonged pregnancy, 125
in self-esteem, 53
in shifting expectations, 54–55
in substance abuse, 386–397
assessment of, 391
and treatment approach, 388, 389
in trauma, 337–338, 340, 348, 449
in domestic violence, 327, 330